Respiratory Distress Syndrome: An Issue of Clinics in Chest Medicine

Respiratory Distress Syndrome: An Issue of Clinics in Chest Medicine

Editor: Alan Reid

AMERICAN
MEDICAL PUBLISHERS
www.americanmedicalpublishers.com

AMERICAN
MEDICAL PUBLISHERS
www.americanmedicalpublishers.com

Cataloging-in-Publication Data

Respiratory distress syndrome : an issue of clinics in chest medicine / edited by Alan Reid.
p. cm.
Includes bibliographical references and index.
ISBN 979-8-88740-578-0
1. Respiratory distress syndrome. 2. Respiratory distress syndrome, Adult. 3. Pulmonary manifestations of general diseases.
4. Chest--Diseases. 5. Chest--Diseases--Diagnosis. 6. Lungs--Diseases--Treatment. I. Reid, Alan.
RC776.R38 R47 2023
616.24--dc23

American Medical Publishers,
41 Flatbush Avenue,
1st Floor, New York,
NY 11217, USA

ISBN 979-8-88740-578-0 (Hardback)

Contents

Preface

Every book is a source of knowledge and this one is no exception. The idea that led to the conceptualization of this book was the fact that the world is advancing rapidly; which makes it crucial to document the progress in every field. I am aware that a lot of data is already available, yet, there is a lot more to learn. Hence, I accepted the responsibility of editing this book and contributing my knowledge to the community.

Respiratory distress syndrome (RDS) refers to a type of breathing disorder that occurs in newborns. Those babies who are born prematurely suffer from this syndrome, as their lungs are not fully developed. This syndrome occurs due to the deficiency of surfactant, a body fluid made by the lungs. There are several symptoms of RDS, such as widening of nostrils while breathing, grunting, fast and shallow breathing, etc. RDS is diagnosed by performing blood tests, lung imaging tests and heart tests. There are various therapies of RDS including mechanical ventilation, nasal continuous positive airway pressure (nCPAP) and surfactant replacement therapy. This book contains a detailed explanation of the various diagnostic and therapeutic techniques associated with respiratory distress syndrome. It aims to shed light on some of the unexplored aspects of this disease. A number of latest researches have been included to keep the readers up-to-date with the global studies on this medical condition.

While editing this book, I had multiple visions for it. Then I finally narrowed down to make every chapter a sole standing text explaining a particular topic, so that they can be used independently. However, the umbrella subject sinews them into a common theme. This makes the book a unique platform of knowledge.

I would like to give the major credit of this book to the experts from every corner of the world, who took the time to share their expertise with us. Also, I owe the completion of this book to the never-ending support of my family, who supported me throughout the project.

Editor

1

Automatic Adjustment of the Inspiratory Trigger and Cycling-Off Criteria Improved Patient-Ventilator Asynchrony During Pressure Support Ventilation

Ling Liu [1], *Yue Yu* [1], *Xiaoting Xu* [1], *Qin Sun* [1], *Haibo Qiu* [1], *Davide Chiumello* [2,3,4†] and *Yi Yang* [1*†]

[1] *Jiangsu Provincial Key Laboratory of Critical Care Medicine, Department of Critical Care Medicine, Zhongda Hospital, School of Medicine, Southeast University, Nanjing, China,* [2] *SC Anesthesia and Resuscitation, San Paolo Hospital—University Campus, ASST Santi Paolo e Carlo, Milan, Italy,* [3] *Department of Health Sciences, University of Milan, Milan, Italy,* [4] *Coordinated Research Center of Respiratory Insufficiency, University of Milan, Milan, Italy*

***Correspondence:**
Yi Yang
yiyiyang2004@163.com

† These authors have contributed equally to this work

Background: Patient-ventilator asynchrony is common during pressure support ventilation (PSV) because of the constant cycling-off criteria and variation of respiratory system mechanical properties in individual patients. Automatic adjustment of inspiratory triggers and cycling-off criteria based on waveforms might be a useful tool to improve patient-ventilator asynchrony during PSV.

Method: Twenty-four patients were enrolled and were ventilated using PSV with different cycling-off criteria of 10% (PS_{10}), 30% (PS_{30}), 50% (PS_{50}), and automatic adjustment PSV (PS_{AUTO}). Patient-ventilator interactions were measured.

Results: The total asynchrony index (AI) and NeuroSync index were consistently lower in PS_{AUTO} when compared with PS_{10}, PS_{30}, and PS_{50}, ($P < 0.05$). The benefit of PS_{AUTO} in reducing the total AI was mainly because of the reduction of the micro-AI but not the macro-AI. PS_{AUTO} significantly improved the relative cycling-off error when compared with prefixed controlled PSV ($P < 0.05$). PS_{AUTO} significantly reduced the trigger error and inspiratory effort for the trigger when compared with a prefixed trigger. However, total inspiratory effort, breathing patterns, and respiratory drive were not different among modes.

Conclusions: When compared with fixed cycling-off criteria, an automatic adjustment system improved patient-ventilator asynchrony without changes in breathing patterns during PSV. The automatic adjustment system could be a useful tool to titrate more personalized mechanical ventilation.

Keywords: automatic adjustment system, pressure support ventilation, patient-ventilator asynchrony, cycling-off, trigger

INTRODUCTION

Pressure support ventilation (PSV) is the most widely used partial mode of assistance to minimize the effort of patients in breathing. During PSV, the assist is delivered by means of a pneumatic signal generated by patient effort and measured in the ventilatory circuit, i.e., flow or pressure (1). The ventilator usually cycles from inspiration to expiration when the inspiratory flow falls to a predetermined fraction of the peak inspiratory flow, which is the cycling-off criterion (2). Ideally, the ventilator trigger and cycling should coincide with the beginning and the end of the inspiratory effort of the patients (3). However, patient-ventilator asynchrony is common during PSV (4, 5), thereby contributing to the increased patient effort, increased duration of mechanical ventilation, and even increased mortality (6).

During PSV, prefixed pneumatic controllers can become progressively less effective, especially when patients have abnormal respiratory mechanics or ventilator over-assist (7). Delayed or missed triggers are sensed as an uncomfortable isometric load leading to increased effort intensity and pronounced dyspnea (8). Moreover, with prefixed cycling-off criteria, such as the default value of 30% peak flow in some ventilators, premature cycling is more frequent in patients with restrictive breathing patterns characterized by low respiratory system compliance and may result in double triggering. Delayed cycling occurs more frequently in patients with an obstructive pattern characterized by high resistance (6, 9). Different approaches for optimal ventilator triggering and cycling have been developed to minimize these problems, such as flow-triggering sensitivity and adjustable flow cycling during PSV.

It has been demonstrated that a noninvasive method based on flow and airway-pressure tracings was effective for detecting asynchrony (10–12). Therefore, an automatic adjustment system (IntelliCycleTM2.0) capable of automatically adjusting, breath by breath, the triggering and cycling-off criteria based on pressure-time and flow-time waveforms during PSV have been developed (see **Supplementary Material**).

The objective of our study was to show a reduction in patient-ventilator asynchrony with the use of an automatic adjustment system as compared with prefixed trigger and cycling-off criteria in patients with PSV.

METHODS

This unblinded crossover study was conducted in a 60-bed general intensive care unit of a teaching hospital affiliated with Southeast University in China. The protocol was approved by the Institutional Ethics Committee of Zhongda Hospital (number 2016ZDSYLL067-P01). Written informed consent was obtained from the legal primary decision-maker, which was the spouse of the patient or the parent or child if no spouse. The trial was registered at clinicaltrials.gov (NCT04091269).

Patients

Postoperative (abdominal surgery or orthopedic surgery) or acute respiratory failure patients were eligible when meeting all the following criteria: receiving invasive mechanical ventilation and being able to sustain PSV more than 1 h with inspiratory support $\leq$ 15 cm H_2O. Patients were excluded if (1) age $<$ 18 or $>$85 years; (2) tracheostomy at time of the study; (3) sedation level on the Richmond Agitation–Sedation Scale ≤ -2 or ≥ 2; (4) contraindication for nasogastric tube insertion, e.g., history of esophageal varices, gastroesophageal surgery in the previous 12 months, or gastroesophageal bleeding in the previous 7 days, international standard ratio $>$ 1.5, activated partial thromboplastin time $>$ 44 s, history of leukemia (13); and (5) hemodynamic instability (heart rate $>$ 140 beats/min, vasopressors required with $\geq$ 5 μg/kg/min dopamine/dobutamine, or $\geq$ 0.2 μg/kg/min norepinephrine).

Study Protocol

After obtaining consent, enrolled patients were switched to a Servo-i ventilator (Maquet, Solna, Stockholm, Sweden). A 16-F nasogastric feeding tube (NeuroVent Research Inc., Toronto, ON, Canada) with electrodes measuring the electrical activity of the diaphragm (EAdi) and balloons measuring esophageal (Pes) pressures was inserted through the nose and secured after confirming positioning according to the recommendations of the manufacturer. Static respiratory system compliance (C_{RS}), resistance (R_{RS}), and intrinsic positive end-expiratory pressure (PEEPi) were measured during volume control ventilation (without spontaneous drive) (see **Supplementary Material**).

Then sedation was decreased to maintain light sedation with the Richmond Agitation–Sedation Scale ranging from 0 to −2. As spontaneous breathing and EAdi recovered, patients were switched to an SV800 ventilator with IntelliCycleTM2.0 which can automatically adjust triggering and cycling-off criteria breath-by-breath, (Mindray, Shenzhen, China) and were ventilated by PSV with the pressure support level adjusted to a target tidal volume (V_T) of 6 ml/kg (of predict body weight, PBW). During the entire recording period, PEEPe and a fraction of inspired oxygen (FiO_2) were maintained as set by the clinician in charge of the patient.

During prefixed pneumatically controlled PSV, the inspiratory trigger was set at 1.5 L/min for flow triggering, and the rate of rise in pressure was set to 0.05 s in all patients. The cycling-off criteria were set to 10% (PS_{10}), 30% (PS_{30}), and 50% (PS_{50}). During automatic adjustment PSV, the inspiratory trigger was set as flow-trigger 1.5 L/min, the rate of rise in pressure was set to 0.05 s, and the cycling-off criterion was set to "AUTO" (PS_{AUTO}). Both the trigger and cycling-off criteria were adjusted by the automatic adjustment system according to an established algorithm based on the pressure-time and flow-time waveforms (**Supplementary Figures 1, 2**). First, patients were ventilated with four independent modes (PS_{10}, PS_{30}, PS_{50}, and PS_{AUTO}) applied in randomized order (**Supplementary Table 1**). Each independent condition was maintained for 20 min without washout periods (**Supplementary Figure 3**).

Data Acquisition and Analysis

Flow, airway pressure (P_{aw}), esophageal pressure (P_{es}), and EAdi were acquired during the 20-min time window in each condition at 100 Hz from the ventilator *via* an RS 232 interface connected to a computer. Data were stored for later offline analysis (NeuroVent Research Inc., Toronto, ON, Canada). To quantify patient-ventilator interaction, all variables were calculated manually breath by breath from a stable 3-min period in each condition using customized software (NeuroVent Research Inc., Toronto, ON, Canada) by two independent researchers who were blinded to the patient number and assigned order of crossover treatments, and mean values were calculated. In the event of a mismatch, a third researcher was consulted.

Six types of asynchrony were analyzed as previously described by Thille et al. and Lamouret et al. (6, 14). Macro asynchronies include ineffective triggering, which is defined by the existence of a diaphragmatic signal without a respiratory cycle; auto-triggering is defined by the existence of a ventilator cycle without a diaphragmatic signal; and double triggering is defined by the presence of two successive inspiratory cycles without an intermediate expiration or with an interrupted expiration. Micro-asynchronies are defined by a time difference exceeding 200 ms between the onset of the EAdi and the early initial rise in Paw; between the 70% of peak EAdi and early decrease in airway pressure (the opening of the expiratory valve)-late cycling; and between the decrease in airway pressure and 70% of peak EAdi-premature cycling. For each subtype of asynchrony, a percentage of asynchronies was calculated as follows: the number of asynchrony events divided by the total neural respiratory rate (which corresponds to the total EAdi signals) × 100%. Macro-asynchrony index (AI), micro-AI, and total AI were calculated as the number of macro asynchrony events, micro-asynchrony, or total asynchrony events divided by the neural respiratory rate × 100%.

Triggering and cycling-off errors, which were classified as either too late (positive values) or too early (negative values) (13), breathing pattern, inspiratory effort, and inspiratory effort for triggering were measured (see **Supplementary Material**). To estimate the overall extent of asynchrony and dys-synchrony, the NeuroSync index was calculated by averaging the percentage errors in triggering and cycling-off for all breaths (13). The primary endpoint was the difference in the total AI between PS_{AUTO} and PSV with prefixed triggering and cycling-off criteria (PS_{10}, PS_{30}, and PS_{50}).

Statistical Analysis

All statistical analyses were carried out using SPSS 20 (Chicago, IL, USA). The values are stated as mean ± SD unless specified otherwise. Data from two *post-hoc* subgroups, a restrictive subgroup defined as having C_{RS} < 40 ml/cm H_2O with R_{RS} < 12 cm H_2O/LS, and an obstructive subgroup, defined as having R_{RS} > 12 cm H_2O/LS with C_{RS} > 40 ml/cm H_2O, were analyzed. The normal distribution of continuous variables was assessed by using the Shapiro–Wilk test. Log-transformation was used for skewed data. Variables were compared between modes using repeated-measures ANOVA followed by Bonferroni's *post-hoc* test. Categorical data were compared by the chi-square test followed by Bonferroni's *post-hoc* test. *P*-values <0.05 were considered significant.

TABLE 1 | Patient characteristics.

Parameter	All (*n* = 24)	Obstructive subgroup (*n* = 8)	Restrictive subgroup (*n* = 8)	Other patients (*n* = 8)
Sex, male/female	19/5	5/3	7/1	7/1
Age, year	68 ± 17	75 ± 9	65 ± 17	68 ± 23
APACHE II	17.1 ± 5.3	17.9 ± 4.0	18.7 ± 6.0	14.8 ± 6.5
Main diagnosis				
Pneumonia, *n* (%)	4 (16.7%)	–	4 (50%)	
Extrapulmonary sepsis, *n* (%)	2 (8.3%)	–	2 (25%)	
AECOPD, *n* (%)	8 (33.3%)	8 (100.0%)	–	
Abdominal surgery	4 (16.7%)	–	–	4 (50.0%)
Orthopedic surgery, *n* (%)	4 (16.7%)	–	–	4 (50.0%)
Severe trauma, *n* (%)	2 (8.3%)		2 (25%)	
RASS	0 (−1, 0)	0 (−1, 0)	−1 (−2, 0)	0 (−1, 0)
PBW, Kg	63 ± 8	63 ± 7	59 ± 9	65 ± 7
PaO_2, mm Hg	107 ± 36	96 ± 30	95 ± 16	135 ± 42
PaO_2/FiO_2	276 ± 90	362 ± 78	239 ± 76	227 ± 41
$PaCO_2$, mm Hg	39 ± 11	48 ± 14	36 ± 6	32 ± 4
pH	7.41 ± 0.06	7.39 ± 0.05	7.43 ± 0.03	7.41 ± 0.06
C_{RS}, ml/cm H_2O	45.8 ± 9.7	50.9 ± 5.8	34.1 ± 5.1	52.5 ± 3.5
R_{RS}, cm H_2O/L/S	12.1 ± 4.9	17.9 ± 4.1	9.2 ± 2.1	9.4 ± 1.7
PEEPi, cm H_2O	1.7 ± 2.0	3.6 ± 2.4	0.9 ± 0.2	0.7 ± 0.7

Data are provided as mean ± SD or median (interquartile range).

APACHE II, Acute Physiology and Chronic Health Evaluation II; RASS, Richmond Agitation-Sedation Scale; PBW, predictive body weight; C_{RS}, static compliance of the respiratory system; R_{RS}, resistance of respiratory system; PEEPi, static intrinsic positive end expiratory pressure.

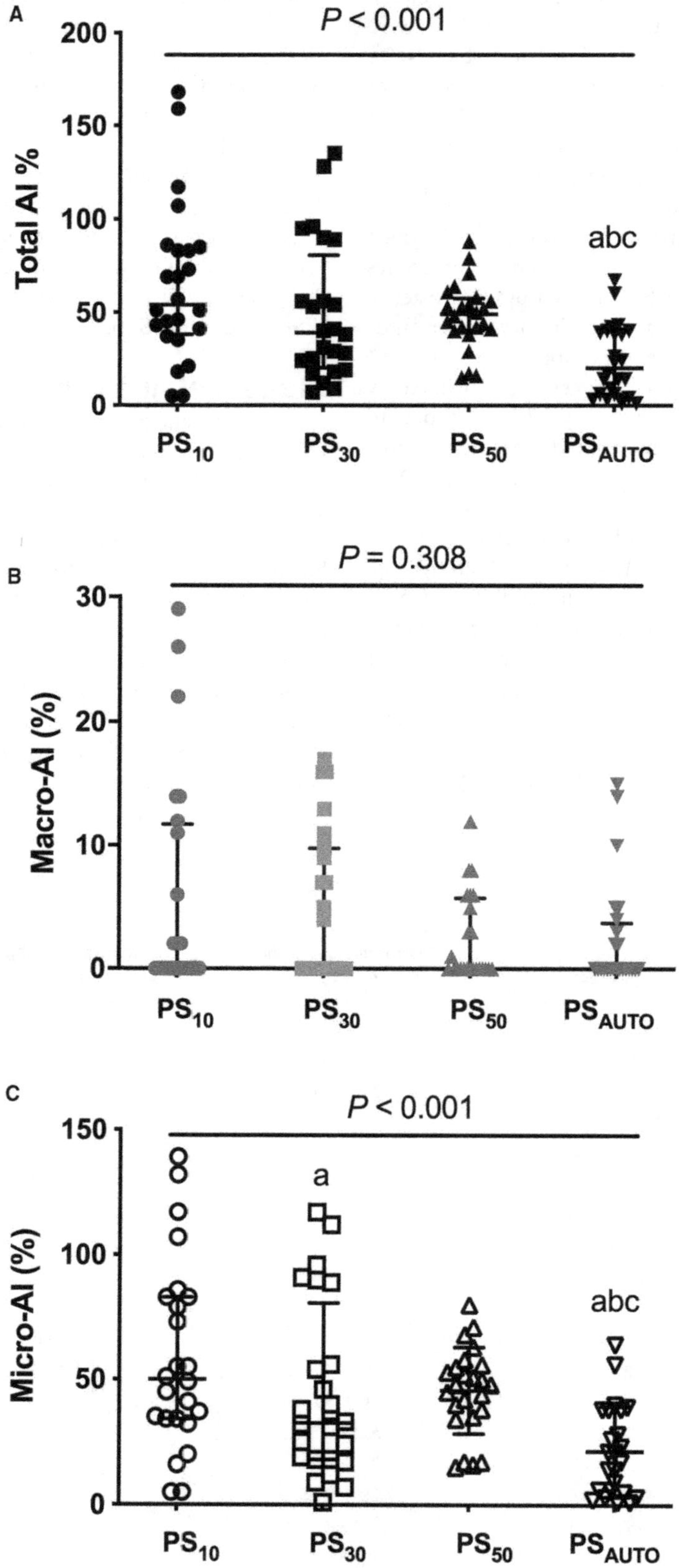

FIGURE 1 | Total AI **(A)**, macro-AI **(B)**, and micro-AI **(C)** in different modes. AI, asynchrony index; PS_{10}, pressure support ventilation with cycling-off criteria set to 10%; PS_{30}, pressure support ventilation with cycling-off criteria set to 30%; PS_{50}, pressure support ventilation with cycling-off criteria set to 50%; PS_{AUTO}, pressure support ventilation with automatic. Gray lines showed median (interquartile range). Compared with PS_{10}, $^{a}P < 0.05$; Compared with PS_{30}, $^{b}P < 0.05$; compared with PS_{50}, $^{c}P < 0.05$.

TABLE 2 | Asynchronies, NeuroSync index, inspiratory effort, and relative timing errors of cycling-off and trigger in different modes.

Parameters	PS_{10}	PS_{30}	PS_{50}	PS_{AUTO}	*P* value
Ineffective triggering, %	0.0 (0.0, 2.3)	0.0 (0.0, 0.0)	0.0 (0.0, 1.0)	0.0 (0.0, 1.4)	0.118
Auto-triggering, %	0.0 (0.0, 0.0)	0.0 (0.0, 3.3)	0.0 (0.0, 0.0)	0.0 (0.0, 0.0)	0.039
Double triggering, %	0.0 (0.0, 6.7)	0.0 (0.0, 0.0)	0.0 (0.0, 0.0)	0.0 (0.0, 0.0)	0.569
Premature cycling-off, %	0.0 (0.0, 2.6)	0.0 (0.0, 1.8)	5.4 (0.0, 22.5)[b]	0.0 (0.0, 1.8)[c]	<0.001
Late cycling-off, %	7.1 (0.0, 28.1)	1.8 (0.0, 20.8)	0.0 (0.0, 0.0)[a]	0.0 (0.0, 0.0)[a]	<0.001
Inspiratory trigger delay, %	38.3 (22.4, 48.9)	25.9 (11.4, 47.1)	30.3 (16.3, 45.6)	19.0 (5.0, 31.3)[abc]	<0.001
NeuroSync index, %	15.3 ± 8.2	13.3 ± 6.7[a]	13.1 ± 4.8	9.7 ± 4.4[abc]	<0.001
"Perfect" synchrony breath, %	18.5 (16.4, 20.7)	21.9 (19.5, 24.2)[a]	19.7 (17.5, 21.9)	42.2 (39.5, 44.9)[abc]	<0.001
"Acceptable" synchrony breath, % (95% CI)	81.1 (78.9, 83.2)	87.9 (86.0, 89.7)[a]	89.5 (87.8, 91.2)[a]	94.8 (93.5, 96.0)[abc]	<0.001
$PTP_{es-Trig}$, $cmH_2O.S.min^{-1}$	−3.1 (−6.0, −1.1)	−2.3 (−4.1, −1.1)	−2.0 (−3.6, −1.1)[a]	−1.9 (−3.7, −0.8)[ab]	<0.001
PTP_{es}, $cmH_2O.S.min^{-1}$	−17.1 (−88.2, −13.1)	−38.7 (−71.3, −10.6)	−40.8 (−58.0, −8.9)	−37.4 (−61.2, −9.1)	0.802

Data are provided as mean ± SD or median (interquartile range).
NeuroSync index is an overall indicator of patient-ventilator interaction, where 0% error, perfect; 100% error, zero patient-ventilator interaction; $PTP_{es-Trig}$, Pre-trigger Pes-time product; PTP_{es}, Pes-time product; PS_{10}, pressure support ventilation with cycling-off criteria set to 10%; PS_{30}, pressure support ventilation with cycling-off criteria set to 30%; PS_{50}, pressure support ventilation with cycling-off criteria set to 50%; PS_{AUTO}, pressure support ventilation with automatic adjustment system; CI, Confidence interval, "perfect" synchrony, relative timing errors of triggering and for cycling-off ≤10% of neural timings, "acceptable" synchrony, relative timing errors of triggering and for cycling-off ≤10% of neural timings.
Compared with PS_{10}, [a]$P < 0.05$; Compared with PS_{30}, [b]$P < 0.05$; Compared with PS_{50}, [c]$P < 0.05$.

RESULTS

The study included 24 patients, such as eight patients in the restrictive subgroup, eight patients in the obstructive subgroup, and eight other patients without obvious acute respiratory failure ($C_{RS} > 40$ ml/cm H_2O with $R_{RS} < 12$ cm H_2O/LS). Patient characteristics and lung mechanism are summarized in **Table 1**.

AI

Total AI was consistently lower in PS_{AUTO} when compared with PS_{10}, PS_{30}, and PS_{50}, ($P < 0.05$). The benefit of PS_{AUTO} in reducing total AI was mainly in the reduction of micro-AI but not macro-AI (**Figure 1**). The percentages of all kinds of asynchronies are reported in **Table 2**. Total AI and micro-AI were lower in PS_{AUTO} when compared with PS_{10} and PS_{30} in the obstructive subgroup and were lower in PS_{AUTO} when compared with PS_{50} in the restrictive subgroup (**Supplementary Table 2**).

NeuroSync Index

The NeuroSync index (average of the percentage errors of triggering and cycling-off) was consistently lower in PS_{AUTO} when compared with PS_{10}, PS_{30}, and PS_{50}, indicating improved patient-ventilator interaction (**Table 2**). **Figure 2** shows a plot of the percentage errors of triggering (*X*-axis) and cycling-off (*Y*-axis) for every breath. We have inserted a small centered box suggesting "perfect" asynchrony to be ≤10% of neural timing and a larger box suggesting "acceptable" asynchrony to be ≤33% of neural timing (15). There were more "Perfect" asynchrony breaths and "Acceptable" asynchrony breaths in PS_{AUTO} than in the fixed cycling-off criteria mode (PS_{10}, PS_{30}, and PS_{50}, all $P < 0.05$; **Figure 2**).

Cycling-Off and Triggering Error

Automatic adjustment PSV significantly improved the relative cycling-off error when compared with PS_{10}, PS_{30}, and PS_{50} in the whole population (**Figure 3**). The relative cycling-off error in PS_{AUTO} was comparable with that in PS_{50} in the obstructive subgroup and was comparable with that in PS_{10} in the restrictive subgroup. PS_{AUTO} significantly shortened the absolute and relative triggering errors when compared with a prefixed trigger (PS_{10}, PS_{30}, or PS_{50}; **Figure 3**). The Absolute and relative triggering errors were significantly lower when compared with PS_{10}, PS_{30}, and PS_{50} in the obstructive subgroup but not in the restrictive subgroup (**Supplementary Figure 4**).

Respiratory Drive and Breathing Pattern

Inspiratory effort for triggering determined by $PTP_{es-trig}$ was significantly lower in PS_{AUTO} when compared in PS_{10} and PS_{30}; however, total inspiratory effort determined by PTP_{es} was not different among modes (**Table 3**). In the obstructive subgroup, $PTP_{es-trig}$ was significantly lower in PS_{AUTO} than in PS_{10}, PS_{30}, and PS_{50} ($P < 0.05$; **Supplementary Table 2**). Peak airway pressure was higher in PS_{10} than in other modes. There was no difference in the respiratory drive between modes (**Table 3**). Breathing patterns and respiratory drive in obstructive and restrictive subgroups are shown in **Supplementary Table 3**.

DISCUSSION

This study showed that when compared with PSV with prefixed pneumatic controllers, an automatic adjustment system decreased total AI and improved patient-ventilator interaction mainly through a decrease of micro-asynchronies. The automatic system was associated with the lower cycling-off error, triggering error, and triggering effort in PSV patients.

AI and NeuroSync Index

Both AI and the NeuroSync index are indicators that reflect the overall patient-ventilator interaction from different perspectives. PS_{AUTO} constantly reduced total AI and the NeuroSync

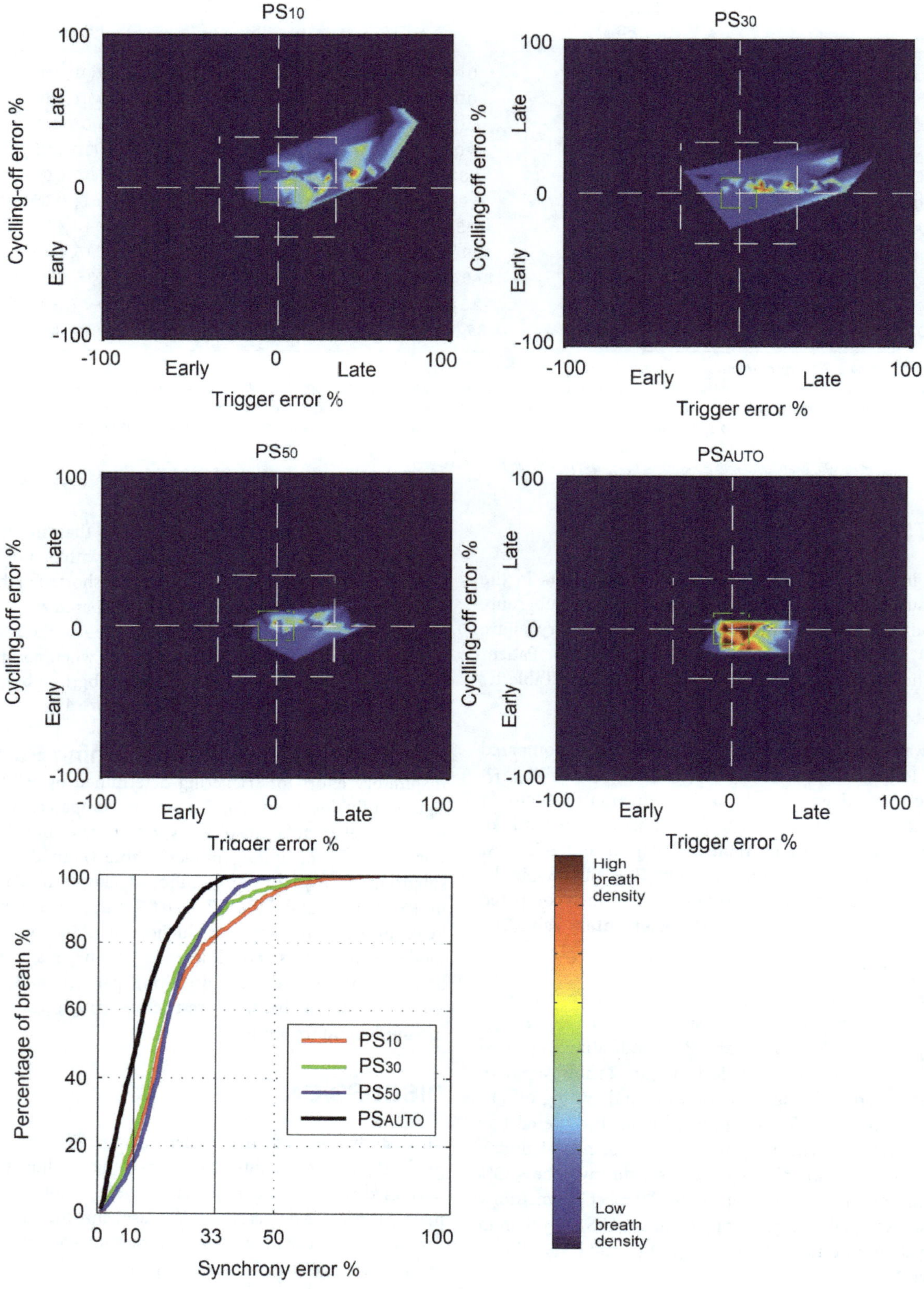

FIGURE 2 | Breath density graph for relative trigger (*X*-axis) and cycling-off (*Y*-axis) errors, for all breaths in all patients, during each ventilator mode. PS_{10}, pressure support ventilation with cycling-off criteria set to 10%; PS_{30}, pressure support ventilation with cycling-off criteria set to 30%; PS_{50}, pressure support ventilation with cycling-off criteria set to 50%; PS_{AUTO}, pressure support ventilation with automatic adjustment system; asynchrony error, breathes inside the box of percentage error of neural timings.

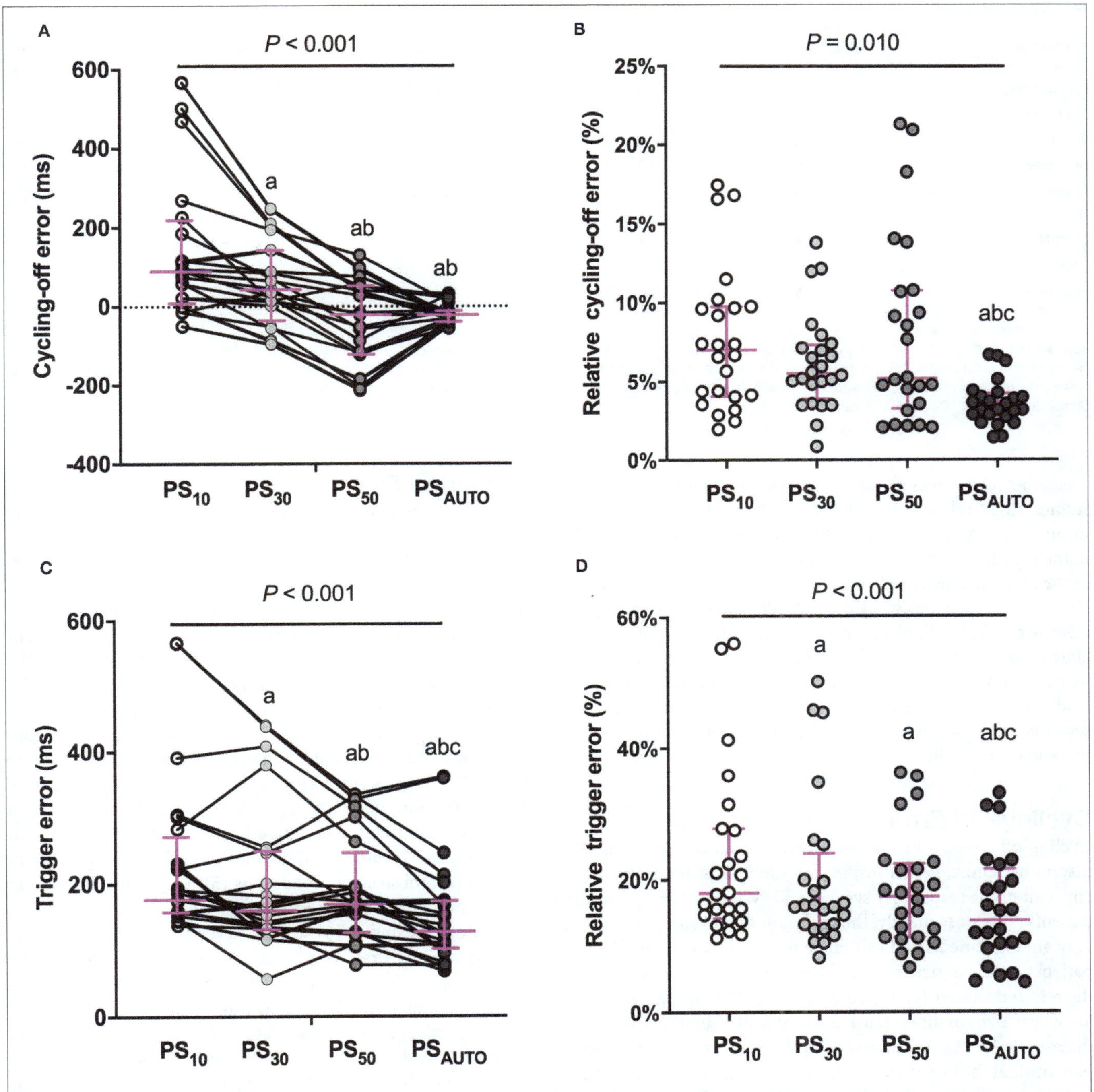

FIGURE 3 | Cycling-off error and trigger error in different modes. **(A)** cycling-off error, **(B)** relative cycling-off error, **(C)** trigger error, and **(D)** relative trigger error, *Y*-axis for cycling-off error: positive values indicate late cycling-off, and negative values indicate early cycling off. Magenta line showed median (interquartile range). ms, millisecond; PS_{10}, pressure support ventilation with cycling-off criteria set to 10%; PS_{30}, pressure support ventilation with cycling-off criteria set to 30%; PS_{50}, pressure support ventilation with cycling-off criteria set to 50%; PS_{AUTO}, pressure support ventilation with automatic. Compared with PS_{10}, $^{a}P < 0.05$; Compared with PS_{30}, $^{b}P < 0.05$; Compared with PS_{50}, $^{c}P < 0.05$.

index when compared with PSV with prefixed pneumatic controllers, indicating improved patient-ventilator interaction. Given that macro-asynchronies were rare, the benefit of PS_{AUTO} in reducing the total AI was mainly due to the reduction of micro-asynchronies. These findings agree with previous work comparing PSV and neurally adjusted ventilatory assist, which showed the difference in AI is found only in micro-asynchronies (14).

The present study showed a higher total AI (median of 23–57% during PS_{10}, PS_{30}, PS_{50}, and PS_{AUTO}) when compared with those in previous studies (range from 0 to 27%) (6, 16, 17). Despite the differences among study patients and ventilators

TABLE 3 | Breathing pattern and respiratory drive in different modes.

Parameter	PS_{10}	PS_{30}	PS_{50}	PS_{AUTO}	*P* value
Ppeak, cmH_2O	16.5 ± 4.2	15.4 ± 4.2[a]	15.4 ± 4.1[a]	14.6 ± 4.1[a]	<0.001
PEEP, cmH_2O	6.2 ± 1.7	6.1 ± 1.6	6.3 ± 1.5	6.6 ± 1.5	0.120
Vt, cmH_2O/kg	6.1 ± 0.2	6.1 ± 0.2	6.1 ± 0.3	6.0 ± 0.1	0.169
RR_N, breath/min	20.1 ± 5.6	19.3 ± 7.7	19.3 ± 5.9	20.5 ± 6.4	0.331
Ti_N, s	1.2 ± 0.0	1.1 ± 0.0	1.2 ± 0.0	1.1 ± 0.0	0.373
Te_N, s	2.2 ± 0.2	2.4 ± 0.2	2.7 ± 0.3	2.4 ± 0.2	0.129
TiN/TtN, %	37.0 ± 1.4	33.4 ± 1.6	35.7 ± 1.7	36.5 ± 1.5	0.042
Peak EAdi, μV	12.9 ± 1.7	12.0 ± 1.5	12.8 ± 1.9	12.4 ± 1.9	0.611
Peak EAdi, μV	8.1 ± 5.5	9.3 ± 6.1	8.0 ± 2.4	6.8 ± 2.0	0.864

Data are provided as mean ± SD.
PS_{10}, pressure support ventilation with cycling-off criteria set to 10%; PS_{30}, pressure support ventilation with cycling-off criteria set to 30%; PS_{50}, pressure support ventilation with cycling-off criteria set to 50%; PS_{AUTO}, pressure support ventilation with automatic adjustment system; Ppeak, peak airway pressure; PEEP, positive end expiratory pressure; Vt, tidal volume; RR, respiratory rate; Ti_N, neural inspiratory time; Te_N, neural expiratory time; Peak EAdi, peak diaphragm electrical activity.
Compared with PS_{10}, $^aP < 0.05$; Compared with PS_{30}.

used, the major reason for the apparent differences between studies might relate to the calculation method for the AI. First, inspiratory trigger delay was included in the calculation of the AI in the present study, which provided about one-third to one-half of the total AI during PSV with prefixed pneumatic controllers. However, the previous study did not calculate inspiratory trigger delay in the AI (6). Second, we defined asynchrony as an error of 200 ms between the origin of the EAdi and ventilator insufflation, which was more sensitive than the threshold used in previous studies (6, 16–18). Therefore, the AI in the present study is more sensitive and comprehensive and therefore not comparable to those in other studies.

Cycling-Off Error

Cycling-off asynchrony is dependent on factors, such as the inspiratory effort, neural inspiratory time, assist levels, the time constant of the respiratory system, and cycling-off criteria of the patients (3). Consequently, the optimum flow cycling-off criteria vary among patients and can range from very low levels (5%) in patients with a restrictive condition (such as acute respiratory distress syndrome) (4, 19) to more than 50% in patients with an obstructive condition (such as chronic obstructive pulmonary disease) (5, 20, 21). A previous study showed in a mixed sample of patients that the use of a variable, real-time-adjusted termination criterion improved some indices of patient-ventilator asynchrony when compared with a fixed termination criterion (5% of peak inspiratory flow) (22). However, a termination criterion of 5% of peak inspiratory flow was not commonly used clinically during PSV. Our results showed a significant improvement in relative cycling-off error during PS_{AUTO} when compared with PSV with prefixed cycling-off criteria of 10%, 30%, and 50%. It was not unexpected that during PSV with prefixed pneumatic controllers, PS_{50} and PS_{10} were the "best" cycling-off settings with the lowest relative cycling-off errors in the obstructive and restrictive subgroups. In each subgroup, relative cycling-off error in PS_{AUTO} was comparable with the "best" cycling-off setting during PSV with a prefixed cycling-off.

Triggering Error

The present study showed the median delay for triggering during PS_{10}, PS_{30}, PS_{50}, and PS_{AUTO} ranged from 187 to 130 ms. These values fall within the 80–540 ms range of values previously reported for PSV (1, 18, 23). Beloncle et al. reported absolute values for trigger delay < 200 ms in almost all patients, which was lower than that reported in the present study (18). The different ventilators and flow-trigger used in different studies might be one reason, and different types of the enrolled patients might be another reason for the difference in trigger delay. During PS_{AUTO}, the algorithm will trigger the ventilator to initiate the inspiratory phase when it detects a sudden increase of flow waveform, which reflects the inspiratory effort, leading to a reduced triggering delay. Furthermore, triggering delay was likely reduced as a consequence of reduced cycling-off delay during PS_{AUTO}, which led to a longer expiration time and lower PEEPi, especially in patients with obstructive conditions (5). Unfortunately, we did not measure PEEPi during each mode.

Of note, a single flow-trigger level in the present study made it hard to draw conclusions regarding the effect of the PS_{AUTO} mode on inspiratory triggering asynchronies when compared with lower flow-triggering (e.g., 1.0 L/min). From this perspective, a fixed flow-trigger of 1.5 L/min might be not sensitive enough. Considering the similar or shorter triggering delay and no obvious auto-triggering during PS_{AUTO}, automatic adjustment of triggering based on waveforms might be a useful tool for making the triggering setting easier.

Inspiratory Effort and Breathing Pattern

Because PS_{AUTO} significantly reduced triggering delay, it was not unexpected that it was associated with lower inspiratory effort for triggering. The present study showed a comparable breathing pattern and respiratory drive between PS_{AUTO} and PSV with prefixed pneumatic controllers. Of interest, neural expiratory time remained unchanged at the various cycling-off settings in the present study. These findings agree with previous work in which expiratory time did not change with the increase in cycling-off criteria in chronic obstructive pulmonary disease patients (5, 20). However, the findings contradict those in previous studies which show an increased expiratory time in the presence of delayed cycling in acute lung injury (24, 25). Therefore, PS_{AUTO} improved the cycling-off criteria, which was demonstrated to affect the inspiratory time only at high-pressure support (20). Peak EAdi around 12 μV confirmed the absence of over-assistance during PSV in the present study.

Limitations

There are some limitations that should be noted. First, our study was conducted in a small group of patients. Second, respiratory mechanics were evaluated in patients under sedation who were not actively breathing, therefore, the results will be different from those measured during PSV. Third, patients were maintained at each mode setting for only 20 min, and steady-state conditions might not have been achieved. However, the duration was in line with that of several studies on the effects of cycling criteria modifications (4, 19).

CONCLUSIONS

An automatic adjustment system based on waveform was associated with less patient-ventilator asynchrony when compared with PSV with prefixed pneumatic controllers. Our results indicated that this system might be a useful tool to titrate more personalized mechanical ventilation, especially in patients with a high risk of patient-ventilator asynchrony.

Hospital. The patients/participants provided their written informed consent to participate in this study.

AUTHOR CONTRIBUTIONS

LL, YYa, DC, and HQ have given substantial contributions to the conception or the design of the manuscript. LL, YYu, XX, and QS to acquisition, analysis, and interpretation of the data. All authors contributed equally to the manuscript and read and approved the final version of the manuscript.

FUNDING

This study was supported by the Clinical Science and Technology Specific Projects of Jiangsu Province [BE2020786 and BE2019749], the National Natural Science Foundation of China [Grant Numbers 81870066 and 81670074], the Natural Science Foundation of Jiangsu Province (BK20171271), Jiangsu Provincial Medical Youth Talent (QNRC 2016807), and Third Level Talents of the 333 High Level Talents Training Project in the fifth phase in Jiangsu (LGY2016051). This study received funding from Mindray (China). The funder was not involved in the study design, collection, analysis, interpretation of data, the writing of this article, or the decision to submit it for publication.

ACKNOWLEDGMENTS

The authors thank Mr. Jinglei Liu, Xiaoyong Zhou, and Jun Chen (Shenzhen Mindray Bio-Medical Electronics Co., Ltd.) for helping to making the figures.

REFERENCES

1. Spahija J, Marchie M, Albert M, Bellemare P, Delisle S, Beck J, et al. Patient-ventilator interaction during pressure support ventilation and neurally adjusted ventilatory assist. *Crit Care Med.* (2010) 38:518–26. doi: 10.1097/CCM.0b013e3181cb0d7b
2. MacIntyre NR. Clinically available new strategies for mechanical ventilatory support. *Chest.* (1993) 104:560–5. doi: 10.1378/chest.104.2.560
3. Yamada Y, Du HL. Analysis of the mechanisms of expiratory asynchrony in pressure support ventilation: a mathematical approach. *J Appl Physiol.* (2000) 88:2143–50. doi: 10.1152/jappl.2000.88.6.2143
4. Tokioka H, Tanaka T, Ishizu T, Fukushima T, Iwaki T, Nakamura Y, et al. The effect of breath termination criterion on breathing patterns and the work of breathing during pressure support ventilation. *Anesth Analg.* (2001) 92:161–5. doi: 10.1097/00000539-200101000-00031
5. Tassaux D, Gainnier M, Battisti A, Jolliet P. Impact of expiratory trigger setting on delayed cycling and inspiratory muscle workload. *Am J Respir Crit Care Med.* (2005) 172:1283–9. doi: 10.1164/rccm.200407-880OC
6. Thille AW, Rodriguez P, Cabello B, Lellouche F, Brochard L. Patient-ventilator asynchrony during assisted mechanical ventilation. *Intensive Care Med.* (2006) 32:1515–22. doi: 10.1007/s00134-006-0301-8
7. Jubran A, Van de Graaff WB, Tobin MJ. Variability of patient-ventilator interaction with pressure support ventilation in patients with chronic obstructive pulmonary disease. *Am J Respir Crit Care Med.* (1995) 152:129–36. doi: 10.1164/ajrccm.152.1.7599811
8. Gilstrap D, MacIntyre N. Patient-ventilator interactions. Implications for clinical management. *Am J Respir Crit Care Med.* (2013) 188:1058–68. doi: 10.1164/rccm.201212-2214CI
9. Garofalo E, Bruni A, Pelaia C, Liparota L, Lombardo N, Longhini F, et al. Recognizing, quantifying and managing patient-ventilator asynchrony in invasive and noninvasive ventilation. *Expert Rev Respir Med.* (2018) 12:557–67. doi: 10.1080/17476348.2018.1480941
10. Thille AW, Brochard L. Promoting patient-ventilator synchrony. *Clin Pulm Med.* (2007) 14:350–9. doi: 10.1097/CPM.0b013e31815b1234
11. Giannouli E, Webster K, Roberts D, Younes M. Response of ventilator-dependent patients to different levels of pressure support and proportional assist. *Am J Respir Crit Care Med.* (1999) 159:1716–25. doi: 10.1164/ajrccm.159.6.9704025
12. Mellott KG, Grap MJ, Munro CL, Sessler CN, Wetzel PA. Patient-ventilator dysasynchrony: clinical significance and implications for practice. *Crit Care Nurse.* (2009) 29:41–55. doi: 10.4037/ccn2009612
13. Liu L, Xia F, Yang Y, Longhini F, Navalesi P, Beck J. Neural versus pneumatic control of pressure support in patients with chronic obstructive pulmonary diseases at different levels of positive end expiratory pressure: a physiological study. *Crit Care.* (2015) 19:244. doi: 10.1186/s13054-015-0971-0
14. Lamouret O, Crognier L, Vardon BF, Conil JM, Dilasser C, Raimondi T, et al. Neurally adjusted ventilatory assist (NAVA) versus pressure support ventilation: patient-ventilator interaction during invasive ventilation delivered by tracheostomy. *Crit. Care.* (2019) 23:22. doi: 10.1186/s13054-018-2288-2
15. Sinderby C, Liu S, Colombo D, Camarotta G, Slutsky AS, Navalesi P, et al. An automated and standardized neural index to quantify patient-ventilator interaction. *Crit Care.* (2013) 17:R239. doi: 10.1186/cc13063

16. Demoule A, Clavel M, Rolland-Debord C, Perbet S, Terzi N, Kouatchet A, et al. Neurally adjusted ventilatory assist as an alternative to pressure support ventilation in adults: a French multicenter randomized trial. *Intensive Care Med.* (2016) 42:1723–32. doi: 10.1007/s00134-016-4447-8
17. Yonis H, Crognier L, Conil JM, Serres I, Rouget A, Virtos M, et al. Patient-ventilator asynchrony in neurally adjusted ventilatory assist (NAVA) and pressure support ventilation (PSV): a prospective observational study. *BMC Anesthesiol.* (2015) 15:117. doi: 10.1186/s12871-015-0091-z
18. Beloncle F, Piquilloud L, Rittayamai N, Sinderby C, Rozé H, et al. A diaphragmatic electrical activity-based optimization strategy during pressure support ventilation improves synchronization but does not impact work of breathing. *Crit Care.* (2017) 21:21. doi: 10.1186/s13054-017-1599-z
19. Chiumello D, Pelosi P, Taccone P, Slutsky A, Gattinoni L. Effect of different inspiratory rise time and cycling off criteria during pressure support ventilation in patients recovering from acute lung injury. *Crit Care Med.* (2003) 31:2604–10. doi: 10.1097/01.CCM.0000089939.11032.36
20. Chiumello D, Polli F, Tallarini F, Chierichetti M, Motta G, Azzari S, et al. Effect of different cycling-off criteria and positive end-expiratory pressure during pressure support ventilation in patients with chronic obstructive pulmonary disease. *Crit. Care Med.* (2007) 35:2547–52. doi: 10.1097/01.CCM.0000287594.80110.34
21. Tassaux D, Michotte JB, Gainnier M, Gratadour P, Fonseca S, Jolliet P. Expiratory trigger setting in pressure support ventilation: from mathematical model to bedside. *Crit Care Med.* (2004) 32:1844–50. doi: 10.1097/01.CCM.0000138561.11634.6F
22. Hoff FC, Tucci MR, Amato MBP, Santos LJ, Victorino JA. Cycling-off modes during pressure support ventilation: effects on breathing pattern, patient effort, and comfort. *J Crit Care.* (2014) 29:380–5. doi: 10.1016/j.jcrc.2014.01.015
23. Meric H, Calabrese P, Pradon D, Lejaille M, Lofaso F, Terzi N. Physiological comparison of breathing patterns with neurally adjusted ventilatory assist (NAVA) and pressure-support ventilation to improve NAVA settings. *Respir Physiol Neurobiol.* (2014) 195:11–8. doi: 10.1016/j.resp.2014.01.021
24. Younes M, Kun J, Webster K, Roberts D. Response of ventilator-dependent patients to delayed opening of exhalation valve. *Am J Respir Crit Care Med.* (2002) 166:21–30. doi: 10.1164/rccm.2107143
25. Kondili E, Prinianakis G, Anastasaki M, Georgopoulos D. Acute effects of ventilator settings on respiratory motor output in patients with acute lung injury. *Intensive Care Med.* (2002) 27:1147–57. doi: 10.1007/s001340101000

2

Sex Differences in Use of Low Tidal Volume Ventilation in COVID-19—Insights from the PRoVENT–COVID Study

Pien Swart [1], Sunny G. L. H. Nijbroek [1,2], Frederique Paulus [1], Ary Serpa Neto [1,3,4] and Marcus J. Schultz [1,5,6] for the 'PRactice of VENTilation in COVID-19' (PRoVENT-COVID) Collaborative Group[†]*

[1] Department of Intensive Care, Amsterdam University Medical Center, Location 'Academic Medical Center', Amsterdam, Netherlands, [2] Department of Anaesthesiology, Amsterdam University Medical Center, Location 'Academic Medical Center', Amsterdam, Netherlands, [3] Australian and New Zealand Intensive Care Research Centre, Monash University, Melbourne, VIC, Australia, [4] Department of Critical Care Medicine, Hospital Israelita Albert Einstein, São Paulo, Brazil, [5] Mahidol Oxford Tropical Medicine Research Unit (MORU), Mahidol University, Bangkok, Thailand, [6] Nuffield Department of Medicine, University of Oxford, Oxford, United Kingdom

***Correspondence:**
Pien Swart
p.swart@amsterdamumc.nl

[†] PRactice of VENTilation in patients with COVID-19; Collaborators are presented at the end of the article

The purpose of this study was to compare and understand differences in the use of low tidal volume ventilation (LTVV) between females and males with acute respiratory distress syndrome (ARDS) related to coronavirus disease 2019 (COVID-19). This is a *post-hoc* analysis of an observational study in invasively ventilated patients with ARDS related to COVID-19 in 22 ICUs in the Netherlands. The primary endpoint was the use of LTVV, defined as having received a median tidal volume (V_T) ≤6 ml/kg predicted body weight (PBW) during controlled ventilation. A mediation analysis was used to investigate the impact of anthropometric factors, next to the impact of sex *per se*. The analysis included 934 patients, 251 females and 683 males. All the patients had ARDS, and there were no differences in ARDS severity between the sexes. On the first day of ventilation, females received ventilation with a higher median V_T compared with males [6.8 (interquartile range (IQR) 6.0–7.6 vs. 6.3 (IQR 5.8–6.9) ml/kg PBW; $p < 0.001$]. Consequently, females received LTVV less often than males (23 vs. 34%; $p = 0.003$). The difference in the use of LTVV became smaller but persisted over the next days (27 vs. 36%; $p = 0.046$ at day 2 and 28 vs. 38%; $p = 0.030$ at day 3). The difference in the use LTVV was significantly mediated by sex *per se* [average direct effect of the female sex, 7.5% (95% CI, 1.7–13.3%); $p = 0.011$] and by differences in the body height [average causal mediation effect, −17.5% (−21.5 to −13.5%); $p < 0.001$], but not by the differences in actual body weight [average causal mediation effect, 0.2% (−0.8 to 1.2%); $p = 0.715$]. In conclusion, in this cohort of patients with ARDS related to COVID-19, females received LTVV less often than males in the first days of invasive ventilation. The difference in the use of LTVV was mainly driven by an anthropometric factor, namely, body height. Use of LTVV may improve by paying attention to correct titration of V_T, which should be based on PBW, which is a function of body height.

Keywords: lung protective ventilation, low tidal volume ventilation (LTVV), sex, gender, COVID-19, intensive care unit, critical care, mechanical ventilation

INTRODUCTION

Coronavirus disease 2019 (COVID-19) pandemic continues to have a relentless impact on the healthcare systems worldwide. Critical care systems are overloaded as many patients with COVID-19 develop acute respiratory failure requiring admission to a hospital for supplementary oxygen. A substantial proportion of these patients need admission to an intensive care unit (ICU) for ventilatory support (1, 2). Lung-protective ventilation, including the use of a low tidal volume (V_T), is recommended in patients with acute respiratory distress syndrome (ARDS) (3, 4) and there is growing evidence that the use of low-V_T ventilation (LTVV) also benefits patients with ARDS related to COVID-19 (5, 6).

Differences between females and males with regard to the use of LTVV have been described in surgery patients during general anesthesia (7–12) as well as critically ill patients in the ICU—and irrespective of the presence of ARDS (13–16, 44). It is uncertain if the sex difference in the use of LTVV also exists in patients with COVID-19. Use of LTVV might be limited in these patients because, due to the large numbers of patients requiring respiratory support, ventilation may need to be provided by healthcare professionals with much less experience in invasive ventilation, and thus also in the use of LTVV—it is uncertain whether this translates into sex differences.

To compare ventilation management with respect to LTVV in females vs. males, we reassessed the database of a conveniently-sized national multicenter study named "PRactice of VENTilation in patients with COVID-19" (PRoVENT-COVID) (5), a study that focused on ventilator settings and ventilation parameters in the first 4 calendar days of ventilation. Next to the hypothesis that the use of LTVV differs between the sexes, we also tested the hypothesis that differences in LTVV use are driven by anthropometric differences, i.e., differences in height and weight between the sexes, more than by sex *per se*.

MATERIALS AND METHODS

Design, Setting, and Participants

Secondary analysis of the database from the PRoVENT-COVID study, an investigator-initiated, national, multicenter, observational study in 22 ICUs in the Netherlands in the first 3 months of the national outbreak (5).

The protocol of the study of PRoVENT-COVID was approved by the institutional review boards of each participating hospital—need for individual patient informed consent was waived seen the observational design of the investigation. The PRoVENT-COVID study was registered at clinicaltrial.gov under the identifier NCT04346342.

Consecutive patients aged 18 years or older were enrolled if admitted to an ICU in one of the participating hospitals and having had received invasive ventilation for acute respiratory failure due to COVID-19, which had to be confirmed by RT-PCR. The PRoVENT-COVID study excluded SARS-CoV-2 infected patients that received ventilation for other reasons than COVID-19, e.g., patients that received ventilation for post-operative ventilation.

Data Collection and Analysis

Demographics, home medication, comorbidities, and disease severity scores were collected at baseline. The Berlin definition for ARDS was used to determine whether a patient had ARDS, and for ARDS severity (17).

Detailed information regarding ventilation management was captured in the first 4 calendar days of invasive ventilation at fixed time points every 8 h. Pulmonary and extrapulmonary events were captured up to hospital discharge, with a maximum of 28 days. Outcomes, such as intubation and life status, were collected till day 90.

We used the following equations:

$$V_T \text{ normalized to predicted body weight (PBW) } (V_{T,PBW}) \text{ [ml/kg]} = \text{absolute } V_T \text{ (ml)/PBW (kg) (18);} \quad (1)$$

$$\text{PBW in females (kg)} = 45.5 + 0.91^{*}(\text{height [cm]} - 152.4); \quad (2a)$$

$$\text{and PBW in males (kg)} = 50.0 + 0.91^{*}(\text{height [cm]} - 152.4); \quad (2b)$$

$$V_T \text{ normalized to actual body weight (ABW) } (V_{T,ABW}) \text{ [ml/kg]} = \text{absolute } V_T \text{ (ml)/ABW (kg)} \quad (3)$$

$$\text{driving pressure } (\Delta P) \text{ [cm } H_2O] = \text{peak pressure (Ppeak) [cm } H_2O] - \text{PEEP [cm } H_2O]\text{; and}$$
$$\text{respiratory system compliance (Crs) [ml/cm } H_2O] = \text{Absolute } V_T \text{ (ml)}/\Delta P[\text{cm } H_2O] \quad (4)$$

Study Endpoints

The primary endpoint was the use of LTVV in the first 4 calendar days of invasive ventilation. Secondary endpoints were other key ventilation parameters, including absolute V_T, $V_{T,ABW}$ and $V_{T,PBW}$, PEEP, ΔP, and Crs.

Power Calculation

The PRoVENT-COVID study contains a conveniently sized cohort of patients. We did not perform a formal power calculation; the sample size was based on the number of patients available in the database. With 1,000 patients, the study has >80% power to detect an absolute difference ranging from 9 and 15% in the use of LTVV considering a use rate of 50% in the female patients as shown previously (16).

Statistical Analysis

No assumptions were made for missing data. As the first calendar day was a flexible day that lasted from the moment of intubation and start of ventilation in the participating ICU and in theory could last from 1 min to 23 h and 59 min, we merged the first and second calendar day, which was then named "day 1." The following calendar days were named "day 2" and "day 3." As the ventilation strategy and settings may vary substantially in the first

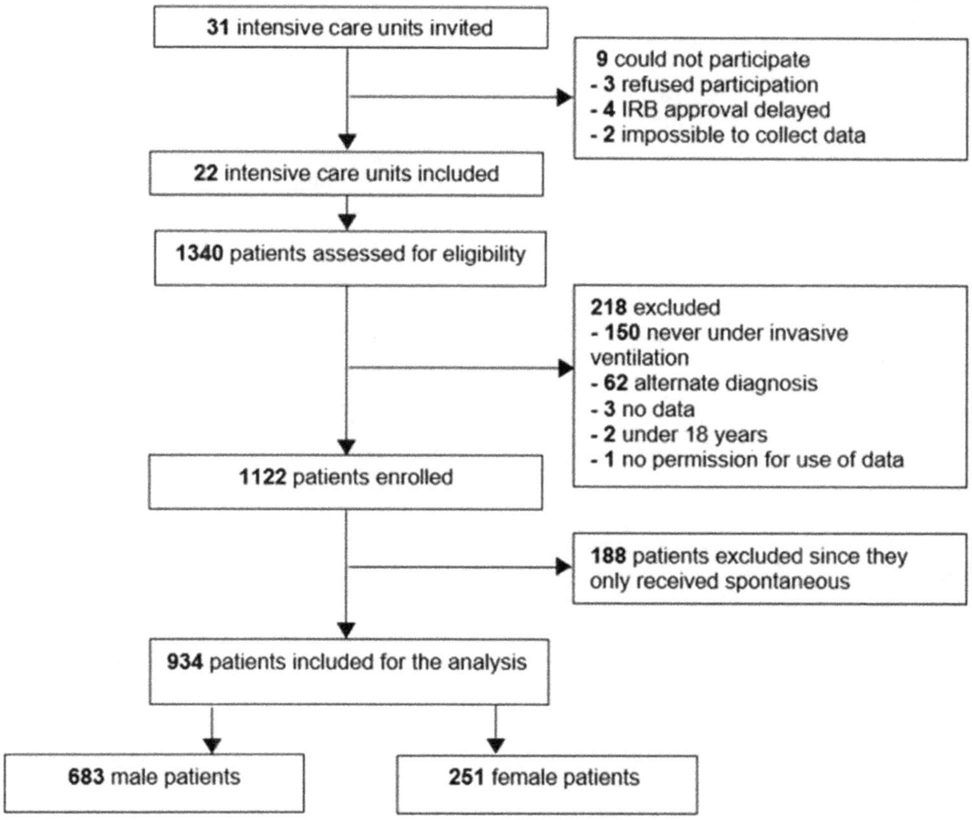

FIGURE 1 | Study flowchart.

hour of intubation, we also ignored the first available V_T, i.e., collected within 1 h of intubation.

Data are reported as numbers and proportions for categorical variables, and as medians with interquartile ranges (IQRs) for continuous variables. In addition, we also provided the 90% range for V_T. For baseline characteristics, the sexes were compared using the Fisher exact test for categorical variables, and the Wilcoxon rank-sum test for continuous variables. In all the analyses, males are used as the reference.

Ventilation parameters per day are presented in cumulative distribution plots, and in line graphs with error bars. In the distribution plots, vertical dotted lines represent the ideal cutoff for each parameter, and horizontal dotted lines the respective proportion of patients reaching each cutoff. All the ventilatory variables were aggregated per day and reported as such. For this, we calculated the mean of each ventilatory parameter per patient per day. In the tables, continuous variables were reported as medians of the means per each patient.

Patients were classified as having received LTVV, if the mean $V_{T,PBW}$ was $\leq$6 ml/kg during the controlled ventilation. For day 1, we ignored the breath in the first hour of ventilation, as this breath could have not been adjusted to achieve LTVV, e.g., in patients who started ventilation in the emergency department. Breaths collected under pressure support ventilation were also ignored, as were a breath that was collected at the moment spontaneous breathing activity was likely. This was the case if the measured (total) RR exceeded the set RR >2 breaths per min.

To further assess if sex is associated with differences in V_T an unadjusted mixed-effects linear regression model was used to extract the risk difference among the sexes. All analyses were performed using multilevel (patients nested in hospitals), mixed modeling with hospitals as a random effect to account for within-center clustering. Two *P*-values were reported in the graphs: (1) *P*-value for sex differences, reflecting the overall test for difference between sex across the days; and (2) *p*-values for the sex × day interaction, evaluating if change over time differed between the sexes.

The proportions of patients having had received LTVV are described and visualized in pie charts. An unadjusted mixed-effect generalized linear model was used to extract the risk difference for LTVV use.

To investigate whether differences in the use of LTVV between females and males are mediated by body height and ABW, a mixed-effect mediation model was used. In the mediation analysis, we assessed the individual impact of body height and ABW as potential mediators for the difference in the use of LTVV between sex. Mediators are variables that are affected by group assignment and that subsequently can affect the outcome.

TABLE 1 | Baseline characteristics of patient.

	Overall	Females	Males	p
Number of patients	934	251	683	
Age, years	65.0 [57.0, 72.0]	64.0 [55.0, 71.5]	65.0 [57.0, 72.0]	0.177
Weight, kg	86.0 [77.3, 96.4]	80.0 [70.0, 90.0]	89.0 [80.0, 98.2]	<0.001
Height, cm	176.0 [170.0, 183.0]	165.0 [162.0, 170.0]	180.0 [174.0, 185.0]	<0.001
BMI, kg/m^2	27.8 [25.2, 30.9]	28.4 [25.9, 32.3]	27.6 [25.2, 30.1]	0.002
Intubation at admission	152 (16.3)	38 (15.1)	114 (16.7)	0.618
NIV before intubation	77 (9.2)	23 (10.0)	54 (8.9)	0.688
Duration of NIV	7.5 [2.0, 18.1]	5.0 [1.8, 11.5]	8.0 [2.2, 24.0]	0.327
CT before intubation	326 (36.2)	97 (40.8)	229 (34.6)	0.099
% affected lung parenchyma on CT				0.682
0%	14 (4.3)	4 (4.1)	10 (4.3)	
25%	103 (31.4)	27 (27.8)	76 (32.9)	
50%	99 (30.2)	35 (36.1)	64 (27.7)	
75%	93 (28.4)	26 (26.8)	67 (29.0)	
100%	19 (5.8)	5 (5.2)	14 (6.1)	
X-ray before intubation	485 (85.7)	122 (85.3)	363 (85.8)	0.891
Number of affected quadrants				0.335
1	38 (7.8)	7 (5.9)	31 (8.5)	
2	114 (23.5)	34 (28.6)	80 (21.9)	
3	135 (27.8)	35 (29.4)	100 (27.3)	
4	198 (40.8)	43 (36.1)	155 (42.3)	
Pneumothorax	4 (1.8)	2 (3.8)	2 (1.2)	0.238
SAPS II	36.0 [29.0, 43.5]	35.0 [31.0, 43.5]	36.0 [29.0, 43.2]	0.573
APACHE II	16.0 [14.0, 21.0]	15.0 [12.0, 20.0]	17.0 [14.0, 22.0]	0.039
APACHE IV	56.0 [45.0, 70.0]	57.0 [46.0, 69.2]	56.0 [44.0, 70.0]	0.460
SOFA	7.0 [6.0, 10.0]	7.0 [6.0, 9.2]	7.0 [6.0, 10.0]	0.160
ARDS severity				0.386
Mild	188 (20.4)	51 (20.7)	137 (20.3)	
Moderate	630 (68.4)	162 (65.9)	468 (69.3)	
Severe	103 (11.2)	33 (13.4)	70 (10.4)	
Co-existing disorders				
Arterial hypertension	310 (33.2)	72 (28.7)	238 (34.8)	0.085
Heart failure	37 (4.0)	7 (2.8)	30 (4.4)	0.345
Diabetes	214 (22.9)	56 (22.3)	158 (23.1)	0.861
Chronic kidney disease	39 (4.2)	10 (4.0)	29 (4.2)	1.000
Baseline creatinine, µmol/L*	77.0 [62.0, 98.5]	63.5 [51.8, 78.0]	82.0 [68.0, 105.0]	<0.001
Liver cirrhosis	3 (0.3)	2 (0.8)	1 (0.1)	0.178
COPD	72 (7.7)	20 (8.0)	52 (7.6)	0.890
Active hematological malignancy	13 (1.4)	3 (1.2)	10 (1.5)	1.000
Active solid tumor malignancy	26 (2.8)	10 (4.0)	16 (2.3)	0.182
Neuromuscular disease	4 (0.4)	2 (0.8)	2 (0.3)	0.294
Immunosuppression	20 (2.1)	5 (2.0)	15 (2.2)	1.000
Home medication				
Systemic corticosteroids	34 (3.6)	8 (3.2)	26 (3.8)	0.844
Inhalation corticosteroids	105 (11.2)	40 (15.9)	65 (9.5)	0.007
ACE inhibitor	155 (16.6)	37 (14.7)	118 (17.3)	0.374
ARB II	106 (11.3)	22 (8.8)	84 (12.3)	0.162
Beta blocker	171 (18.3)	37 (14.7)	134 (19.6)	0.104
Insulin	68 (7.3)	20 (8.0)	48 (7.0)	0.670
Metformin	148 (15.8)	33 (13.1)	115 (16.8)	0.189
Statin	284 (30.4)	62 (24.7)	222 (32.5)	0.025
Calcium channel blocker	165 (17.7)	41 (16.3)	124 (18.2)	0.562

Data are median (quartile 25%–quartile 75%) or no (%). Percentages may not total 100 because of rounding.

**Most recent measurement in 24 h before intubation, or at ICU admission under invasive ventilation.*

APACHE, Acute Physiology and Chronic Health Evaluation; SAPS, Simplified Acute Physiology Score; SOFA, Sequential Organ Failure Assessment; ARDS, acute respiratory distress syndrome.

Therefore, mediators are on the causal pathway of the relation between group and outcome, at least partly explaining the effects of the group on the outcome. For the mediation models, the following estimates are described: (1) the total effect (estimates the total effect of sex on ventilation); (2) the average causal mediation effect [ACME, explains how much of the effect of sex on ventilation is explained by the mediator (height or weight)]; and (3) the average direct effect (ADE, explains how much of the effect of sex on ventilation is still explained by sex after considering the effect of the mediator). For this model, Quasi-Bayesian 95% CI were estimated after 10,000 simulations. The mediation models included day and centers as a random effects.

All the analyses were done in R version 4.0.2 and the significance level was set at 0.05.

RESULTS

Patients

Of 1,122 eligible patients, 188 patients did not receive controlled ventilation at any time point data were collected for this study, leaving us with 934 fully analyzable patients, 251 females and 683 males (**Figure 1**). Males had a higher median body height and also a higher median ABW. Aside from differences in baseline APACHE II scores, plasma creatinine, and use of statins and inhalation corticosteroids at home, there were no differences at baseline between the sexes (**Table 1**). Other severity scores and ARDS severity were comparable between females and males (**Table 1**). Compared with females, males had a higher mortality rate and a longer duration of ventilation (**Table 2**).

Ventilation Parameters

On day 1, females received a higher median $V_{T,PBW}$ than males [6.8 (IQR 6.0–7.6, 90% range 5.4–8.8) vs. 6.3 (IQR 5.8–6.9, 90% range 5.0–8.0) ml/kg PBW; $p < 0.001$; **Figures 2, 3** and **Table 3**]. This sex difference became smaller at day 2 [6.4 (IQR 5.9–7.1, 9% range 5.0–8.4) vs. 6.3 (IQR 5.8–7.0, 90% range 5.0–7.9) ml/kg PBW; $p = 0.046$] and at day 3 [6.5 (IQR 6.0–7.1, 90% range 5.1–8.2) vs. 6.2 (IQR 5.6–6.9; 90% range 4.9–7.8) ml/kg PBW; $p = 0.001$; **Supplementary Figures 1, 2** and **Supplementary Tables 1, 2**]. On day 1, females received ventilation with a slightly lower median PEEP and a higher median ΔP (**Figures 2, 3** and **Table 3**). These differences became smaller on days 2 and 3 (**Supplementary Figures 1, 2** and **Supplementary Tables 1, 2**). Median Crs was lower in females at all 3 days.

Use of LTVV

Low tidal volume ventilation was generally underused, with only a third of patients receiving ventilation with a median $V_{T,PBW}$ ≤6 ml/kg PBW–at day 1, females received LTVV less often than males (23 vs. 34%; $p = 0.003$; **Figure 4**). The sex difference in use

TABLE 2 | Outcome.

	Overall	Females	Males	*p*
Number of patients	934	251	683	
Ventilatory free days at 28 days	2.0 [0.0, 16.0]	9.0 [0.0, 18.0]	0.0 [0.0, 15.0]	0.001
Extubation	545 (58.8)	159 (63.3)	386 (57.1)	0.098
Duration of ventilation, days	14.0 [8.0, 23.0]	12.0 [7.0, 20.8]	15.0 [8.0, 24.0]	0.012
Duration of ventilation in survivors at day 28	16.0 [10.0, 28.0]	13.0 [9.0, 23.0]	17.0 [10.0, 29.0]	0.003
Tracheostomy	154 (16.6)	32 (12.8)	122 (18.1)	0.059
Reintubation	118 (12.8)	38 (15.3)	80 (11.9)	0.184
Pneumothorax	8 (0.9)	1 (0.4)	7 (1.1)	0.690
Thromboembolic complications*	266 (28.5)	65 (25.9)	201 (29.4)	0.326
Acute kidney injury**	421 (45.2)	100 (40.0)	321 (47.1)	0.054
Renal replacement therapy	173 (18.5)	35 (13.9)	138 (20.2)	0.029
ICU length of stay, days	15.0 [9.0, 27.0]	14.0 [9.0, 24.0]	16.0 [9.0, 27.5]	0.094
In survivors, days	18.0 [11.0, 30.0]	16.0 [10.0, 27.0]	18.0 [11.0, 31.0]	0.067
Hospital length of stay, days	24.0 [14.0, 37.0]	22.0 [14.0, 36.0]	24.0 [14.0, 39.0]	0.408
In survivors, days	29.5 [20.0, 44.0]	27.0 [20.0, 39.0]	30.0 [20.0, 46.0]	0.062
ICU mortality	301 (33.0)	66 (27.2)	235 (35.2)	0.026
Hospital mortality	310 (36.1)	67 (29.9)	243 (38.3)	0.029
d7 mortality	97 (10.5)	27 (10.9)	70 (10.3)	0.809
d28 mortality	266 (28.9)	60 (24.6)	206 (30.5)	0.084
d90 mortality	323 (37.9)	70 (31.1)	253 (40.3)	0.016

Data are median (quartile 25%–quartile 75%) or no (%). Percentages may not total 100 because of rounding.

**Pulmonary embolism was defined when confirmed by chest CT angiography or when highly suspicious according to clinical assessment and treated accordingly by the attending the physician.*

***Acute kidney injury was defined when one of the following criteria was met at any point within 28 days after intubation: (1) a 1.5-fold increase of creatinine compared with baseline; and/or (2) an absolute creatinine increase of 26.5 μmol/L compared with baseline; and/or (3) a urinary output <0.5 ml/kg per h for more than 6 h.*

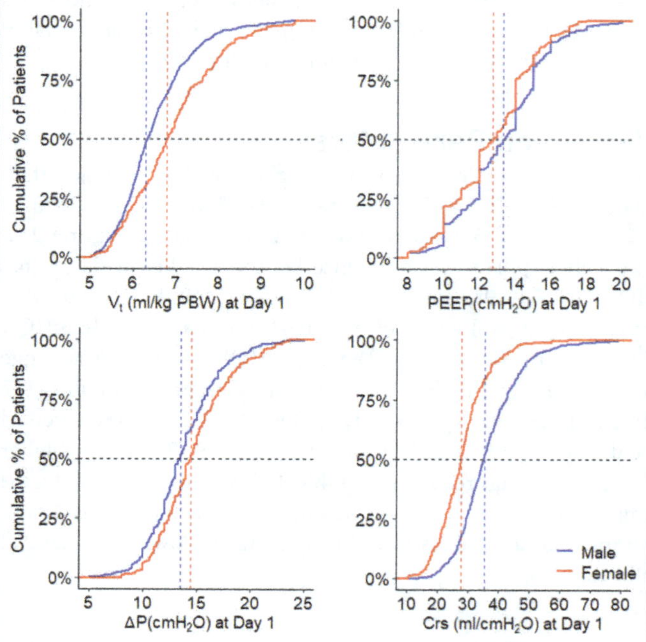

FIGURE 2 | Ventilation parameters during the first day. Cumulative frequency distribution of tidal volume, PEEP, driving pressure, and respiratory system compliance. Vertical dotted lines represent the median on the first calendar day of ventilation for each variable, and horizontal dotted lines show the respective proportion of patients reaching each cutoff. V_T, tidal volume; PEEP, positive end expiratory pressure; ΔP, driving pressure; Crs, respiratory system compliance; PBW, predicted body weight. The *p*-value for the sex reflects the overall test for difference between sex over the days, the *p*-value for the sex × year interaction evaluates if change over time differed by sex.

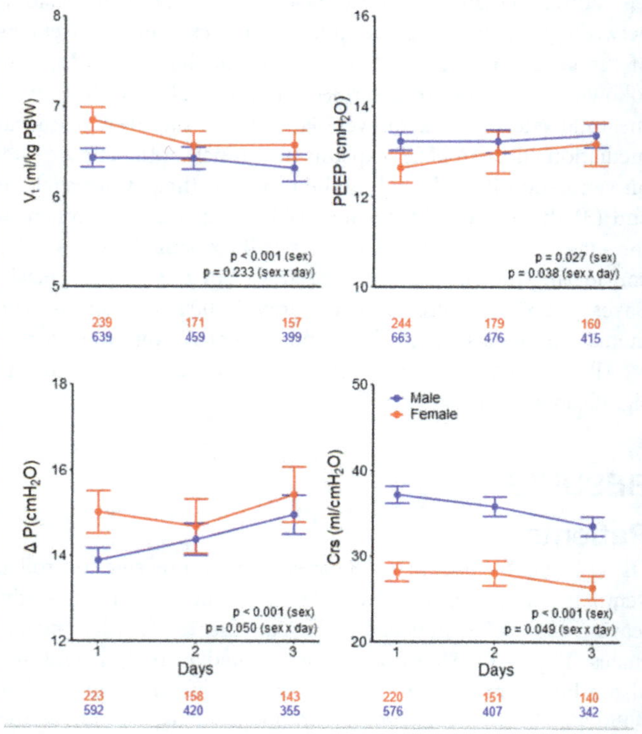

FIGURE 3 | Ventilatory variables over the days. Line graphs with error bars of tidal volume, PEEP, driving pressure, and respiratory system compliance. The numbers under the x-axis indicate the number of patients. V_T, tidal volume; PEEP, positive end-expiratory pressure; ΔP, driving pressure; Crs, respiratory system compliance; PBW, predicted body weight. The *p*-value for the sex reflects the overall test for difference between sex over the days, the *p*-value for the sex × year interaction evaluates if change over time differed by sex.

of LTVV persisted at day 2 (27 vs. 36%; $p = 0.046$) and at day 3 (28 vs. 38%; $p = 0.030$; **Figure 4** and **Supplementary Tables 1, 2**).

Mediation Analysis

The difference in the use of LTVV between females and males was significantly mediated by sex [average causal mediation effect 7.5% (95% CI 1.7–13.3%); $p = 0.011$] but more by body height [average causal mediation effect −17.5% (95% CI −21.5 to −13.5%); $p < 0.001$; **Table 4**]. The difference was also significantly mediated by ABW in the model that only used this factor [average causal mediation effect −1.7% (95% CI −2.7 to −1.0); $p < 0.001$], but not in a model that also used body height, meaning that the difference in the use of LTVV was mainly mediated by differences in height, and not by weight.

DISCUSSION

The results of this analysis of a large cohort of critically ill patients with ARDS related to COVID-19 who received invasive ventilation in the ICU during the first wave of the national outbreak in the Netherlands can be summarized as follows: (1) females were at a higher risk of not receiving LTVV at all 4 days of ventilation; (2) PEEP was lower and ΔP was higher, but only at day 1; and (3) females had a lower Crs, a difference that did not change over the days. In addition, the mediation analysis suggests that (4) differences are partly explained by sex *per se*; (5) but are mostly explained by the differences in body height.

Our study has several strengths. The PRoVENT–COVID study is one of the largest multicenter studies that collected ventilator data at several time points per day, allowing a better insight into ventilation practice, and differences herein between females and males. This study involved more than one-third of all invasively ventilated patients with ARDS related to COVID-19 in the first wave of the outbreak in the Netherlands. Furthermore, we enrolled patients in 22 centers included university hospitals, non-university teaching as well as non-teaching hospitals, accounting for around one-fourth of the ICUs in the Netherlands. This all increases the generalizability of the findings. The design of PRoVENT–COVID assured completeness of data collection and the short timeframe within which data were gathered, avoiding the effect of practice changes over time. At last, we followed the analysis plan strictly and used sophisticated mediation analysis to determine which factors determine the sex difference in the use of LTVV.

The differences in V_T between females and males may seem small, especially when focusing on the median V_T, PBW. However, the 90% range clearly shows that V_T differs between the sexes–for instance, 16% of female patients received ventilation with a $V_{T,PBW}$ >8 ml/kg, while only 5% of male patients received

TABLE 3 | Ventilatory variables during the first day.

	Overall	Females	Males	p
Number of patients	908*	244	664	
V_T, Absolute, mL	451.0 [406.1, 500.0]	396.5 [343.8, 440.5]	468.5 [427.2, 514.8]	<0.001
V_T, mL/kg ABW	5.2 [4.6, 5.9]	4.9 [4.2, 5.8]	5.3 [4.6, 6.0]	<0.001
90% range	3.4–7.1	3.3–7.0	3.8–7.2	
V_T, mL/kg PBW	6.4 [5.9, 7.1]	6.8 [6.0, 7.6]	6.3 [5.8, 6.9]	<0.001
90% range	5.1–8.4	5.4–8.8	5.0–8.0	
V_T, PBW ≤6 mL/kg, %	272 (31.0)	56 (23.4)	216 (33.8)	0.003
V_T, PBW ≤8 mL/kg, %	808 (92.0)	202 (84.5)	606 (94.8)	<0.001
V_T, PBW ≤10 mL/kg, %	874 (99.5)	238 (99.6)	636 (99.5)	1.000
PEEP, cmH_2O	13.2 [11.3, 15.0]	12.7 [10.7, 14.0]	13.3 [11.7, 15.0]	0.002
Peak pressure, cmH_2O	27.0 [24.0, 30.0]	27.2 [24.7, 30.2]	27.0 [24.0, 30.0]	0.116
Driving pressure, cmH_2O	13.8 [12.0, 16.0]	14.5 [12.4, 16.9]	13.5 [11.8, 15.8]	<0.001
Mechanical power, J/min	18.9 [15.5, 22.9]	16.8 [14.0, 20.0]	19.8 [16.5, 23.7]	<0.001
Compliance, mL/ cmH_2O	32.9 [27.5, 40.1]	27.6 [22.6, 32.2]	35.2 [29.6, 42.7]	<0.001
Respiratory rate, bpm	22.0 [20.0, 24.2]	22.0 [20.0, 25.0]	22.0 [20.0, 24.0]	0.257
FiO_2, %	0.5 [0.4, 0.6]	0.5 [0.4, 0.6]	0.5 [0.4, 0.6]	0.505
SpO_2, %	95.0 [93.6, 96.4]	95.0 [93.5, 96.2]	95.0 [93.7, 96.5]	0.588
$etCO_2$, mmHg	37.5 [33.1, 42.4]	37.0 [32.4, 42.1]	37.5 [33.4, 42.6]	0.351
Heart rate, beats per min	81.0 [70.0, 93.0]	80.4 [71.0, 93.8]	81.1 [69.7, 93.0]	0.713
Mean arterial pressure, mmHg	76.4 [71.5, 82.3]	76.2 [71.9, 82.0]	76.5 [71.3, 82.5]	0.930
pH	7.4 [7.3, 7.4]	7.4 [7.3, 7.4]	7.4 [7.3, 7.4]	0.259
Lactate, mmol/L	1.2 [1.0, 1.5]	1.2 [1.0, 1.5]	1.2 [1.0, 1.5]	0.755
PaO_2	80.0 [72.9, 90.7]	79.8 [72.2, 91.1]	80.1 [73.0, 89.9]	0.823
P/F ratio	174.2 [142.9, 208.6]	172.7 [135.6, 210.0]	174.6 [145.0, 208.0]	0.549
$PaCO_2$, mmHg	45.1 [40.5, 51.2]	44.0 [40.0, 50.1]	45.4 [41.0, 51.8]	0.056
Prone positioning	325 (47.6)	95 (49.2)	230 (46.9)	0.610
Duration of prone positioning	15.0 [11.0, 22.0]	16.0 [11.0, 23.0]	14.0 [11.0, 20.0]	0.129
Minute ventilation	9.7 [8.5, 11.2]	8.6 [7.5, 9.7]	10.2 [8.9, 11.5]	<0.001
Ventilatory ratio	1.7 [1.4, 2.0]	1.7 [1.4, 2.1]	1.7 [1.4, 2.0]	0.030
Recruitment maneuver	16 (2.8)	4 (2.3)	12 (3.0)	0.787

Data are median (quartile 25%–quartile 75%) or no (%). Percentages may not total 100 because of rounding.
PEEP, positive end-expiratory pressure; FiO_2, fraction of inspired oxygen; SpO_2, oxygen saturation; $PaCO_2$, partial pressure of arterial carbon dioxide; PaO_2, partial pressure of arterial oxygen.
Of 934 patients who received controlled ventilation on at least one timepoint of data collection, 908 received controlled ventilation at day 1.

ventilation with a $V_{T,PBW}$ above this upper threshold of what is generally accepted as safe. The use of a high V_T is associated with a higher mortality and morbidity in ICU patients (5, 6, 13–15, 19–21). An earlier analysis showed that a one SD increases in $V_{T,PBW}$ meant an increase of 28% in 28-day mortality (5). The finding that females received ventilation with a higher median V_T than males in this cohort is in line with results from several investigations originating from before the COVID-19 pandemic (13–16, 44). It interesting to note that V_T, in both females and males, was lower than in those previous cohorts, suggesting a temporal trend toward the use of lower V_T in critically ill patients (16). Despite the improved use of LTVV, however, differences between females and males persist.

Several reports on ventilated in patients with COVID-19 show a higher mortality in male patients (5, 22–30). This was also found in the current cohort. Interestingly, another study reported that the mortality of severely ill premenopausal but not post-menopausal female patients with COVID-19 are lower than age-matched male patients (31). The LUNG SAFE study, before COVID-19, did not find sex differences in mortality, but in that cohort, females had a shorter duration of invasive ventilation and a lower length of ICU stay (15). The reasons why male patients with COVID-19 have higher mortality remains uncertain. Biological factors, hormone factors such as estrogen, and factors related to the activity of X-linked genes have been suggested (31–34) and also sociocultural factors could play a role (34). It could also be interesting to look into the possible benefit of inhalation corticosteroids. In the current cohort, female patients had a significantly higher usage of inhalation corticosteroids as home medication. A total of 2 randomized clinical trials showed that using intravenous corticosteroids could reduce mortality (35, 36). These findings are confirmed in a recent meta-analysis (37). However, it is important to point out the difference between administration, i.e., intravenous vs. inhalation, and setting, i.e., during hospital admission vs. home medication.

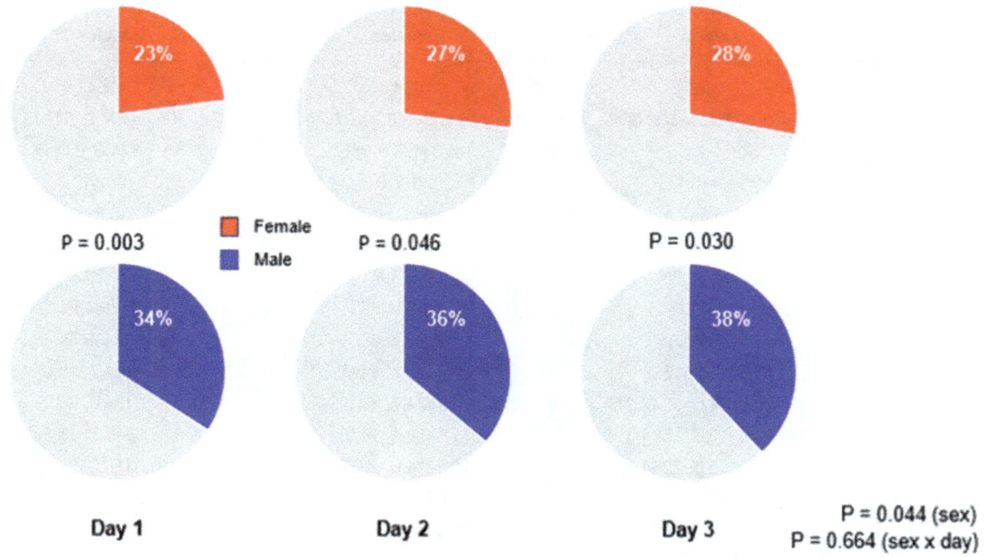

FIGURE 4 | Percentages of patients receiving low tidal volume ventilation. Significant *p*-value for the sex reflects the overall test for difference between sex over the days, while the *p*-value for the sex × year interaction evaluates if change over time differed by sex.

TABLE 4 | Mediation analysis.

	Adjusted absolute difference (95% CI)[a]	*p-value*
Univariable mediation model		
Body height as mediator		
Total effect of sex	−10.0 (−14.3 to −6.0)	<0.001
Average causal mediation effect of body height	−16.0 (−19.0 to −13.0)	<0.001
Average direct effect of female sex	6.0 (1.0 to 11.0)	0.018
Body weight as mediator		
Total effect of sex	−10.0 (−14.3 to −6.0)	<0.001
Average causal mediation effect of body weight	−1.7 (−2.7 to −1.0)	<0.001
Average direct effect of female sex	−8.4 (−12.7 to −4.0)	<0.001
Body height and weight as mediators*		
Total effect of sex	−9.8 (−13.6 to −6.0)	<0.001
Average causal mediation effect of body height	−17.5 (−21.5 to −13.5)	<0.001
Average causal mediation effect of body weight	0.2 (−0.8 to 1.2)	0.715
Average direct effect of female sex	7.5 (1.7 to 13.3)	0.011

[a]*All estimated were generated after 10,000 simulations.*
**CI estimated from robust clustered standard errors.*

The outcome advantage of female patients, however, should not withhold ICU doctors and nurses from using a correct V_T, seen the advantage of LTVV that has been found in pre-COVID-19 studies and in COVID-19 studies. In fact, this could increase the outcome differences between females and males.

Several studies in patients with non-COVID-19 have shown sex differences in important aspects of care in critically ill patients (7, 38–41). For instance—among patients with sepsis or shock, females are less likely to receive deep venous thrombosis prophylaxis or invasive ventilation, but are more likely to receive red blood cell transfusions (40). On the contrary, males receive "more intense" care, including placement of the central catheters for infusion of vasoactive medication (38) and invasive ventilation (38, 39). It is uncertain if similar differences, i.e., in non-ventilatory care, exist in patients with COVID-19 as well.

Of note, while $V_{T,PWB}$ was higher in the female patients, $V_{T,ABW}$ was higher in the male patients. It should be noticed, however, that the male patients had a significantly higher body mass index (BMI) compared with the females.

Next to the finding that female patients are ventilated with higher $V_{T,PBW}$, it is seen that PEEP was lower and ΔP was higher. These differences were rather small, and probably, therefore, less meaningful, and were only present at day 1. There was a remarkable difference in median Crs between the sexes. This finding is in line with the results of the earlier studies in patients with ARDS before COVID-19 (15, 42). The difference in Crs might be explained by differences in height (42). Further research may reveal associations between other anthropometric factors and Crs.

The findings of the mediation analysis are in line with findings of the previous studies in patients in the ICU (16) and in the operating room (12). In contrary to previous findings, we see that differences are only partly explained by sex *per se*. The actual body weight mediated the sex inequality in the use of LTVV in a model as a single factor, but not in the model using also body height.

Our findings point out the importance of using reliable methods to measure the height of the patients.

This analysis has some limitations; first, we only collected data during the first 4 calendar days of ventilation, and we cannot exclude the possibility that ventilation practices beyond these days remain different. Seen the observational nature of the study, we could not control for the unmeasured confounders. Also, the knowledge that ventilation data were being captured could have interfered with daily practice. The selection of ICUs was based on the personal contacts, which could have resulted in an overrepresentation of ICUs with more experience in lung-protective ventilation, including the use of LTVV, and the willingness to participate could have led to selection bias. Another limitation is that because this study was a national study, its worldwide generalizability is uncertain. Finally, the PRoVENT–COVID study did not collect the type of oxygen support before intubation. Early application of HFNC (high-flow nasal cannula) in the mild stage of ARDS may reduce mortality in the elderly patients with severe COVID-19 pneumonia (43). Further research should look into the influence of HFNC and should consider grouping the patients by age to see the impact of age on the use of LTVV in general and in female patients.

CONCLUSION

In this cohort of patients with ARDS related to COVID-19 who required invasive ventilation in the first wave of the national outbreak in the Netherlands, females received LTVV less often than males. Alike in the previous studies, in this cohort, the difference in the use of LTVV was driven by the anthropometric factors more than by sex *per se*. This information could be helpful in the proper titration of V_T in critically ill patients with COVID-19 and beyond.

AUTHOR CONTRIBUTIONS

PS, MS, and FP were involved in the conceptualization, methodology, and worked with drafting of the manuscript. Acquisition, analysis, or interpretation of data was done by all the authors. Critical revision of the manuscript for important intellectual content by all the other authors. Statistical analysis was done by PS and AN. Administrative, technical, or material support was done by MS. MS, FP, and AN supervised the work.

THE PROVENT–COVID COLLABORATIVE GROUP

Investigators (in alphabetic order) J. P. van Akkeren; A. G. Algera; C. K. Algoe; R. B. van Amstel; O. L. Baur; P. van de Berg; D. C. J. J. Bergmans; D. I. van den Bersselaar; F. A. Bertens; A. J. G. H. Bindels; M. M. de Boer; S. den Boer; L. S. Boers; M. Bogerd; L. D. J. Bos; M. Botta; J. S. Breel; H. de Bruin; S. de Bruin; C. L. Bruna; L. A. Buiteman–Kruizinga; O. Cremer; R. M. Determann; W. Dieperink; D. A. Dongelmans; H. S. Franke; M. S. Galek Aldridge; M. J. de Graaff; L. A. Hagens; J. J. Haringman; N. F. L. Heijnen; S. Hiel; S. T. van der Heide; P. L. J. van der Heiden; L. L. Hoeijmakers; L. Hol; M. W. Hollmann; M. E. Hoogendoorn; J. Horn; R. van der Horst; E. L. K. Ie; D. Ivanov; N. P. Juffermans; E. Kho; E. S. de Klerk; A. W. M. Koopman; M. Koopmans; S. Kucukcelebi; M. A. Kuiper; D. W. de Lange; D. M. van Meenen; Ignacio Martin–Loeches, Guido Mazzinari; N. van Mourik; S. G. Nijbroek; M. Onrust; E. A. N. Oostdijk; F. Paulus; C. J. Pennartz; J. Pillay; L. Pisani; I. M. Purmer; T. C. D. Rettig; J. P Roozeman; M. T. U. Schuijt; M. J. Schultz; A. Serpa Neto; M. E. Sleeswijk; M. R. Smit; P. E. Spronk; W. Stilma; A. C. Strang; A. M. Tsonas; P. R Tuinman; C. M. A. Valk; F. L. Veen; A. P. J. Vlaar; L. I. Veldhuis; P. van Velzen; W. H. van der Ven; P. van Vliet; P. van der Voort; H. H. van der Wier; L. van Welie; H. J. F. T. Wesselink; B. van Wijk; T. Winters; W. Y. Wong; and A. R. H. van Zanten.

REFERENCES

1. Wu C, Chen X, Cai Y, Xia J, Zhou X, Xu S, et al. Risk factors associated with acute respiratory distress syndrome and death in patients with coronavirus disease 2019 pneumonia in Wuhan, China. *JAMA Intern Med.* (2020) 180:934–43. doi: 10.1001/jamainternmed.2020.0994
2. Bennett S, Tafuro J, Mayer J, Darlington D, Wong CW, Muntean EA, et al. Clinical features and outcomes of adults with coronavirus disease 2019: a systematic review and pooled analysis of the literature. *Int J Clin Pract.* (2021) 75:e13725. doi: 10.1111/ijcp.13725
3. Brower RG, Matthay MA, Morris A, Schoenfeld D, Thompson BT, Wheeler A. Ventilation with lower tidal volumes as compared with traditional tidal volumes for acute lung injury and the acute respiratory distress syndrome. *N Engl J Med.* (2000) 342:1301–8. doi: 10.1056/nejm200005043421801
4. Griffiths MJD, Mcauley DF, Perkins GD, Barrett N, Blackwood B, Boyle A, et al. Guidelines on the management of acute respiratory distress syndrome. *BMJ Open Respir Res.* (2019) 6:e000420. doi: 10.1136/bmjresp-2019-000420
5. Botta M, Tsonas AM, Pillay J, Boers LS, Algera AG, Bos LDJ, et al. Ventilation management and clinical outcomes in invasively ventilated patients with COVID-19 (PRoVENT-COVID): a national, multicentre, observational cohort study. *Lancet Respir Med.* (2020) 9:139–48. doi: 10.1016/s2213-2600(20)30459-8
6. Ferreira JC, Ho Y-L, Besen BAMP, Malbouisson LMS, Taniguchi LU, Mendes PV, et al. Protective ventilation and outcomes of critically ill patients with COVID-19: a cohort study. *Ann Intensive Care.* (2021) 11:92. doi: 10.1186/s13613-021-00882-w
7. Fernandez-Bustamante A, Wood CL, Tran ZV, Moine P. Intraoperative ventilation: incidence and risk factors for receiving large tidal volumes during general anesthesia. *BMC Anesthesiol.* (2011) 11:22. doi: 10.1186/1471-2253-11-22
8. Karalapillai D, Weinberg L, Galtieri J, Glassford N, Eastwood G, Darvall J, et al. Current ventilation practice during general anaesthesia: a prospective audit in Melbourne, Australia. *BMC Anesthesiol.* (2014) 14:85. doi: 10.1186/1471-2253-14-85
9. Bender SP, Paganelli WC, Gerety LP, Tharp WG, Shanks AM, Housey M et al. Intraoperative lung-protective ventilation trends and practice patterns: a report from the multicenter perioperative outcomes group. *Anesth Analg.* (2015) 121:1231–9. doi: 10.1213/ane.0000000000000940
10. Wanderer JP, Ehrenfeld JM, Epstein RH, Kor DJ, Bartz RR, Fernandez-Bustamante A, et al. Temporal trends and current practice patterns for intraoperative ventilation at U.S. academic medical centers: a retrospective study. *BMC Anesthesiol.* (2015) 15:40. doi: 10.1186/s12871-015-0010-3
11. Kowa CY, Jin Z, Longbottom R, Cullinger B, Walker P. Risk factors for excessive tidal volumes delivered during intraoperative mechanical ventilation, a retrospective study. *Int J Physiol Pathophysiol Pharmacol.* (2020) 12:51–7.

12. Nijbroek SG, Hol L, Swart P, Hemmes SNT, Serpa Neto A, Binnekade JM, et al. Sex difference and intra-operative tidal volume: insights from the LAS VEGAS study. *Eur J Anaesthesiol.* (2021) 38:1034–41. doi: 10.1097/eja.0000000000001476
13. Gajic O, Dara SI, Mendez JL, Adesanya AO, Festic E, Caples SM, et al. Ventilator-associated lung injury in patients without acute lung injury at the onset of mechanical ventilation. *Crit Care Med.* (2004) 32:1817–24. doi: 10.1097/01.ccm.0000133019.52531.30
14. Lellouche F, Dionne S, Simard S, Bussieres J, Dagenais F. High tidal volumes in mechanically ventilated patients increase organ dysfunction after cardiac surgery. *Anesthesiology.* (2012) 116:1072–82. doi: 10.1097/ALN.0b013e3182522df5
15. McNicholas BA, Madotto F, Pham T, Rezoagli E, Masterson CH, Horie S, et al. Demographics, management and outcome of females and males with acute respiratory distress syndrome in the LUNG SAFE prospective cohort study. *Eur Respir J.* (2019) 54:1900609. doi: 10.1183/13993003.00609-2019
16. Swart P, Deliberato RO, Johnson AEW, Pollard TJ, Bulgarelli L, Pelosi P, et al. Impact of sex on use of low tidal volume ventilation in invasively ventilated ICU patients—a mediation analysis using two observational cohorts. *PLoS ONE.* (2021) 16:e0253933. doi: 10.1371/journal.pone.0253933
17. Ranieri VM, Rubenfeld GD, Thompson BT, Ferguson ND, Caldwell E, Fan E, et al. Acute respiratory distress syndrome: the Berlin definition. *JAMA.* (2012) 307:2526–33. doi: 10.1001/jama.2012.5669
18. Angus DC, Derde L, Al-Beidh F, Annane D, Arabi Y, Beane A, et al. Effect of hydrocortisone on mortality and organ support in patients with severe COVID-19: the REMAP-CAP COVID-19 corticosteroid domain randomized clinical trial. *JAMA.* (2020) 324:1317–29. doi: 10.1001/jama.2020.17022
19. Serpa Neto A, Hemmes SN, Barbas CS, Beiderlinden M, Biehl M, Binnekade JM, et al. Protective versus conventional ventilation for surgery: a systematic review and individual patient data meta-analysis. *Anesthesiology.* (2015) 123:66–78. doi: 10.1097/aln.0000000000000706
20. Madotto F, Pham T, Bellani G, Bos LD, Simonis FD, Fan E, et al. Resolved versus confirmed ARDS after 24 h: insights from the LUNG SAFE study. *Intensive Care Med.* (2018) 44:564–77. doi: 10.1007/s00134-018-5152-6
21. Lanspa MJ, Peltan ID, Jacobs JR, Sorensen JS, Carpenter L, Ferraro JP, et al. Driving pressure is not associated with mortality in mechanically ventilated patients without ARDS. *Crit Care.* (2019) 23:424. doi: 10.1186/s13054-019-2698-9
22. Azzolina D, Magnani C, Gallo E, Ferrante D, Gregori D. [Gender and age factors affecting the mortality during the COVID-19 epidemic in Italy]. *Epidemiol Prev.* (2020) 44:252–9. doi: 10.19191/ep20.5-6.S2.125
23. Chen J, Bai H, Liu J, Chen G, Liao Q, Yang J, et al. Distinct clinical characteristics and risk factors for mortality in female inpatients with coronavirus disease 2019 (COVID-19): a sex-stratified, large-scale cohort study in Wuhan, China. *Clin Infect Dis.* (2020) 71:3188–95. doi: 10.1093/cid/ciaa920
24. Jin JM, Bai P, He W, Wu F, Liu XF, Han DM, et al. Gender differences in patients with COVID-19: focus on severity and mortality. *Front Public Health.* (2020) 8:152. doi: 10.3389/fpubh.2020.00152
25. Kragholm K, Andersen MP, Gerds TA, Butt JH, Østergaard L, Polcwiartek C, et al. Association between male sex and outcomes of coronavirus disease 2019 (Covid-19) - a Danish nationwide, register-based study. *Clin Infect Dis.* (2020) 73:e4025–30. doi: 10.1093/cid/ciaa924
26. Nasiri MJ, Haddadi S, Tahvildari A, Farsi Y, Arbabi M, Hasanzadeh S, et al. COVID-19 clinical characteristics, and sex-specific risk of mortality: systematic review and meta-analysis. *Front Med.* (2020) 7:459. doi: 10.3389/fmed.2020.00459
27. Takahashi T, Ellingson MK, Wong P, Israelow B, Lucas C, Klein J, et al. Sex differences in immune responses that underlie COVID-19 disease outcomes. *Nature.* (2020) 588:315–20. doi: 10.1038/s41586-020-2700-3
28. Pijls BG, Jolani S, Atherley A, Derckx RT, Dijkstra JIR, Franssen GHL, et al. Demographic risk factors for COVID-19 infection, severity, ICU admission and death: a meta-analysis of 59 studies. *BMJ Open.* (2021) 11:e044640. doi: 10.1136/bmjopen-2020-044640
29. Tejpal A, Gianos E, Cerise J, Hirsch JS, Rosen S, Kohn N, et al. Sex-based differences in COVID-19 outcomes. *J Womens Health.* (2021) 30:492–501. doi: 10.1089/jwh.2020.8974
30. Vahidy FS, Pan AP, Ahnstedt H, Munshi Y, Choi HA, Tiruneh Y, et al. Sex differences in susceptibility, severity, and outcomes of coronavirus disease 2019: cross-sectional analysis from a diverse US metropolitan area. *PLoS ONE.* (2021) 16:e0245556. doi: 10.1371/journal.pone.0245556
31. Liu D, Ding HL, Chen Y, Chen DH, Yang C, Yang LM, et al. Comparison of the clinical characteristics and mortalities of severe COVID-19 patients between pre- and post-menopause women and age-matched men. *Aging.* (2021) 13:21903–13. doi: 10.18632/aging.203532
32. Ambrosino I, Barbagelata E, Corbi G, Ciarambino T, Politi C, Moretti AM. Gender differences in treatment of coronavirus disease-2019. *Monaldi Arch Chest Dis.* (2020) 90:646–56. doi: 10.4081/monaldi.2020.1508
33. Van Zeggeren IE, Boelen A, Van De Beek D, Heijboer AC, Vlaar APJ, Brouwer MC. Sex steroid hormones are associated with mortality in COVID-19 patients: level of sex hormones in severe COVID-19. *Medicine.* (2021) 100:e27072. doi: 10.1097/md.0000000000027072
34. Viveiros A, Rasmuson J, Vu J, Mulvagh SL, Yip CYY, Norris CM, et al. Sex differences in COVID-19: candidate pathways, genetics of ACE2, and sex hormones. *Am J Physiol Heart Circ Physiol.* (2021) 320:H296–304. doi: 10.1152/ajpheart.00755.2020
35. Edalatifard M, Akhtari M, Salehi M, Naderi Z, Jamshidi A, Mostafaei S, et al. Intravenous methylprednisolone pulse as a treatment for hospitalised severe COVID-19 patients: results from a randomised controlled clinical trial. *Eur Respir J.* (2020) 56:2002808. doi: 10.1183/13993003.02808-2020
36. Horby P, Lim WS, Emberson JR, Mafham M, Bell JL, Linsell L, et al. Dexamethasone in hospitalized patients with covid-19. *N Engl J Med.* (2021) 384:693–704. doi: 10.1056/NEJMoa2021436
37. Yu GQ, Jiang ZH, Yang ZB, Jiang SQ, Quan XQ. The effect of glucocorticoids on mortality in severe COVID-19 patients: evidence from 13 studies involving 6612 cases. *Medicine.* (2021) 100:e27373. doi: 10.1097/md.0000000000027373
38. Valentin A, Jordan B, Lang T, Hiesmayr M, Metnitz PG. Gender-related differences in intensive care: a multiple-center cohort study of therapeutic interventions and outcome in critically ill patients. *Crit Care Med.* (2003) 31:1901–7. doi: 10.1097/01.Ccm.0000069347.78151.50
39. Fowler RA, Sabur N, Li P, Juurlink DN, Pinto R, Hladunewich MA, et al. Sex- and age-based differences in the delivery and outcomes of critical care. *CMAJ.* (2007) 177:1513–9. doi: 10.1503/cmaj.071112
40. Pietropaoli AP, Glance LG, Oakes D, Fisher SG. Gender differences in mortality in patients with severe sepsis or septic shock. *Gend Med.* (2010) 7:422–37. doi: 10.1016/j.genm.2010.09.005
41. Chapa J, Nonas S. Differences in lung protective ventilation use in female vs male organ donors. *Chest.* (2018) 154:1101A. doi: 10.1016/j.chest.2018.08.1001
42. Vandenbunder B, Ehrmann S, Piagnerelli M, Sauneuf B, Serck N, Soumagne T, et al. Static compliance of the respiratory system in COVID-19 related ARDS: an international multicenter study. *Crit Care.* (2021) 25:52. doi: 10.1186/s13054-020-03433-0
43. Deng L, Lei S, Wang X, Jiang F, Lubarsky DA, Zhang L, et al. Course of illness and outcomes in older COVID-19 patients treated with HFNC: a retrospective analysis. *Aging.* (2021) 13:15801–14. doi: 10.18632/aging.203224
44. (2018). ESICM LIVES 2018: Paris, France. 20-24 October 2018. *Intensive Care Med Exp* 6:40. doi: 10.1186/s40635-018-0201-6

3

Early Immunomodulatory Effects of Different Natural Surfactant Preparations in Preterms with Respiratory Distress

Mehmet Yalaz[1], *Sema Tanriverdi*[2*], *Özgün Uygur*[3], *Özge Altun Köroğlu*[1], *Elif Azarsiz*[4], *Guzide Aksu*[4] *and Nilgün Kültürsay*[1]

[1] Department of Pediatrics, Division of Neonatology, Ege University Medical School, Izmir, Turkey, [2] Department of Pediatrics, Division of Neonatology, Manisa Celal Bayar University Medical School, Manisa, Turkey, [3] Department of Pediatrics, Division of Neonatology, Izmir Tepecik Training and Research Hospital, Izmir, Turkey, [4] Department of Pediatrics, Division of Pediatric Immunology, Ege University Medical School, Izmir, Turkey

Correspondence:
Sema Tanriverdi
drsemarala@yahoo.com

Background: Respiratory distress syndrome (RDS) is the most common respiratory disease in premature infants. Exogenous natural surfactant preparations are used in the treatment of RDS. In recent years, it has become increasingly evident that surfactant plays an immunoregulatory role.

Objectives: The aim of this study was to evaluate cytokine and chemokine response following three different regimens of natural surfactant treatment in preterm newborns with RDS.

Methods: Premature newborns below 32 weeks of gestation who were intubated for RDS and given early surfactant rescue therapy were included in the study. Newborns were randomly divided into three groups and Beractant 100 mg/kg (B-100), Poractant alfa 100 mg/kg (Pα-100) and Poractant alfa 200 mg/kg (Pα-200) were administered intratracheally. Blood samples and transtracheal aspirates (TA) were collected just before and 4–6 h after the surfactant treatment. Total eosinophil count, inducible T Cell alpha chemoattractant (ITaC), macrophage inflammatory protein 3 beta (MIP3b), interleukins (IL) 5, 8, 9, 10, 13, immunoglobulin E (IgE), interferon gamma (IFN-γ), eotaxin and tumor necrosis factor beta-1 (TGF-β1) were measured from blood and tracheal aspirate samples.

Results: A total of 45 infants, 15 in each group, were included in the study. Mean gestational age, birth weight, antenatal, demographic and clinical characteristics of the study groups were similar. IFNγ concentration and eosinophil counts in TA decreased after surfactant replacement in all groups, especially in the infants treated with Pα-100 and Pα-200. Eotaxin, TGF beta and IL-8 concentrations in TA increased significantly in the infants treated with Pα-100 and Pα-200. IL-9 levels in TA decreased in the B-100 group but increased in the Pα-100 and Pα-200 groups. Blood levels of cytokines and chemokines showed significantly decreased levels of ITaC and MIP3b only in the B-100 group, but no significant change was observed in the Pα-100 and Pα-200 groups.

Conclusion: In our study, the different immunomodulatory effects of natural surfactant preparations on newborn lung is proven. We found that Poractant α, one of the natural surfactant preparations, shifted the lung immune system toward TH2.

Keywords: surfactant, prematurity, respiratory distress syndrome, immune response, newborn

INTRODUCTION

Respiratory distress syndrome (RDS) is a disease that can result in serious morbidities and death in premature infants. It is mainly caused by alveolar surfactant deficiency accompanying structural immaturity in the lung. Surfactant, which is a phospholipid-protein mixture (90% lipids, 5–10% proteins), reduces the surface tension keeping the alveoli open (1, 2). It is well known that natural exogenous surfactant treatment reduces mortality and morbidity in premature infants with RDS (3). Natural exogenous surfactant preparations, which have been shown to be more effective in infants with RDS, should be preferred in the treatment. Natural exogenous surfactant preparations are obtained by bronchopulmonary lavage or from mincing the lung tissue and extraction with organic solvents; it can then be purified by chromatography or supplemented with active ingredients. All surfactant preparations contain all the phospholipids found in endogenous lung surfactant; surfactant protein B and C also form part of the chemical composition.

Poractant alpha (Poractant α), one of the natural surfactant preparations available in our country, is produced by the lipid separation and purification of minced pork lung tissue by liquid gel chromatography. Its phospholipid concentration is 76 mg/ml, and protein concentration is 1 mg/ml (0.45 mg/ml surfactant protein B and 0.55 mg/ml surfactant protein C). Another natural surfactant preparation, Beractant, is produced from minced bovine lung tissue by lipid cleavage, and supplemented with dipalmitoylphosphatidylcholine, palmitic acid and tripalmitin. Its phospholipid concentration is 25 mg/ml and protein concentration is <1 mg/ml (surfactant protein B and C). As is seen, both preparations exhibit differences per dose and content. However, surfactant A and D proteins are not present in preparations available in the market (4). In addition to their roles in surfactant homeostasis, surfactant A and D proteins are known to be crucial host defense components against respiratory pathogens and allergens, play immunomodulatory roles (5).

Surfactant is an important component of the innate and adaptive immune system of the lung. It is necessary to regulate the immune response of the lung (6). Knowledge on the immunomodulatory effects of natural exogenous surfactant preparations in newborns is limited. RDS is characterized by intense inflammation along with the influx of neutrophils, monocytes, and macrophages within the alveoli and their released cytokines and chemokines such as interleukin 1 (IL-1), interleukin 8 (IL-8), interleukin 12 (IL-12), interferon-gamma (IFN-γ) and tumor necrosis factor alpha (TNF-α). The increase in the concentrations of these cytokines and chemokines were associated with severity of RDS. This inflammation significantly damages the lung parenchyma (7, 8). These proinflammatory mechanisms may cause secondary surfactant inactivation (7, 9). *In vitro* studies showed that, in cell cultures that have been exposed to inflammatory stimuli, Poractant α suppressed TNF-α synthesis and TNF-α receptors (10), Beractant was found to inhibit IL-1 beta and suppress the synthesis of Macrophage inflammatory protein 1 (MIP-1) (11). *In vivo* studies have also confirmed that surfactant applied intratracheally suppresses cytokine release (12). In a study comparing two surfactant preparations of 200 mg/kg Poractant α and 100 mg/kg Beractant treatment doses, it was shown that it did not affect the airway inflammatory response and there was no significant difference between IL-6 and IL-8 values in the tracheal aspirate (13). In this study, cytokine and chemokine responses were investigated in preterm infants with RDS following three different natural surfactant treatment protocols.

MATERIALS AND METHODS

Premature infants below 32 weeks of gestation who were intubated in our hospital for RDS and were treated with early surfactant rescue were included in our study. Surfactant replacement therapy should be administered as soon as possible (within 1–2 h after birth) in infants with RDS symptoms and a need for surfactant, which is the current strategy recommended for lung protection (1). The study was carried out with the approval of the Ege University Clinical Research Ethics Committee (12-1.1/15) and the financial support of the Ege University Scientific Research Projects Unit (MY-13-TIP-030).

Intubated premature infants with clinical findings of RDS were randomized according to their hospitalization protocol numbers and divided into three groups. Intubation was performed and intratracheal 100 mg/kg Beractant (B-100), 100 mg/kg Poractant alfa (Pα-100) and 200 mg/kg Poractant alfa (Pα-200) was administered to the infants in the 1st group, the 2nd group and the 3rd group, respectively.

Infants who needed mechanical ventilation for non-pulmonary conditions (congenital malformations such as cardiac defects, gastrointestinal defects such as abdominal wall defects and diaphragmatic hernia) were excluded from the study. Demographic and clinical features of newborns (intraventricular hemorrhage, patent ductus arteriosus, bronchopulmonary dyplasia, retinopathy of prematurity, pneumothorax, early and late onset sepsis, mortality) were recorded. During hospitalization, blood culture samples were obtained from the umbilical catheter and treated with ampicillin and gentamicin. Appropriate total parenteral fluid support was started, and minimal enteral nutrition was initiated for all newborn babies within the first 24 h of life.

In our neonatal unit, according to international guidelines, mechanical ventilation therapy was performed using the Babylog 8000 plus (Draeger, Lübeck, Germany) synchronized intermittent positive pressure ventilation-volume guarantee (SIPPV-VG) ventilation mode. Initial ventilator settings; were set to tidal volume (VT): 4 mL/kg, positive end-expiratory pressure (PEEP): 5 cm H_2O, peak inspiratory pressure (PIP) 2–3 cm H_2O higher than minimum pressure to achieve target VT, respiratory rate: 40–60/min, inspiratory time: 0.30-0.3 and fraction of inspired oxygen (FiO_2) was adjusted to provide a saturation of 90–95%. Respiration rate, VT, and FiO_2 were adjusted during weaning from the mechanical ventilator.

Sample Collection

Blood and tracheal aspirate fluid samples were collected just before and 6 h after surfactant administration. Tracheal aspirate was taken from the endotracheal tube after 1 cc of saline was given and positive pressure was applied 5 times, and negative pressure was applied with a sterile aspiration catheter. Eosinophil counts from blood and tracheal aspirate samples were immediately done with an instant Abbott Cell DYN 3700 counter. Other tracheal aspirate fluid and blood samples were centrifuged at 10,000 rpm and the obtained samples were stored at −80°C until batch analysis. After all samples were collected, inducible T Cell alpha chemoattractant (ITaC), macrophage inflammatory protein 3 beta (MIP3b), eotaxin, IL-5, IL-8, IL-9, IL-10, IL-13, immunoglobulin E (IgE), IFN-γ, tumor necrosis factor beta-1 (TGF-β1) levels were measured by ELISA method in Ege University Medical Faculty Immunology Laboratory. The results of serum and tracheal aspirate samples in the three surfactant treatment protocols were compared. All cases in the study groups were monitored prospectively in terms of clinical findings, short term morbidity and mortality.

Statistical Analysis

Statistical analysis was performed using the SPSS for Windows statistical package (SPSS version 21.0 for Windows, IBM Corp., US). The difference between two groups was examined by independent samples *t*-test for normally distributed variables and the Mann–Whitney U-test for non-normally distributed variables. Differences among more than two groups were examined by ANOVA with repeated measures. A paired *t*-test was used to compare the arithmetic averages of two independent groups. The chi-square was used to compare categorical variables between groups. The Kolmogorov–Smirnov test was used to evaluate the normal distribution assumption for numerical variables. A *p*-value of <0.05 was considered statistically significant.

RESULTS

Forty-five premature infants with clinical signs of RDS who were intubated were randomized into three groups. Fifteen preterm infants in group 1 were on B-100, 15 preterm infants in group 2 were on Pα-100, and 15 preterm infants in group 3 were on Pα-200. The mean gestational age of the groups (B-100 Group: 28.13 ± 2.55 weeks; Pα-100 Group: 28.80 ± 2.56 weeks; Pα-200 Group: 27.46 ± 3.64 weeks) and birth weights (B-100 Group: 1212.33 ± 382.82 grams; Pα-100 Group: 1319, 80 ± 390.95 grams; Pα-200 Group: 1127.07 ± 840.00 grams), demographic and antenatal characteristics showed no difference among the groups (**Table 1**).

There was no difference in terms of the hours of surfactant administered as early rescue therapy among the groups. There was no significant difference among the three groups with regard to mechanical ventilation need, mechanical ventilation duration, oxygen index (OI), nasal continuous positive airway pressure (nCPAP), and pneumothorax frequency (**Table 2**).

In the clinical follow-up of the cases, no significant difference was found among the groups in terms of sepsis, patent ductus arteriosus (PDA), retinopathy of prematurity (ROP), necrotizing enterocolitis (NEC), bronchopulmonary dysplasia (BPD), length of hospital stay and mortality. However, intraventricular hemorrhage (IVH) and hydrocephalus rates were found to be significantly higher in group 3 (**Table 3**).

Chemokine and cytokine responses of three surfactant treatment protocols (B-100, Pα-100 and Pα-200) in preterm infants with RDS were evaluated in tracheal aspirate (TA) samples before and after surfactant administration (**Table 4**). Eosinophil ratios and IFN-γ levels decreased significantly in three groups after surfactant therapy ($p < 0.05$). Eotaxin and TGF-β1 levels decreased significantly in the B-100 group after surfactant, and eotaxin and TGF-β1 levels increased significantly in the Pα-100 and Pα-200 groups ($p < 0.05$). IL-8 levels increased significant ly in all three groups after treatment ($p > 0.05$). There were no significant changes in ITaC, MIP3b, IgE, IL-5, IL-9, IL-10, IL-13 levels in the three groups (**Figure 1**).

Chemokine and cytokine responses of three surfactant treatment protocols (B-100, Pα-100, Pα-200) in preterm infants with RDS were evaluated in blood serum samples before and after surfactant administration (**Table 5**). Only ITaC and MIP3b levels showed a significant decrease in the B-100 group, while no significant change was seen in the Pα-100 and Pα-200 groups (**Table 5**).

DISCUSSION

Our results show that natural exogenous surfactant administration in preterm infants with RDS may cause some quantitative changes in local and systemic immune mediators which may have a possible short and/or long-term effects, although we were unable to predict long-term outcomes. Pulmonary surfactant is a lipoprotein complex that performs two main functions. It reduces surface tension at the air-liquid interface of the lung and it plays a role in host defense against infection and inflammation (14). The literature of the last 20 years has revealed that endogenous pulmonary surfactant has immunoregulatory abilities that can alter the function of the innate and acquired immune system (15). Surfactant has the potential to interact with a variety of immune system cells that regulate allergen- or pathogen-induced airway inflammatory events. Surfactant modulates airway physiology and immunology in inflammatory conditions (6).

TABLE 1 | Comparison of demographic characteristics of the groups.

Groups	B-100 *(n = 15)*	Pα-100 *(n = 15)*	Pα-200 *(n = 15)*	*P*-value
Gestational age (week) (mean ± SD)	28.13 ± 2.55 (25–32)	28.80 ± 2.56 (23–32)	27.46 ± 3.64 (22–32)	0.475
Birth weight (g) (mean ± SD)	1212.33 ± 382.82 (760–1940)	1319.80 ± 390.95 (800–1880)	1127.07 ± 840.00 (630–1880)	0.471
Cesarean section (*n*, %)	15 (%100)	13 (%86.7)	11 (%73.4)	0.099
Male gender (*n*, %)	8 (%53.4)	8 (%53.4)	7 (%46.6)	0.915
Antenatal steroid treatment* (*n*, %)	7 (%46.6)	11 (%73.4)	10 (%66.6)	0.293
Chorioamnionitis** (*n*, %)	1 (%6.6)	3 (%20)	5 (%33.3)	0.189
PROM*** (*n*, %)	5 (%33.3)	7 (%46.6)	7 (%46.6)	0.695
Apgar score at 1st min (median)	5 (3–8)	5 (4–8)	5 (4–8)	0.586
Apgar score at 5th min (median)	7 (6–10)	7 (6–10)	7 (6–10)	0.378

**Antenatal steroid therapy was considered to be given if mother received two doses of 12 mg of betamethasone intramuscularly 24 h apart at any time prior to delivery. **Chorioamnionitis was diagnosed by if two or more of the following were present: maternal fever equal to or higher than 37.8°C, with no alternative source; white blood cell count above 15,000 cells/mm3; uterine fundal tenderness; fetal tachycardia and vaginal discharge with purulent or foul odor. ***PROM, premature rupture of membranes.*

TABLE 2 | Comparison of respiratory follow-up of the groups.

Groups	B-100 *(n = 15)*	Pα-100) *(n = 15)*	Pα-200) *(n = 15)*	*P*-value
Mechanical ventilation duration (day) (mean ± SD)	14.07 ± 19.00 (1–70)	10.40 ± 14.21 (1–57)	35.26 ± 64.59 (2–260)	0.209
Oxygen index (before)	6.89 (10.8)	8.5 (7.5)	8.6 (15.1)	0.454
Oxygen index (after)	5.76 (3.6)	5.6 (12.4)	6.14 (3.3)	0.315
nCPAP* duration (day) (mean ± SD)	9.60 ± 9.20 (1–21)	11.71 ± 11.54 (2–33)	12.25 ± 13.25 (1–39)	0.922
Oxygen treatment duration (day) (mean ± SD)	22.76 ± 26.24 (1–80)	21.06 ± 36.37 (1–149)	47.86 ± 69.46 (4-280)	0.257
Pneumothorax (*n*, %)	2 (%13.3)	3 (%20)	6 (%40)	0.209
Surfactant administration time after birth (hour)	1.53 (1.12)	1.93 (1.33)	2.07 (1.43)	0.513

**nCPAP, Nasal Continuous Positive Airway Pressure.*

The main risk factors for pulmonary pathophysiological sequelae from RDS in premature infants include immature lung tissue, decreased host defense and antioxidant systems, volutrauma and barotrauma due to mechanical ventilation, oxidant damage and infection from supplemental oxygen exposure (16). A common finding among these risk factors is that they are known to cause an undesirable inflammatory response in the lung. Events that lead to inflammation in the lung and subsequent remodeling of the lung structure result in the inflammatory response immediately after birth even if lung protective respiratory strategies are used (17). Surfactant-treated preterm lambs and baboons with RDS develop BPD associated with elevation of proinflammatory cytokines in the lungs (18, 19). These findings have also been reported in newborn infants who subsequently developed BPD (20, 21). These relationships support the claim that inflammation in the lung is an important precursor in the development of BPD (16).

Surfactant consists of four different types of proteins: SP-A, SP-B, SP-C and SP-D. The hydrophilic proteins i.e., SP-A and SP-D are members of the collectin protein family that have the ability to opsonize pathogens and facilitate phagocytosis by macrophages and monocytes (22). The immunoregulatory property of surfactant is provided by surfactant proteins A and D (23). They regulate the production of inflammatory mediators (24). At the onset of allergic inflammation, SP-A and SP-D inhibit T lymphocyte proliferation (25). Interestingly, SP-A increased TGF-β secretion and increased the frequency of regulatory T lymphocytes (26). Both SP-A and SP-D inhibit IgE binding to allergens, suppress histamine release from mast cells, suppress TH2 cells and decrease TH2 cytokine levels, increase TH1 cytokine level, and stimulate anti-inflammatory TGF-β1 secretion (27).

In recent years, SP-A and SP-D have attracted more and more attention because of their role in host defense and lung immune responses (23). In experimental asthma models, it has been shown that acute allergic airway inflammation is more severe as a result of increased eosinophil infiltration and abnormal activation of lymphocytes, which leads to the production of TH2 cytokines in SP-A or SP-D deficient mice (28). On the contrary, inflammatory cytokines released during allergic inflammation lead to impaired pulmonary surfactant function (29, 30). It has been shown that administration of synthetic surfactant preparations (without SP A and SP-D) in asthmatic patients

TABLE 3 | Comparison of short morbidity and mortality of the groups.

Groups	B-100 *(n = 15)*	Pα-100 *(n = 15)*	Pα-200 *(n = 15)*	*P*-value
Hemodynamically significant PDA* (*n*, %)	6 (%40)	8 (%53.3)	7 (%46.6)	0.765
BPD (*n*, %)**				0.185
None	9 (%60)	11 (%73.3)	8 (%53.3)	
Mild	3 (%20)	2 (%13.3)	0 (%0)	
Moderate	0 (%0)	0 (%0)	2 (%13.3)	
Severe	3 (%20)	2 (%13.3)	5 (%33.3)	
BPD**-postnatal steroid usage (*n*, %)	3 (%20)	5 (%33.3)	5 (%33.3)	0.548
Pulmonary hypertension (*n*, %)***	1 (%6.6)	4 (%26.6)	3 (%20)	0.345
Pulmonary hemorrhage (*n*, %)	2 (%13.3)	4 (%26.6)	3 (%20)	0.659
Sepsis (*n*, %)				0.624
None	3 (%20)	1 (%6.6)	2 (%13.3)	
Clinical	9 (% 60)	10 (%66.6)	7 (%46.6)	
Proven	3 (%20)	4 (%26.6)	6 (%40)	
Early sepsis (*n*, %)				0.175
None	7 (%46.6)	4 (%26.6)	3 (%20)	
Clinical	8 (%53.3)	11 (%73.3)	10 (%66.6)	
Proven	0 (%0)	0 (%0)	2 (%13.3)	
Late sepsis (*n*, %)				0.827
None	7 (%46.6)	8 (%53.3)	6 (%40)	
Clinical	6 (%40)	5 (%33.3)	7 (%46.6)	
Proven	2 (%13.3)	2 (%13.3)	2 (%13.3)	
ROP** (*n*, %)**				0.823
No	13 (%86.6)	12 (%80)	12 (%80)	
Yes	2 (%13.3)	3 (%20)	3 (%20)	
ROP****-laser treatment (*n*, %)	0 (%0)	1 (%6.6)	1 (%6.6)	0.518
IVH*** (*n*, %)**				**0.027**
None	10 (%66.6)	5 (%33.3)	4 (%26.6)	
Stage 1	2 (%13.3)	4 (%26.6)	1 (%6.6)	
Stage 2	0 (%0)	1 (%6.6)	0 (%0)	
Stage 3	0 (%0)	4 (%26.6)	8 (%53.3)	
Stage 4	3 (%20)	1 (%6.6)	2 (%13.3)	
Hydrocephalus (*n*, %)	3 (%20)	2 (%13.3)	8 (%53.3)	**0.046**
NEC**** (*n*, %)**				0.933
None	9 (%60)	7 (%46.6)	8 (%53.3)	
Stage 1	1 (%6.6)	2 (%13.3)	2 (%13.3)	
Stage 2	2 (%13.3)	3 (%20)	1 (%6.6)	
Stage 3	3 (%20)	3 (%20)	4 (%26.6)	
NEC****** surgery (*n*, %)	3 (%20)	3 (%20)	3 (%20)	1
Mortality (*n*, %)	7 (%46.6)	7 (%46.6)	6 (%40)	0.914
Length of hospital stay (day) (mean ± SD)	31.08 ± 31.64 (1-107)	40.27 ± 46.83 (1-149)	58.40 ± 68.55 (4-280)	0.373

**PDA, patent ductus arteriosus; **BPD, bronchopulmonary dysplasia; ****ROP, retinopathy of prematurity; *****IVH, intraventricular hemorrhage; ******NEC, necrotizing enterocolitis. ***Pulmonary hypertension was diagnosed in the patients with clinical signs by pediatric cardiology echocardiography. The bold values are statistically significant.*

improves lung function; however it also worsens the underlying allergic immune response (6).

Recent studies have shown that phospholipids and hydrophobic proteins SP-B and SP-C, which are essential for biophysical functions, also have anti-inflammatory and antibacterial functions and contribute to immunomodulation (31, 32). It has been demonstrated that SP-B and SP-C reduce the activation of neutrophil granulocytes, can also affect other immunological cells such as macrophages, and reduce lipopolysaccharide-induced inflammation via their anti-inflammatory properties (33, 34). It has been found that SP-C binds to lipopolysaccharide through its N-terminal shadow and contributes to immunomodulation as a result of its effect (31, 32, 35). CHF5633, a new synthetic surfactant preparation

TABLE 4 | Comparison of cytokine and chemokine levels before and after surfactant in tracheal aspirate samples of three groups.

Groups	B-100 (n = 15)			Pα-100 (n = 15)			Pα-200 (n = 15)		
	Before	After	p-value	Before	After	p-value	Before	After	p-value
Eosinophil ratio (%)	57	44	*	62	43	*	55	38	*
IFN-γ (mean ± SD)	0.28 ± 0.14	0.05 ± 0.03	*	0.29 ± 0.14	0.07 ± 0.17	*	0.33 ± 0.01	0.09 ± 0.07	*
Eotaxin (mean ± SD)	44.92 ± 84.79	32.75 ± 50.03	*	6.98 ± 4.56	31.26 ± 29.03	*	8.25 ± 5.33	14.87 ± 8.11	*
TGF-β1 (mean ± SD)	3548.46 ± 1257.13	2922.58 ± 1670.26	*	3347.88 ± 1993.56	4190.92 ± 1950.93	*	2794.88 ± 1625.88	3850.17 ± 1793.02	*
IL8 (mean ± SD)	616.51 ± 840.69	1036.10 ± 784.12	*	541.66 ± 804.63	1024.01 ± 852.40	*	714.16 ± 862.73	1071.86 ± 869.02	*
IL9 (mean ± SD)	0.17 ± 0.13	0.15 ± 0.14	**	0.18 ± 0.14	0.22 ± 0.12	**	0.28 ± 0.14	0.32 ± 0.12	**
ITaC (mean ± SD)	1753.64 ± 615.40	1324.15 ± 292.75	**	1744.74 ± 462.51	1823.57 ± 302.96	**	1758.16 ± 691.23	1857.83 ± 607.60	**
MIP 3b (mean ± SD)	48.86 ± 64.98	38.08 ± 45.80	**	47.04 ± 54.58	57.84 ± 52.05	**	49.65 ± 47.95	55.92 ± 90.85	**
IgE (mean ± SD)	16.28 ± 5.92	3.80 ± 6.10	**	14.97 ± 4.77	3.98 ± 2.35	**	4.52 ± 7.73	9.60 ± 2.09	**
IL5 (mean ± SD)	0.467 ± 0.076	0.328 ± 0.077	**	0.458 ± 0.058	0.680 ± 0.077	**	0.211 ± 0.076	0.210 ± 0.077	**
IL10 (mean ± SD)	0.258 ± 0.261	1.741 ± 0.143	**	0.322 ± 0.229	1.038 ± 0.227	**	0.423 ± 0.183	0.630 ± 0.214	**
IL13 (mean ± SD)	16.97 ± 50.67	15.72 ± 46.06	**	14.43 ± 26.89	14.43 ± 35.50	**	15.58 ± 60.40	18.34 ± 17.81	**

*$p < 0.05$; **$p > 0.05$.

containing SP-B and SP-C analogs, has been shown to reduce lipopolysaccharide-induced TNF-α and IL-1 beta cytokine production in human neonatal monocytes (36).

It was reported that SP-B deficiency results in reversible pulmonary inflammation and leads to neutrophil migration to the lung (37). Mice lacking SP-C have an excessive and persistent immune response of macrophages to viral and bacterial lung infections, suggesting that SP-C is a factor that minimizes inflammation (35). Unlike SP-A and SP-D, SP-C does not opsonize pathogens, while the absence of SP-C results in impaired phagocytosis by alveolar macrophages (38).

Natural and synthetic surfactant preparations have been used successfully in the treatment of RDS (39). Natural surfactant preparations contain all the phospholipids found in endogenous lung surfactant, SP-B and SP-C proteins; however, SP-A and SP-D proteins are lacking (40).

Surfactant proteins of natural surfactant preparations, phospholipids of natural and synthetic surfactant preparations, as well as artificial components are antigenic (41). Whether there is a risk of immunological sensitization in infants administered exogenous surfactant is still a matter of debate. Furthermore, surfactant and its components modulate the initiation of the inflammatory response by changing the immune function of the lung (42). *In vitro* studies have documented an interaction between alveolar macrophages and surfactant in immunological defense during inflammatory processes in the lungs. It has been suggested that the change in surfactant phospholipids in various pathological conditions may cause an increase in macrophage accumulation in the alveolar space (43). The mechanisms by which exogenous surfactants or phospholipids modulate the inflammatory cascade in alveolar macrophage are unclear (44). Probably cytokines play a central role in the immune response and pathogenesis (45). It has been shown that synthetic surfactant reduces the level of inflammatory cytokines in human alveolar macrophages and suppresses cytokine production in TH1 (46).

In the study conducted in preterm lambs, the synthetic surfactant lucinactant (the amount of KL4 peptide similar to SP B in its structure is 3 times higher than that of Beractant and Poractant α) showed that lung and systemic inflammation was less severe, and lung structural integrity was preserved compared to natural animal-derived Beractant and Poractant α (47). It is a key component of SP-B's ability to reduce alveolar surface tension, maintain surfactant structure, and protect against lung injury (48). These protective effects increase with the higher concentration of SP-B-like KL4 peptide in lucinactant (47). CHF5633, a new generation synthetic surfactant containing SP-B and SP-C synthetic analogs, is a surfactant preparation that also has no proinflammatory effect, balances pro- and anti-inflammatory cytokine response (49). Bezerra et al. (50) showed that proinflammatory markers IL 17 and TNF-α were reduced after the administration of Poractant α to adult mice with ARDS. Van Rensburg et al. (51) compared the immunogenic effects of three surfactant preparations (synthetic surfactant Synsurf, natural porcine lung surfactant Poractant α and bovine lung surfactant Liposurf in which the phospholipid concentrations were standardized as 500–1,500 μg/ml. They found that the

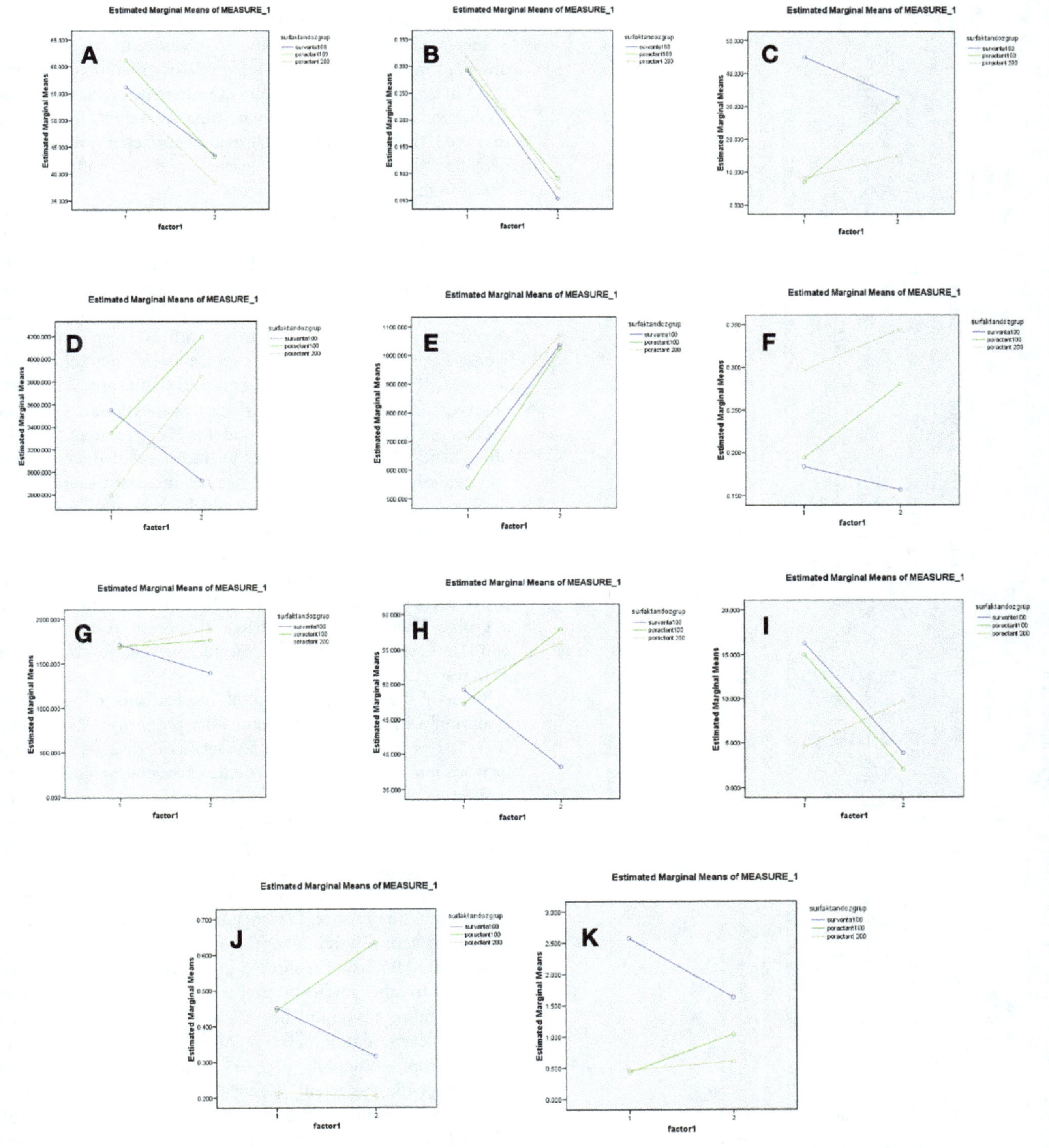

FIGURE 1 | Levels of intratracheal chemokines and cytokines before and after surfactants administration in all three groups **(A)** TA [Eosinophil (%)] **(B)** TA (IFN-γ) **(C)** TA (8Eotaxin) **(D)** TA (TGF beta) **(E)** TA (IL-8) **(F)** TA (IL-9) **(G)** TA (ITaC) **(H)** TA (MIP) **(I)** TA (IgE) **(J)** TA (IL-5) **(K)** TA (IL-10).

proinflammatory markers IL-8, TNF-α and IFN-γ levels were significantly decreased in the bronchoalveolar lavage samples taken after administration of all three surfactant preparations in sick children. It was stated that there was a significant increase in the levels of anti-inflammatory markers IL-10 and IL-12. These changes were more pronounced in the Poractant α group (51).

In our study, when the lung inflammatory response to intratracheal exogenous natural surfactant preparation

TABLE 5 | Comparison of cytokine and chemokine levels before and after surfactant in blood samples of three groups.

Groups	B-100 (n = 15)			Pα-100 (n = 15)			Pα-200 (n = 15)		
	Before	After	p-value	Before	After	p-value	Before	After	P-value
IFN-γ (mean ± SD)	0.52 ± 1.26	0.57 ± 0.88	**	0.41 ± 0.78	0.60 ± 0.89	**	0.66 ± 1.14	0.47 ± 027	**
Eotaxin (mean ± SD)	71.186 ± 47.70	58.17 ± 20.65	**	86.053 ± 51.52	87.06 ± 47.74	**	50.59 ± 29.25	58.53 ± 43.20	**
TGF-β1 (mean ± SD)	29583.00 ± 9111.39	24914.20 ± 3942.51	**	28950.20 ± 15095.30	27513.40 ± 15619.05	**	26928 ± 12708.01	21018.21 ± 11875.05	**
IL8 (mean ± SD)	684.11 ± 537.26	718.77 ± 570.61	**	847.88 ± 688.37	1012.96 ± 571.47	**	600.83 ± 429.86	696.35 ± 462.32	**
IL9 (mean ± SD)	1.26 ± 0.30	1.25 ± 0.24	**	1.29 ± 0.32	1.30 ± 0.22	**	1.35 ± 0.65	1.36 ± 0.58	**
ITaC (mean ± SD)	1715.14 ± 927.30	1388.29 ± 805.12	*	1691.85 ± 1039.44	1760.46 ± 1017.68	**	1685.58 ± 1024.27	1785.66 ± 1086.92	**
MIP3b (mean ± SD)	165.53 ± 43.18	138 ± 30.95	*	172.57 ± 55.46	170.52 ± 58.87	**	191.72 ± 53.24	232.58 ± 116.61	**
IgE (mean ± SD)	12.30 ± 3.10	12.43 ± 4.30	**	13.77 ± 4.28	13.48 ± 4.88	**	13.11 ± 2.47	13.25 ± 3.24	**

*$p < 0.05$; **$p > 0.05$.

was evaluated in intubated preterm infants with RDS, as proinflammatory markers IFN-γ decreased significantly, IL-8 increased significantly while no significant changes were observed in the levels of anti-inflammatory markers IL-10 and IL-13 in tracheal aspirate samples examined before and after the application of porcine and bovine lung surfactant. It was seen that Pα-100, Pα-200, and B-100 natural surfactant preparations had no significant proinflammatory and anti-inflammatory effects in the lung.

However, it was seen that eosinophil ratio, IFN-γ, eotaxin and TGF-β1 levels decreased significantly, and IL-8 levels increased significantly in tracheal aspirate samples after B-100 administration. Eosinophil ratio and IFN-γ level decreased significantly, and eotaxin, TGF-β1 and IL8 levels increased significantly after administration of both 100 mg/kg and 200 mg/kg doses of Poractant α. As an important marker of TH1 response, IFN-γ level decreased, while no significant change was observed in the level of ITaC, which was measured to evaluate chemotaxis only after Pα-100 and Pα-200 treatment. On the other hand, IL-8 level, which is an indicator of inflammation and oxidative stress and a TH2 marker, increased significantly. Besides the level of eotaxin, which evaluates eosinophil migration and allergic response increased significantly. All these findings suggested a TH2 shift as the immunological response to Poractant α. The IL-9 level, which evaluates bronchial hyperreactivity, was also insignificantly elevated in the Poractant α group. There was no consistent change in IL-5 and IL-10 and IL-13 cytokine levels, which were measured to evaluate the TH2 response.

One of the pathophysiological mechanisms of asthma is associated with the immunomodulatory properties of surfactant (52). It has been shown that Poractant α given after allergy provocation in asthmatic patients accelerates eosinophilic infiltration, eotaxin and IL-5 cytokine levels, which indicate the TH2 response in the bronchoalveolar lavage fluid, increase, and IFN-α levels decrease (53). Dry powder surfactant (Pumactant) inhalation administered after allergen provocation in patients with allergic asthma abolished the early phase response of asthma, but did not affect the late phase response (54). In a study comparing natural porcine, bovine and synthetic surfactants in *in vitro* studies, Poractant α showed higher eosinophil chemotaxis compared to other surfactant preparations, but lower eosinophil viability, more eosinophil necrosis and apoptosis, and higher cytokine levels, eosinophilic cationic protein (ECP) eotaxin released from eosinophils (53, 55). These findings indicate that the therapeutic surfactant, especially Poractant α, may affect allergic inflammation in the lung by acting on eosinophils (56). When the interaction between TH2 and surfactant proteins were investigated in animal studies, it has been shown that SP-D levels are significantly higher in the lungs of mice with high IL-4, IL-5, IL-13 cytokine levels (57, 58). SP-D, which is not found in natural surfactant preparations, has been shown to be an immune molecule that plays a protective role against allergies, asthma and inflammation. In experimental studies, it has been shown that SP-D inhibits the allergen-IgE interaction, suppresses histamine release from mast cells and specific IgE production. It can also shift the TH2 response to the TH1 response in allergic stimulation. Interestingly, it is known that Surfactant D deficient mice have excessive IL-13 secretion and IL-13 plays a role in the development of asthma (59).

It is known that exogenous surfactant treatment reduces mortality and morbidity in premature infants with RDS. In studies comparing surfactant treatment with placebo, it has been shown that the severity of RDS, mortality, mid-long-term pulmonary morbidities such as BPD, and pneumothorax are reduced. When poractant alfa is administered at an initial dose of 200 mg/kg, it has been shown to be associated with lower mortality than the same preparation at a dose of 100 mg/kg or beractant 100 mg/kg. However, it is not clear whether this relationship is dependent on the dose or the application of different surfactant preparations (3, 60, 61). In our study, the clinical follow-up of the cases, no significant difference was found among the groups in terms of BPD, pneumothorax and mortality.

CONCLUSION

In conclusion, natural surfactant preparations continue to be used successfully in the treatment of RDS in the neonatal period, but it is still a matter of debate whether there is a risk of immunological sensitization in patients given surfactant preparations. In our study, we found that Poractant α, one of the natural surfactant preparations, shifted the lung immune system toward TH2, which made us think that due to this immunomodulatory feature of surfactant, it may predispose to allergic inflammatory conditions such as asthma and bronchial hyperreactivity in older ages. SP-A and SP-D, which are not found in natural surfactant preparations, are known to reduce allergic inflammation and bronchial hypersensitivity. Therefore, the biological importance of Surfactant protein A and D against various lung diseases is increasingly recognized. The use of surfactant preparations supplemented with SP-A and SP-D in the treatment of RDS, which is the most common lung disease in preterm infants, seems to be promising due to early or late-term immune response regulation that may occur in the lung.

Limitations

The size of the population sample is limited. We did not compare immunological response to synthetic surfactants in this study.

ETHICS STATEMENT

The studies involving human participants were reviewed and approved by Ege University Clinical Research Ethics Committee (12-1.1/15). Written informed consent to participate in this study was provided by the participants' legal guardian/next of kin. Written informed consent was obtained from the minor(s)' legal guardian/next of kin for the publication of any potentially identifiable images or data included in this article.

AUTHOR CONTRIBUTIONS

All authors listed have made a substantial, direct, and intellectual contribution to the work and approved it for publication.

REFERENCES

1. Sweet DG, Carnielli V, Greisen G, Hallman M, Ozek E, Pas AT, et al. European consensus guidelines on the management of respiratory distress syndrome – 2019 update. *Neonatology.* (2019) 115:432–50. doi: 10.1159/000499361
2. Wiingreen R, Greisen G, Ebbesen F, Petersen JP, Zachariassen G, Henriksen TB, et al. Surfactant need by gestation for very preterm babies initiated on early nasal CPAP: a danish observational multicentre study of 6,628 infants born 2000-2013. *Neonatology.* (2017) 111:331–6. doi: 10.1159/000451021
3. Singh N, Halliday HL, Stevens TP, Suresh G, Soll R, Rojas-Reyes MX, et al. Comparison of animal- derived surfactants for the prevention and treatment of respiratory distress syndrome in preterm infants. *Cochrane Database Syst Rev.* (2015) 21:CD010249. doi: 10.1002/14651858.CD010249.pub2
4. Blanco O, Perez-Gil J. Biochemical and pharmacological differences between preparations of exogenous natural surfactant used to treat respiratory distress syndrome: role of the different components in an efficient pulmonary surfactant. *Eur J Pharmacol.* (2007) 568:1–15. doi: 10.1016/j.ejphar.2007.04.035
5. Kishore U, Greenhough TJ, Waters P, Shrive AK, Ghai R, Kamran MF, et al. Surfactant proteins SP-A and SP-D: structure, function and receptors. *Mol Immunol.* (2006) 43:1293–315. doi: 10.1016/j.molimm.2005.08.004
6. Winkler C, Hohlfeld JM. Surfactant and allergic airway inflammation. *Swiss Med Wkly.* (2003) 143:w13818. doi: 10.4414/smw.2013.13818
7. Speer CP. Neonatal respiratory distress syndrome: an inflammatory disease? *Neonatology.* (2011) 99:316–9. doi: 10.1159/000326619
8. Robertson B. Background to neonatal respiratory distress syndrome and treatment with exogenous surfactant. *Dev Pharmacol Therapeut.* (1989) 13:159–63. doi: 10.1159/000457599
9. Speer CP. Inflammation and bronchopulmonary dysplasia: a continuing story. *Semin Fetal Neonatal Med.* (2006) 11:354–62. doi: 10.1016/j.siny.2006.03.004
10. Speer CP, Götze B, Curstedt T, Robertson B. Phagocytic functions and tumor necrosis factor secretion of human monocytes exposed to natural porcine surfactant (Curosurf). *Pediatr Res.* (1991) 30:69–74. doi: 10.1203/00006450-199107000-00015
11. Geertsma MF, Teeuw WL, Nibbering PH, van Furth R. Pulmonary surfactant inhibits activation of human monocytes by recombinant interferon-[gamma]. *Immunology.* (1994) 82:450–6.
12. Mittal N, Sanyal SN. In vivo effect of surfactant on inflammatory cytokines during endotoxin- induced lung injury in rodents. *J Immunotoxicol.* (2011) 8:274–83. doi: 10.3109/1547691X.2011.591294
13. Mercado VV, Cristea I, Ali N, Pham CC, Buescher E, Yang J, et al. Does surfactant type cause a differential proinflammatory response in preterm infants with respiratory distress syndrome? *Adv Ther.* (2010) 27:476–82. doi: 10.1007/s12325-010-0044-3
14. Wright JR. Pulmonary surfactant: a front line of lung host defense. *J Clin Invest.* (2003) 111:1453–5. doi: 10.1172/JCI200318650
15. Schulz A, Raluy LP, Kolman JP, Königs I, Trochimiuk M, Appl B, et al. The inhibitory effect of curosurf and alveofact on the formation of neutrophil extracellular traps. *Front Immunol.* (2021) 11:582895. doi: 10.3389/fimmu.2020.582895
16. Jobe AH, Ikegami M. Prevention of bronchopulmonary dysplasia. *Curr Opin Pediatr.* (2001) 13:124–9. doi: 10.1097/00008480-200104000-00006
17. Wallace MJ, Probyn ME, Zahra VA, Crossley K, Cole TJ, Davis PG, et al. Early biomarkers and potential mediators of ventilation- induced lung injury in very

preterm lambs. *Respir Res.* (2009) 10:19. doi: 10.1186/1465-9921-10-19

18. Albertine KH, Jones GP, Starcher BC, Bohnsack JF, Davis PL, Cho SC, et al. Chronic lung injury in preterm lambs. disordered respiratory tract development. *Am J Respir Crit Care Med.* (1999) 159:945–58. doi: 10.1164/ajrccm.159.3.9804027
19. Coalson JJ, Winter VT, Siler-Khodr T, Yoder BA. Neonatal chronic lung disease in extremely immature baboons. *Am J Respir Crit Care Med.* (1999) 160:1333–46. doi: 10.1164/ajrccm.160.4.9810071
20. Groneck P, Speer CP. Inflammatory mediators and bronchopulmonary dysplasia. *Arch Dis Child Fetal Neonatal Ed.* (1995) 73:1-3. doi: 10.1136/fn.73.1.F1
21. Bose CL, Dammann CE, Laughon MM. Bronchopulmonary dysplasia and inflammatory biomarkers in the premature neonate. *Arch Dis Child Fetal Neonatal Ed.* (2008) 93:455–61. doi: 10.1136/adc.2007.121327
22. Whitsett JA, Nogee LM, Weaver TE, Horowitz AD. Human sur- factant protein B: structure, function, regulation and genetic disease. *Physiol Rev.* (1995) 75:749–57. doi: 10.1152/physrev.1995.75.4.749
23. Wright JR. Immunoregulatory functions of surfactant proteins. *Nat Rev Immunol.* (2005) 5:58–68. doi: 10.1038/nri1528
24. Wright JR. Immunomodulatory functions of surfactant. *Physiol Rev.* (1997) 77:931–62. doi: 10.1152/physrev.1997.77.4.931
25. Borron P, Veldhuizen RA, Lewis JF, Possmayer F, Caveney A, Inchley K, et al. Surfactant associated protein-A inhibits human lymphocyte proliferation and IL-2 production. *Am J Respir Cell Mol Biol.* (1996) 15:115–21. doi: 10.1165/ajrcmb.15.1.8679215
26. Mukherjee S, Giamberardino C, Thomas JM, Gowdy K, Pastva AM, Wright JR. Surfactant protein a modulates induction of regulatory T cells via TGF-beta. *J Immunol.* (2012) 188:4376–84. doi: 10.4049/jimmunol.1101775
27. Kishore U, Bernal AL, Kamran MF, Saxena S, Singh M, Sarma PU, et al. Surfactant protein SP-A and SP-D in human health and disease. *Arch Immunol Ther Exp.* (2005) 53:399–417.
28. Madan T, Reid KB, Singh M, Sarma PU, Kishore U. Susceptibility of mice genetically deficient in the surfactant protein (SP)-A or SP-D gene to pulmonary hypersensitivity induced by antigens and allergens of Aspergillus fumigatus. *J Immunol.* (2005) 174:6943–54. doi: 10.4049/jimmunol.174.11.6943
29. Atochina-Vasserman EN, Beers MF, Gow AJ. Review: chemical and structural modifications of pulmonary collectins and their functional consequences. *Innate Immun.* (2010) 16:175–82. doi: 10.1177/1753425910368871
30. Atochina-Vasserman EN, Winkler C, Abramova H, Schaumann F, Krug N, Gow AJ, et al. Segmental allergen challenge alters multimeric struc- ture and function of surfactant protein D in humans. *Am J Respir Crit Care Med.* (2011) 183:856–64. doi: 10.1164/rccm.201004-0654OC
31. Mulugeta S, Beers MF. Surfactant protein C: its unique properties and emerging immunomodulatory role in the lung. *Microbes Infect.* (2006) 8:2317–23. doi: 10.1016/j.micinf.2006.04.009
32. Kuronuma K, Mitsuzawa H, Takeda K, Nishitani C, Chan ED, Kuroki Y, et al. Anionic pulmonary surfactant phospholipids inhibit inflammatory responses from alveolar macrophages and U937 cells by binding the lipopolysaccharide-interacting proteins CD14 and MD-2. *J Biol Chem.* (2009) 284:25488–500. doi: 10.1074/jbc.M109.040832
33. Epaud R, Ikegami M, Whitsett JA, Jobe AH, Weaver TE, Akinbi HT. Surfactant protein B inhibits endotoxin-induced lung inflammation. *Am J Respir Cell Mol Biol.* (2003) 28:373–8. doi: 10.1165/rcmb.2002-0071OC
34. Garcia-Verdugo I, Garcia de Paco E, Espinassous Q, Gonzalez-Horta A, Synguelakis M, Kanellopoulos J, et al. Synthetic peptides representing the N- terminal segment of surfactant protein C modulate LPS-stimulated TNF- alpha production by macrophages. *Innate Immun.* (2009) 15:53–62. doi: 10.1177/1753425908100500
35. Arroyo R, Khan MA, Echaide M, Pérez-Gil J, Palaniyar N. SP-D attenuates LPS-induced formation of human neutrophil extracellular traps (NETs), protecting pulmonary surfactant inactivation by NETs. *Commun Biol.* (2019) 2:470. doi: 10.1038/s42003-019-0662-5
36. Glaser K, Fehrholz M, Papsdorf M, Curstedt T, Kunzmann S, Speer CP. The new generation synthetic reconstituted surfactant CHF5633 suppresses LPS-induced cytokine responses in human neonatal monocytes. *Cytokine.* (2016) 86:119–23. doi: 10.1016/j.cyto.2016.08.004
37. Ikegami M, Whitsett JA, Martis PC, Weaver TE. Reversibility of lung inflammation caused by SP-B deficiency. *Am J Physiol Lung Cell Mol Physiol.* (2005) 289:L962–970. doi: 10.1152/ajplung.00214.2005
38. Glasser SW, Senft AP, Whitsett JA, Maxfield MD, Ross GF, Richardson TR, et al. Macrophage dysfunction and susceptibility to pulmonary Pseudomonas aeruginosa infection in surfactant protein C-deficient mice. *J Immunol.* (2008) 181:621–8. doi: 10.4049/jimmunol.181.1.621
39. Jobe AH. Which surfactant for treatment of respiratory-distress syndrome? *Lancet.* (2000) 355:1380–1. doi: 10.1016/S0140-6736(00)02130-9
40. Blanco O, Lugones Y, Fernandez O, Faure R. An update on clinical surfactant preparations and respiratory disease. *Biotecnologia Aplicada.* (2012) 29:53–9.
41. Strayer D. Immunogenecity of pulmonary surfactant preparations. *Clin Immunother.* (1994) 1:441–8. doi: 10.1007/BF03259036
42. Kremlev SG, Umstead TM, Phelps DS. Surfactant protein A regu- lates cytokine production in the monocytic cell line THP-1. *Am J Physiol.* (1997) 272:L996–1004. doi: 10.1152/ajplung.1997.272.5.L996
43. Mithal 8. Schwartz LW, Christman CA. Alveolar macrophage migration. Influence of lung lining material and acute lung insult. *Am Rev Respir Dis.* (1979) 128:429–39.
44. Kerecman J, Mustafa SB, Vasquez MM, Dixon PS, Catro R. Immunosuppressive properties of surfactant in alveolar macrophage NR8383. *Inflamm Res.* (2008) 57:118–25. doi: 10.1007/s00011-007-7212-1
45. Ahvazi BC, Jacobs P, Stevenson MM. Role of macrophage-derived nitric oxide in suppression of lymphocyte proliferation during blood-stage malaria. *J Leuko Biol.* (1995) 58:23–31. doi: 10.1002/jlb.58.1.23
46. Mittal N, Sanyal SN. Immunomodulatory properties of exogenous surfactant in adult rat alveolar macrophages. *Immunopharmacol Immunotoxicol.* (2010) 32:153–9. doi: 10.3109/08923970903225119
47. Wolfson MR, Wu J, Hubbert TL, Gregory TJ, Mazela J, Shaffer TH. Lucinactant attenuates pulmonary inflammatory response, preserves lung structure, and improves physiologic outcomes in a preterm lamb model of RDS. *Pediatr Res.* (2012) 72:375–83. doi: 10.1038/pr.2012.96
48. Cochrane CG, Revak SD. Pulmonary surfactant protein B (SP-B): structure-function relationships. *Science.* (1991) 254:566–8. doi: 10.1126/science.1948032
49. Fehrholz M, Glaser K, Seidenspinner S, Ottensmeier B, Curstedt T, Speer CP, et al. Impact of the New generation reconstituted surfactant CHF5633 on human CD4 lymphocytes. *PLoS ONE.* (2016) 11:e0153578. doi: 10.1371/journal.pone.0153578
50. Bezerra FS, Ramos CO, Castro TF, Araujo N, de Souza ABF, Bandeira ACB, et al. Exogenous surfactant prevents hyperoxia-induced lung injury in adult mice. *Intens Care Med Exp.* (2019) 7:19. doi: 10.1186/s40635-019-0233-6
51. van Rensburg L, van Zyl JM, Smith J, Goussard P. Effect of exogenous surfactant on paediatric bronchoalveolar lavage derived macrophages' cytokine secretion. *BMC Pulm Med.* (2019) 19:236. doi: 10.1186/s12890-019-1006-4
52. Djukanovic R, Roche WR, Wilson JW, Beasley CR, Twentyman OP, Howarth RH, et al. Mucosal inflammation in asthma. *Am Rev Respir Dis.* (1990) 142:434–57. doi: 10.1164/ajrccm/142.2.434
53. Erpenbeck VJ, Hagenberg A, Dulkys Y, Elsner J, Balder R, Krentel H, et al. Natural porcine surfactant augments airway inflammation after al- lergen challenge in patients with asthma. *Am J Respir Crit Care Med.* (2004) 169:578–86. doi: 10.1164/rccm.200301-104OC
54. Babu KS, Woodcock DA, Smith SE, Staniforth JN, Holgate ST, Conway JH. Inhaled synthetic surfactant abolishes the early allergen-induced response in asthma. *Eur Respir J.* (2003) 21:1046–9. doi: 10.1183/09031936.03.00069202
55. Erpenbeck VJ, Fischer I, Wiese K, Schaumann F, Schmiedl A, Nassen- stein C, et al. Therapeutic surfactants modulate the viability of eosino phils and induce inflammatory mediator release. *Int Arch Allergy Immunol.* (2009) 149:333–42. doi: 10.1159/000205579
56. Erpenbeck VJ, Krug N, Hohlfeld JM. Therapeutic use of surfactant components in allergic asthma. *Naunyn-Schmiedeberg's Arch Pharmacol.* (2009) 379:217–24. doi: 10.1007/s00210-008-0354-z
57. Homer RJ, Zheng T, Chupp G, He S, Zhu Z, Chen Q, et al. Pulmonary type II cell ypertrophy and pulmonary lipoproteinosis are features of chronic IL-13 exposure. *Am J Physiol Lung Cell Mol Physiol.* (2002) 283:52–

9. doi: 10.1152/ajplung.00438.2001

58. Jain-Vora S, Wert SE, Temann UA, Rankin JA, Whitsett JA. Interleukin-4 alters epithelial cell differentiation and surfactant homeostasis in the postnatal mouse lung. *Am J Respir Cell Mol Biol.* (1997) 17:541–51. doi: 10.1165/ajrcmb.17.5.2883
59. Qaseem AS, Sonar S, Mahajan L, Madan T, Sorensen GL, Shamji MH, et al. Linking surfactant protein SP-D and IL-13: implications in asthma and allergy. *Mol Immunol.* (2013) 54:98–107. doi: 10.1016/j.molimm.2012.10.039
60. Rojas-Reyes MX, Morley CJ, Soll R. Prophylactic versus selective use of surfactant in preventing morbidity and mortality in preterm infants. *Cochrane Database Syst Rev.* (2012) 3:CD000510. doi: 10.1002/14651858.CD000510.pub2
61. Bahadue FL, Soll R. Early versus delayed selective surfactant treatment for neonatal respiratory distress syndrome. *Cochrane Database Syst Rev.* (2012) 11:CD001456. doi: 10.1002/14651858.CD001456.pub2

4

Implementation of Nurse-Led, Goal-Directed Lung Physiotherapy for Older Patients with Sepsis and Pneumonia in the ICU

Jianhua Sun [1†], Na Cui [1], Wen Han [1†], Qi Li [1*], Hao Wang [2*], Zunzhu Li [1], Wei Cheng [1], Hongbo Luo [1] and Mingxi Zhao [1]*

[1] Department of Critical Care Medicine, State Key Laboratory of Complex Severe and Rare Diseases, Peking Union Medical College Hospital, Peking Union Medical College, Chinese Academy of Medical Science, Beijing, China, [2] Department of Critical Care Medicine, Beijing Jishuitan Hospital, Beijing, China

***Correspondence:**
Na Cui
pumchcn@163.com
Qi Li
18612671394@163.com
Hao Wang
newwanghao@hotmail.com

† These authors have contributed equally to this work

Objectives: This study aimed to investigate the effect of nurse-led, goal-directed lung physiotherapy (GDLPT) on the prognosis of older patients with sepsis caused by pneumonia in the intensive care unit.

Methods: We conducted a prospective, two-phase (before-and-after) study over 3 years called the GDLPT study. All patients received standard lung therapy for sepsis caused by pneumonia and patients in phase 2 also received GDLPT. In this study, 253 older patients (age $\geq$ 65 years) with sepsis and pneumonia were retrospectively analyzed. The main outcome was 28 day mortality.

Results: Among 742 patients with sepsis, 253 older patients with pneumonia were divided into the control group and the treatment group. Patients in the treatment group had a significantly shorter duration of mechanical ventilation [5 (4, 6) vs. 5 (4, 8) days; $P = 0.045$], and a lower risk of intensive care unit (ICU) mortality [14.5% (24/166) vs. 28.7% (25/87); $P = 0.008$] and 28 day mortality [15.1% (25/166) vs. 31% (27/87); $P = 0.005$] compared with those in the control group. GDLPT was an independent risk factor for 28 day mortality [odds ratio (OR), 0.379; 95% confidence interval (CI), 0.187–0.766; $P = 0.007$].

Conclusions: Nurse-led GDLPT shortens the duration of mechanical ventilation, decreases ICU and 28-day mortality, and improves the prognosis of older patients with sepsis and pneumonia in the ICU.

Keywords: goal-directed lung physiotherapy, older patients, sepsis, pneumonia, intensive care unit

INTRODUCTION

Aging of the population is a critical worldwide trend. The proportion of individuals older than 60 years has tripled over the last 50 years and will triple again before 2050. This aging has major consequences on the health system, including the intensive care unit (ICU). In the USA, almost half (48.7%) of the patients admitted to an ICU are aged 65 years or older, and patients aged 85 years or older account for 7 to 25% of the admission rate (1, 2). The rate of pneumonia increases rapidly with age. Approximately 19% of adults hospitalized with pneumonia have an ICU admission, including 60.7% of patients aged 65 years or older (3). Pneumonia in older patients can lead to cardiopulmonary failure, sepsis, and even systemic multiple organ failure, and they have a high mortality rate (4). Older people with pneumonia are at risk for a longer hospital stay, extended antibiotic therapy, and higher healthcare costs (5, 6). Therefore, an appropriate treatment protocol for pneumonia in older patients needs to be determined.

Because of age-related changes in the body, comorbidity, and malnutrition, the onset of pneumonia is insidious, rapid, and critical, and clinical treatment is difficult in older patients (2, 7, 8). Lung physiotherapy plays an important role in treatment of older patients with pneumonia (2, 7, 8). Lung physiotherapy can help patients in reducing the accumulation of airway secretion, clearing the respiratory tract, preventing a collapsed lung, improving lung compliance, and reducing comorbidities (9, 10). Nurses are responsible for most respiratory treatment in China. However, there is little evidence for the effect of nurse-led GDLPT on the prognosis of pneumonia in older patients with sepsis. In a previous study, we found that nurse-led GDLPT improved the outcomes in patients with sepsis and pneumonia (11). In this study, we carried out a retrospective analysis of older patients (age ≥ 65 years) with sepsis and pneumonia to evaluate whether GDLPT affects the clinical outcome.

MATERIALS AND METHODS

Study Design and Patients

The GDLPT study was a prospective, two-phase (before-and-after) study conducted in Peking Union Medical College Hospital of China from January 2017 to January 2020. Details of this study, including the inclusion and exclusion criteria, have been published previously (11). The study period was divided into two stages of phase 1 and phase 2. During phase 1 (January to December 2017), patients received standard physiotherapy for pneumonia, and patients in phase 2 (February 2018 to January 2020) also received GDLPT. The two study periods were separated by a 1 month washout period that was dedicated to teaching the GDLPT protocol to all nursing and medical staff. The study protocol was approved by the ethics committee of Peking Union Medical College Hospital (approval number: JS-1170). All family members agreed to participating in the study and signed an informed consent form, and the study was registered at chictr.org.cn (identifier: ChiCTR-ROC-17010750).

Figure 1 shows a flow diagram of patient screening and selection for this study. In the nurse-led GDLPT study, 609 of 742 patients were diagnosed with sepsis caused by pneumonia, of whom 253 (41.5%) were older than 65 years. Demographics, comorbidities, clinical parameters, and laboratory data were analyzed.

Intervention and Comparisons

The protocols for pneumonia in the pre- and post-protocol groups are shown in **Figure 2**. Details of this study, including study details such as the intervention objective, methods, and intervention frequency, were the same as those in our previous study (11). The **Supplementary File** provides additional evidence relevant to the intervention and comparisons.

Data Collection

Baseline data of the patients, including sex, age, underlying diseases, the Sequential Organ Failure Assessment (SOFA) score, the Acute Physiology and Chronic Health Evaluation

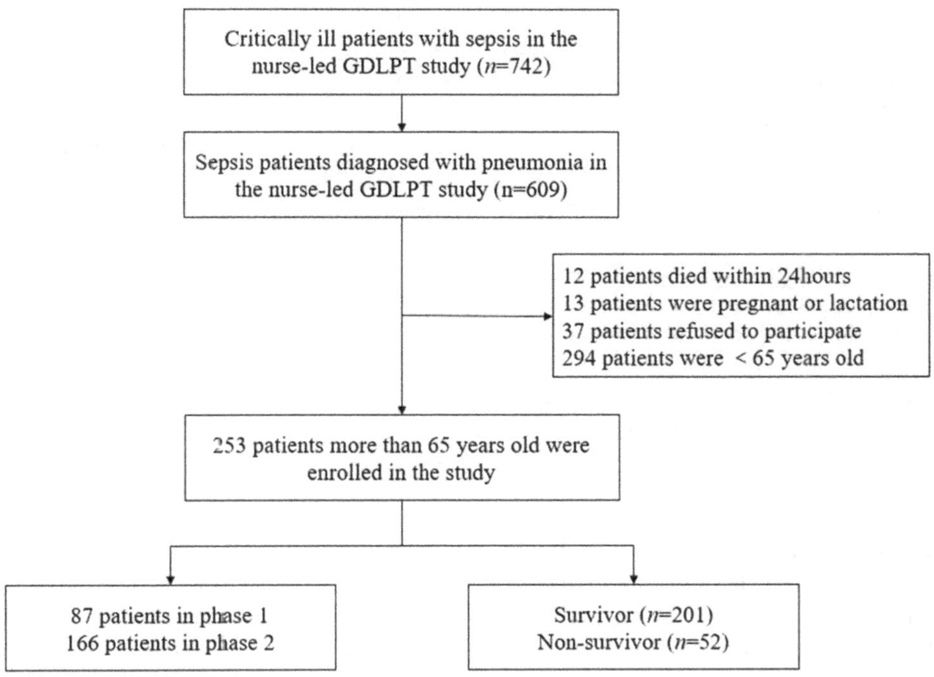

FIGURE 1 | The flowchart of patients screening and selection in this study.

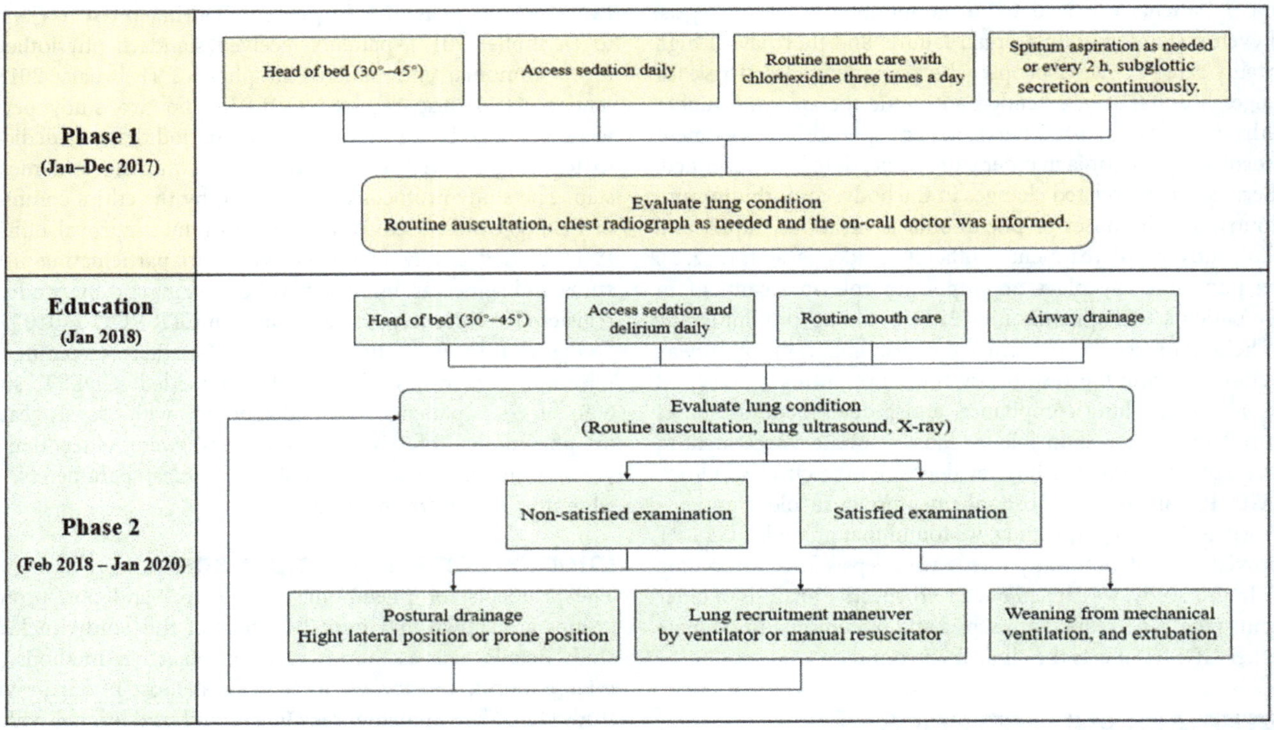

FIGURE 2 | The protocols for pneumonia in the pre- and post-protocol groups.

(APACHE) II score, and the Clinical Pulmonary Infection Score (CPIS), were analyzed. Vital signs, laboratory parameters, arterial blood gases, ventilatory parameters, life-sustaining treatments, and infection-related data during admission were also included. The data used in this study were the worst values in the first 24 h after ICU admission. The primary outcomes of this study were 28 day mortality. The secondary outcomes were the duration of ventilation, the length of the ICU stay, and the ICU mortality rate.

Statistical Analysis

Data were analyzed by IBM SPSS version 21.0 (IBM Corp., Armonk, NY, USA). The frequency and percentage and mean and standard deviation were calculated for descriptive statistics. Bivariate analysis was performed using the chi-square test for categorical variables and the t test or one-way analysis of variance for continuous variables. Logistic regression analysis was performed with 28 day mortality as the dependent factor, which was significant ($p < 0.2$) in univariate analysis.

RESULTS

Baseline Characteristics

Among 742 patients with sepsis, 253 patients who were older than 65 years were included in this study. **Table 1** shows the clinical characteristics of the patients who were enrolled in this study. The median age of the patients was 72 years (interquartile range: 68–78 years) and 62.1% (157/253) were men. At admission to the ICU, the mean SOFA score was 11.49 ± 3.95, the median APACHE II score was 18 (12–18), and the median CPIS score was 6 (5–8). Ninety-two (36.4%) patients had heart failure, 19 (7.5%) had chronic obstructive pulmonary disease, 74 (29.2%) had diabetes mellitus, 3 (1.2%) had liver cirrhosis, 44(17.4%) with tumors, and 18 (7.1%) had chronic renal failure. There were no significant differences in age, sex, underlying diseases, source of admission, disease severity scores (APACHE II, SOFA, and CPIS scores), vital signs (heart rate, respiratory rate, and mean arterial pressure), ventilatory parameters, arterial blood gases, clinical laboratory evaluation, life-sustaining treatments, coexisting pathogens, or drug therapy between the two groups after ICU admission.

There was no significant difference in the ICU duration between the groups. Patients in the treatment group had a significantly shorter duration of mechanical ventilation [5 (4, 6) vs. 5 (4, 8) days, $P = 0.045$], and a lower ICU mortality [14.5% (24/166) vs. 28.7% (25/87); $P = 0.008$] and 28 day mortality [15.1% (25/166) vs. 31% (27/87); $P = 0.005$] compared with those in the control group.

Clinical Differences Between Survivors and Non-survivors

The clinical characteristics of all patients and for survivors and non-survivors (28 day) are shown in **Table 2**. Non-survivors had a higher APACHE II score, higher CPIS score, faster respiratory rate, higher carbon dioxide partial pressure on ICU admission, and longer mechanical ventilation compared with survivors (all $P < 0.05$). The rates of heart failure and chronic renal failure

TABLE 1 | Characteristics of patients in the control and treatment groups at ICU admission.

Variables	Sepsis ($n = 253$)	Control ($n = 87$)	Treatment ($n = 166$)	*P*-value
Age (years)	72 (68,78)	72 (68,79)	72 (68,77)	0.512
Sex (male)	157 (62.1)	55 (63.2)	102 (61.4)	0.892
Underlying diseases, *n* (%)				
Chronic obstructive pulmonary disease	19 (7.5)	7 (8)	12 (7.2)	0.806
Heart failure	92 (36.4)	39 (44.8)	53 (31.9)	0.054
Diabetic mellitus	74 (29.2)	25 (28.7)	49 (29.5)	1
Liver Cirrhosis	3 (1.2)	1 (1.1)	2 (1.2)	1
Tumor	44 (17.4)	10 (11.5)	34 (20.5)	0.082
Chronic renal failure	18 (7.1)	8 (9.2)	10 (6)	0.44
Source of admission, *n* (%)				
Internal medicine	40 (15.8)	16 (18.4)	24 (14.5)	0.469
Surgery	75 (29.6)	23 (26.4)	52 (31.3)	0.47
Emergency	62 (24.5)	18 (20.7)	44 (26.5)	0.357
Outside hospital	76 (30.0)	24 (27.6)	52 (31.3)	0.567
Disease severity scores				
APACHE II score	18 (16,22)	18 (15,21)	19 (16,22.25)	0.373
Sequential organ failure score	11.49 ± 3.95	11.23 ± 3.88	11.62 ± 4	0.457
Clinical pulmonary infection score	6 (5,8)	8 (6,9)	8 (6,9.3)	0.789
Vital signs				
Heart rate (beats/min)	99 (86.5,115.5)	101 (90,115)	98 (85,116)	0.38
Respiratory rate (breaths/min)	22 (17,27)	22 (17,26)	22 (18,27)	0.748
Mean artery pressure (mm Hg)	88.02 ± 12.64	88.32 ± 12.82	87.86 ± 12.58	0.781
Ventilator parameters				
Tide volume (ml)	420 (390,480)	430 (400,480)	410 (390,482.5)	0.192
Inhalation oxygen concentration (%)	0.35 (0.3,0.4)	0.35 (0.28,0.40)	0.35 (0.31,0.4)	0.064
Artery blood gas				
Lactic acid (mmol/L)	2 (1,2)	2 (1,2)	2 (1,2)	0.673
Arterial oxygen pressure (mm Hg)	95.7 (78.45,116.84)	94.76 (80.7,116.8)	96 (77.87,116.97)	0.706
Carbon dioxide partial pressure (mm Hg)	39 (35.7,43.45)	39 (35.6,42.1)	38.95 (35.85,44.03)	0.742
Oxygen index	284 (207.5,360.5)	287 (227,380)	277.5 (202.75,348.5)	0.203
Clinical laboratory evaluation				
Creatinine (umol/L)	86 (67.5,146)	107 (73,169)	81 (61.5,144.25)	0.086
Albumin level (g/L)	32 (29,35)	32 (28,35)	31.5 (29,34)	0.597
Total bilirubin (umol/L)	16.7 (14.1,24.35)	16.5 (13.4,24.2)	16.7 (14.38,24.73)	0.247
Life-sustaining treatments, *n* (%)				
Need for mechanism ventilation	238 (94.1)	83 (95.4)	155 (93.4)	0.589
Need for vasopressor	163 (64.4)	53 (60.9)	110 (66.3)	0.41
Need for RRT	53 (20.9)	14 (16.1)	39 (23.5)	0.195
Coexisting pathogens, *n* (%)				
Bacteria	216 (85.4)	78 (89.7)	138 (83.1)	0.192
Fungal	26 (10.3)	7 (8)	19 (11.4)	0.515
Else	5 (2)	0 (0)	5 (3)	0.168
Drug therapy, *n* (%)				
Antibiotics for GNB	189 (74.7)	64(73.6)	125 (75.3)	0.763
Antibiotics for GPB	237 (93.7)	83(95.4)	154 (92.8)	0.588
Antifungal drugs	85 (33.6)	31(35.6)	54 (32.5)	0.675
Outcomes				
Ventilation day (days)	5 (4,7)	5 (4,8)	5 (4,6)	0.045
ICU duration (days)	10 (5,19)	9 (6,20)	10 (4,18.25)	0.699
ICU mortality, *n* (%)	49 (19.4)	25 (28.7)	24 (14.5)	0.008
28 day mortality, *n* (%)	52 (20.6)	27 (31)	25 (15.1)	0.005

Continuous variables are expressed as mean ± standard deviation or median (interquartile range). P-values reflect comparisons between the control and treatment groups. ICU, intensive care unit; APACHE II, Acute Physiology and Chronic Health Evaluation II; oxygen index, (partial pressure of oxygen) / (fraction of inspirated oxygen); RRT, continuous renal replacement therapy; GPB, Gram-positive bacteria; GNB, Gram-negative bacteria.

TABLE 2 | Characteristics of the study population in survivors and non-survivors according to 28 day mortality.

Variables	Sepsis (*n* = 253)	Non-Survival (*n* = 52)	Survival group (*n* = 201)	*P*-value
Age (years)	72 (68,78)	73 (69,78)	71 (68,78)	0.214
Sex (male)	157 (62.1)	34 (65.4)	123 (61.2)	0.633
Underlying diseases, *n* (%)				
Chronic obstructive pulmonary disease	19 (7.5)	7 (13.5)	12 (6.0)	0.079
Heart failure	92 (36.4)	28 (53.8)	64 (31.8)	0.006
Diabetic mellitus	74 (29.2)	20 (38.5)	54 (26.9)	0.124
Liver Cirrhosis	3 (1.2)	1 (1.9)	2 (1.0)	0.5
Tumor	44 (17.4)	13 (25.0)	31 (15.4)	0.149
Chronic renal failure	18 (7.1)	10 (19.2)	8 (4.0)	0.001
Source of admission, *n* (%)				
Internal medicine	40 (15.8)	6 (11.5)	34 (16.9)	0.348
Surgery	75 (29.6)	16 (30.8)	59 (29.4)	0.866
Emergency	62 (24.5)	12 (23.1)	50 (24.9)	0.858
Outside hospital	76 (30.0)	16 (30.8)	60 (29.9)	1
Disease severity scores				
APACHE II score	18 (16, 22)	21.5 (17, 26)	18 (15, 21)	0.001
Sequential organ failure score	11.49 ± 3.95	12.33 ± 3.82	11.27 ± 3.97	0.085
Clinical pulmonary infection score	6 (5, 8)	8 (6, 9)	6 (5, 8)	0.0001
Vital signs				
Heart rate (beats/min)	99 (86.5,115.5)	105 (90,119.75)	98 (85,114)	0.064
Respiratory rate (breaths/min)	22 (17,27)	24 (20,28)	21 (17,27)	0.039
Mean artery pressure (mm Hg)	88.02 ± 12.64	86.58 ± 13.63	88.39 ± 12.38	0.358
Ventilator parameters				
Tide volume (ml)	420 (390,480)	410 (392.5,480)	420 (390,490)	0.425
Inhalation oxygen concentration (%)	0.35 (0.3,0.4)	0.37 (0.32,0.42)	0.35 (0.3,0.4)	0.188
Artery blood gas				
Lactic acid (mmol/L)	2 (1, 2)	2 (1, 2)	2 (1, 2)	0.727
Arterial oxygen pressure (mm Hg)	95.7 (78.45,116.84)	103.35 (78.28,118.69)	93.31 (78.83,115.44)	0.125
Carbon dioxide partial pressure (mm Hg)	39 (35.7,43.45)	41 (36.25,46.23)	38.8 (35.5,42.85)	0.035
Oxygen index	284 (207.5,360.5)	282.5 (218.25,365.75)	284 (206.5,360.5)	0.952
Clinical laboratory evaluation				
Creatinine (umol/L)	86 (67.5,146)	114 (74.25,146.25)	83 (62,146)	0.103
Albumin level (g/L)	32 (29,35)	31 (29,33)	32 (28.5,35)	0.375
Total bilirubin (umol/L)	16.7 (14.1,24.35)	17.2 (12.73,40.63)	16.5 (14.2,23.5)	0.957
Life-sustaining treatments, *n* (%)				
Need for mechanism ventilation	238 (94.1)	51 (98.1)	187 (93)	0.319
Need for vasopressor	163 (64.4)	35 (67.3)	128 (63.7)	0.745
Need for RRT	53 (20.9)	17 (32.7)	36 (17.9)	0.034
Coexisting pathogens, *n* (%)				
Bacteria	216 (85.4)	47 (90.4)	169 (84.1)	0.377
Fungal	26 (10.3)	7 (13.5)	19 (9.5)	0.442
Else	5 (2)	0 (0)	5 (2.5)	0.587
Drug therapy, *n* (%)				
Antibiotics for GNB	189 (74.7)	37 (71.2)	152 (75.6)	0.591
Antibiotics for GPB	237 (93.7)	51 (98.1)	186 (92.5)	0.205
Antifungal drugs	85 (33.6)	21 (40.4)	64 (31.8)	0.253
Received nurse-led GDLPT	166 (65.6)	25 (48.1)	141 (70.1)	0.005
Outcomes				
Mechanical ventilation days (days)	5 (4, 7)	5.5 (5, 12)	5 (4, 6)	0.0001
ICU duration (days)	10 (5, 19)	11 (7, 20)	9 (5, 19)	0.22

Continuous variables are expressed as mean ± standard deviation or median (interquartile range). P-values reflect comparisons between the survivor and non-survivor groups. ICU, intensive care unit; APACHE II, Acute Physiology and Chronic Health Evaluation II; oxygen index, (partial pressure of oxygen) / (fraction of inspirated oxygen); RRT, continuous renal replacement therapy; GPB, Gram-positive bacteria; GNB, Gram-negative bacteria; GDLPT, goal-directed lung physiotherapy.

TABLE 3 | Multivariate logistic regression analysis for predicting 28 day mortality in older patients with sepsis and pneumonia.

Parameters	OR	95% CI	p-value
Heart failure	2.779	1.360–5.679	0.005
Tumor	2.825	1.181–6.757	0.020
Inhalation oxygen concentration	2.438	0.094–63.291	0.592
Creatinine	0.999	0.995–1.003	0.564
Need for continuous renal replacement therapy	2.450	1.122–5.351	0.025
Received nurse-led GDLPT	0.379	0.187–0.766	0.007
Mechanical ventilation days	1.147	1.055–1.247	0.001

GDLPT, goal-directed lung physical therapy; OR, odds ratio; CI, confidence interval.

were significantly higher in non-survivors than in survivors (both $P < 0.05$). The requirement for renal replacement therapy was significantly more frequent in the in non-survivors compared with survivors (32.7 vs. 17.9%, $P = 0.034$). Importantly, more patients received nurse-led GDLPT in survivors than in non-survivors (70.1 vs. 48.1%, $P = 0.005$).

Risk Factors for 28 Day Mortality in Older Patients With Sepsis Caused by Pneumonia

Multivariate logistic regression analysis identified five factors that independently predicted 28-day mortality in patients with sepsis who were diagnosed with pneumonia. These factors were nurse-led GDLPT [odds ratio (OR), 0.379; 95% confidence interval (CI), 0.187–0.766; $P = 0.007$], heart failure (OR, 2.779; 95% CI, 1.360–5.679; $P = 0.005$), tumor (OR, 2.825; 95% CI, 1.181–6.757; $P = 0.02$), need for renal replacement therapy (OR, 2.450; 95% CI, 1.122–5.351; $P = 0.025$), and mechanical ventilation days (OR, 1.147; 95% CI, 1.055–1.247; $P = 0.001$). GDLPT was a protective factor for 28 day mortality (**Table 3**).

DISCUSSION

Pneumonia is frequently encountered in older patients admitted to the ICU, with an incidence rate of >60% in those with sepsis (6). In numerous clinical studies, lung physiotherapy was analyzed in patients with various critical diseases (12, 13, 19). However, little is known about nurses providing lung physiotherapy to older patients with sepsis and pneumonia. Furthermore, the effect of lung physiotherapy on the prognosis of these patients is unclear. In this study, we found that nurse-led GLDPT was associated with shorter ventilation days, and reduced ICU mortality and 28 day mortality rates.

With aging, there are significant changes in the anatomical and physiological function of the lungs. Older people are more likely to develop pulmonary complications and underlying diseases, including COPD, aspiration, pneumonia, tumor, heart failure, chronic renal failure, and have a poor prognosis (14). The GDLPT protocol has several advantages over conventional physiotherapy. One advantage is that the frequency of oral care is determined by the Beck Oral Assessment Scale score and mucosal-plaque score. Another advantage is that enhancement of airway drainage is conducted every 4 h for 20 to 30 min each time, with a vibration frequency of 20 to 30 Hz. Additionally, the cough strength is evaluated every 6 h. Older people with a weak cough are more likely to have nosocomial pneumonia and aspiration pneumonia (15). In the USA, the incidence of aspiration pneumonia in older patients is 30.9 cases per 10,000 people, which is twice that in patients aged < 65 years (16). A further advantage is that airway humidification is evaluated regularly to maintain humidification at degree II (17). For patients with specific pulmonary consolidation, goal-directed patient positioning is actively used. The frequency of turning over is adjusted, and a lung recruitment maneuver is also performed through mechanical ventilation or a manual resuscitator. Therefore, as a non-invasive intervention strategy, nurse-led GDLPT is useful for older patients with pneumonia.

In this nurse-led GDLPT study, pain assessment, delirium assessment, and active early activities were carried out every 6 h by nurses. Delirium varies from 11 to 42% in older patients and has adverse outcomes and high health care costs (18). Up to 60% of delirious patients were unrecognized unless actively screened, and sedative medications and deeper sedation are associated with the development of delirium (20). According to the patient's delirium status, early activities were carried out, such as sitting at the wheel and early walking. Frailty in older patients is also a risk of a longer ICU stay, prolonged ventilation duration, and increased mortality. Early exercise is the most effective intervention for debilitating syndrome and significantly improves muscle strength. In this nurse-led GDLPT study, old patients without delirium were able to get out of bed into a wheelchair early or walk early after therapy. Additionally, patients with intermittent delirium were able to perform bedside wheelchair activity, and patients with continuous delirium were able to receive passive movement in bed or sitting upon the bed. The nurse-led GDLPT protocol was formulated in the critical clinical setting and designed using more than 20 years of clinical experience, with specific items and strong operability. This therapy enabled good management of older patients.

In this study, nurse-led GDLPT significantly shortened the duration of ventilation. Prolonged mechanical ventilation might result in an increased incidence of ventilator-associated pneumonia, which is clinically meaningful, especially for older patients with pneumonia. A high frequency of antibiotic use and antibiotic resistance in patients is caused by ventilator-associated pneumonia. The prevalence of multidrug resistance is increasing, and ventilator-associated pneumonia caused by multidrug resistance is often fatal in the ICU (21). Several factors such as the CPIS score, and the APACHE II score contribute to a high percentage of multidrug resistance in the ICU and are important reasons for the poor prognosis of older patients with sepsis and pneumonia (22).

At present, older patients with a critical illness are frequently admitted in the ICU. However, data on older patients with pneumonia are relatively rare, and there have been few evidence-based medical reports (23). This study was a retrospective analysis based on data from a previous nurse-led GDLPT study. All collected data, including vital signs, ventilatory parameters, and laboratory indicators, were obtained from electronic information systems. Data were double checked to minimize the risk of data entry errors and there were missing data. Therefore, prospective, randomized, controlled trials are required to further investigate the role of nurse-led GDLPT on older patients with pneumonia. The nurse-led GDLPT study was a prospective, before-and-after study in a single center. Therefore, a multicenter study needs to be performed to further examine the details of GDLPT and validate its wide applicability in older patients with pneumonia.

CONCLUSIONS

Managing pneumonia in critically ill older patients is a complex issue. Aging, comorbidities, frailty, and other factors in older patients significantly increase the management requirements and risks for those with critical illness. Nurse-led GDLPT significantly shortens the duration of ventilation and improves the 28 day mortality rate in older patients with sepsis and pneumonia. Nurse-led GDLPT is a new clinical intervention for the refined management of older patients with pneumonia, and it promotes the recovery of older patients with severe pneumonia.

Union Medical College Hospital (No. JS-1170). The study was registered at chictr.org.cn (identifier: ChiCTR1900025850). The patients/participants provided their written informed consent to participate in this study.

AUTHOR CONTRIBUTIONS

NC, QL, HW, and JS contributed to the conception of the study, data interpretation, and drafted the manuscript. WH, HL, and MZ contributed to the data collection and data analysis. WC and ZL contributed to data collection and interpretation and critically revised the manuscript for important intellectual content. All authors approved the final version of the manuscript.

FUNDING

The work was supported by National Natural Science Foundation of China (No. 82072226), Beijing Municipal Science and Technology Commission (No. Z201100005520049), Fundamental Research Funds for the Central Universities (No. 3332021018), Non-profit Central Research Institute Fund of Chinese Academy of Medical Sciences (No. 2019XK320040), Tibet Natural Science Foundation (No. XZ2019ZR-ZY12(Z)), and Excellence Program of Key Clinical Specialty of Beijing in 2020 (No. ZK128001).

REFERENCES

1. Fuchs L, Chronaki CE, Park S, Novack V, Baumfeld Y, Scott D. S. ICU admission characteristics and mortality rates among elderly and very elderly patients. *Intensive Care Med.* (2012) 38:1654–61. doi: 10.1007/s00134-012-2629-6
2. Esme M, Topeli A, Yavuz BB, Akova M. Infections in the elderly critically-Ill patients. *Front Med.* (2019) 6:118. doi: 10.3389/fmed.2019.00118
3. Storms AD, Chen J, Jackson LA, Nordin JD, Naleway AL, Glanz JM, et al. Rates and risk factors associated with hospitalization for pneumonia with ICU admission among adults. *BMC Pulm Med.* (2017) 17:208. doi: 10.1186/s12890-017-0552-x
4. Corrales-Medina VF, Musher DM, Shachkina S, Chirinos JA. Acute pneumonia and the cardiovascular system. *Lancet.* (2013) 381:496–505. doi: 10.1016/S0140-6736(12)61266-5
5. Restrepo MI, Faverio P, Anzueto A. Long-term prognosis in community-acquired pneumonia. *Curr Opin Infect Dis.* (2013) 26:151–8. doi: 10.1097/QCO.0b013e32835ebc6d
6. Vincent JL, Rello J, Marshall J, Silva E, Anzueto A, Martin CD, et al. International study of the prevalence and outcomes of infection in intensive care units. *JAMA.* (2009) 302:2323–9. doi: 10.1001/jama.2009.1754
7. Dyer C, Pugh L. Lung health in older adults. *Age Ageing.* (2019) 48:319–22. doi: 10.1093/ageing/afz008
8. Valley TS, Sjoding MW, Ryan AM, Iwashyna TJ, Cooke CR. Association of intensive care unit admission with mortality among older patients with pneumonia. *JAMA.* (2015) 314:1272–9. doi: 10.1001/jama.2015.11068
9. Belli S, Prince I, Savio G, Paracchini E, Cattaneo D, Bianchi M, et al. Airway clearance techniques: the right choice for the right patient. *Frontiers in medicine.* (2021) 8:544826–544826. doi: 10.3389/fmed.2021.544826
10. Wang TH, Wu CP, Wang LY. Chest physiotherapy with early mobilization may improve extubation outcome in critically ill patients in the intensive care units. *Clin Respir J.* (2018) 12:2613–21. doi: 10.1111/crj.12965
11. Sun J, Han W, Cui N, Li Q, Wang H, Li Z, et al. Effect of nurse-led goal-directed lung physical therapy on the prognosis of pneumonia in sepsis patients in the icu: a prospective cohort study. *J Intensive Care Med.* (2021). doi: 10.1177./0885066620987200. [Epub ahead of print].
12. Newman A, Gravesande J, Rotella S, Wu SS, Topp-Nguyen N, Kho ME, et al. Physiotherapy in the neurotrauma intensive care unit: a scoping review. *J Crit Care.* (2018) 48:390–406. doi: 10.1016/j.jcrc.09, 037.
13. Battaglini D, Robba C, Caiffa S, Ball L, Brunetti I, Loconte M, et al. Chest physiotherapy: an important adjuvant in critically ill mechanically ventilated patients with COVID-19. *Respir Physiol Neurobiol.* (2020) 282:103529. doi: 10.1016/j.resp.2020.103529
14. Sharma G, Goodwin J. Effect of aging on respiratory system physiology and immunology. *Clin Interv Aging.* (2006) 1:253–60. doi: 10.2147/ciia.1, 3.253
15. Torres A, Gatell JM, Aznar E, El-Ebiary M, Puig DLBJ, González J, et al. Re-intubation increases the risk of nosocomial pneumonia in patients needing mechanical ventilation. *Am J Respir Crit Care Med.* (1995) 152:137–41. doi: 10.1164/ajrccm.152.1.7599812
16. Wu CP, Chen YW, Wang MJ, Pinelis E. National trends in admission for aspiration pneumonia in the United States, 2002-2012. *Ann Am Thorac Soc.* (2017) 14:874–9. doi: 10.1513/AnnalsATS.201611-867OC
17. Yang M, Song Y, Pan L, Xie X. Evaluation of the effect of two active warming and humidifying high-flow oxygen therapy systems in patients with tracheotomy. *Biomed Rep.* (2019) 11:31–7. doi: 10.3892/br.2019.1219
18. Li D, Zhang J, Bai G, Chen J, Cheng W, Cui N. Lymphocyte and NK cell counts can predict sepsis-associated delirium in elderly patients. *Front Aging Neurosci.* (2021) 12:621298–621298. doi: 10.3389/fnagi.2020.621298
19. Do ABM, Timenetsky K. Chest physiotherapy and outcomes in ICU. *Intensive Care Med.* (2007) 33:2232. doi: 10.1007/s00134-007-0893-7
20. Maxine D, Fan J, Yennu S, Tanco K, Shin SH, Wu J, et al. The frequency of missed delirium in patients referred to palliative care in a comprehensive cancer center. *Support Care Cancer.* (2015) 23:2427–33. doi: 10.1007/s00520-015-2610-3
21. Petty NK, Ben ZN, Stanton-Cook M, Skippington E, Totsika M, Forde

BM, et al. Global dissemination of a multidrug resistant Escherichia coli clone. *Proc Natl Acad Sci U S A.* (2014) 111:5694–9. doi: 10.1073/pnas.1322678111

22. Paramythiotou E, Routsi C. Association between infections caused by multidrug-resistant gram-negative bacteria and mortality in critically ill patients. *World J Crit Care Med.* (2016) 5:111–20. doi: 10.5492/wjccm.v5.i2.111
23. Ding X, Lian H, Wang X, Chinese CUSG. Management of very old patients in intensive care units. *Aging Dis.* (2021) 12:614–24. doi: 10.14336/AD.2020.0914

5

Incidence and Mortality of Acute Respiratory Distress Syndrome in Patients with Burns

Baoli Wang [1,2,3†], Wei Chenru [1†], Yong Jiang [1†], Lunyang Hu [1], He Fang [1], Feng Zhu [1], Qing Yu [1], Banghui Zhu [1], Guosheng Wu [1], Yu Sun [1*] and Zhaofan Xia [1,3*]*

[1] Department of Burn Surgery, The First Affiliated Hospital of Naval Medical University, Shanghai, China, [2] Department of Burns and Plastic Surgery, General Hospital of Central Theater Command of Chinese People's Liberation Army, Shanghai, China, [3] Research Unit of Key Techniques for Treatment of Burns and Combined Burns and Trauma Injury, Chinese Academy of Medical Sciences, Shanghai, China

Correspondence:
Guosheng Wu
18019359841@163.com
Yu Sun
littlefish0916@126.com
Zhaofan Xia
xiazhaofan_smmu@163.com

† These authors have contributed equally to this work

Objective: We conducted a systematic review and meta-analysis to comprehensively estimate the incidence and mortality of acute respiratory distress syndrome (ARDS) in overall and subgroups of patients with burns.

Data sources: Pubmed, Embase, the Cochrane Library, CINAHL databases, and China National Knowledge Infrastructure database were searched until September 1, 2021.

Study selection: Articles that report study data on incidence or mortality of ARDS in patients with burns were selected.

Data extraction: Two researchers independently screened the literature, extracted data, and assessed the quality. We performed a meta-analysis of the incidence and mortality of ARDS in patients with burns using a random effects model, which made subgroup analysis according to the study type, inclusion (mechanical ventilation, minimal burn surface), definitions of ARDS, geographic location, mean age, burn severity, and inhalation injury. Primary outcomes were the incidence and mortality of burns patients with ARDS, and secondary outcomes were incidence for different subgroups.

Data synthesis: Pooled weighted estimate of the incidence and mortality of ARDS in patients with burns was 0.24 [95% confidence interval (CI)0.2–0.28] and 0.31 [95% CI 0.18–0.44]. Incidences of ARDS were obviously higher in patients on mechanical ventilation (incidence = 0.37), diagnosed by Berlin definition (incidence = 0.35), and with over 50% inhalation injury proportion (incidence = 0.41) than in overall patients with burns. Patients with burns who came from western countries and with inhalation injury have a significantly higher incidence of ARDS compared with those who came from Asian/African countries (0.28 vs. 0.25) and without inhalation injury (0.41 vs. 0.24).

Conclusion: This systematic review and meta-analysis revealed that the incidence of ARDS in patients with burns is 24% and that mortality is as high as 31%. The incidence rates are related to mechanical ventilation, location, and inhalation injury. The patients with burns from western countries and with inhalation injury have a significantly higher incidence than patients from Asian/African countries and without inhalation injury.

Systematic Review Registration: identifier: CRD42021144888.

Keywords: ARDS, incidence, mortality, burn patients, meta

INTRODUCTION

Acute respiratory distress syndrome is very common in critically ill patients. After years of basic and clinical research, its diagnosis and treatment are improving daily, but the associated mortality rate is still as high as 30% (30-day mortality) (1). The causes of ARDS are diverse and, excluding cardiac-induced conditions, can include severe infection, shock, trauma, and burns. These injuries can induce diffuse pulmonary interstitial and alveolar edema, resulting in acute hypoxic respiratory insufficiency or failure (2). Among the causes of ARDS, severe burns can also cause a series of pathophysiological changes in various organs of the body. Among them, the lung is one of the earliest organs to be damaged, and damage to the lung is one of the main causes of death in severely burned patients (3). Although many studies have reported the incidence, treatment, and outcome of ARDS, there is no meta-analysis of ARDS in patients with burns. Our objective is to comprehensively collect published literature on ARDS in patients with burns and assess the incidence/mortality in overall and subgroups of the patient with burns.

METHODS

Literature Search

We retrieved studies from Pubmed, Embase, the Cochrane Library, CINAHL databases, and the China National Knowledge Infrastructure database. The retrieval time for each database is from the formation of the database to September 1, 2021. We searched the databases by combining subject words and free words. Search terms included "Respiratory Distress Syndrome, Adult," AND "incidence OR Mortality," AND "burn." Detailed search strategies are provided in **Appendix 1**. We evaluated the qualifications of the identified publications and independently extracted data from the studies selected. Differences were resolved through a consensus.

Study Selection

Inclusion criteria were as follows: (1) study type was an observational study, case-control study, cohort study, or randomized controlled trial; (2) subjects were patients with burns; (3) incidence or mortality of ARDS was reported; (4) articles were written in English or Chinese. Exclusion criteria were as follows: (1) studies with obvious abnormal and incomplete data sets; (2) repeated publishing of the same batch of data by multiple articles; (3) sample size of the study was <20; (4) research subjects were special populations, such as children or pregnant women; (5) research subjects were only patients with inhalation injury; (6) any limitation in the length of stay and death; (7) comments, reviews, or lectures.

Data Extraction

We extracted the characteristics of the study (author, publication year, study type, study area and centers, sample size, and study quality), basic characteristics of the research subject (average age, total body surface area (TBSA), full-thickness burn injury, inhalation injury), ARDS cases, and ARDS-related deaths. Two researchers separately collected the data and cross-checked the sampling of the other.

Quality Assessment

Methodological quality assessment studies were also conducted by two separate researchers. We took the same type of meta-analysis "Incidence and Mortality of Acute Respiratory Distress Syndrome in Children: A Systematic Review and Meta-Analysis" as a reference, and used the evaluation tools of the research for evaluation. Our study refers to the quality evaluation in the relevant literature, and the quality of each method (bias risk) was based on a list of 13 items (4). The list of 13 items is provided in **Appendix 2**.

Quantitative Data Synthesis

Statistical Pooling and Evaluation of Heterogeneity

We conducted a meta-analysis with the Meta package (metaprop, version R3.5.3). The data were converted with four estimation methods, and a normality test was performed on the data before the meta-analysis. In accordance with the test results, the method closest to a normal distribution was selected. Then, we combined the data (ARDS incidence and mortality) and performed a heterogeneity analysis. The confidence interval (CI) was 95%, and the statistical heterogeneity was judged by calculating I^2. We choose a fixed effects model or a random effects model based on p-value and I^2. A sensitivity analysis was performed to investigate the stability of the meta-analysis. The funnel plot method was used to judge publication bias.

Subgroup Analyses

We performed a subgroup meta-analysis to obtain the rate of special groups of patients with burns and explore potential sources of heterogeneity. We assessed factors, including the study type, inclusion (mechanical ventilation, minimal burn surface), definitions of ARDS, geographic location, mean age, burn severity, and inhalation injury. Divided by these factors, the combined weighted estimates were used to derive the incidence and mortality of ARDS in different subgroups. The statistical tests were all two-sided with a level of $\alpha = 0.1$.

RESULTS

Study Characteristics

The search identified 712 reports potentially pertaining to the morbidity and mortality of ARDS in patients with burns. After screening, 35 publications on incidence (5–39) and 9 on mortality (5, 7, 9, 11, 24, 32–34, 38) were considered to be eligible (**Figure 1**). The basic characteristics of the included studies, with respect to incidence and mortality, are shown in **Supplementary Tables 1**, **2**. Most of the studies were conducted in a single center. The research population of "Incidence" was 10,899 and that of "Mortality" was 2,771. These data were from multiple countries on multiple continents; however, most of the studies were carried out in the United States, Canada, China, and Spain. The research time window of all the included studies was from 1978 to 2021. The study subjects were patients with burn,

---

Abbreviations: ARDS, acute respiratory distress syndrome; TBSA, total body surface area; AECC, American-European Consensus Conference.

with ARDS-related records. In most of the publications, the age limit of the patients was over 18 years. In 1994, the American-European Consensus Conference (AECC) definition of ARDS was published, which had problems with lack of a criterion for acute onset, the need for a pulmonary artery catheter, and difficult hypoxemia criteria. Therefore, a new definition of ARDS, called the Berlin definition, was published, in 2012 (40). Since the definition of ARDS was constantly being adjusted with the development of clinical guidelines and practice, some studies continued to clarify the criteria used in the definition of ARDS. Most studies provide burn-related data, such as mean TBSA (%), mean full-thickness burn injury (%), and proportion with inhalation injury (%).

Quality Assessment

The methodological quality of the study was good (average score of "Incidence" 77.1 [50–88]; the average score of "Mortality" 80.6 [69–86]). The detailed quality assessment is shown in **Supplementary Tables 3, 4.**

Quantitative Data Synthesis

Overall Incidence and Mortality of ARDS in Patients With Burns

The incidence of pooled weighted ARDS in patients with burns was 0.24 [95% CI 0.2–0.28] (**Figure 2**). Patients with burns had a pooled weighted ARDS mortality of 0.31 [95% CI 0.18–0.44] (**Figure 3**). Studies assessing burn patient incidence (I^2 = 98%) and burn patient mortality (I^2 = 99%) showed significant heterogeneity. The heterogeneity of "incidence" and "mortality" is so high that they challenge the relevance of the studies, and they could come from the differences in the inclusion criteria of patients (such as mechanical ventilation and minimal burn surface), definitions of ARDS, geographic location, mean age, burn severity, and inhalation injury, so we made the subgroup analysis to get the accurate incidence of special burn patients. Due to the number of studies included in mortality analysis being only 9, we did not divide these studies into subgroups.

Incidence of ARDS in Patients With Burns by Different Study Type

Considering the type of study that may influence the incidence of ARDS in patients with burns, we divided the studies into two types (retrospective and prospective). There are 15 retrospective studies and 3 prospective studies; the "retrospective" subgroup has 6,685 patients in total, and the "prospective" subgroup has 245 patients. For patients with burns in the retrospective studies, the incidence of ARDS was 0.24 [95% CI 0.18–0.3], while that for burns patients in the retrospective studies, the incidence of 0.15 [95% CI 0.06–0.39]. I^2 was 99 and 86%, respectively. No statistical difference was noted between them (p = 0.33) (**Supplementary Figure 1; Table 1**).

Incidence of ARDS in Patients With Burns and on Mechanical Ventilation

We found a total of eight studies containing mechanical ventilation in the inclusion criteria. The number of patients with burns and mechanical ventilation was 2,630, and for these patients, the incidence of ARDS was 0.37 [95% CI 0.29–0.44], and the heterogeneity was decreased to 93% (**Supplementary Figure 2; Table 1**).

Incidence of ARDS in Patients With Burns and TBSA ≥20%

Some "incidence" studies used TBSA (%) as an inclusion criterion, which included TBSA ≥1, 20, 30%, and so on. There were nine studies that set TBSA to ≥20% as an inclusion criterion, two studies set TBSA to ≥30%, and one study set TBSA to ≥50%. The minima burn surfaces of all these patients (n = 1127) were over 20%. The incidence of ARDS in these patients was 0.32 [95% CI 0.21–0.42], and heterogeneity was 92% (**Supplementary Figure 3; Table 1**).

Incidence of ARDS Defined by AECC and Berlin Definition

We found nine studies that defined ARDS by the Berlin definition and six studies by the AECC definition, and the number of patients was 2,738 and 1,989, respectively. The incidence of ARDS defined by the Berlin definition was 0.35, and the incidence of ARDS defined by the AECC definition (41) was 0.3 (**Supplementary Figure 4**). There was no significant difference between these subgroups (p = 0.61; **Table 1**).

Incidence of ARDS in Patients With Burns by Location

We divided the studies into Western research projects and Asian-African groups based on geography. The incidence of ARDS in burn patients in Western countries was 0.28 ([95% CI 0.27–0.33], I^2 = 99%, N = 22), and the incidence in Asian and African countries was 0.25 ([95% CI 0.22–0.29], I^2 = 95%, N = 13) (**Supplementary Figure 5**). There was no difference between the subgroups (P = 0.38; **Table 1**).

Incidence of ARDS in Patients With Burns by Mean Age

For studies where the average age of patients was 20–39 years, we combined the incidence of ARDS, and the outcome was 0.25 [95% CI 0.14–0.36]. For the subgroups with ages of 40–59 years, the incidence was 0.27 [95% CI 0.21–0.33] (**Supplementary Figure 6**). No statistical difference was found in this comparison (P = 0.73; **Table 1**).

Incidence of ARDS in Patients With Burns by Mean TBSA (%)

The incidence of ARDS in the TBSA ≥ 30% burn group is a little bit higher than the TBSA < 30% (**Table 1**). The results were mean TBSA ≥ 30%,0.26 [95% CI 0.21–0.31], N = 21, I^2 = 95% vs. mean TBSA < 30%0.22 [95% CI 0.15–0.29], N = 9, I^2 = 99% (**Supplementary Figure 7**).

Incidence of ARDS in Patients With Burns by Average Full-Thickness (%)

The incidence of ARDS in patients with burns and an average full-thickness of over 10% was 0.24 ([95% CI 0.17–0.35], N = 14, I^2 = 98%). Those with an average full-thickness ≤10% had an incidence of 0.19 ([95% CI 0.05–0.7], N = 2, I^2 = 94%;

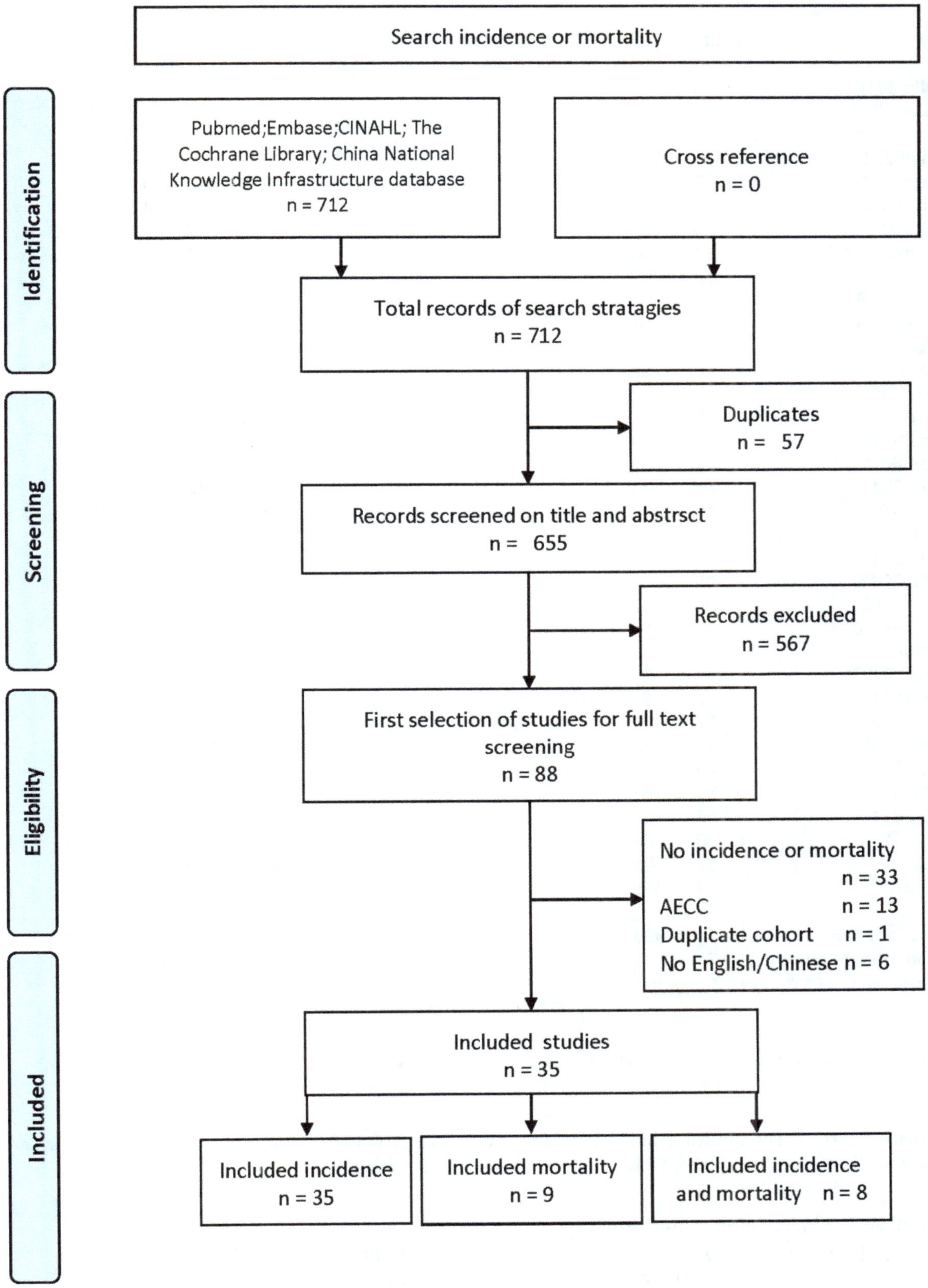

FIGURE 1 | Flowchart of literature searching and inclusion.

Study	Events	Total	Proportion	95%-CI	Weight (fixed)	Weight (random)
Cartotto 2016	70	162	0.43	[0.35; 0.51]	0.4%	2.9%
Clemens 2016	299	830	0.36	[0.33; 0.39]	1.9%	3.2%
Waters 2015	304	891	0.34	[0.31; 0.37]	2.1%	3.2%
Jeschke 2015	116	573	0.20	[0.17; 0.24]	1.9%	3.2%
Belenkiy 2014	95	291	0.33	[0.27; 0.38]	0.7%	3.1%
Béchir 2013	12	45	0.27	[0.15; 0.42]	0.1%	2.4%
Liffner 2005	36	91	0.40	[0.29; 0.50]	0.2%	2.7%
McCormick 2003	18	84	0.21	[0.13; 0.32]	0.3%	2.8%
Chen 2002	34	339	0.10	[0.07; 0.14]	2.0%	3.2%
Aharoni 1989	12	482	0.02	[0.01; 0.04]	10.6%	3.3%
Cakirca 2019	6	61	0.10	[0.04; 0.20]	0.4%	2.9%
Chong 2018	42	202	0.21	[0.15; 0.27]	0.7%	3.1%
Lin 2018	16	53	0.30	[0.18; 0.44]	0.1%	2.5%
Yeong 2018	4	33	0.12	[0.03; 0.28]	0.2%	2.6%
Liu 2018	9	92	0.10	[0.05; 0.18]	0.6%	3.0%
Wang 2019	32	72	0.44	[0.33; 0.57]	0.2%	2.5%
Ziolkowski 2017	49	983	0.05	[0.04; 0.07]	11.1%	3.3%
Herrero 2015	11	143	0.08	[0.04; 0.13]	1.1%	3.1%
Mokline 2015	10	20	0.50	[0.27; 0.73]	0.0%	1.6%
Li 2014	70	147	0.48	[0.39; 0.56]	0.3%	2.9%
Castilla 2014	9	25	0.36	[0.18; 0.57]	0.1%	1.8%
Thamm 2013	35	1637	0.02	[0.01; 0.03]	41.9%	3.3%
Guallar 2012	38	362	0.10	[0.08; 0.14]	2.1%	3.2%
Cachafeiro 2012	20	64	0.31	[0.20; 0.44]	0.2%	2.6%
Klein 2007	25	72	0.35	[0.24; 0.47]	0.2%	2.6%
Cochran 2007	104	202	0.51	[0.44; 0.59]	0.4%	3.0%
Cartotto 2003	5	38	0.13	[0.04; 0.28]	0.2%	2.6%
Dancey 1999	67	126	0.53	[0.44; 0.62]	0.3%	2.8%
Haddadi 2021	19	392	0.05	[0.03; 0.07]	4.6%	3.2%
Klein 2021	29	90	0.32	[0.23; 0.43]	0.2%	2.7%
Ren 2021	54	131	0.41	[0.33; 0.50]	0.3%	2.8%
Zhang 2014	62	922	0.07	[0.05; 0.09]	7.9%	3.3%
Chen 2020	20	48	0.42	[0.28; 0.57]	0.1%	2.3%
Li 2009	62	581	0.11	[0.08; 0.13]	3.3%	3.2%
Tang 2017	64	615	0.10	[0.08; 0.13]	3.5%	3.2%
Fixed effect model		**10899**	**0.07**	**[0.07; 0.08]**	**100.0%**	--
Random effects model			**0.24**	**[0.20; 0.28]**	--	**100.0%**

Heterogeneity: $I^2 = 98\%$, $\tau^2 = 0.0119$, $p = 0$

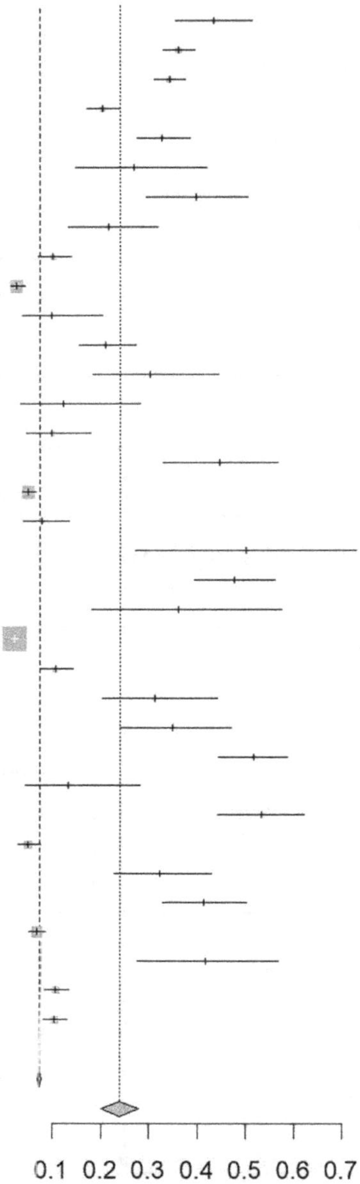

FIGURE 2 | Forest plot showing the overall incidence of acute respiratory distress syndrome in patients with burns.

Supplementary Figure 8). The incidence was not significantly different between these groups ($P = 0.74$; **Table 1**).

Incidence of ARDS in Patients With Burns by Inhalation Injury Proportion (%)

The incidence rate in the subgroup with over 50%inhalation injury proportion in patients with burns were 0.41 ([95% CI 0.34–0.48], $N = 4$, $I^2 = 49\%$), which is significantly higher than that of the subgroup with <50% inhalation injury proportion (0.24 [95% CI 0.17–0.3], $N = 18$, $I^2 = 99\%$ (**Supplementary Figure 9**). There was a significant difference between these subgroups ($p < 0.01$; **Table 1**).

Publication Bias and Sensitivity Analysis

We used a funnel plot to test for publication bias in 35 incidence and 9 mortality studies. The inverted funnel plot suggested there was a little bit of bias in studies reporting incidence and no obvious publication bias in mortality (**Supplementary Figures 10, 11**). To assess whether

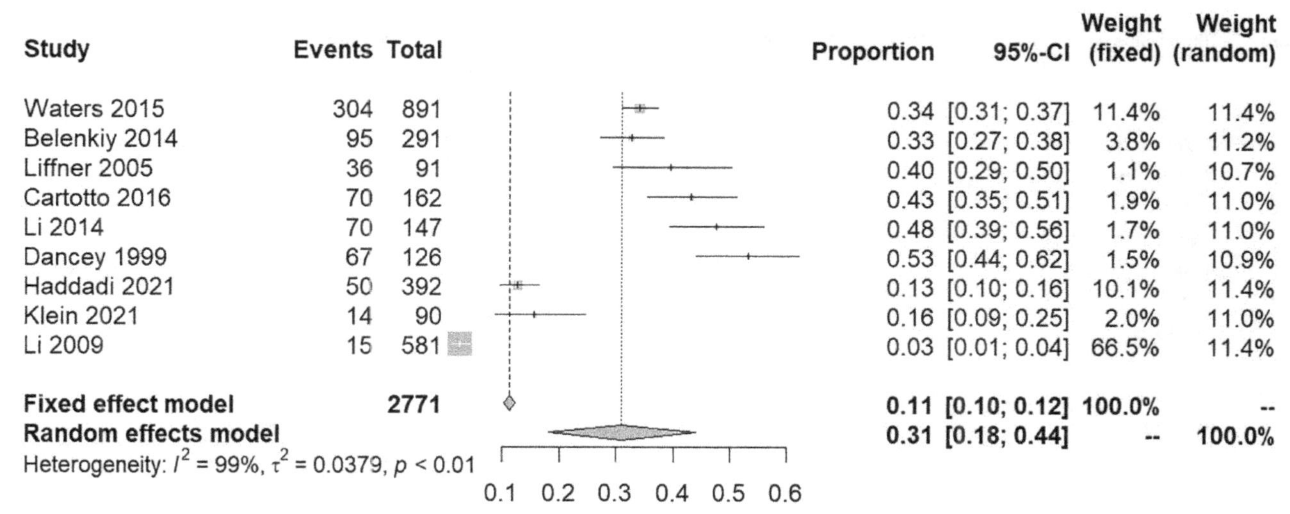

FIGURE 3 | Forest plot showing the overall mortality of acute respiratory distress syndrome in patients with burns.

the pooled incidence or mortality of ARDS in this meta-analysis was stable, a sensitivity analysis was performed. The effect estimation of sensitivity analysis showed that regardless of pooled incidence or pooled mortality, the results were stable (**Supplementary Figures 12, 13**).

DISCUSSION

This systematic review and meta-analysis included the first large-scale analysis of the incidence and mortality rates of ARDS in patients with burns. We calculated the pooled incidence and mortality of ARDS in patients with burns, as well as those in subgroups with alternative definitions, average age, TBSA, full-thickness burn injury, and inhalation injury proportion. These findings can help guide clinicians in assessing and diagnosing ARDS in patients with burns in the future and play an important role in the allocation of medical resources for disease and its prevention.

We selected several influencing factors related to ARDS which are common in most studies on the condition. These were used in the subgroup analysis and included study type, mechanical ventilation, minima burn surface within inclusion criteria, ARDS definition, geographic location, age, TBSA, full-thickness burn injury, and inhalation injury. We compared the rates and found that the "prospective-study type" might prevent ARDS from happening (incidence = 0.15), which may be caused by different types of treatment and healthcare. The incidences of ARDS were obviously higher in patients who is with mechanical ventilation (incidence = 0.37), whose minima burn surface were over 20% (incidence = 0.32), and which subgroup is with over 50% inhalation injury proportion (incidence = 0.41) than the common burn patients (incidence = 0.24). What is more, I^2 decreases while the rate increases, which makes the incidence more credible. In our result, mechanical ventilation, location, and inhalation injury were, again, identified as risk factors of ARDS.

We found that the more severe the inhalation injury, the higher the incidence, which is in line with the majority of previous research conclusions. The patients with burns and inhalation injury have a significantly higher incidence of ARDS compared with those without inhalation injury. As such, it can be concluded that inhalation injury was an independent risk factor for ARDS. However, using the new Berlin definition of ARDS (incidence = 0.35), it was clear the rates were higher than when using the older AECC definition (incidence = 0.30). From the perspective of diagnostic criteria, The PaO_2/FiO_2 requirements of Berlin are higher (40). The reason why the incidence of Berlin is higher than that of AECC is that the level of medical treatment has improved significantly with the development of time. The development of sophisticated testing equipment has enabled physicians to discover more patients with potential ARDS. The result shows that ARDS was more common in the subgroup of burns patients aged 40–59 years (incidence = 0.27) than the subgroup of burns patients aged 20–39 years (incidence = 0.25). However, the number of 40–59 years group studies (N = 18, n = 7,542) is higher than 20–39 years group (N = 10, n = 3,970), which means burns are common in 20–39 years group, but ARDS was common in 40–59 years group. Although the results are surprising, they should not be a problem. We can design a large targeted prospective study to prove this result further.

As this article is a meta-analysis of a single-group rate, we encountered the common problem of high heterogeneity. The I^2 of incidence was > 80%, regardless of whether heterogeneity was calculated for the "incidence" rates or the "mortality" rates. As a result, we chose to use a random effects model in the analysis. We explored the possible sources of heterogeneity in the studies of incidence by subgroup meta-analysis. Although we tried a lot of factors that may cause high levels of heterogeneity, including study type, inclusion, definition, location, mean age, TBSA, etc., we could not find a single model to account for these factors together. In the series of "incidence" studies, except

TABLE 1 | Pooled estimation of incidence of acute respiratory distress syndrome in burn patients and its subgroup.

Factors	Subgroups	Studies, *n*	No. of patients	Proportion [95% CI][a]	I^2[b]	*P*-value for heterogeneity	*P*-value for subgroup differences
Study type	Retrospective	15	6,685	0.24 [0.18–0.30]	99%	<0.01	0.33
	Prospective	3	245	0.15 [0.06–0.39]	86%	<0.01	
Inclusion	With mechanical ventilation	8	2,630	0.37 [0.29–0.44]	93%	<0.01	–[g]
	minima burn surface ≥20%	9	1,127	0.32 [0.21–0.42]	92%	<0.01	–
Definition[c]	Berlin	9	2,738	0.35 [0.31–0.40]	81%	<0.01	0.61
	AECC	6	1,989	0.30 [0.08–0.51]	98%	<0.01	
Location	Western	22	9,100	0.28 [0.27–0.33]	99%	<0.01	**0.01**
	Asian/African	13	12,659	0.25 [0.22–0.29]	95%	<0.01	
Mean age	20y–39y	10	3,097	0.25 [0.14–0.36]	98%	<0.01	0.73
	40y–59y	18	7,542	0.27 [0.21–0.33]	97%	<0.01	
TBSA[d]	<30%	9	4,763	0.22 [0.15–0.29]	99%	<0.01	0.22
	≥30%	21	3,877	0.28 [0.22–0.34]	95%	<0.01	
FT[e]	≤10%	3	970	0.29 [0.09–0.49]	97%	<0.01	0.91
	>10%	15	5,691	0.30 [0.23–0.37]	99%	<0.01	
II[f]	<50%	18	6,909	0.24 [0.17–0.30]	99%	<0.01	**<0.01**
	≥50%	4	387	0.41 [0.34–0.48]	49%	0.12	

(a) 95% CI: 95% confidence interval.
(b) I^2: heterogeneity of the studies.
(c) Definition: which definition of acute respiratory distress syndrome used in the studies, the American-European Consensus Conference (AECC) definition or the Berlin definition.
(d) TBSA, total body surface area.
(e) FT, full-thickness (FT) burn injury.
(f) II: the proportion of patients combined inhalation injury of the total sample.
(g) "–" means the date is not available.
Bold values mean statistically significant.

for the "study style- prospective," "definition- Berlin" subgroups, and "inhalation injury-≥50%" whose heterogeneity was slightly reduced ($I^2 < 90$), the remaining studies were more than 90% heterogeneous, with the vast majority being over 95%. When we compared the I^2 with other "a single-group rate" meta-analysis (28, 42), we found that high heterogeneity was common. Therefore, it might be acceptable that I^2 was 99% for the "mortality" study. For the subgroup of patients with burns and over 50% inhalation injury proportion, the incidence of ARDS (0.41) was precise because $I^2 = 49\%$. In addition to the heterogeneous sources suggested by the statistical results, we speculate that the inclusion criteria for each study could also be a main source of heterogeneity. We included diversiform literature, which were recording data related to ARDS and "burns." Patients with burns in some of the studies had different therapeutic schedules. Besides, some studies only analyzed mechanically ventilated patients with burns. The funnel plots showed that the distribution of "incidence" was asymmetric. The bias was very strong ($p = 0.01$). These variations in methodology and patient sampling may be the reason for the high heterogeneity. The distribution for "mortality" was visually symmetrical based on the results of the funnel plot. Furthermore, after sensitivity testing, the aggregated weighted ARDS morbidity and mortality were stable.

This meta-analysis has several advantages. First, this is the first comprehensive systematic analysis of ARDS in patients with burns. Most of the previous studies on the subject were based on specific groups (large area burns, burns with inhalation injuries, etc.). Comparing the findings here with previous studies, we note that this study is more thorough in including overall types of patients with burns. This leads to a more comprehensive and accurate assessment of the incidence and mortality rates of ARDS. Second, we use a rigorous screening method to exclude studies from different subject areas conducted by the same authors, while conducting detailed quality assessments of the articles included. Third, we made the most of the more than 8,000 samples; refining the study population classification according to different indicators, obtaining the incidence rates of different subgroups, and determining the relevant risk factors for ARDS. However, there are also some limitations in our research. First, our target population includes overall patients with burns. While the sensitivity analysis shows that the incidence and mortality rates are stable, we do recognize that there are many influencing factors, such as mechanical ventilation, definition, geographic location, inclusion criteria, age, burn severity, and inhalation injury in ARDS. The influence of all these various factors causes a substantial amount of heterogeneity in the data. Second, we were unable to retrieve data on individual patients and only conducted a meta-analysis on the results of each study. We used these data to determine the risk factors of ARDS based on the rate of events and characteristics of the study population. In subsequent studies, it would be advantageous to arrange a large and multicenter cohort of burn victims to address these issues.

CONCLUSION

This systematic review and meta-analysis revealed that the incidence of ARDS in patients with burns is 24% and that mortality is as high as 31%. The incidence rates are related to mechanical ventilation, location, and inhalation injury. Patients with burns from western countries and with inhalation injury have a significantly higher incidence than patients from Asian/African countries and without inhalation injury.

AUTHOR CONTRIBUTIONS

BW, ZX, YS, and GW: substantial contributions to the conception and design of the study. BW, WC, YJ, LH, and GW: acquisition, analysis, and interpretation of data for the study. BW, WC, YJ, HF, FZ, QY, and BZ: drafting of the article. BW, GW, YS, and ZX: revising the article critically for important intellectual content. GW, YS, and ZX: final approval of the version submitted for publication. All authors contributed to the article and approved the submitted version.

SUPPLEMENTARY MATERIAL

Supplementary Figure 1 | Forest plot: incidence for the retrospective and prospective subgroups.

Supplementary Figure 2 | Forest plot showing the incidence of acute respiratory distress syndrome in patients with burns and on mechanical ventilation.

Supplementary Figure 3 | Forest plot showing the incidence of acute respiratory distress syndrome in patients with burn and TBSA $\geq$ 20%.

Supplementary Figure 4 | Forest plot: incidence for the subgroups of American-European Consensus Conference definition and Berlin definition.

Supplementary Figure 5 | Forest plot: incidence for the subgroups of Western countries and Asian and African countries.

Supplementary Figure 6 | Forest plot: incidence for the subgroups of 20–39- and 40–59-year-olds.

Supplementary Figure 7 | Forest plot: incidence for the subgroups of mean total body surface area <30 and $\geq$30%.

Supplementary Figure 8 | Forest plot: incidence for the subgroups of inclusion of full-thickness burn injury $\leq$10 and >10%.

Supplementary Figure 9 | Forest plot: incidence for the subgroups of patients with combined inhalation injury <50 and $\geq$50%.

Supplementary Figure 10 | Funnel plot of incidence studies.

Supplementary Figure 11 | Funnel plot of mortality studies.

Supplementary Figure 12 | Sensitive analysis for incidence of acute respiratory distress syndrome in patients with burns.

Supplementary Figure 13 | Sensitive analysis for the mortality of acute respiratory distress syndrome in patients with burns.

Supplementary Table 1 | Characteristic of studies included in meta-analysis of incidence in burn patients.

Supplementary Table 2 | Characteristic of studies included in meta-analysis of mortality in burn patients.

Supplementary Table 3 | Quality assessment of the included studies on incidence of acute respiratory distress syndrome in burn patient with full-text.

Supplementary Table 4 | Quality assessment of the included studies on mortality of acute respiratory distress syndrome in burn patient with full-text.

Appendix 1 | Search strategies of PubMed, Embase, CINAHL databases, and China National Knowledge Infrastructure database.

Appendix 2 | Quality assessment of the included studies.

REFERENCES

1. Shaw TD, McAuley DF, O'Kane CM. Emerging drugs for treating the acute respiratory distress syndrome. *Expert Opin Emerg Drugs.* (2019) 24:29–41. doi: 10.1080/14728214.2019.1591369
2. Bittner EA, Shank E, Woodson L, Martyn JA. Acute and perioperative care of the burn-injured patient. *Anesthesiology.* (2015) 122:448–64. doi: 10.1097/ALN.0000000000000559
3. Nielson CB, Duethman NC, Howard JM, Moncure M, Wood JG. Burns: pathophysiology of systemic complications and current management. *J Burn Care Res.* (2017) 38:e469–81. doi: 10.1097/BCR.0000000000000355
4. Schouten LR, Veltkamp F, Bos AP, van Woensel JB, Serpa Neto A, Schultz MJ, et al. Incidence and mortality of acute respiratory distress syndrome in children: a systematic review and meta-analysis. *Crit Care Med.* (2016) 44:819–29. doi: 10.1097/CCM.0000000000001388
5. Cartotto R, Li Z, Hanna S, Spano S, Wood D, Chung K, et al. The Acute Respiratory Distress Syndrome (ARDS) in mechanically ventilated burn patients: an analysis of risk factors, clinical features, and outcomes using the Berlin ARDS definition. *Burns.* (2016) 42:1423–32. doi: 10.1016/j.burns.2016.01.031
6. Clemens MS, Stewart IJ, Sosnov JA, Howard JT, Belenkiy SM, Sine CR, et al. Reciprocal risk of acute kidney injury and acute respiratory distress syndrome in critically ill burn patients. *Crit Care Med.* (2016) 44:e915–22. doi: 10.1097/CCM.0000000000001812
7. Waters JA, Lundy JB, Aden JK, Sine CR, Buel AR, Henderson JL, et al. A comparison of acute respiratory distress syndrome outcomes between military and civilian burn patients. *Mil Med.* (2015) 180:56–9. doi: 10.7205/MILMED-D-14-00390
8. Jeschke MG, Pinto R, Kraft R, Nathens AB, Finnerty CC, Gamelli RL, et al. Morbidity and survival probability in burn patients in modern burn care. *Crit Care Med.* (2015) 43:808–15. doi: 10.1097/CCM.0000000000000790
9. Belenkiy SM, Buel AR, Cannon JW, Sine CR, Aden JK, Henderson JL, et al. Acute respiratory distress syndrome in wartime military burns: application of the Berlin criteria. *J Trauma Acute Care Surg.* (2014) 76:821–7. doi: 10.1097/TA.0b013e3182aa2d21
10. Bechir M, Puhan MA, Fasshauer M, Schuepbach RA, Stocker R, Neff TA. Early fluid resuscitation with hydroxyethyl starch 130/0.4 (6%) in severe burn injury: a randomized, controlled, double-blind clinical trial. *Crit Care.* (2013) 17:R299. doi: 10.1186/cc13168
11. Liffner G, Bak Z, Reske A, Sjoberg F. Inhalation injury assessed by score does not contribute to the development of acute respiratory distress syndrome in burn victims. *Burns.* (2005) 31:263–8. doi: 10.1016/j.burns.2004.11.003
12. McCormick JT, O'Mara MS, Wakefield W, Goldfarb IW, Slater H, Caushaj PF. Effect of diagnosis and treatment of sinusitis in critically ill burn victims. *Burns.* (2003) 29:79–81. doi: 10.1016/S0305-4179(02)00233-4

13. Chen XL, Wang YJ, Wang CR, Hu DL, Sun YX, Li SS. Burns due to gunpowder explosions in fireworks factory: a 13-year retrospective study. *Burns.* (2002) 28:245–9. doi: 10.1016/S0305-4179(01)00122-X
14. Aharoni A, Moscona R, Kremerman S, Paltieli Y, Hirshowitz B. Pulmonary complications in burn patients resuscitated with a low-volume colloid solution. *Burns.* (1989) 15:281–4. doi: 10.1016/0305-4179(89)90001-6
15. Cakirca M, Sozen I, Tozlu Bindal G, Baydar M, Yasti AC. Relationship between the albumin level and the anesthesia method and the effect on clinical course in patients with major burns. *Ulus Travma Acil Cerrahi Derg.* (2019) 25:55–9. doi: 10.5505/tjtes.2018.71278
16. Chong SJ, Kok YO, Tay RXY, Ramesh DS, Tan KC, Tan BK. Quantifying the impact of inhalational burns: a prospective study. *Burns Trauma.* (2018) 6:26. doi: 10.1186/s41038-018-0126-z
17. Lin KH, Chu CM, Lin YK, Chiao HY, Pu TW, Tsai YM, et al. The abbreviated burn severity index as a predictor of acute respiratory distress syndrome in young individuals with severe flammable starch-based powder burn. *Burns.* (2018) 44:1573–8. doi: 10.1016/j.burns.2018.01.006
18. Yeong EK, O'Boyle CP, Huang HF, Tai HC, Hsu YC, Chuang SY, et al. Response of a local hospital to a burn disaster: contributory factors leading to zero mortality outcomes. *Burns.* (2018) 44:1083–90. doi: 10.1016/j.burns.2018.03.019
19. Liu K, Wood D, Cartotto R. Mechanical ventilation of burn patients who do not have the acute respiratory distress syndrome (ARDS). *J Burn Care Res.* (2018) 39:S68. doi: 10.1093/jbcr/iry006.127
20. Wang W, Yu X, Zuo F, Yu S, Luo Z, Liu J, et al. Risk factors and th associated limit values for abnormal elevation of extravascular lung water in severely burned adults. *Burns.* (2019) 45:849–59. doi: 10.1016/j.burns.2018.11.007
21. Ziolkowski N, Rogers AD, Xiong W, Hong B, Patel S, Trull B, et al. The impact of operative time and hypothermia in acute burn surgery. *Burns.* (2017) 43:1673–81. doi: 10.1016/j.burns.2017.10.001
22. Herrero EH, Sánchez M, Cachafeiro L, Agrifoglio A, Galván B, Asensio MJ, et al. Lactate in the burn patient. *Crit Care.* (2015) 19:S50. doi: 10.1186/cc14225
23. Mokline A, Rahmani I, Gharsallah L, Hachani A, Tlaili S, Hammouda R, et al. Intraabdominal hypertension in burn patients. *Crit Care.* (2015) 19:S136. doi: 10.1186/cc14467
24. Li Z, Chung K, Cartotto R. Application of the new berlin definition of Acute Respiratory Distress Syndrome (ARDS) to burn patients. *J Burn Care Res.* (2014) 35:S65. doi: 10.1097/01.bcr.0000445188.61189.d4
25. Ruiz-Castilla M, Barret JP, Sanz D, Aguilera J, Serracanta J, Garcia V, et al. Analysis of intra-abdominal hypertension in severe burned patients: the Vall d'Hebron experience. *Burns.* (2014) 40:719–24. doi: 10.1016/j.burns.2013.09.021
26. Thamm OC, Perbix W, Zinser MJ, Koenen P, Wafaisade A, Maegele M, et al. Early single-shot intravenous steroids do not affect pulmonary complications and mortality in burned or scalded patients. *Burns.* (2013) 39:935–41. doi: 10.1016/j.burns.2012.10.007
27. Guallar C, Saénchez M, Cachafeiro L, Herrero E, Asensio MJ, Hernandez M, et al. An epidemiologic study of burn patients admitted in a burn intensive care unit. *Intensive Care Med.* (2012) 38:S84–5. doi: 10.1007/s00134-012-2683-0
28. Cachafeiro L, Sanchez M, Herrero E, Camacho J, Hernandez M, Agrifoglio A, et al. Epidemiological study of critical burn patients in an ICU. *Crit Care.* (2012) 16:S164–5. doi: 10.1186/cc11070
29. Klein MB, Hayden D, Elson C, Nathens AB, Gamelli RL, Gibran NS, et al. The association between fluid administration and outcome following major burn: a multicenter study. *Ann Surg.* (2007) 245:622–8. doi: 10.1097/01.sla.0000252572.50684.49
30. Cochran A, Morris SE, Edelman LS, Saffle JR. Burn patient characteristics and outcomes following resuscitation with albumin. *Burns.* (2007) 33:25–30. doi: 10.1016/j.burns.2006.10.005
31. Cartotto R, Choi J, Gomez M, Cooper A. A prospective study on the implications of a base deficit during fluid resuscitation. *J Burn Care Rehabil.* (2003) 24:75–84. doi: 10.1097/01.BCR.0000054177.24411.13
32. Dancey DR, Hayes J, Gomez M, Schouten D, Fish J, Peters W, et al. ARDS in patients with thermal injury. *Intensive Care Med.* (1999) 25:1231–6. doi: 10.1007/PL00003763
33. Haddadi S, Parvizi A, Niknama R, Nemati S, Farzan R, Kazemnejad E. Baseline characteristics and outcomes of patients with head and neck burn injuries; a cross-sectional study of 2181 cases. *Arch Acad Emerg Med.* (2021) 9:e8. doi: 10.22037/aem.v9i1.948
34. Klein HJ, Rittirsch D, Buehler PK, Schweizer R, Giovanoli P, Cinelli P, et al. Response of routine inflammatory biomarkers and novel Pancreatic Stone Protein to inhalation injury and its interference with sepsis detection in severely burned patients. *Burns.* (2021) 47:338–48. doi: 10.1016/j.burns.2020.04.039
35. Ren HT, Chen HQ, Han CM. Establishment of a predictive model for acute respiratory distress syndrome and analysis of its predictive value in critical burn patients. *Zhonghua Shao Shang Za Zhi.* (2021) 37:333–9. doi: 10.3760/cma.j.cn501120-20200301-00109
36. Zhang T, Li X, Deng Z, Zhang Z, Tang W, Chen B, et al. Analysis of respiratory complications in 922 severely burned patients. *Zhonghua Shao Shang Za Zhi.* (2014) 30:199–202.
37. Chen JY, Liu SX. Influence of directed restrictive fluid management strategy on patients with severe burns complicated by inhalation injury. *Zhongguo Shaoshang Chuangyang Za Zi.* (2020) 32:340–51. Available online at: https://kns.cnki.net/kcms/detail/detail.aspx?FileName=SSCS202005010&DbName=CJFQ2020
38. Li XJ, Zhang Z, Huo LZ, Liang DR, Liang R, Zhong XM, et al. Respiratory system complications and treatment of severe burns patients. *China Acad J Electr Publ House.* (2009) 1:283–4. Available online at: https://kns.cnki.net/kcms/detail/detail.aspx?FileName=SSWK200911001511&DbName=CPFD2010
39. Tang Y, Wang LX, Xie WG, Shen ZA, Guo GH, Chen JJ, et al. [Multicenter epidemiological investigation of hospitalized elderly, young and middle-aged patients with severe burn]. *Zhonghua Shao Shang Za Zhi.* (2017) 33:537–44. doi: 10.3760/cma.j.issn.1009-2587.2017.09.003
40. Lam NN, Hung TD, Hung DK. Acute respiratory distress syndrome among severe burn patients in a developing country: application result of the berlin definition. *Ann Burns Fire Disasters.* (2018) 31:9–12.
41. Sine CR, Belenkiy SM, Buel AR, Waters JA, Lundy JB, Henderson JL, et al. Acute respiratory distress syndrome in burn patients: a comparison of the berlin and american-european definitions. *J Burn Care Res.* (2016) 37:e461–9. doi: 10.1097/BCR.0000000000000348
42. Hirsch L, Jette N, Frolkis A, Steeves T, Pringsheim T. The incidence of parkinson's disease: a systematic review and meta-analysis. *Neuroepidemiology.* (2016) 46:292–300. doi: 10.1159/000445751

6

Time Interval from Early-Term Antenatal Corticosteroids Administration to Delivery and the Impact on Neonatal Outcomes

*Jing Li, Jing Zhang, Qingfei Hao, Yanna Du, Jie Lu, Haoming Chen and Xiuyong Cheng**

Department of Neonatology, The First Affiliated Hospital of Zheng Zhou University, Zhengzhou, China

Correspondence:
Xiuyong Cheng
fccchengxy@zzu.edu.cn

Objectives: To determine the association between the time interval from antenatal corticosteroids administration to delivery and neonatal complications in diabetic mothers undergoing early term (37+0 to 38+6 weeks) scheduled cesarean section (ETSCS).

Study Design: A retrospective cohort study of women with any form of diabetes in pregnancy undergoing ETSCS was included. Cases were stratified into the following groups based on the time interval from the first dose of corticosteroids administration to delivery: <2, 2–7, and >7 days. Women undergoing ETSCS, who did not receive corticosteroids were included as controls. We assessed the association between the time interval and neonatal outcomes in a multivariate regression model that controlled for potential confounders. Primary outcomes were the incidence of respiratory distress syndrome (RDS)/transient tachypnea of the newborn (TTN) and neonatal hypoglycemia.

Results: The study cohort comprised 1,165 neonates. Of those, 159 (13.6%) were delivered within 2 days of maternal corticosteroids administration, 131 (11.2%) were delivered within 2–7 days after maternal corticosteroids administration, and 137 (11.8%) delivered more than 7 days after maternal corticosteroids administration. The remaining 738 (63.3%) were not exposed to corticosteroids. Multivariate analysis demonstrated that delivery within any time of antenatal corticosteroids administration was not associated with decreased risks of RDS/TTN. The risk of neonatal hypoglycemia was highest in the delivery of <2 days group (adjusted odds ratio [aOR]: 2.684, 95% confidence interval [CI]: 1.647–4.374 for control group; aOR: 2.827, 95% CI: 1.250–6.392 for delivery 2–7 days group; aOR:2.975, 95% CI: 1.265–6.996 for delivery >7 days group).

Conclusions: Corticosteroids treatment for diabetic mothers undergoing ETSCS was not associated with beneficial neonatal respiratory outcomes. In addition, delivery, <2 days after antenatal corticosteroids administration was associated with an increased risk of neonatal hypoglycemia.

Keywords: antenatal corticosteroids, gestational diabetes mellitus, neonatal respiratory distress, early term scheduled cesarean section, hypoglycemia

INTRODUCTION

Infants born by elective cesarean delivery at term are at increased risk for developing respiratory complications compared with those born by vaginal delivery, particularly if born *via* cesarean section (CS) at 37+0 to 38+6 weeks of gestation (1–3). Gestational diabetes mellitus (GDM) is a common complication of pregnancy, and the prevalence of GDM in mainland China is 14.8%, with an increasing trend in recent years (4). Neonates to diabetic mothers are also subjected to a higher risk of respiratory morbidity than neonates of non-diabetic mothers (5–8). Such situations raise the question of the place of antenatal corticosteroids (ACS) in pregnant women with GDM or diabetes in pregnancy (DIP) undergoing an early term scheduled cesarean section (ETSCS) (9).

In pregnancies uncomplicated by diabetes, ACS treatment before term elective CS reduces the incidence of respiratory distress syndrome (RDS) and transient tachypnea of the newborn (TTN) and has been proposed as a way of reducing adverse neonatal outcomes in this population (10–12). Whereas, there appears to be insufficient evidence regarding the benefit of ACS in the early term period in pregnancies complicated by diabetes, it is because women with diabetes have largely been excluded (13), remained unidentified (11), or were included only in small numbers (6/819 women with GDM) (10) in studies investigating the efficacy of ACS. Recently, two retrospective studies investigating the efficacy and safety of ACS in women with GDM undergoing a term CS obtained inconsistent findings (14, 15). The time interval between corticosteroids administration and CS in one study ranged from 1 to 46 days (14), which may dilute the benefit of ACS treatment given that the optimal intervention timing is when delivery occurs within 2–7 days of administration (16). The corticosteroids administration timing was not specified in the other study, which found a reduction of respiratory complications (15). It is unclear whether exposure to ACS at different time points for these early-term infants is beneficial or may lead to some harm. The aim of our study, therefore, was to investigate whether the time interval from early-term corticosteroids administration to delivery is associated with a change in the likelihood of RDS/TTN, and neonatal hypoglycemia.

MATERIALS AND METHODS

We conducted a retrospective cohort study of all women who were diagnosed with GDM, DIP, or pre-existing DIP undergoing an early term (37^{+0} to 38^{+6}) elective cesarean section in the First Affiliated Hospital of Zhengzhou University, Zhengzhou, China, between 2016 and 2021. Exclusion criteria included multiple gestations, major fetal anomaly or fetal chromosomal abnormalities, and women who underwent an emergency CS. Cases were stratified into the following 4 groups based on the time interval from the first dose of antenatal corticosteroid administration to delivery: <2, 2–7, >7 days, and control group (corticosteroids not administered).

The following demographic and obstetrical variables were recorded: type of diabetes, ways of glycemic control, maternal age ≥35 years, hypertensive disorders, body mass index (BMI), indications to initiate treatment with ACS, and glycated hemoglobin (HbA1c) in the second or third trimester. The neonatal baseline data collected included the following: gestational age, birth weight, small/large for gestational age, male sex, and 1-min Apgar score <7. The primary outcomes of interest were RDS/TTN and neonatal hypoglycemia. Secondary outcomes included neonatal intensive care unit (NICU) admissions and length of stay in NICU.

The GDM or DIP is diagnosed based on one or more abnormal glucose values: (GDM: fasting blood glucose ≥5.1 mmol/L; 1-h post 75 g OGTT≥10 mmol/L; and 2-h post 75 g OGTT≥8.5 mmol/L, DIP: fasting glucose ≥7 mmol/L, 2-h glucose ≥11.1 mmol/L, following World Health Organization criteria) (17). The diagnosis of emergency cesarean delivery referred to the literature (18). The birth weight percentile was calculated using the Fenton curves in 2013 (19). Diagnostic criteria for RDS include the following: (1) representative clinical manifestations, including progressive respiratory distress occurring shortly after birth, tachypnea, flaring of the nostrils, expiratory grunting, cyanosis, positive three-concave sign, reduced or absent breathing sounds, and severe dyspnea, require continuous positive pressure ventilatory support for at least 72 h; (2) typical chest X-ray findings, such as fine granular densities, ground-glass opacity, air bronchogram sign, or white lungs; (3) arterial blood gas analysis showing hypoxia, hypercapnia, and oxygen tension/fraction of inspired oxygen ratio (PaO_2/FiO_2) ≤200 mmHg (20). The chest X-ray findings of TTN are mainly interstitial, alveolar, and interlobular pleural effusion. Neonatal hypoglycemia was defined as glucose levels ≤2.2 mmol/L within 24 h post-delivery (21). All neonates with a glucose level of ≤2.6 mmol/L were subsequently treated using a regimen that included intravenous dextrose therapy and surveillance in our unit.

Newborn exposure to ACS was defined as the administration of at least 1 of the 4 doses of 6 mg dexamethasone, given intramuscularly 12 h apart, as part of an antenatal corticosteroids course. The indications for ACS administration in this cohort were classified in a hierarchical classification system as one of the following: (1) preterm labor defined as regular uterine contractions causing cervical changes; (2) preterm pre-labor rupture of membranes (PPROM); (3) fetal indications (such as intrauterine growth restriction, oligohydramnios, or placental insufficiency); (4) maternal indications (such as hypertensive disorders, GDM, or DIP); (5) abnormal vaginal bleeding (such as placental abruption and placenta previa); (6) asymptomatic changes of the cervix (cervical length of <15 mm and/or dilation of >4 cm). However, the decision to administer ACS was ultimately left to the discretion of the obstetrician.

Statistical Analysis

Data analysis was performed with the SPSS version 22.0 software. Continuous variables were compared among groups using the ANOVA test. The LSD test (for homogeneity of variance) or the Tamhane's test (heterogeneity of variance) was used for comparison between any two groups. The chi-square test with Bonferroni correction was used for categorical variables. Differences were considered significant when the *p*-value was <

0.05. Multivariable logistic regression analysis was performed to evaluate the association between the time interval and neonatal outcomes while adjusting for potential confounders.

RESULTS

A total of 9,121 parturients with GDM or DIP were identified during the study period, and 1,165 of them were included in the study (**Figure 1**). Of those, 159 (13.6%) delivered within 2 days of ACS administration, 131 (11.2%) delivered within 2–7 days after ACS administration, and 137 (11.8%) delivered more than 7 days after ACS administration. Characteristics of the included infants and their mothers are shown in **Table 1**. There were statistically significant differences in the baseline characteristics, such as maternal hypertensive disorders, doses of ACS treatment, gestational age at delivery, birth weight, and the percentage of small for gestational age among the 4 groups (**Table 1**). The proportion of maternal age ≥35 years, type of diabetes, ways of glycemic control, BMI, HbA1c in the second or third trimester, neonatal sex, and the proportion of 1-m Apgar score of <7 were all similar among the 4 groups (**Table 1**). Women with an ACS-delivery interval of <2 and 2–7 days were more likely to have received ACS for maternal indications rather than for fetal indications (**Table 2**).

Multivariate analysis showed that the incidences of RDS/TTN were similar among the 4 groups (**Tables 3–5**). The associated risk for neonatal hypoglycemia was highest in the delivery with <2 days group (adjusted odds ratio [aOR]: 2.684, 95% confidence interval [CI]: 1.647–4.374 for control group; aOR: 2.827, 95% CI: 1.250–6.392 for delivery 2–7 days group; aOR:2.975, 95% CI: 1.265–6.996 for delivery >7 days group) (**Tables 3–5**). Of the 159 neonates who were delivered within 2 days of ACS administration, 73 were delivered within 24 h and 86 were delivered between 24 and 48 h after administration. The incidence of RDS/TTN was similar between the 2 groups, while the incidence of hypoglycemia was significantly lower (11 vs. 32.6%; $P = 0.001$) among neonates who were delivered within 24 h of ACS administration than among those who were delivered between 24 and 48 h after administration (**Table 6**).

DISCUSSION

In this cohort, ACS treatment in ETSCS among women with GDM or DIP, regardless of the time interval to delivery, was not associated with a reduction of RDS/TTN but increased the risk of neonatal hypoglycemia when delivery occurred within 2 days after administration.

Similar to previous studies (14, 22, 23), we found that ACS administration did not reduce respiratory morbidity in early term infants of mothers with any form of diabetes, despite there being some differences in the gestational age of infants and the timing of ACS treatment among studies. In addition, the secondary analysis of a large cohort study found that ACS did not improve neonatal outcomes even when applied to mothers with diabetes between 23^{+0} and 33+6 weeks of gestation (24). While ACS treatment accelerates neonatal pulmonary maturity, it is also well-known that ACS causes maternal hyperglycemia and subsequent fetal hyperinsulinemia, which contribute to delayed pulmonary maturity (25–28). Thus, it is possible that neonates born to women with GDM or DIP do not receive the same benefit from ACS, compared with those of mothers uncomplicated by diabetes, because of the maternal and fetal metabolic side effects

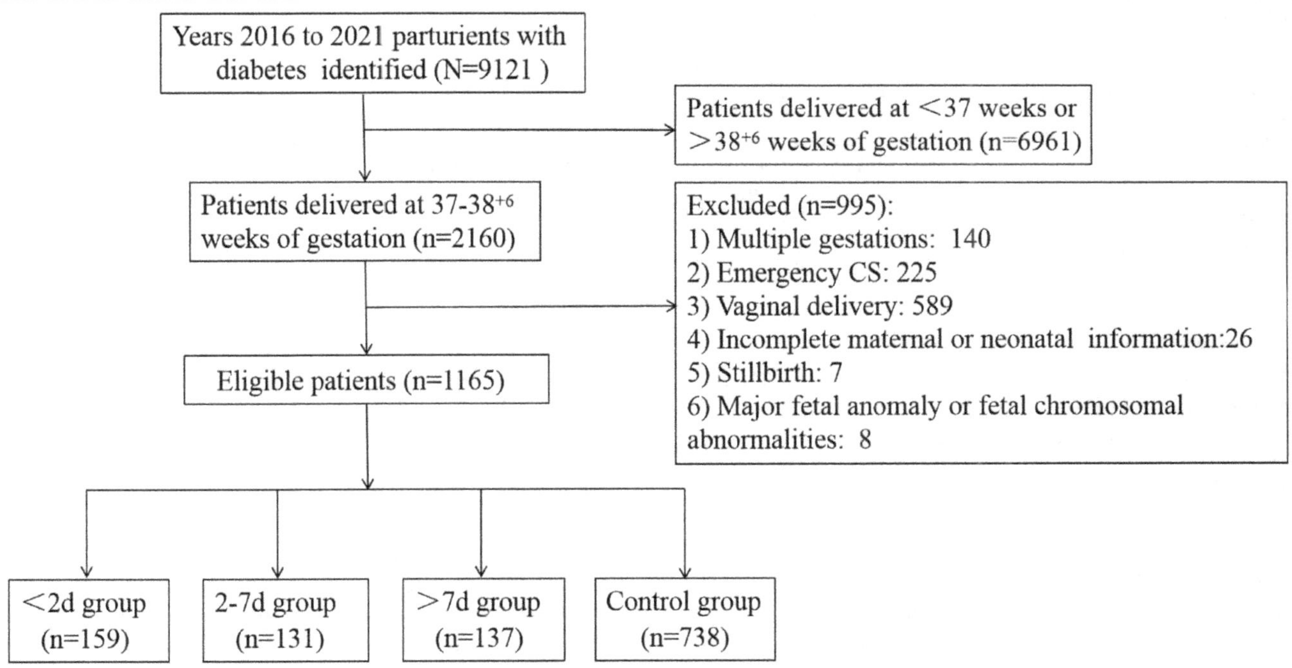

FIGURE 1 | Flow chart of included patients.

TABLE 1 | Characteristics of the studied groups.

Variables	Delivered <2 d after ACS administration ($n = 159$)	Delivered 2–7 d after ACS administration ($n = 131$)	Delivered >7 d after ACS administration ($n = 137$)	ACS not administerd ($n = 738$)	*P-value*
Type of diabetes, *n* (%)					0.337
GDM	152 (95.6)	120 (91.6)	132 (96.4)	696 (94.3)	
DIP	7 (4.4)	11 (8.4)	5 (3.6)	42 (5.7)	
Ways of glycemic control, *n* (%)					0.101[f]
Diet only	110 (69.6)	77 (59.7)	74 (54.4)[a]	477 (64.7)	
Insulin and diet	48 (30.4)	52 (40.3)	62 (45.6)[a]	258 (35.0)	
Medication and diet	0	0	0	2 (0.3)	
Maternal age≥35 years, *n* (%)	53 (33.3)	48 (36.6)	60 (43.8)	270 (36.6)	0.298
Hypertensive disorders, *n* (%)	16 (10.1)	14 (10.7)	26 (19.0)	73 (9.9)[c]	**0.019**
HbA1c in second or third trimester, %, median (Range), *n*	5.5 (4.9–6.9) 102	5.7 (4.5–9.3) 87	5.6 (2.7–7.6) 87	5.6 (1.7–8.4) 405	0.392
BMI (kg/m^2), mean ± SD	28.6 ± 4.0	29.8 ± 5.0[a]	28.6 ± 5.0	28.9 ± 4.4	0.165
Full course of ACS, *n* (%)	50 (31.4)	125 (95.4)[a]	132 (97.1)[a]	0[bc]	**<0.001**
Gestational age, mean ± SD	37.8 ± 0.5	37.8 ± 0.5	38.0 ± 0.6[b]	38.3 ± 0.6[abc]	**<0.001**
Birth weight (g), mean ± SD	3251.1 ± 477.2	3173.8 ± 521.7	3177.9 ± 500.2	3404.2 ± 486.9[abc]	**<0.001**
Small for gestational age, *n* (%)	3 (1.9)	5 (3.8)	4 (2.9)	2 (0.3)[abc]	**0.001**
Large for gestational age, *n* (%)	2 (1.3)	2 (1.5)	2 (1.5)	10 (1.4)	1.000
Male sex, *n* (%)	91 (57.2)	79 (60.3)	71 (51.8)	424 (57.5)	0.541
1-min Apgar score<7, *n* (%)	1 (0.6)	1 (0.8)	3 (2.2)	4 (0.5)	0.514
RDS (including TTN), *n* (%)	4 (2.5)	0	2 (1.5)	14 (1.9)	0.154
Serum glucose level, median (Range)	2.5 (0.8–5.2)	2.8 (1.2–8.5)	2.7 (1.7–6.0)	2.8 (1.1–6.2)[a]	**0.024**
Neonatal hypoglycemia, n (%)	36 (22.6)	15 (11.5)	13 (9.5)[a]	62 (8.4)[a]	**<0.001**
Times of hypoglycemia, median (Range)	1 (1–3)	1 (1–2)	1 (1–1)[b]	1 (1–2)	**0.013**
NICU admission, *n* (%)	37 (23.3)	33 (25.2)	26 (19.0)	117 (15.9)[a]	**0.023**
Days in NICU, median (Range)	5.5 (1–23)	5.5 (2–24)	6 (1–22)	6 (1–38)	0.846

PROM, premature rupture of membranes; ACS, antenatal corticosteroids. Bold indicate statistically signifcant.
Post-hoc method by Bonferroni: [a]*Means vs. Delivered <2 d after ACS administration group.*
[b]*Means vs. Delivered 2–7 d after ACS administration group.*
[c]*Means vs. Delivered >7 d after ACS administration group. Bold values are statistically significant.*

TABLE 2 | Comparison of indications for antenatal corticosteroids administration among groups.

Variables	Delivered <2 d after ACS administration ($n = 159$)	Delivered 2–7 d after ACS administration ($n = 131$)	Delivered >7 d after ACS administration ($n = 137$)	P-value
Indications for ACS, *n* (%)				**<0.001**
Preterm labor, *n* (%)	2 (1.3)	0	24 (17.5)	
PROM, *n* (%)	13 (8.2)	3 (2.3)	1 (0.7)	
Fetal indications, *n* (%)	17 (10.7)	21 (16.0)	46 (33.6)	
Maternal indications, *n* (%)	127 (79.9)	104 (79.4)	54 (39.4)	
Abnormal vaginal bleeding, *n* (%)	0	2 (1.5)	11 (8.0)	
Asymptomatic changes of the cervix, *n* (%)	0	1 (0.8)	1 (0.7)	

PROM, premature rupture of membranes; ACS, antenatal corticosteroids. Bold values are statistically significant.

of corticosteroids exposure, as well as the underlying glycemic metabolism disorders (24).

We observed an increased likelihood of neonatal hypoglycemia among neonates born within 2 days of ACS administration, which was consistent with findings of other's research (14, 29). Gupta et al. (14) found that ACS administration in ETSCS among women with GDM or DIP is associated with more neonatal hypoglycemia (24.2 vs. 4.4%; aOR, 18.96; 95% CI, 2.18–165.23), although they made the presumption that ACS administered at different time points before delivery would confer equal risk to neonatal hypoglycemia. A recently large cohort study (115/1,248 women with GDM) demonstrated that

TABLE 3 | Association between time interval from antenatal corticosteroids administration to delivery and adverse neonatal outcomes.

Outcome	Adjusted OR (95%CI)	*P*-value
RDS (including TTN)		
<2 d after ACS	1.308 (0.410, 4.170)	0.650
2–7 d after ACS	–	0.996
>7 d after ACS	0.943 (0.565, 1.575)	0.823
ACS not administerd	Ref	
Hypoglycemia		
<2 d after ACS	2.684 (1.647–4.374)	**<0.001**
2–7 d after ACS	1.128 (0.822–1.548)	0.455
>7 d after ACS	0.986 (0.791–1.229)	0.902
ACS not administerd	Ref	

Adjusted for hypertensive disorders, gestational age, birth weight, small for gestational age. OR, odds ratio; CI, confidence interval; ACS, antenatal corticosteroids; RDS, respiratory distress syndrome; TTN, transient tachypnea of the newborn; Ref, reference. Bold values are statistically significant.

TABLE 4 | Association between time interval from antenatal corticosteroids administration to delivery and adverse neonatal outcomes.

Outcome	Adjusted OR (95%CI)	*P*-value
RDS (including TTN)		
<2 d after ACS	–	0.996
2-7 d after ACS	Ref	
>7 d after ACS	–	0.993
Hypoglycemia		
<2 d after ACS	2.827 (1.250, 6.392)	**0.013**
2-7 d after ACS	Ref	
>7 d after ACS	0.960 (0.735, 1.253)	0.763

Adjusted for hypertensive disorders, gestational age, birth weight, small for gestational age, and number of antenatal corticosteroid doses (1~3 or 4). OR, odds ratio; CI, confidence interval; ACS, antenatal corticosteroids; RDS, respiratory distress syndrome; TTN, transient tachypnea of the newborn; Ref, reference. Bold values are statistically significant.

TABLE 5 | Association between time interval from antenatal corticosteroids administration to delivery and adverse neonatal outcomes.

Outcome	Adjusted OR (95%CI)	*P*-value
RDS (including TTN)		
<2 d after ACS	1.727 (0.134, 22.278)	0.675
2–7 d after ACS		0.993
>7 d after ACS	Ref	
Hypoglycemia		
<2 d after ACS	2.975 (1.265, 6.996)	**0.012**
2–7 d after ACS	1.063 (0.713, 1.586)	0.763
>7 d after ACS	Ref	

Adjusted for hypertensive disorders, gestational age, birth weight, small for gestational age and number of antenatal corticosteroid doses (1~3 or 4). OR, odds ratio; CI, confidence interval; ACS, antenatal corticosteroids; RDS, respiratory distress syndrome; TTN, transient tachypnea of the newborn; Ref, reference. Bold values are statistically significant.

TABLE 6 | Comparison of neonatal outcomes between newborns delivered within 24 h and those deliveries between 24 and 48 h after early-term antenatal corticosteroid administration.

Neonatal outcome	Delivered <24 h after ACS administration (*n* = 73)	Delivered 24–48 h after ACS Administration (*n* = 86)	*P*-value
RDS (including TTN), *n* (%)	1 (1.4)	3 (3.5)	0.732
Neonatal hypoglycemia, *n* (%)	8 (11.0)	28 (32.6)	**0.001**

ACS, antenatal corticosteroids; RDS, respiratory distress syndrome; TTN, transient tachypnea of the newborn. Bold values are statistically significant.

late preterm infants' risk of hypoglycemia decreased as the time interval from ACS administration to delivery increased, and the risk for hypoglycemia was highest in the delivery of <2 days group (29). Reports have suggested that even mild hypoglycemia which responds to treatment is still associated with poor neurocognitive and developmental outcomes (30). Currently, there is a lack of uniform opinions about whether the use of ACS should extend beyond 34 weeks of gestation among women with diabetes (31). Based on the results of this study, we suggest that ACS may be safely omitted in women with any form of diabetes in pregnancy undergoing ETSCS.

There are several strengths to this study. We evaluated the association between different time intervals from the administration of ACS to delivery and adverse neonatal outcomes in women with any form of diabetes undergoing ETSCS for the first time; a specific and unique population not thoroughly investigated previously. Another strength of this study is our sample size, which included 1,165 early-term neonates from singleton pregnancies exposed to ACS, is among the largest reported in the literature.

This study also has several limitations. This was a single-center retrospective cohort study. The HbA1c in the second or third trimester of some women was unavailable, which is a known risk factor for neonatal hypoglycemia (**Table 2**) (32), but there was no significant difference among groups based on current data. Although adjusted for in our multivariable analyses, there were some significant differences in the baseline characteristics among the 4 study groups, such as indications for ACS administration, doses of ACS treatment, gestational age, etc., which have been independently associated with adverse neonatal outcomes and may have contributed to our findings. Finally, we do not have data on whether neonates diagnosed with hypoglycemia had any related adverse events, especially impaired neurocognitive development. Therefore, a larger, randomized controlled trial is required to further confirm these findings and assess the long-term impact of hypoglycemia on neonates.

In conclusion, our findings suggest that ACS treatment for women, with any form of diabetes in pregnancy undergoing ETSCS, is not associated with improved neonatal respiratory outcomes, and may increase the incidence of neonatal hypoglycemia, especially when delivery occurred <2 days after ACS treatment. Therefore, we do not recommend administration in this population until further evidence regarding the safety of ACS is available.

AUTHOR CONTRIBUTIONS

JLi and JZ conceived the idea. JLi and QH analyzed the data. JLi wrote the manuscript. JZ, QH, YD, JLu, HC, and XC reviewed and edited the manuscript.

REFERENCES

1. Zanardo V, Simbi AK, Franzoi M, Solda G, Salvadori A, Trevisanuto D. Neonatal respiratory morbidity risk and mode of delivery at term: influence of timing of elective caesarean delivery. *Acta Paediatr.* (2004) 93:643–7. doi: 10.1111/j.1651-2227.2004.tb02990.x
2. Brown MJ, Olver RE, Ramsden CA, Strang LB, Walters DV. Effects of adrenaline and of spontaneous labour on the secretion and absorption of lung liquid in the fetal lamb. *J Physiol.* (1983) 344:137–52. doi: 10.1113/jphysiol.1983.sp014929
3. Irestedt L, Lagercrantz H, Belfrage P. Causes and consequences of maternal and fetal sympathoadrenal activation during parturition. *Acta Obstet Gynecol Scand Suppl.* (1984) 118:111–5. doi: 10.3109/00016348409157136
4. Gao C, Sun X, Lu L, Liu F, Yuan J. Prevalence of gestational diabetes mellitus in mainland China: a systematic review and meta-analysis. *J Diabetes Investig.* (2019) 10:154–62. doi: 10.1111/jdi.12854
5. Becquet O, El KF, Alberti C, Mohamed D, Blachier A, Biran V, et al. Insulin treatment of maternal diabetes mellitus and respiratory outcome in late-preterm and term singletons. *Bmj Open.* (2015) 5:e8192. doi: 10.1136/bmjopen-2015-008192
6. Hiersch L, Berger H, Okby R, Ray JG, Geary M, McDonald SD, et al. Gestational diabetes mellitus is associated with adverse outcomes in twin pregnancies. *Am J Obstet Gynecol.* (2019) 220:101–2. doi: 10.1016/j.ajog.2018.10.027
7. Mrudhula TG, Samanth J, Vasudeva A, Lewis L, Kumar P, Nayak K, et al. Fetal echocardiography at term in diabetic pregnancies helps predict the adverse neonatal outcome - results of a prospective observational study from South India. *Indian Heart J.* (2020) 72:576–81. doi: 10.1016/j.ihj.2020.09.017
8. Eidem I, Vangen S, Hanssen KF, Vollset SE, Henriksen T, Joner G, et al. Perinatal and infant mortality in term and preterm births among women with type 1 diabetes. *Diabetologia.* (2011) 54:2771–8. doi: 10.1007/s00125-011-2281-7
9. Jain L, Dudell GG. Respiratory transition in infants delivered by cesarean section. *Semin Perinatol.* (2006) 30:296–304. doi: 10.1053/j.semperi.2006.07.011
10. Stutchfield P, Whitaker R, Russell I. Antenatal betamethasone and incidence of neonatal respiratory distress after elective caesarean section: pragmatic randomised trial. *BMJ.* (2005) 331:662. doi: 10.1136/bmj.38547.416493.06
11. Ahmed MR, Sayed AW, Mohammed TY. Antenatal steroids at 37 weeks, does it reduce neonatal respiratory morbidity? A randomized trial. *J Matern Fetal Neonatal Med.* (2015) 28:1486–90. doi: 10.3109/14767058.2014.958461
12. Saccone G, Berghella V. Antenatal corticosteroids for maturity of term or near term fetuses: systematic review and meta-analysis of randomized controlled trials. *BMJ.* (2016) 355:i5044. doi: 10.1136/bmj.i5044
13. Amiya RM, Mlunde LB, Ota E, Swa T, Oladapo OT, Mori R. Antenatal corticosteroids for reducing adverse maternal and child outcomes in special populations of women at risk of imminent preterm birth: a systematic review and meta-analysis. *PLoS ONE.* (2016) 11:e147604. doi: 10.1371/journal.pone.0147604
14. Gupta K, Rajagopal R, King F, Simmons D. Complications of antenatal corticosteroids in infants born by early term scheduled cesarean section. *Diabetes Care.* (2020) 43:906–8. doi: 10.2337/dc19-2126
15. Paul R, Murugesh C, Chepulis L, Tamatea J, Wolmarans L. Should antenatal corticosteroids be considered in women with gestational diabetes before planned late gestation caesarean section. *Aust N Z J Obstet Gynaecol.* (2019) 59:463–6. doi: 10.1111/ajo.12963
16. Committee Opinion No. 713. Antenatal corticosteroid therapy for fetal maturation. *Obstet Gynecol.* (2017) 130:e102–9. doi: 10.1097/AOG.0000000000002237
17. WHO Reproductive Health Library. *WHO Recommendation on the Diagnosis of Gestational Diabetes in Pregnancy.* Geneva: World Health Organization, (2018).
18. Lucas DN, Yentis SM, Kinsella SM, Holdcroft A, May AE, Wee M, et al. Urgency of caesarean section: a new classification. *J R Soc Med.* (2000) 93:346–50. doi: 10.1177/014107680009300703
19. Fenton TR, Kim JH. A systematic review and meta-analysis to revise the Fenton growth chart for preterm infants. *Bmc Pediatr.* (2013) 13:59. doi: 10.1186/1471-2431-13-59
20. Liu J, Shi Y, Dong JY, Zheng T, Li JY, Lu LL, et al. Clinical characteristics, diagnosis and management of respiratory distress syndrome in full-term neonates. *Chin Med J.* (2010) 123:2640–4.
21. Persson M, Shah PS, Rusconi F, Reichman B, Modi N, Kusuda S, et al. Association of maternal diabetes with neonatal outcomes of very preterm and very low-birth-weight infants: an international cohort study. *JAMA Pediatr.* (2018) 172:867–75. doi: 10.1001/jamapediatrics.2018.1811
22. Krispin E, Hochberg A, Chen R, Wiznitzer A, Hadar E, Borovich A. Neonatal outcome in gestational-diabetic mothers treated with antenatal corticosteroids delivering at the late preterm and term. *Arch Gynecol Obstet.* (2018) 298:689–95. doi: 10.1007/s00404-018-4848-8
23. Ali H, Salama H, Robertson N, Olukade T, Al-Obaidly S, Al-Qubaisi M, et al. Antenatal corticosteroids and short-term neonatal outcomes in term and near-term infants of diabetic mothers. analysis of the Qatar PEARL-peristat registry. *J Perinat Med.* (2021) 49:377–82. doi: 10.1515/jpm-2020-0249
24. Battarbee AN, Sandoval G, Grobman WA, Bailit JL, Reddy UM, Wapner RJ, et al. Antenatal corticosteroids and preterm neonatal morbidity and mortality among women with and without diabetes in pregnancy. *Am J Perinatol.* (2020) 39:67–74. doi: 10.1055/s-0040-1714391
25. McGillick EV, Morrison JL, McMillen IC, Orgeig S. Intrafetal glucose infusion alters glucocorticoid signaling and reduces surfactant protein mRNA expression in the lung of the late-gestation sheep fetus. *Am J Physiol Regul Integr Comp Physiol.* (2014) 307:R538–45. doi: 10.1152/ajpregu.00053.2014
26. Moore TR. A comparison of amniotic fluid fetal pulmonary phospholipids in normal and diabetic pregnancy. *Am J Obstet Gynecol.* (2002) 186:641–50. doi: 10.1067/mob.2002.122851
27. Piper JM, Xenakis EM, Langer O. Delayed appearance of pulmonary maturation markers is associated with poor glucose control in diabetic pregnancies. *J Matern Fetal Med.* (1998) 7:148–53. doi: 10.1002/(SICI)1520-6661(199805/06)7:3<148::AID-MFM9>3.0.CO;2-K
28. Sifianou P, Thanou V, Karga H. Metabolic and hormonal effects of antenatal betamethasone after 35 weeks of gestation. *J Pediatr Pharmacol Ther.* (2015) 20:138–43. doi: 10.5863/1551-6776-20.2.138
29. Gulersen M, Gyamfi-Bannerman C, Greenman M, Lenchner E, Rochelson B, Bornstein E. Time interval from late preterm antenatal corticosteroid administration to delivery and the impact on neonatal outcomes. *Am J Obstet Gynecol MFM.* (2021) 3:100426. doi: 10.1016/j.ajogmf.2021.100426
30. Burns CM, Rutherford MA, Boardman JP, Cowan FM. Patterns of cerebral injury and neurodevelopmental outcomes after symptomatic

neonatal hypoglycemia. *Pediatrics.* (2008) 122:65–74. doi: 10.1542/peds.2007-2822

31. Kamath-Rayne BD, Rozance PJ, Goldenberg RL, Jobe AH. Antenatal corticosteroids beyond 34 weeks gestation: what do we do now? *Am J Obstet Gynecol.* (2016) 215:423–30. doi: 10.1016/j.ajog.2016.06.023
32. Kumar N, Kumar P, Harris N, Monga R, Sampath V. Impact of maternal HbA1c levels </=6% and race in nondiabetic pregnancies on birthweight and early neonatal hypoglycemia. *J Pediatr.* (2020) 227:121–7. doi: 10.1016/j.jpeds.2020.08.026

7

Early Alterations of Lymphocyte Subsets in Acute Respiratory Distress Syndrome Caused by *Acinetobacter baumannii* Pneumonia

Wei Cheng[1], *Jiahui Zhang*[1], *Dongkai Li*[1], *Guangxu Bai*[1], *Wen Han*[1], *Jianwei Chen*[1], *Hao Wang*[2*] *and Na Cui*[1*]

[1] State Key Laboratory of Complex Severe and Rare Diseases, Department of Critical Care Medicine, Peking Union Medical College Hospital, Chinese Academy of Medical Science and Peking Union Medical College, Beijing, China, [2] Department of Critical Care Medicine, Beijing Jishuitan Hospital, Beijing, China

***Correspondence:**
Hao Wang
newwanghao@hotmail.com
Na Cui
pumchcn@163.com

Background: To prospectively observe the early alterations of lymphocyte subsets in ARDS caused by Acinetobacter *baumannii*.

Methods: ARDS patients admitted to our ICU between January 1, 2017 and May 30, 2020 were selected. We enrolled all the pulmonary ARDS caused by Acinetobacter *baumannii* pneumonia who required mechanical ventilation or vasopressors. All the available clinical data, follow up information and lymphocyte subsets were recorded.

Results: Eighty-seven of all the 576 ARDS patients were enrolled. The 28-day mortality of the enrolled patients was 20.7% (18/87). The T lymphocyte count (452 vs. 729 cells/ul, $P = 0.004$), especially the $CD8^+$ T lymphocyte count (104 vs. 253 cells/ul, $P = 0.002$) was significantly lower in non-survivors, as were counts of the activated T cell subsets ($CD8^+CD28^+$ and $CD8^+CD38^+$). The $CD8^+$ T cell count was an independent risk factor for 28-day mortality, and a cutoff value of 123 cells/ul was a good indicator to predict the prognosis of ARDS caused by Acinetobacter *baumannii* pneumonia, with sensitivity of 74.6% and specificity of 83.3% (AUC 0.812, $P < 0.0001$).

Conclusions: Lower $CD8^+$ T cell count was associated with higher severity and early mortality in ARDS patients caused by Acinetobacter *baumannii* pneumonia, which could be valuable for outcome prediction.

Keywords: Acinetobacter *baumannii*, lymphocyte subset counts, acute respiratory distress syndrome, prognosis, ARDS

BACKGROUND

Acinetobacter baumannii (A. baumannii) is an opportunistic pathogen and one of the most common causes of hospital-acquired pneumonia, resulting from the increasingly serious occurrence of antibiotic resistance (1). Acute respiratory distress syndrome (ARDS) caused by *A. baumannii* pneumonia has significantly high mortality (2). It follows that there has been growing interest in identifying biological sub-phenotypes of ARDS patients (3). Measuring plasma biomarkers in ARDS can help find subgroups of patients those share important host-response features and/or those have worse clinical outcomes. Li et al. (4) found that neutrophil to lymphocyte ratio (NLR) was significantly associated with 28-day mortality in patients with ARDS, and NLR was related to the severity of ARDS. However, how the lymphocyte counts changed in NLR and their correlation with prognosis were not clearly illustrated.

Traditionally, *A. baumannii* was thought to cause extracellular infection, and innate immunity played a vital role in the defense against *A. baumannii* infection. Monocytes release tumor necrosis factor (TNF) to recruit granulocytes, which phagocytize bacteria or produce reactive oxygen species. Immature dendritic cells (DCs) capture and process antigens with high efficiency. $CD4^+$ T cells differentiate toward a Th_1-polarizing phenotype through the activation of DCs (5). However, A. baumannii has been shown to cause facultative intracellular infection recently, and many studies have confirmed its ability to invade lung epithelial cells and macrophages (1, 6–8). Therefore, many immune cells and cytokines that act against intracellular and extracellular infection might be involved in the immune response against *A. baumannii* infection, which is worth of further study. There have been few clinical studies on the changes and specific roles of lymphocyte subsets in the pathogenesis of ARDS caused by *A. baumannii* pneumonia. In this study we aimed to explore the role of lymphocyte subsets in ARDS caused by *A. baumannii* and its correlation with prognosis.

METHODS

We screened all the ARDS patients according to the 2012 Berlin definition (9) admitted to the intensive care unit (ICU) of Peking Union Medical College Hospital (PUMCH) between January 1, 2017 and May 30, 2020. Pulmonary ARDS caused by *A. baumannii* pneumonia and required mechanical ventilation or vasopressors were enrolled in our study. All eligible patients needed to be over 18 years old, ICU stays for 48 h and met none of the exclusion criteria. Exclusion criteria were: (1) any condition causing neutropenia as receiving corticosteroids or immunosuppression; (2) pregnancy or lactation; (3) any condition causing primary or acquired immunodeficiency, such as HIV infection, active autoimmune disease, hematopathy, or malignant tumors receiving chemotherapy within the previous 3 months; and (4) life expectancy <48 h. This study was approved by the Institutional Review Board of PUMCH (approval number: JS-1170), and all methods were performed in accordance with the relevant guidelines and regulations. Informed consent was obtained from all patients, and the study was registered at chictr.org.cn (identifier ChiCTR-ROC-17010750).

The Berlin definition of ARDS included 4 aspects (9): (1) Timing: newly onset or worsening respiratory syndrome within 1 week of known clinical insults; (2) Chest imaging: Bilateral opacities—not fully explained by effusion, lobar/lung collapse, or nodules; (3) Origin of edeme: respiratory failure that can not be fully explained by cardiac failure or fluid overload and need objective assessment to exclude hydrostatic edema if no risk factors present, such as echocardiography; (4) Oxygenation: Mild ARDS 200 mm Hg < PaO_2/FIO_2 ≤300 mm Hg with PEEP or CPAP ≥5 cm H_2O, Moderate ARDS 100 mm Hg < PaO_2/FIO_2 ≤200 mm Hg with PEEP≥5 cm H_2O, Severe ARDS PaO_2/FIO_2 ≤100 mm Hg with PEEP ≥5 cm H_2O.

Clinical diagnostic criteria of pneumonia (10–12): Pneumonia was diagnosed pulmonary infiltrates caused by infection, and at least two of the following findings: fever with a body temperature >38°C or hypothermia with a temperature <36°C; leukocytosis (>12,000 cells/mm^3) or leukopenia (<4,000 cells/mm^3); presence of newly purulent tracheal secretions; and a decrease in oxygenation.

Microbiological methods to diagnose pneumonia (12): lower respiratory tract specimens were obtained immediately after ICU admission and were sent to the PUMCH Clinical Microbiology Laboratory. Samples were obtained using non-invasive sampling and cultured semi-quantitatively. Endotracheal aspirates with >25 neutrophils on Gram's stain with <10 epithelial cells per high-power field were required for culture. If qualified samples of suputum were difficult to obtain or diagnose pneumonia, invasive respiratory sampling with bronchoalveolar lavage, protected specimen brush and blind bronchial sampling could be used. The Clinical Microbiology Laboratory determined antimicrobial susceptibility of isolated bacteria by means of the microdilution method (MicroScan System; Baxter health Care, West Sacramento, CA, USA). Results were interpreted according to breakpoints defined by the National Committee for Clinical Laboratory Standards (13). *A. baumannii* had to be the only pathogenic bacterium isolated from the enrolled patients. Bacterial colonization and ventilator-associated tracheobronchitis was carefully excluded by more than two intensivists, and other infections were cautiously excluded.

After enrollment, the following baseline information was collected: age, sex, comorbidities, treatment strategies, ventilator parameters, antibiotics, lymphocyte subsets, cytokines, and other laboratory data. SOFA score, Acute Physiology and Chronic Health Evaluation II (APACHE II) score and Clinical Pulmonary Infection Score (CPIS) within 24 h of admission were calculated, as well as the duration of mechanical ventilation, ICU stay and hospital stay, and 28-day mortality.

Lymphocyte subsets were evaluated in the Infection Laboratory. Peripheral blood mononuclear cells were stained with fluorescent monoclonal antibodies, then subjected to flow cytometric analysis (3-Color EPICS-XL Flow Cytometer; Beckman Coulter, Brea, CA, USA) to detect T cells ($CD3^+$),

Abbreviations: ARDS, acute respiratory distress syndrome; *A. baumannii*, Acinetobacter *baumannii*; ICU, intensive care unit; NLR, neutrophil to lymphocyte ratio; TNF, tumor necrosis factor; DCs, dendritic cells; NK, natural killer cells; SOFA, sequential organ failure assessment score; CPIS, clinical pulmonary infection score; Ig, immunoglobulin; IQR, interquartile range; ROC, Receiver operating characteristic curve; OR, odds ratio; AUC, area under the curve; P/F, ratio PaO_a: FiO_2; BALF, bronchoalveolar lavage fluid.

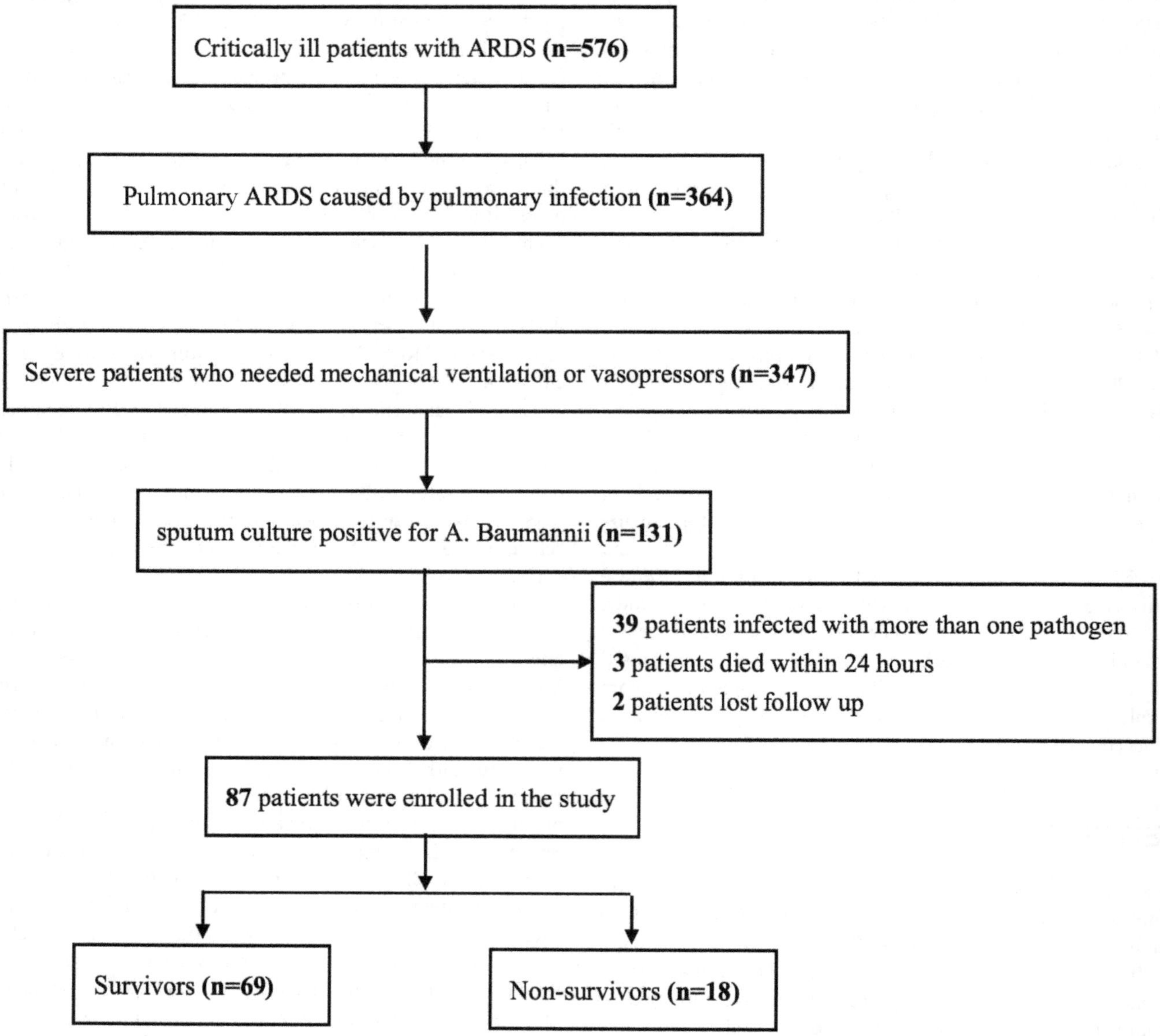

FIGURE 1 | Enrollment flowchart. *A. baumanni, Acinetobacter baumannii.*

$CD4^+$ T cell subgroups, $CD8^+$ T cell subgroups, B cells ($CD19^+$), and NK cells ($CD3^+CD16^+CD56^+$). Rate nephelometry (Array 360; Beckman Coulter) was used to measure serum levels of IgA, IgG, and IgM and complement factors C3 and C4.

Initial and targeted antibiotics: initial antibiotics were those given empirically at admission. Targeted antibiotics were those sensitive to *A. baumannii* in *in vitro* sensitivity tests, commonly including ampicillin/sulbactam, cefoperazone sulbactam, amikacin, ceftazidime averbatan, minocycline, carbapenems, tigecycline, and polymyxins.

The study protocol did not call for a standardized approach to critical care, and all treatment measures and drug selections were decided by the intensivists. As circulatory failure happened in most of patients, ECMO was not commonly used in this group.

Statistical Analysis

Normally distributed data were expressed as the mean and standard deviation and were compared using Students' *t*-test. Non-normally distributed data were presented as median and interquartile range (IQR) and were analyzed using the non-parametric Mann–Whitney *U*-test. Categorical variables were expressed as number and percentage and were compared with the chi-square or Fisher's exact test. A Cox proportional hazards model were performed successively to determine the association between lymphocyte subsets and outcome. Receiver operating characteristic (ROC) curve analysis was performed to determine the discriminatory ability of parameters for predicting 28-day mortality. Youden's index was defined for points along the ROC curve, and the reliability was assessed by sensitivity and

TABLE 1 | Baseline characters of ARDS patients caused by *A. baumannii* pneumonia.

	All (n = 87)	Survivors (N = 69)	Non-survivors (N = 18)	*P*-value
Baseline characteristics				
Sex (male%)	61 (70.1%)	51 (73.9%)	10 (55.6%)	0.13
Age (years) (M, IQR)	66 (57, 71)	66 (57, 71)	64.5 (58, 73)	0.846
Comorbidities				
Chronic pulmonary disease	3 (3.4%)	2 (2.9%)	1 (5.6%)	0.582
Diabetes mellitus	33 (37.9%)	23 (33.3%)	10 (55.6%)	0.084
Cardiovascular disease	45 (51.7%)	38 (55.1%)	7 (38.9%)	0.241
Chronic kidney disease	6 (6.9%)	5 (7.2%)	1 (5.6%)	0.801
Autoimmune disease	4 (4.6%)	3 (4.3%)	1 (5.6%)	0.828
Hepatopathy	2 (2.3%)	2 (2.9%)	0	0.465
Malignant tumor	10 (11.5%)	8 (11.6%)	2 (11.1%)	0.954
SOFA score	11.5 (9.75, 14)	11 (9, 14)	12 (10, 15.5)	0.339
Apache II score	19 (15, 22)	19 (15, 22)	21 (13.5, 26)	0.815
CPIS score	6 (5, 8)	6 (5, 8)	7 (5.5, 9)	0.345
Prognosis related parameters				
Ventilation day (days)	6.1 (2.6, 10.6)	7 (2.5, 10.5)	4.2 (3.8, 11)	0.797
ICU stay (days)	16 (10, 27)	20 (11, 29)	10 (4, 17.3)	0.004
Hospital stay (days)	20 (10, 28.5)	21 (12, 32)	11.5 (4, 21.3)	0.005

ARDS, acute respiratory distress syndrome; A. baumannii, Acinetobacter baumannii; M, Median; IQR, inter quartile range; SOFA, sequential organ failure assessment; Apache II Score, acute physiology and chronic health evaluation II score; CPIS, clinical pulmonary infection score; ICU, intensive care unit.
P-value for the comparison of survivors and non-survivors according to 28-day mortality.

specificity. $P < 0.05$ was considered statistically significant. The results were expressed as P-value and hazard ratio (OR) with 95% confidence interval (CI). IBM SPSS 23.0 software was used for all statistical analyses (IBM Corp., Armonk, NY, USA).

RESULTS

A total of 576 ARDS patients based on the Berlin definition were admitted to our ICU during the study period. There were 364 ARDS patients caused by pulmonary infection; 347 of which were severe enough to receive mechanical ventilation or vasopressor treatment. Cultures from the lower respiratory tract of 131 patients were positive for *A. baumannii*. Among the 131 patients with pulmonary ARDS, 39 were infected with more than one pathogen, three died within 24 h after admission, and two were lost to follow-up. Finally, 87 pulmonary ARDS patients caused by *A. baumannii* pneumonia were enrolled in the study (**Figure 1**).

Baseline Characteristics of Pulmonary ARDS Patients Caused by *A. baumannii*

The median age of these ARDS patients caused by *A. baumannii* was 66 years (IQR 57–71 years), with males accounting for 70.1% (61/87). The 28-day mortality of these patients was 20.7% (18/87), and there were no significant differences in sex, age, and comorbidities between survivors and non-survivors. According to the 28-day mortality, the severity of the disease was slightly higher in non-survival group than that of survival group, as the differences in SOFA core, APACHE II score, and CPIS score at admission were not significant. The ICU and hospital stays were significantly longer in the survivors (20 vs. 10 days, $P = 0.004$, and 21 vs. 11.5 days, $P = 0.005$, respectively) (**Table 1**).

Clinical Characteristics of ARDS Patients Caused by *A. baumannii* Pneumonia

According to the 28-day mortality, there were no significant differences in vital signs and laboratory results between survivors and non-survivors. In terms of respiratory parameters, the PaO_2: FiO_2 (P/F) ratio (198 vs. 178, $P = 0.173$) was lower, the driving pressure (12 vs. 13 cmH_2O, $P = 0.083$) was higher, and the peak airway pressure (21 vs. 24 cmH_2O, $P = 0.016$) was significantly higher in the non-survivor group. As for treatment, the non-survivors received more renal replacement therapy and glucocorticoids (23.2 vs. 55.6%, $P = 0.008$ and 11.6 vs. 33.3%, $P = 0.025$, respectively). There was no significant difference between the two groups in the initial empirical antibiotic treatment, including the use of effective antibiotics against *A. baumannii* and the subsequent targeted anti-infective treatment. There was also no significant difference in the time interval from the empirical treatment to the targeted treatment. One patient in each group changed antibiotics because of adverse effects, which had no effect on the final statistical analysis (**Table 2**).

Comparison of Inflammatory and Immune Parameters in ARDS Caused by *A. baumannii* Pneumonia

According to the 28-day mortality, there was no significant differences in procalcitonin, (1,3)-β-D Glucan, interleukin, Tumor necrosis factor-α and other inflammatory markers, as well as complement and immunoglobulin between the two groups.

TABLE 2 | Clinical characteristics of ARDS caused by *A. baumannii* pneumonia.

	All (*N* = 87)	Survivors (*N* = 69)	Non-survivors (*N* = 18)	*P*
Vital signs at admission				
Temperature (°C)	37.5 ± 0.7	37.6 ± 0.7	37.4 ± 0.9	0.345
Heart rate (per minute)	108 ± 19	107 ± 19	109 ± 21	0.728
MAP (mmHg)	84 ± 13	84 ± 14	86 ± 8	0.453
CVP (mmHg)	9 ± 3	9 ± 3	9 ± 2	0.813
Laboratory test at admission				
Platelet (*10^9/L)	160 ± 69	166 ± 69	91 ± 46	0.319
Creatinine (umol/L)	114 ± 56	117 ± 57	102 ± 53	0.323
TBil (umol/L)	23.9 ± 13.2	23.6 ± 13.0	25.4 ± 13.9	0.601
Albumin (g/L)	33 ± 4	33 ± 4	33 ± 4	0.649
cTnI (ug/L)	3.4 ± 5.7	3.3 ± 5.9	3.5 ± 4.7	0.963
Nt-ProBNP (pg/ml)	6658 ± 8615	6944 ± 9036	5372 ± 6625	0.606
PT (seconds)	16.7 ± 4.9	16.6 ± 5.0	16.9 ± 4.8	0.784
APTT-R	1.8 ± 3.8	1.9 ± 4.3	1.4 ± 0.4	0.555
Lactate (mmol/L)	2.0 ± 2.0	1.9 ± 2.1	2.6 ± 1.9	0.205
ScvO2 (%)	71 ± 8.1	71 ± 7.8	71 ± 9.6	0.956
NLR	12.3 (7.4–19.5)	11.8 (7.4–18.5)	17.4 (8.3–25.6)	0.224
Respiratory parameters at admission				
Tidal volume (ml)	410 (390–440)	410 (400–440)	400 (380–450)	0.4
$PaCO_2$ (mmHg)	39 (34–42)	39 (34.4–42)	38 (31.8–42.3)	0.602
P/F ratio	191 (160–228)	198 (165–229)	178 (155–207)	0.173
PEEP (cmH_2O)	8 (5–10)	8 (5–10)	8 (6–10)	0.324
Ppeak (cmH_2O)	22 (18–24)	21 (18–23)	24 (21.5–26.5)	0.016
Driving pressure (cmH_2O)	12 (10–15)	12 (10–14)	13 (11.5–17.5)	0.083
RR (per minute)	15 (15–18)	15 (15–18)	15 (15–17)	0.642
Treatment strategies				
Vasopressor	73(83.9%)	57 (82.6%)	16 (88.9%)	0.518
RRT	26 (29.9%)	16 (23.2%)	10 (55.6%)	0.008
ECMO	2 (2.3%)	2 (2.9%)	0	0.465
Neuroblockade agent	4 (4.6%)	2 (2.9%)	2 (11.1%)	0.138
RM	13 (14.9%)	10 (14.5%)	3 (16.7%)	0.818
Prone position	29 (33.3%)	24 (34.8%)	5 (27.8%)	0.574
GCs	14 (16.1%)	8 (11.6%)	6 (33.3%)	0.025
Immunosuppressor	1 (1.1%)	1 (1.4%)	0	0.607
Initial empiral antibiotics				
Antibiotics for GNB	84 (96.6%)	67 (97.1%)	17 (94.4%)	0.582
Effective for A.B.	51 (58.6%)	39 (56.5%)	12 (66.7%)	0.436
Antibiotics for GPB	61 (70.1%)	49 (71%)	12 (66.7%)	0.72
Anti-fungal drugs	30 (34.5%)	21 (30.4%)	9 (50%)	0.12
Antiviral drugs	6 (6.9%)	5 (7.2%)	1 (5.6%)	0.801
Virus co-exist	6 (6.9%)	4 (5.8%)	2 (11.1%)	0.428
Candida co-exist	4 (4.6%)	3 (4.3%)	1 (5.6%)	0.828
Target antibiotics				0.671
Tigercycline	56 (64.4%)	43 (62.3%)	13 (72.2%)	
Polymyxins	8 (9.2%)	6 (8.7%)	2 (11.1%)	
Other drugs*	19 (21.8%)	17 (24.6%)	2 (11.1%)	
Duration from admission to target antibiotics (hours)	15 (11–22)	16 (12–22)	12.5 (10.8–23.5)	0.463

ARDS, acute respiratory distress syndrome; A. baumannii (A. B.), Acinetobacter baumannii; MAP, mean arterial blood pressure; CVP, central venous pressure; TBil, total Bilirubin; cTnI, cardiac troponin I; Nt-ProBNP, N-terminal pro brain natriuretic peptide; PT, prothrombin time; APTT-R, activated partial thromboplastin time ratio; ScvO$_2$, Central venous oxygen saturation; NLR, neutrophil to lymphocyte ratio; PaCO$_2$, arterial partial pressure of carbon dioxide; P/F, ratio PaO$_2$/FiO$_2$; PEEP, positive end expiratory pressure; Ppeak, peak pressure; RR, respiratory rate; RRT, renal replacement therapy; ECMO, extracorporeal membrane oxygenation; RM, recruitment maneuver; GCs, glucocorticoids; GNB, gram negative bacteria; GPB, gram positive bacteria.

**Antibiotics that were effective for AB in vitro besides Tigercycline and Polymyxins, such as Ampicillin sulbactam, Cefoperazone sulbactam, Amikacin, Ceftazidime averbatan, Minocycline, Carbapenems et al.*

P-value for the comparison of survivors and non-survivors according to 28-day mortality.

TABLE 3 | Inflammatory and immune related markers of ARDS caused by *A. baumannii* pneumonia.

	All	Survivors ($n = 69$)	Non-survivors ($n = 18$)	P
Inflammatory markers				
PCT (ng/ml)	8.8 ± 13.7	7.8 ± 12.6	12.9 ± 17.1	0.165
BDG (pg/ml)	160 ± 326	155.3 ± 344	180.8 ± 246.8	0.729
GM test (pg/ml)	0.52 ± 0.87	0.55 ± 0.98	0.43 ± 0.21	0.606
hsCRP (mg/L)	106.9 ± 85.8	111.1 ± 86.4	92.8 ± 84.6	0.443
IL-6 (pg/ml)	100.9 ± 179.6	99.6 ± 193.2	105.5 ± 127.7	0.921
IL-8 (pg/ml)	225.4 ± 343.2	249.7 ± 379.7	138.2 ± 129.9	0.324
IL-10 (pg/ml)	17.2 ± 22.8	15.7 ± 23.4	22.3 ± 20.7	0.38
TNF-a (pg/ml)	28.6 ± 37.2	31.5 ± 40.8	16.7 ± 10.9	0.319
Immune parameters				
C3 (g/L)	0.80 ± 0.23	0.79 ± 0.23	0.85 ± 0.22	0.307
C4 (g/L)	0.18 ± 0.07	0.17 ± 0.07	0.20 ± 0.09	0.132
IgG (g/L)	10.8 ± 3.9	10.7 ± 3.6	11.1 ± 4.8	0.719
IgA (g/L)	2.6 ± 1.2	2.6 ± 1.3	2.8 ± 0.9	0.429
IgM (g/L)	0.95 ± 0.53	0.92 ± 0.5	1.1 ± 0.6	0.297
Lymphocyte subsets (cells/ul)				
White blood cell	13474 ± 8080	13584 ± 8743	13061 ± 5059	0.809
Neutrophil	11769 ± 7665	11659 ± 8170	12194 ± 5475	0.794
Monocyte	580 ± 372	559 ± 349	668 ± 459	0.299
Lymphocyte	963 ± 532	1016 ± 526	765 ± 525	0.084
B lymphocyte	206 ± 250	193 ± 221	252 ± 341	0.375
NK T cell	77 ± 72	84 ± 75	51 ± 49	0.087
T lymphocyte	671 ± 372	729 ± 364	452 ± 322	0.004
$CD4^{+}$ T cell	419 ± 252	443 ± 250	332 ± 245	0.095
$CD4^{+}CD28^{+}$ T cell	404 ± 245	427 ± 248	318 ± 221	0.097
$CD8^{+}$ T cell	221 ± 185	253 ± 191	104 ± 94	0.002
$CD8^{+}CD28^{+}$ T cell	117 ± 83	132 ± 83	59 ± 58	0.001
Memory $CD4^{+}$ T	292 ± 169	311 ± 162	221 ± 182	0.067
$45RA^{+}CD4^{+}$ T	126 ± 114	132 ± 119	103 ± 89	0.348
Naïve $CD4^{+}$ T	118 ± 106	124 ± 111	96 ± 88	0.324
$CD8^{+}DR^{+}$ T	131 ± 161	151 ± 174	58 ± 61.9	0.029
$CD8^{+}CD38^{+}$ T	128 ± 159	151 ± 172	44 ± 36	0.011
$CD4^{+}$ T/$CD8^{+}$ T	2.9 ± 1.4	2.5 ± 2.2	4.0 ± 2.8	0.018

ARDS, acute respiratory distress syndrome; A. baumannii, Acinetobacter baumannii; PCT, procalcitonin; BDG, (1,3)-β-D Glucan; GM, test Galactomannan test; hsCRP, hypersensitive C-reactive protein; IL, interleukin; TNF-a, tumor necrosis factor-a; C3, complement 3; Ig, immunoglobulin; NK T cell, natural killer T cell.
P-value for the comparison of survivors and non-survivors according to 28-day mortality.

TABLE 4 | Cox regression of lymphocyte subsets related parameters and survival.

	B	SE	Wald	OR	95%CI	P-value
$CD8^{+}$ T cell count (cells/ul)	1.3	0.438	8.789	3.667	1.553, 8.659	0.003
$CD8^{+}CD28^{+}$ T count (cells/ul)	2.043	0.723	7.992	7.714	1.871, 31.801	0.005
$CD8^{+}CD38^{+}$ T count (cells/ul)	0.995	0.436	5.222	2.705	1.152, 6.353	0.022

SE, standard error of the mean; OR, odds ratio; 95% CI, 95% confidence interval.

As for lymphocyte subsets: there was no significant difference in the total number of leukocytes and neutrophils between the two groups. The number of T cells (452 ± 322 vs. 729 ± 364/μl, $P =$ 0.004), especially $CD8^{+}$ T cells (104 ± 94 vs. 253 ± 191/μl, $P =$ 0.002) was significantly lower in non-survivors than in survivors. The total number of lymphocytes and $CD4^{+}$ T cells was also lower in non-survivors (765 ± 525 vs. 1,016 ± 526/μl, $P = 0.084$ and 332 ± 245 vs. 729 ± 364/μl, $P = 0.011$ respectively) (**Table 3**).

Parameters Associated With 28-Day Mortality

To clarify the factors independently associated with 28-day mortality, A cox proportional hazards model were performed. SOFA score, lactate level, P/F ratio and driving pressure that had been confirmed to be related to survival were included in the model as well as the parameters that were significantly different between the survivors and non-survivors in our study (Ppeak,

RRT and Glucocorticoids use). Lymphocyte related parameters were also included in the model separately. $CD8^+$ T cell count and its subtypes were independent factors associated with 28-day mortality of ARDS caused by *A. baumannii* pneumonia ($CD8^+$ T cell count: OR 3.667, 95% CI 1.553–8.659, $P = 0.003$; $CD8^+CD28^+$ T cell count: OR 2.043, 95% CI 1.871–31.801, $P = 0.005$; $CD8^+CD38^+$ T cell count: OR 2.705, 95% CI 1.152–6.353, $P = 0.022$) (**Table 4**).

To further analyze the influence of lymphocyte subsets related parameters that differed significantly between survivors and non-survivors in the univariate analysis on prognosis, ROC curve analysis was performed. The $CD8^+$ T cell count had the greatest discriminatory ability, with an area under the curve of 0.812. A cutoff value of 123 cells/μl at ICU admission was predictive of 28-day mortality for ARDS caused by *A. baumannii* with a sensitivity of 74.6% and specificity of 83.3% ($P < 0.0001$) (**Figure 2**).

Furthermore, we divided these ARDS patients into two groups according to the $CD8^+$ T cell count (<123 and ≥123 cells/μl). the accumulative survival rate from the Kaplan-Meier curve was significantly lower and ventilation free day was significantly shorter (14.5 vs. 21 days, $P = 0.001$) in patients with a lower $CD8^+$ T cell count, while 28-day mortality was significantly higher than that in patients with a higher $CD8^+$ T cell count (46.9 vs. 5.7%, $P < 0.0001$). The patients with lower $CD8^+$ T cell counts had lower P/F ratio, higher driving pressure at admission. The NLR, PCT level and CPIS at admission were also higher in patients with a lower $CD8^+$ T cell count (**Table 5, Figures 3A–E**). We divided the cohort into different severity of ARDS according to admission P/F ratio and found that patients with increasing severity of ARDS had progressively lower $CD8^+$ T cell counts (**Figure 4**).

DISCUSSION

To our knowledge, this is the first clinical study exploring the early alterations of lymphocyte subsets in ARDS caused by *A. baumannii* pneumonia. 28-day mortality of these patients was 20.7%. The T cell count, especially for $CD8^+$ T cells, at admission was independently associated with 28-day mortality. The $CD8^+$ T cell count was an early predictive marker for prognosis. So far, studies about *A. baumannii* and immunity have been limited to basic research, and there are limited data for clinical use. Our study first confirmed that T cell immunity might play an important role in ARDS caused by *A. baumannii* pneumonia, which could be important for clinical practice.

Immune disorder is the characteristic manifestation of sepsis, and increasing evidence shows that the immune system plays a bridging role between severe infection, organ damage and prognosis. However, the current view of how the two most complex syndromes, systemic inflammatory response syndrome and immune response syndrome, affect each other is still rudimentary (14, 15). The first step is to clarify the relationship between certain diseases and immune responses. There is a profound relationship between NLR and sepsis, NLR and ARDS, the $CD4^+$ T cell count and carbapenem-resistant Enterobacteriaceae (CRE) infection (16), and there has been growing interest in identifying biological sub-phenotypes of ARDS patients with similar host-response features for prognostic enrichment (3). Basic immunological research into *A. baumannii* infection is in full swing, along with research into the mechanism of host defense against the infection. For example, there has been in-depth study of outer membrane protein A (5, 17). However, there has been little clinical research on the relationship between immunity to *A. baumannii* infection and prognosis. In this study, we found that the $CD8^+$ and $CD8^+CD28^+$ T cell counts were independently associated with 28-day mortality in ARDS patients caused by *A. baumannii*. Clinically, this is the first-time providing evidence of Acinetobacter baumannii causing intracellular infection, which makes the understanding of this aspect go further.

A variety of immune cells are involved in resistance to ARDS caused by *A. baumannii* pneumonia (18). Large numbers of *A. baumannii* are taken up by alveolar macrophages as early as 4 h after infection. NK T cells are another cell type that act during the immune response against *A. baumannii*. Depletion of NK T cells in a murine pneumonia model caused impaired bacterial clearance and increased mortality. We found that the NK T cell count in non-survivors was lower than in survivors, which was consistent with previous research (19). DCs are the bridge between innate and adaptive immune responses, $CD4^+$ T cells differentiate toward a Th_1-polarizing phenotype through the activation of DCs (5). Subsequently, $CD4^+$ T-helper cells support the production of specific antibodies by B cells and promote the bactericidal activity of phagocytes that together clear the infection. Our previous study also illustrated that the $CD4^+CD28^+$ T cell count was a useful marker for early diagnosis of CRE infection and outcome prediction (16). It was not surprising to see that innate immune cells were involved in the defense against *A. baumannii*, but with the ability to cause intracellular infection, *A. baumannii* pneumonia should induce cellular immunity response. However, the relationship between the $CD8^+$ T cell count and *A. baumannii* has rarely been studied before (6). For the first time, our study illustrated the association between $CD8^+$ T cells and ARDS caused by *A. baumannii* pneumonia. The possible mechanisms were as follows: (1) *A. baumannii* directly invaded alveolar epithelial cells, and cytotoxic $CD8^+$ T cells directly recognized and killed infected epithelial cells (8); and (2) in addition to $CD8^+$ T cells, the $CD8^+CD38^+$ T cells also differed significantly between survivors and non-survivors with *A. baumannii* infection. Inflammatory reaction, antigen exposure and environmental factors have been shown to allow differentiation of the NK-like $CD8^+$ T cells. Therefore, $CD8^+$ cells may also act indirectly against *A. baumannii* infection, which could be important for improving protective immunity (20). Further laboratory and clinical studies are needed to explore the specific mechanism of $CD8^+$ T cells in *A. baumannii* infection.

Our study showed that the $CD8^+$ T cell count was an independent risk factor for 28-day mortality of ARDS caused by *A. baumannii* pneumonia, which could be explained by the difference in physical and biological sub-phenotypes

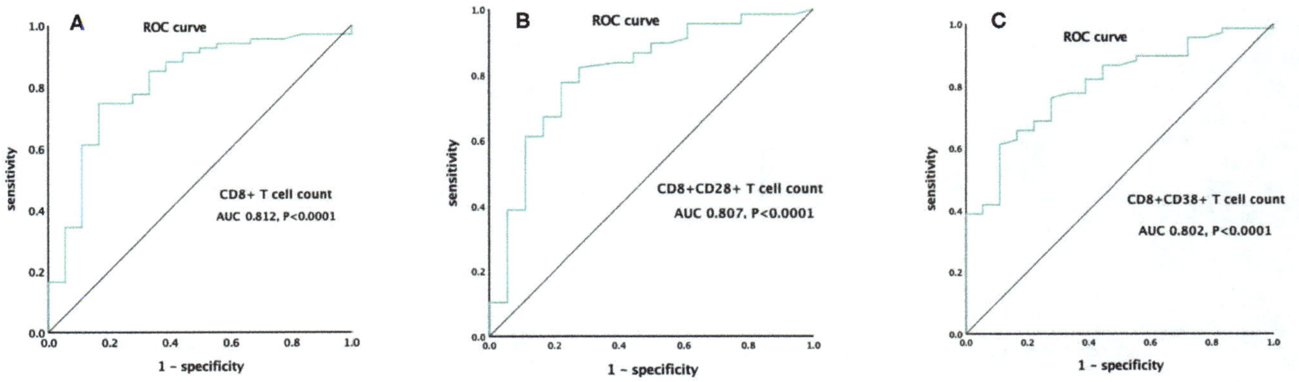

FIGURE 2 | ROC curve of $CD8^+$ T cell count **(A)**, $CD8^+CD28^+$ T cell count **(B)**, and $CD8^+CD38^+$ T cell count **(C)** for the prediction of 28-day mortality.

TABLE 5 | Comparison of ARDS patients with different $CD8^+$ T cell counts.

	$CD8^+$ T cell ≥123 (*n* = 53)	$CD8^+$ T cell<123 (*n* = 32)	*P*
Respiratory parameters of D1			
Tidal volume (ml)	410 (392–448)	400 (380–440)	0.428
PEEP (cmH_2O)	8 (5–9.5)	8 (6–10)	0.222
Ppeak (cmH_2O)	20.5 (18–23)	23 (20–25)	0.002
Driving pressure (cmH_2O)	11 (10–13)	14 (12–17)	<0.0001
RR (per minute)	21 (18–23)	23 (20–25)	0.018
P/F ratio	198 (171–235)	178 (157–212)	0.104
$PaCO_2$ (mmHg)	38 (34–42)	39 (33–42)	0.978
Inflammatory markers of D1			
NLR	10.1 (5.9–15.1)	19.2 (12.5–29.1)	<0.0001
PCT (ng/ml)	5.8 ± 11.3	12.8 ± 15.5	0.022
IL-6 (pg/ml)	120.4 ± 219.7	72.3 ± 96.1	0.35
IL-8 (pg/ml)	211.4 ± 317.2	234.3 ± 391	0.814
IL-10 (pg/ml)	18.3 ± 26.8	15.7 ± 15.6	0.692
TNF-a (pg/ml)	33.4 ± 44.6	19.3 ± 19.9	0.256
Other parameters			
CPIS	6 (4–7)	8 (7–9)	<0.0001
SOFA	11 (9–14)	12 (10–14)	0.271
Apache II score	18 (15–22)	20.5 (14–25.3)	0.774
Ventilation day (days)	5.5 (2.5–11)	6.6 (4–10.3)	0.586
28-day ventilation free day (days)	21 (16–25.5)	14.5 (0–20.9)	0.001
28-day Mortality	3 (5.7%)	15 (46.9%)	<0.0001

ARDS, acute respiratory distress syndrome; D1, the day at admission; D3, 3 days after admission; PEEP, positive end expiratory pressure; Ppeak, peak pressure; RR, respiratory rate; P/F ratio, PaO_2:FiO_2; PaCO2 arterial partial pressure of carbon dioxide; NLR, neutrophil to lymphocyte ratio; PCT, procalcitonin; IL, interleukin; TNF-a, tumor necrosis factor-a; CPIS, clinical pulmonary infection score; SOFA, sequential organ failure assessment; Apache II, Score acute physiology and chronic health evaluation II score.
P-value for the comparison of patients with higher (≥123cells/ul) and lower (<123cells/ul) $CD8^+$ T cell count.

of ARDS patients (3). From the perspective of biological phenotype, multiple large clinical ARDS trials used P/F ratio and driving pressure for prognostic enrichment. The $CD8^+$ T cell count was significantly associated with P/F ratio in ARDS caused by *A. baumannii* pneumonia and stratified according to P/F ratio. The proportion of patients with a lower $CD8^+$ T cell count was significantly higher in severe ARDS patients. The $CD8^+$ T cell count was also significantly associated with driving pressure, and patients with a lower T cell count needed higher driving pressure. Both severity of ARDS and driving pressure were strongly associated with survival rate (2, 21). From the perspective of biological phenotype, this might be related to the intensity of local inflammatory response. T cells, especially $CD8^+$ T cells, were significantly decreased in non-survivors, resulting in a significant increase in NLR. The adaptive immune response to *A. baumannii* was reduced, while the non-specific innate immunity mainly composed of neutrophils was enhanced, which

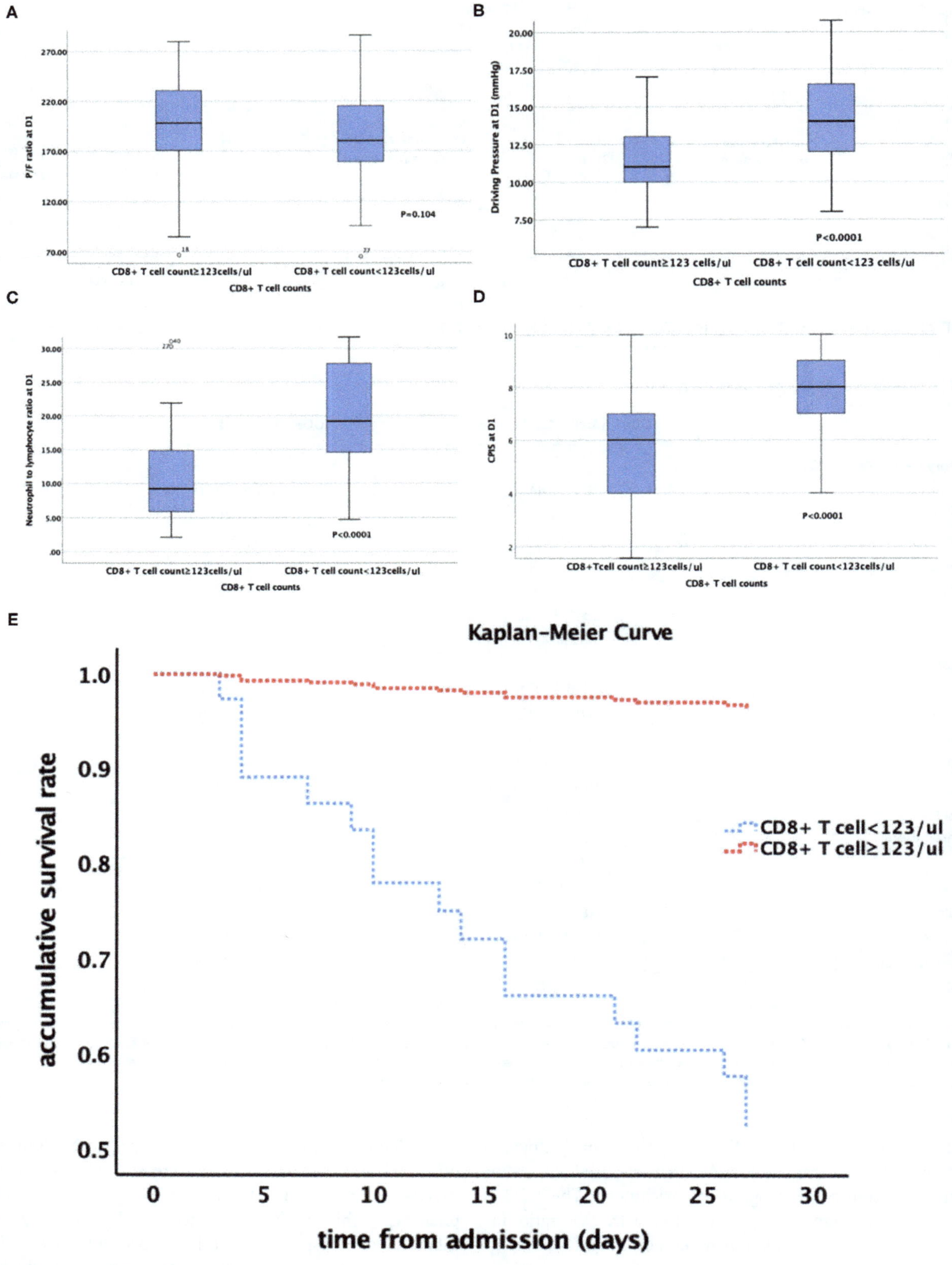

FIGURE 3 | (A–E) relationship between $CD8^+$ T cell count and **(A)** P/F ratio; **(B)** Driving Pressure; **(C)** Neutrophil to lymphocyte ratio; **(D)** CPIS. **(E)** the Kaplan-Meier curve of patients with different $CD8^+$ T cell counts. P/F ratio at D1 PaO_2:FiO_2 at admission; CPIS, clinical pulmonary infection score.

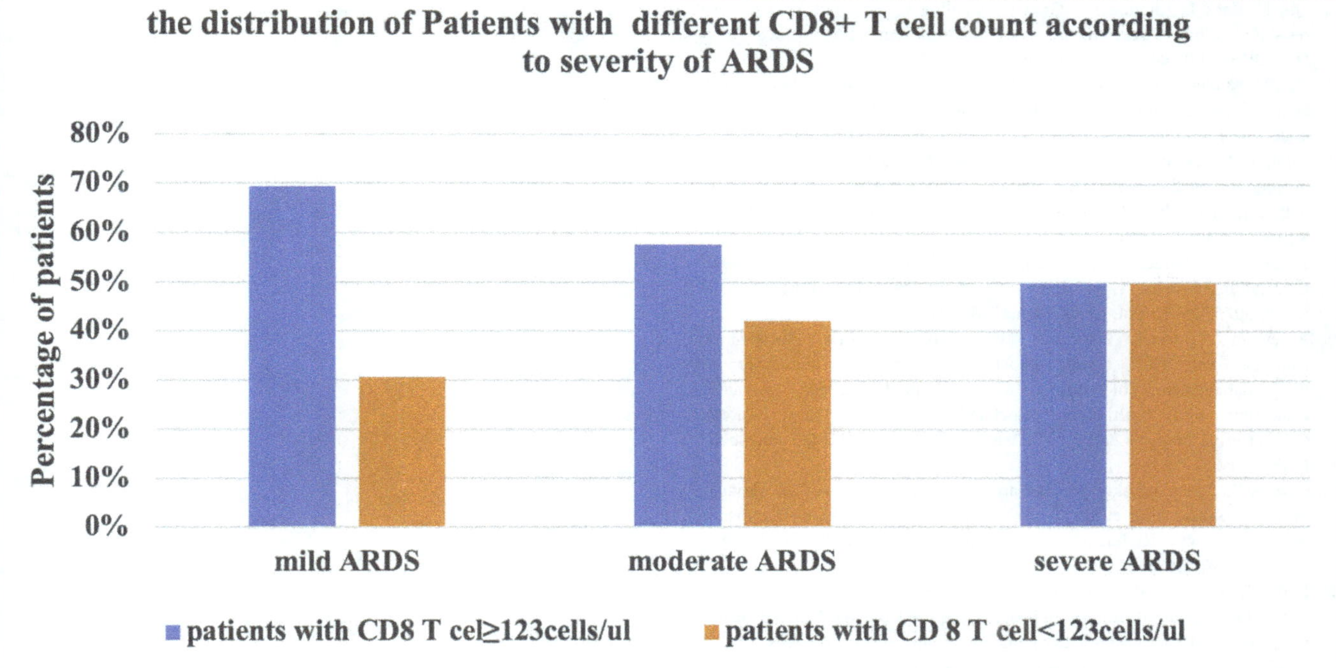

FIGURE 4 | The relationship between the severity of ARDS and the CD8+ T cell counts. ARDS, acute respiratory distress syndrome.

led to enhancement of the local pro-inflammatory response, manifesting as higher CPIS.

There were several limitations to this study. First, the study lasted almost 3 years with extremely strict inclusion criteria. Only septic patients with ARDS whose only pathogen was *A. baumannii* were enrolled, and they needed to receive mechanical ventilation or vasopressor treatment for enrollment. Despite the relatively small sample size, it was large enough to illustrate the role of lymphocytes, especially $CD8^+$ T cells in patients with ARDS caused by *A. baumannii*. Second, the serum lymphocyte count might not be able to reflect the local infection situation. We need to further study the cell subgroup analysis of bronchoalveolar lavage fluid (BALF). However, there are challenges because, at present, the cell classification of BALF cannot be quantified as in routine blood tests, and there is no normal reference range for the cell classification; both of which need further research. Last, one key element that stands out from the existing studies is how much strain-to-strain variation of *A. baumannii* influences the interaction with host cells and observed phenotypes *in vivo*. A deeper understanding of the virulence factors of *A. baumannii* that are important for *in vivo* pathogenesis is needed (1).

CONCLUSIONS

Lower CD8+ T cell count was associated with higher severity and early mortality in ARDS patients caused by A. *baumannii* pneumonia, which could be valuable for outcome prediction.

AUTHOR CONTRIBUTIONS

WC and NC contributed to the conception of the study, data interpretation, and drafted the manuscript. HW, JZ, DL, GB, WH, and JC contributed to data collection and critically revised the manuscript for important intellectual content. All authors approved the final version of the manuscript.

REFERENCES

1. Pires S, Parker D. Innate immune responses to Acinetobacter *baumannii* in the airway. *J Interferon Cytokine Res.* (2019) 39:441–4. doi: 10.1089/jir.2019.0008
2. Thompson BT, Chambers RC, Liu KD. Acute respiratory distress syndrome. *N Engl J Med.* (2017) 377:562–72. doi: 10.1056/NEJMra1608077
3. Wilson JG, Calfee CS. ARDS subphenotypes: understanding a heterogeneous syndrome. *Crit Care.* (2020) 24:102. doi: 10.1186/s13054-020-2778-x
4. Li WJ, Xiaolin A, Yuenan N, Zengpanpan Y, Zongan L. The association between the neutrophil-to-lymphocyte ratio and mortality in patients with acute respiratory distress syndrome: a retrospective cohort study. *Shock.* (2019) 51:161–7. doi: 10.1097/SHK.0000000000001136
5. Lee JS, Lee JC, Lee CM, Jung ID, Jeong YI, Seong EY, et al. Outer membrane protein A of Acinetobacter *baumannii* induces differentiation of $CD4^+$ T cells toward a Th_1 polarizing phenotype through the activation of dendritic cells. *Biochem Pharmacol.* (2007) 74:86–97. doi: 10.1016/j.bcp.2007.02.012

6. Qiu H, Zack L, Rhonda KL, Greg H, Xiaoling G, Hongbin Y, et al. Host resistance to intranasal Acinetobacter *baumannii* reinfection in mice. *Pathog Dis.* (2016) 74:ftw048. doi: 10.1093/femspd/ftw048
7. Qiu, H, Kuolee R, Harris G, Chen W. Role of NADPH phagocyte oxidase in host defense against acute respiratory Acinetobacter *baumannii* infection in mice. *Infect Immun.* (2009) 77:1015–21. doi: 10.1128/IAI.01029-08
8. Choi, CH, Lee JS, Lee YC, Park TI, Lee JC. Acinetobacter *baumannii* invades epithelial cells and outer membrane protein A mediates interactions with epithelial cells. *BMC Microbiol.* (2008) 8:216. doi: 10.1186/1471-2180-8-216
9. Force ARDT, Ranieri VM, Rubenfeld GD, Thompson BT, Ferguson ND Caldwell E. Acute respiratory distress syndrome: the berlin definition. *JAMA* (2012) 307:2526–33. doi: 10.1001/jama.2012.5669
10. American Thoracic Society, Infectious Diseases Society of America. Infectious diseases society of america: guidelines for the management of adults with hospital-acquired, ventilator-associated, and healthcare- associated pneumonia. *Am J Respir Crit Care Med.* (2005) 171:388–416. doi: 10.1164/rccm.200405-644ST
11. Ceccato A, Panagiotarakou M, Ranzani OT, Martin-Fernandez M, Almansa-Mora R, Gabarrus A, et al. Lymphocytopenia as a predictor of mortality in patients with ICU-acquired pneumonia. *J Clin Med.* (2019) 8:843. doi: 10.3390/jcm8060843
12. Kalil AC, Metersky ML, Klompas M, Muscedere J, Sweeney DA, Palmer LB, et al., Management of adults with hospital-acquired and ventilator-associated pneumonia: 2016 clinical practice guidelines by the infectious diseases society of america and the american thoracic society. *Clin Infect Dis.* (2016) 3:e61–111. doi: 10.1093/cid/ciw353
13. Melvin PW. *Methods for Dilution Antimicrobial Susceptibility Tests for Bacteria That Grow Aerobically*, 11th edition. Clinical and Laboratory Standards Institute (2018). Available online at: https://clsi.org/standards/products/microbiology/documents/m07/
14. Rubio I, Osuchowski MF, Shankar-Hari M, Skirecki T, Winkler MS, Lachmann G, et al., Current gaps in sepsis immunology: new opportunities for translational research. *Lancet Infect Dis.* (2019) 19:E422–36. doi: 10.1016/S1473-3099(19)30567-5
15. Singer M, Deutschman CS, Seymour CW, Shankar-Hari M, Annane D, Bauer M, et al. The third international consensus definitions for sepsis and septic shock (Sepsis-3). *JAMA.* (2016) 315:801–10. doi: 10.1001/jama.2016.0287
16. Cheng W, Wang H, Zhang J, Bai G, Han W, Chen J, et al. Lymphocyte subset counts as diagnostic and prognostic markers for carbapenem-resistant Enterobacteriaceae (CRE) infection in critically ill patients. *Int J Infect Dis.* (2020) 96:315–22. doi: 10.1016/j.ijid.2020.04.072
17. Gaddy JA, Tomaras AP, Actis LA. The Acinetobacter *baumannii* 19606 OmpA protein plays a role in biofilm formation on abiotic surfaces and in the interaction of this pathogen with eukaryotic cells. *Infect Immun.* (2009) 77:3150–60. doi: 10.1128/IAI.00096-09
18. Qiu H, KuoLee R, Harris G, Van Rooijen N, Patel GB, Chen W. Role of macrophages in early host resistance to respiratory Acinetobacter *baumannii* infection. *PLoS ONE.* (2012) 7:e40019. doi: 10.1371/journal.pone.0040019
19. Tsuchiya T, Nakao N, Yamamoto S, Hirai Y, Miyamoto K, Tsujibo H. NK1.1$^{(+)}$ cells regulate neutrophil migration in mice with Acinetobacter *baumannii* pneumonia. *Microbiol Immunol.* (2012) 56:107–16. doi: 10.1111/j.1348-0421.2011.00402.x
20. Pita-López ML, Pera A, Solana R. Adaptive memory of human NK-like CD8$^{(+)}$ T-cells to aging, and viral and tumor antigens. *Front Immunol.* (2016) 7:616. doi: 10.3389/fimmu.2016.00616
21. Amato MB, Meade MO, Slutsky AS, Brochard L, Costa EL, Schoenfeld DA, et al. Driving pressure and survival in the acute respiratory distress syndrome. *N Engl J Med.* (2015) 372:747–55. doi: 10.1056/NEJMsa1410639

8

Clinical Risk Factors for Mortality Among Critically Ill Mexican Patients with COVID-19

Carmen M. Hernández-Cárdenas[1], *José Alberto Choreño-Parra*[2,3], *Carlos Torruco-Sotelo*[1], *Felipe Jurado*[1], *Héctor Serna-Secundino*[1], *Cristina Aguilar*[1], *José G. García-Olazarán*[1], *Diana Hernández-García*[1], *Eduardo M. Choreño-Parra*[4], *Joaquín Zúñiga*[2,5]* *and Gustavo Lugo-Goytia*[1]*

[1] Respiratory Intensive Care Unit, Instituto Nacional de Enfermedades Respiratorias Ismael Cosío Villegas, Mexico City, Mexico, [2] Laboratory of Immunobiology and Genetics, Instituto Nacional de Enfermedades Respiratorias Ismael Cosío Villegas, Mexico City, Mexico, [3] Escuela Nacional de Ciencias Biológicas, Instituto Politécnico Nacional, Mexico City, Mexico, [4] Posgrado en Ciencias Biológicas, Universidad Nacional Autónoma de México, Mexico City, Mexico, [5] Tecnologico de Monterrey, Escuela de Medicina y Ciencias de la Salud, Mexico City, Mexico

***Correspondence:**
Joaquín Zúñiga
joazu@yahoo.com
Gustavo Lugo-Goytia
lugogoy@yahoo.com.mx

Little literature exists about critically ill patients with coronavirus disease 2019 (COVID-19) from Latin America. Here, we aimed to describe the clinical characteristics and mortality risk factors in mechanically ventilated COVID-19 patients from Mexico. For this purpose, we recruited 67 consecutive mechanically ventilated COVID-19 patients which were grouped according to their clinical outcome (survival vs. death). Clinical risk factors for mortality were identified by machine-learning and logistic regression models. The median age of participants was 42 years and 65% were men. The most common comorbidity observed was obesity (49.2%). Fever was the most frequent symptom of illness (88%), followed by dyspnea (84%). Multilobe ground-glass opacities were observed in 76% of patients by thoracic computed tomography (CT) scan. Fifty-two percent of study participants were ventilated in prone position, and 59% required cardiovascular support with norepinephrine. Furthermore, 49% of participants were coinfected with a second pathogen. Two-thirds of COVID-19 patients developed acute kidney injury (AKIN). The mortality of our cohort was 44.7%. AKIN, uric acid, lactate dehydrogenase (LDH), and a longitudinal increase in the ventilatory ratio were associated with mortality. Baseline PaO2/FiO2 values and a longitudinal recovery of lymphocytes were protective factors against mortality. Our study provides reference data about the clinical phenotype and risk factors for mortality in mechanically ventilated Mexican patients with COVID-19.

Keywords: COVID-19, SARS-CoV-2, ARDS, risk factors, mortality

INTRODUCTION

The novel severe acute respiratory syndrome coronavirus 2 (SARS-CoV-2), the causative agent of the coronavirus disease 2019 (COVID-19), has rapidly spread worldwide. Although most infected individuals develop mild disease, the spectrum of COVID-19 encompasses severe manifestations that represent up to 5% of cases (1, 2). These forms are characterized by a severe pulmonary inflammation with exudative diffuse alveolar damage and massive capillary congestion accompanied by microthrombi (3, 4). Physiologically, these alterations result in ventilation-perfusion inequalities and severe acute hypoxemic respiratory failure leading to mechanical ventilation (MV) requirement. The exuberant immune response elicited by SARS-CoV-2, together with endothelial dysfunction (5), coagulation disorders (6), and extrapulmonary viral dissemination (7), also precipitate multiorgan failure in a significant proportion of severe COVID-19 cases.

The global case fatality rate (CFR) of COVID-19 varies from 0.2 to 10.5%, depending on several factors, such as age, comorbidities, and geographical region (8). Of note, mortality rates can be as high as 80% among cases admitted to the intensive care unit (ICU) (1). Several clinical and immunological parameters impact on COVID-19-associated morbidity and mortality (2, 9–15). However, most prognostic factors that are currently being used by clinicians have been identified in heterogeneous cohorts of COVID-19 patients with mild to severe manifestations. To what extent those factors independently associated with poor clinical outcomes in the overall population of COVID-19 patients remain informative among individuals in critical condition is not well understood.

The experience with critically ill COVID-19 patients from China, Europe, and the United States has been widely reported in the literature (1, 16–18). However, there is limited information available from Latin America, one of the larger epicenters of the COVID-19 pandemic. Here, we describe the clinical features and outcomes of critically ill COVID-19 patients admitted to the respiratory intensive care unit (RICU) of a national reference center for respiratory diseases in Mexico City. Using a machine-learning algorithm and traditional logistic regression analyses, we also identified clinical risk factors for severe COVID-19-associated mortality. Our results provide reference data about the clinical phenotype of severe COVID-19 among non-Caucasian Hispanic patients from Latin America. Furthermore, our study contributes to a better understanding of the frequency and importance of specific clinical characteristics that determine the risk of mortality in COVID-19 among populations from different geographic regions.

METHODS

Study Design and Participants

We conducted a prospective cohort study in patients with acute respiratory distress syndrome (ARDS) admitted to the RICU of the Instituto Nacional de Enfermedades Respiratorias Ismael Cosío Villegas (INER) in Mexico City, during the period from March to June of 2020. Individuals that tested positive for SARS-CoV-2 infection in swab samples, bronchial aspirates (BA), or bronchoalveolar lavage (BAL) specimens were eligible. Detection of SARS-CoV-2 was performed by real-time polymerase chain reaction (RT-PCR), as described before (19). None of the participants was coinfected with the human immunodeficiency virus (HIV).

Data Retrieval and Definitions

Microsoft Excel (MS Excel 365) was used for data collection. Clinical and demographic data were retrieved from patients' medical records, including age, gender, anthropometrics, comorbidities, symptoms, thoracic computed tomography (CT) scan findings, and initial laboratory tests. Initial laboratory tests were defined as the first test results available, typically within 24 h of hospital admission, and included white blood cell counts, liver and kidney function, serum electrolytes, metabolic panel, gasometrical and ventilatory parameters, tissue-injury biomarkers, coagulation parameters, and the severity of disease scores Sequential Organ Failure Assessment (SOFA) and Acute Physiology and Chronic Health disease Classification System II (APACHE-II). Some laboratory parameters, including lymphocyte counts and ventilatory ratio (VR), were monitored continuously, and the last available test results were retrieved for analysis. The primary endpoint of the study was mortality.

ARDS was diagnosed in accordance with the Berlin definition (20). Acute kidney injury (AKIN) was diagnosed in accordance with the Kidney Disease: Improving Global Outcomes (KDIGO) clinical practice guidelines (21). Body mass index (BMI) was calculated as follows: weight (kg)/height $(m)^2$. Obesity was defined as a BMI ≥ 30 kg/m^2. Bacterial coinfection was defined as a positive culture and consistent clinical data. In cases where the cultures were negative, coinfection was defined based on the presence of persistent fever, leukocytosis, neutrophilia, increased procalcitonin levels, and hemodynamic instability for more than 48 h. Static respiratory-system compliance (Cstat) was calculated as the ratio of the tidal volume to the difference between inspiratory plateau pressure (Pplat) and the positive end-expiratory pressure (PEEP). Driving pressure was calculated as the difference between the Pplat and PEEP. VR was calculated as follows: VR = [minute ventilation (mL/min) × PCO2 (mmHg)]/[predicted body weight × 100 (mL/min) × 37.5 (mmHg)]. Fold changes in variables that were continuously monitored (lymphocyte counts and VR, hereinafter referred to as follow-up parameters) were calculated as the ratio of the difference between values at discharge/death and admission divided by the values of the variables of interest at admission.

Study Approval

The Institutional Review Board of the INER in Mexico City approved the study. All participants or their legal guardians provided written informed consent in accordance with the Declaration of Helsinki for Human Research. Clinical data were managed according to the Mexican Constitution law NOM-012-SSA3-2012, which establishes the criteria for the execution of clinical investigations in humans.

Statistical Analysis

Descriptive statistics were used to characterize the study population clinically. Frequencies and proportions were calculated for categorical data. Means, medians, standard deviations (SD), interquartile ranges (IQR), and 95% confidence intervals were used for continuous variables. Differences in categorical variables between groups were assessed by the Fisher exact or Chi-square test. For comparisons of continuous variables, we used the Student T-test or the Mann-Whitney *U*-test, as appropriate. The *K*-means algorithm was used for clustering study participant characteristics according to their clinical outcome (survival or fatality). Before data

TABLE 1 | Cumulative survival rates in patients with severe COVID-19.

Time after hospital admission	Survival (%)	95% CI
7 days	82.0	70.6–89.4
14 days	56.2	41.6–68.5
21 days	47.6	31.1–62.3
28 days	42.3	25.1–58.5

Survival rates and their 95% confidence interval (95% CI) were estimated using the Kaplan-Meyer method and the log-rank test.

visualization, clinical features and laboratory parameters were scaled and centered.

All clinical variables were included in a random forest analysis. For this purpose, and considering that the small sample size of the study could impact the performance of the model, 1,000 classification and regression trees (CARTs) were conducted to minimize the prediction error of the analysis measured in terms of Out-of-bag (OOB) error (22). The variables with the highest mean Gini decrease values were considered as having the highest impact on mortality and used as covariates for binomial logistic regression analyses. The accuracy of the selected mortality risk factors identified by random forest and logistic regression models was further evaluated with the area under the Receiver Operating Characteristic (ROC) curve (AUC). In addition, Kaplan–Meier curves were constructed to look for differences in survival according to these variables dichotomized by the ROC curve threshold with the highest diagnostic accuracy estimated using the Youden index. For random forest and logistic regression analyses, patients with any missing value in the variables of interest were excluded. All analyses were conducted using GraphPad Prism 8 (La Jolla, CA) and R Statistical Software (Foundation for Statistical Computing, Vienna, Austria). Specific tests are also mentioned in figure legends. Two-sided p-values ≤ 0.05 were considered as significant: $^{*}p \leq 0.05$, $^{**}p \leq 0.01$, $^{***}p \leq 0.001$, $^{****}p \leq 0.0001$.

RESULTS

Clinical Characteristics of Participants

Data from 67 consecutive COVID-19 patients admitted to the RICU were analyzed. Thirty-seven patients survived, and 30 died (44.7%). Survival rates at different time points after admission are shown in **Table 1**. Most fatality cases occurred during the second week after RICU admission. The median age of study participants was 42 years (range 23–73), with no differences between survivors and deceased patients (**Table 2**). Sixty-five percent of participants were men, and the proportion of males was significantly higher in the group of dead patients compared to survivors (80 vs. 54%, $p < 0.05$). Also, the BMI of deceased patients tended to be higher than in survivors. The main comorbidity observed in our study was obesity (49.2%), followed by diabetes (20.8%), and systemic arterial hypertension (SAH; 11.9%). These conditions were similarly distributed across participant groups. Fever was the most frequent manifestation of illness (88%), followed by dyspnea (84%), cough (62%), myalgia (50%), and headache (46%). Only 20% of patients reported diarrhea. The frequency of dyspnea was significantly higher among patients that died.

Thorax CT scan revealed multilobe ground-glass opacities in 76% of COVID-19 patients, whereas focal consolidations and a crazing-paving pattern were observed in 44% and 4% of participants, respectively. The overall median of days of stay in the RICU was 10 days. All patients required invasive MV, and most of them were intubated within the first 24 h after hospitalization. Fifty-two percent of patients were ventilated in the prone position, and 59% required norepinephrine for cardiovascular support. Of note, a higher proportion of patients that succumbed to COVID-19 required norepinephrine than survivors (76 vs. 45%, $p < 0.05$). Strikingly, up to two-thirds of COVID-19 patients admitted to the RICU developed AKIN, mostly of KDIGO stage 1. However, the percentage of individuals with AKIN was significantly much higher in the group of deceased patients than in survivors (96 vs. 40%, $p < 0.0001$). Furthermore, 49% of participants got coinfected with a second pathogen, and the frequency of coinfection tended to be higher in patients that died of COVID-19 (**Table 2**).

Laboratory Parameters of Severely Ill COVID-19 Patients

Most laboratory test results and respiratory parameters at hospital admission were similar in the two groups of COVID-19 patients admitted to the RICU (**Table 3**). Indeed, in unsupervised clustering analysis, patients with a similar clinical outcome did not cluster together according to their baseline laboratory parameters (**Supplementary Figure 1**). This finding reflects the high clinical heterogeneity of our entire cohort of severely ill COVID-19 patients admitted to the RICU. Only uric acid, creatinine (Cr), and bilirubin levels, as well as SOFA score, were significantly higher among deceased patients as compared to survivors (**Table 3**). Procalcitonin levels were also higher in patients that succumbed to the infection than in survivors, but the difference did not reach statistical significance ($p = 0.0576$). In contrast, patients who survived differ significantly from deceased individuals with respect to higher PaO_2/FiO_2 values at admission.

We also monitored lymphocyte counts and VR in all COVID-19 patients. Remarkably, the group of survivors showed a significant recuperation of lymphocyte counts at discharge from the RICU with respect to the baseline (**Table 3**). Conversely, deceased patients showed minimal recovery and even displayed depletion of lymphocytes before death. Finally, patients who died showed a significant increase in VR values, whereas survivors were characterized by a decrease in VR at discharge from the RICU. Fold changes in lymphocytes and VR were significantly different between groups (**Table 3**).

Mortality Risk Factors in Patients With Severe COVID-19

We next investigated clinical risk factors for mortality in our cohort of critically ill COVID-19 patients. For this purpose, we performed a random forest analysis using baseline clinical and laboratory characteristics, as well as follow-up parameters

TABLE 2 | Clinical characteristics of critically ill COVID-19 patients.

Characteristic	Total N = 67	Survivors N = 37	Deceased N = 30	p-value
Age (years), median (range)	42 (23–73)	37 (23–65)	45 (27–73)	0.2336
Males	44 (65.67)	20 (54.0)	24 (80)	0.0383
BMI	30.5 (26.7–37.5)	29.7 (26.4–34.4)	33.8 (27.4–39.5)	0.0748
Comorbidities				
Obesity	33 (49.2)	16 (43.2)	17 (56.6)	0.3302
Diabetes	14 (20.8)	10 (27.0)	4 (13.3)	0.2314
SAH	8 (11.9)	2 (5.4)	6 (20)	0.1264
Symptoms at onset				
Fever	44/50 (88)	23/27 (85.1)	21/23 (91.3)	0.674
Cough	31/50 (62)	17/27 (62.9)	14/23 (60.8)	>0.9999
Dyspnea	42/50 (84)	19/27 (70.3)	23/23 (100)	0.005
Myalgia	25/50 (50)	15/27 (55.5)	10/23 (43.4)	0.5709
Headache	23/50 (46)	12/27 (44.4)	11/23 (47.8)	>0.9999
Diarrhea	10/50 (20)	6/27 (22.2)	4/23 (17.3)	0.7356
CT scan findings				
Ground glass opacities	38/50 (76)	22/27 (81.4)	16/23 (69.5)	0.5077
Crazing paving pattern	2/50 (4)	2/27 (7.4)	0/23 (0)	0.4931
Consolidation	22/50 (44)	9/27 (33.3)	13/23 (56.5)	0.1532
RICU stay (days)	10 (8–17)	13 (9–18)	8 (6–13)	0.003
Supportive interventions				
MV	67 (100)	37 (100)	30 (100)	>0.9999
Prone position	35 (52.2)	17 (45.9)	18 (60)	0.3271
Norepinephrine	40 (59.7)	17 (45.9)	23 (76.6)	0.0133
Complications				
AKIN	44 (65.6)	15 (40.5)	29 (96.6)	<0.0001
Stage 1	20 (29.8)	10 (27.0)	10 (33.3)	0.6019
Stage 2	12 (17.9)	1 (2.7)	11 (36.6)	0.0007
Stage 3	12 (17.9)	4 (10.8)	8 (26.6)	0.1165
Coinfection	33 (49.2)	14 (37.8)	19 (63.3)	0.0506

Data are displayed as n (%), n/N (%), or median (IQR). N is the total number of patients with available data. AKIN, acute kidney injury; BMI, body mass index; CT, computed tomography; IQR, interquartile range; MV, mechanical ventilation; RICU, respiratory intensive care unit; SAH, systemic arterial hypertension. Differences in continuous variables were estimated using the Student T–test or the Mann Whitney U-test. Differences in categorical variables were calculated using the Fisher's exact or the Chi-square test as appropriate.

of study participants. This is a machine-learning algorithm that accurately estimates the importance of each variable from a dataset for the occurrence of a dichotomous variable (i.e., mortality) (22). The results showed that fold change in VR, fold change in lymphocytes, AKIN, uric acid, bilirubin, Cr, activated partial thromboplastin time (aPTT), BMI, lactate dehydrogenase (LDH), age, and PaO_2/FiO_2 were the most explicative variables for mortality, all of them with importance above the overall mean importance of the model (**Figure 1**).

From these variables identified in the random forest analysis, only fold change in VR, AKIN, uric acid, and LDH were independent mortality risk factors in binomial logistic regression analyses. Meanwhile, baseline PaO_2/FiO_2 values and fold change in lymphocytes were protective factors (**Table 4**). In fact, patients with an increase in VR (fold change ≥-0.0351 from baseline), AKIN, high uric acid (≥3.085 mg/dL), and elevated LDH levels (≥528.5 U/L), showed significantly lower survival rates at 28 days after admission to the RICU (**Table 5; Figure 2**). In contrast, patients with a longitudinal increase in lymphocyte counts (fold change ≥0.127 from baseline) and higher PaO2/FiO2 (≥157.5) values at admission had lower mortality rates.

Finally, a binomial regression analysis of the variables not identified as important for mortality by random forest analysis showed that male gender, use of norepinephrine, and SOFA score were independently associated with mortality. In contrast, the neutrophil to lymphocyte ratio (NLR) was a protective factor (**Supplementary Table 1**). From these, only norepinephrine usage was associated with significantly lower survival rates in the Kaplan-Meier and log-rank test analysis (**Supplementary Figure 2**). However, in a second random forest model using all the independent mortality risk and protective factors identified only by binomial logistic regression, none of these additional factors showed to be explicative for mortality (**Supplementary Figure 3**).

TABLE 3 | Laboratory parameters of critically ill COVID-19 patients.

Characteristic	Total $N = 67$	Survivors $N = 37$	Deceased $N = 30$	*p*-value
Blood count				
White blood cells (10^9/L)	9.4 (7.3–13.03)	9.3 (7.2–12.4)	10.2 (7.3–14)	0.7857
Neutrophils (10^9/L)	7.9 (5.7–11.4)	7.9 (5.9–10.5)	8.2 (5.3–12.7)	0.9515
Lymphocytes (10^9/L)	0.8 (0.5–1.02)	0.7 (0.5–1.0)	0.9 (0.6–1.2)	0.1188
NLR	11.2 (6.4–16.2)	11.5 (6.7–17.9)	10.2 (5.6–16)	0.3784
Hgb (g/dL)	13.9 (13.1–15.2)	13.8 (12.7–15.1)	14.0 (13.2–15.4)	0.4139
Platelets (10^9/L)	243 (188.8–308.8)	252 (202–326.5)	213 (150.8–307)	0.1473
Metabolic parameters				
Glucose (mg/dL)	141.2 (108–185)	142.6 (114.5–211)	138.9 (106.5–170.5)	0.4729
Uric acid (mg/dL)	4.0 (2.5–5.0)	3.5 (1.6–4.6)	4.6 (3.6–5.6)	0.0069
Na (mmol/L)	141.2(138.2–143.6)	141 (138.5–143)	141.5(137.8–144.5)	0.4553
K (mmol/L)	4.3 (3.9–4.7)	4.2 (3.9–4.6)	4.3 (3.9–4.7)	0.7808
Total proteins (g/dL)	5.9 (5.5–6.4)	5.8 (5.4–6.3)	6.0 (5.6–6.5)	0.1663
Albumin (g/dL)	2.9 (2.6–3.3)	2.9 (2.6–3.5)	2.9 (2.6–3.2)	0.5667
Renal function				
Cr (mg/dL)	0.9 (0.7–1.4)	0.8 (0.6–1.2)	1.2 (0.8–1.8)	0.0105
BUN (mg/dL)	19.6 (13.9–31.5)	19.8 (14.1–28.9)	19.6 (13.7–36.7)	0.3579
Liver function				
Total bilirubin (mg/dL)	0.5 (0.4–0–6)	0.4 (0.3–0.5)	0.5 (0.4–0.6)	0.036
AST (U/L)	47.3 (30–76)	42.5 (26.8–69.7)	49.5 (31.9–108.8)	0.1981
ALT (U/L)	39.6 (27.9–67.4)	45.4 (28.1–68.5)	37.4 (25.6–62.6)	0.5368
Coagulation parameters				
D dimer (mg/L)	1.0 (0.7–2.1)	1.0 (0.7–2.4)	1.1 (0.7–2.2)	0.6052
INR	1.0 (1.0–1.1)	1.0 (1.0–1.0)	1.0 (0.9–1.1)	0.5146
PT (sec)	15.1 (14.5–16.5)	14.9 (14.6–16.5)	15.4 (14.2–16.5)	0.8317
aPTT (sec)	38.4 (34.6–44.8)	38.5 (35.9–42.1)	37.6 (33.5–49.5)	0.7963
Other biomarkers				
LDH (U/L)	494 (357–711)	450 (356.5–589)	566.5 (358.8–738.3)	0.2009
ALP (U/L)	81.6 (64–96.8)	81.8 (59.1–94)	81.6 (66.3–128.6)	0.3252
CPK (U/L)	152.5 (62.3–900)	180.4 (52.2–964)	146.2 (72.5–1016)	0.694
Procalcitonin (ng/mL)	0.16 (0.1–0.37)	0.12 (0.07–0.2)	0.2 (0.1–0.69)	0.0576
Respiratory parameters				
SO_2%	73 (50–85)	73 (41.5–84.5)	71.5 (57.5–85)	0.8582
PCO_2 (mmHg)	47 (38–56)	49 (41–58)	46 (37.5–52.2)	0.1853
PaO_2/FiO_2 (mmHg)	141 (96–177)	158 (110.5–188.5)	121 (88–157.3)	0.0109
DP (cm H2O)	12 (10–14)	12 (10–14.5)	12 (10.6–14.2)	0.4978
Cstat (ml/cm H2O)	33.6 (27–40.9)	33.3 (26.2–40.9)	35.0 (29.6–40.9)	0.4424
VR	2.0 (1.6–2.4)	2.0 (1.7–2.6)	2.0 (1.6–2.3)	0.3483
Severity of disease				
SOFA score	5 (4–7)	4 (3–7)	6 (4–8)	0.0155
APACHE-II score	10 (6–17)	9 (5–14)	12 (6–17)	0.2706
Follow-up parameters				
Fold change in lymphocytes	0.32 (−0.23–1.12)	0.87 (0.21–1.83)	−0.11 (−0.41–0.68)	<0.0001
Fold change in VR	−0.22 (−0.40–0.22)	−0.35 (−0.45–0.19)	0.15 (−0.23–0.59)	<0.0001

Data are displayed as n (%) or median (IQR). N is the total number of patients with available data. ALP, alkaline phosphatase; ALT, alanine aminotransferase; APACHE-II, Acute Physiology and Chronic Health disease Classification System II; aPTT, activated partial thromboplastin time; AST, aspartate aminotransferase; Cstat, static compliance; BUN, blood ureic nitrogen; CPK, creatine phosphokinase; Cr, creatinine; DP, driving pressure; FiO2, fraction of inspired oxygen; Hgb, hemoglobin; INR, international normalized ratio; IQR, interquartile range; K, potassium; LDH, lactate dehydrogenase; Na, sodium; NLR, neutrophil/lymphocyte ratio; PaO2, partial pressure of oxygen in arterial blood; PCO_2, partial pressure of carbon dioxide in the blood; PT, prothrombin time; SO_2%, oxygen saturation; SOFA, Sequential Organ Failure Assessment; VR, ventilatory ratio. Differences in continuous variables were estimated using the Student T-test or the Mann Whitney U-test. Differences in categorical variables were calculated using the Fisher's exact or the Chi-square test as appropriate. Fold changes were calculated as the ratio of the difference between values at discharge/death and values at admission divided by the initial values of the variables of interest (lymphocyte counts and VR).

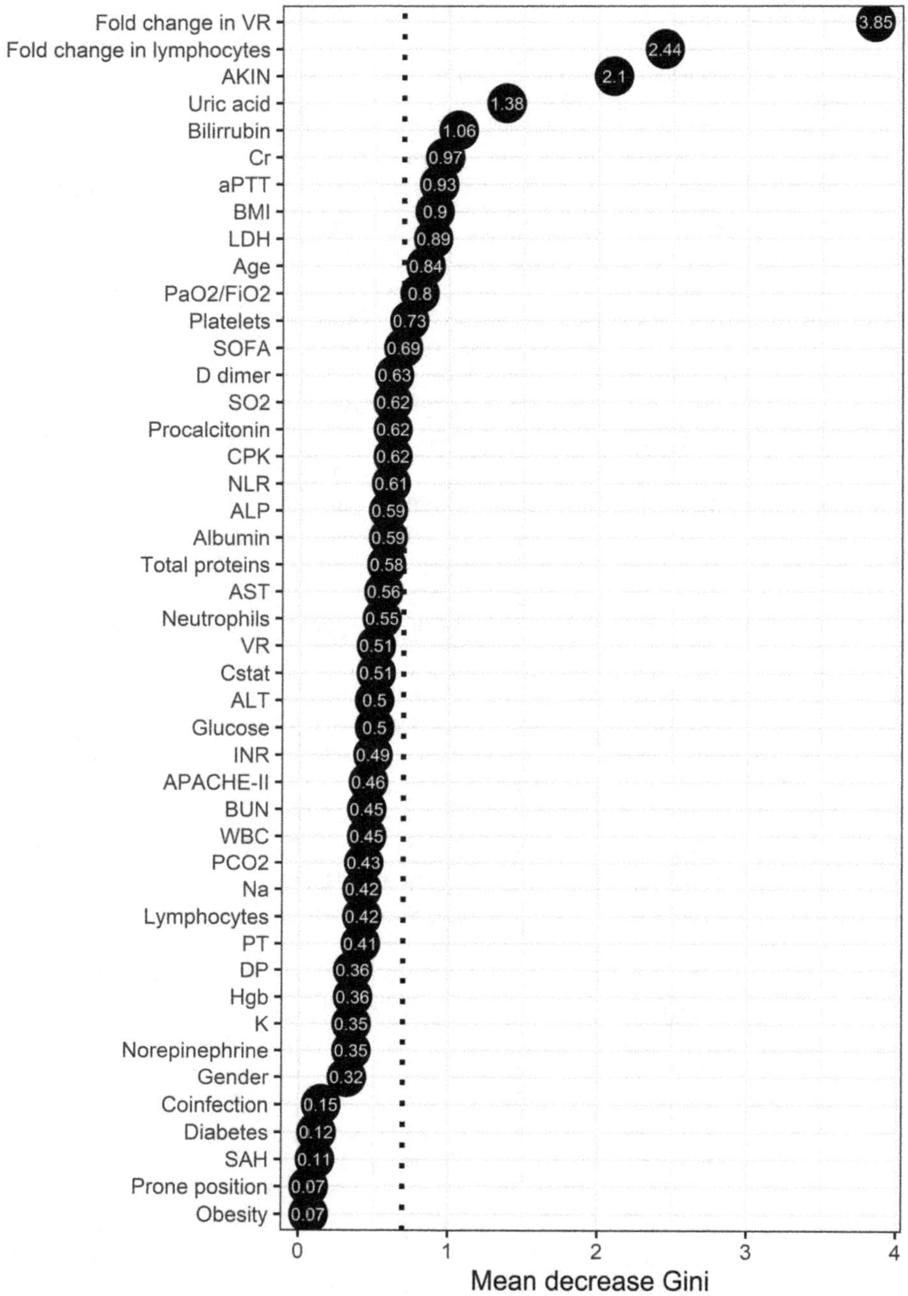

FIGURE 1 | Random forest analysis of the clinical characteristics associated with mortality in critically ill COVID-19 patients. The points represent the mean decrease Gini values, indicative of the importance of each variable to mortality. Variables with mean decease Gini values above the mean importance of the model (discontinuous vertical line) were considered as the most explicative variables of severe COVID-19-associated mortality in our cohort.

DISCUSSION

In the current study, we report the clinical characteristics of a cohort of critically ill patients with COVID-19 that were admitted to the RICU of a national reference center for respiratory diseases in Mexico City. Our analyses showed that most demographic, clinical, radiological, and biochemical characteristics of Mexican patients with severe SARS-CoV-2 infection resemble those reported previously by other groups from China, Europe, and the United States. Furthermore, we determined which factors were independently associated with mortality using a non-conventional statistical approach that included machine-learning algorithms and traditional regression analyses. This strategy of analysis allowed us to identify six variables that had the

TABLE 4 | Logistic regression analysis of risk factors for COVID-19-associated mortality.

Variable	OR	95% CI	*p*-value
Fold change in VR	50.20	8.187–548.3	<0.0001
Fold change in lymphocytes	0.226	0.08815–0.4747	<0.0001
AKIN	36.73	6.631–692.1	<0.0001
Uric acid (mg/dL)	1.237	1.003–1.587	0.0463
Total bilirubin (mg/dL)	3.533	0.3235–45.64	0.3023
Cr (mg/dL)	1.086	0.7491–1.613	0.6568
aPTT (sec)	1.040	0.9702–1.120	0.2696
BMI	1.068	0.9930–1.162	0.0778
LDH (U/L)	1.002	1.000–1.005	0.0360
Age (years)	1.019	0.9778–1.063	0.3768
PaO_2/FiO_2 (mmHg)	0.9872	0.9751–0.9984	0.0241

95% CI, 95% confidence interval; AKIN, acute kidney injury; aPTT, activated partial thromboplastin time; BMI, body mass index; Cr, creatinine; FiO_2, fraction of inspired oxygen; LDH, lactate dehydrogenase; OR, odds ratio; PaO_2, partial pressure of oxygen in arterial blood; VR, ventilatory ratio. Fold changes in lymphocyte counts and VR are defined as the ratio of the difference between values at discharge/death and values at admission divided by the initial values of these variables.

highest impact on the mortality of our cohort: fold change in VR, fold change in lymphocyte counts, AKIN, uric acid, LDH, and PaO^2/FiO^2. From these, fold change in lymphocytes and PaO^2/FiO^2 at admission acted as independent protective factors.

A dramatic depletion of total lymphocytes, as well as of CD8+ and CD4+ T-cells, has been reported in patients with SARS-CoV-2 infection (23–25). This phenomenon is the expression of a dysregulated immune response elicited by the virus that favors immunosuppression and is associated with a high risk of secondary bacterial infection, septic shock, and organ dysfunction (26). Indeed, lymphopenia has been described as a marker of severity and a predictor of mortality in COVID-19 (27). In our cohort, baseline lymphocyte counts were extremely low in all patients, with no differences between survivors and non-survivors. These data may indicate that despite lymphopenia is a readout of severity in the overall population of COVID-19 patients, this marker is not further informative when used only among critically ill individuals. Thus, lymphocyte counts on admission should be used only in the decision-making for patients with mild-to-moderate forms of the disease to predict the progression to severe COVID-19.

Recovery of the adaptive immune system with an increase in the number of circulating T lymphocytes is necessary to eliminate the virus (28). Notably, we also found that longitudinal increases in the number of circulating lymphocytes (here expressed as a fold change in lymphocytes) have a strong protective effect against mortality. In other words, a longitudinal increase in lymphocytes associates with a decreased mortality risk, while a decrease in lymphocytes correlates with a significant increase in the risk of death. This result is consistent with the rapid and dramatic restoration of peripheral T lymphocytes observed in patients who recovered from SARS-CoV-2 infection (28). Hence, our results indicate that changes in the lymphocyte counts could be used as a parameter to guide therapeutic decisions for critically ill COVID-19 patients. For instance, this parameter could determine which patients would benefit from steroids use. These drugs could have both favorable and unfavorable consequences. For example, in patients with an exaggerated inflammatory response, steroids may reduce organ damage. In contrast, in patients with severe immunosuppression, steroids could accentuate this defect, increasing the risk of sepsis and mortality; applying treatments that stimulate the immune system could be useful in these patients (29).

VR is governed by the production of carbon dioxide (CO_2) and the ventilatory efficiency (1-(Vd/Ve)) and can be easily calculated at the patient's bedside using ventilation and blood gas parameters. It correlates with the percentage of dead space and is also associated with an increased risk of mortality (30–32). Previous studies on patients with ARDS and COVID-19 have reported a significant association between the VR at admission and mortality (33). In our patients, we did not observe this association upon admission to the RICU. However, we observed that a longitudinal increase in VR was a marker of poor clinical outcome in our cohort of patients with ARDS due to COVID-19. This result is consistent with other reports that demonstrated that an increase in the fraction of dead space during the first weeks of ARDS is an independent predictor of mortality (30–32). In summary, the worsening of the VR in our cohort was independently associated with an increased risk of mortality. Similar to the tidal volume adjusted for the predicted weight, plateau pressure, DP, and PaO2/FiO2 ratio, the VR should be monitored daily and used to make adjustments to the ventilatory parameters, always taking into account the variables mentioned above.

The most striking mortality risk factor identified in our study population was the incidence of AKIN. The injury of the kidney has been widely reported in patients with sepsis and severe ARDS associated with other respiratory pathogens, such as influenza viruses (34–36). Indeed, AKIN is a well-recognized mortality risk factor in patients with severe pneumonia caused by the pandemic influenza A(H1N1)pdm09 virus (37). Similarly, a high incidence of AKIN has been reported in patients with COVID-19. For instance, Hirsch et al. reported an incidence of 36.6% in a cohort of 5,449 patients with COVID-19 (38). However, in patients with respiratory failure who required invasive MV, the incidence of AKIN was 89.7%, and in those who required hemodialysis the mortality was 55% (38). In our cohort, up to 65% of the patients developed AKIN, and its incidence had a strong effect on mortality. Several mechanisms could contribute to the development of AKIN among patients with severe COVID-19, including direct injury driven by the virus and detrimental effects of the high levels of circulating proinflammatory mediators, endothelial dysfunction, and micro-thrombosis of renal blood vessels. Independently of the causative mechanism, the implementation of the KDIGO supportive care guidelines to avoid AKIN or to prevent progression to more advanced stages must be a priority in critically ill patients with COVID-19 (21).

Uric acid, LDH, and PaO_2/FiO_2 also impacted on mortality of our study population. Interestingly, little evidence exists about

TABLE 5 | Survival rates of severely ill COVID-19 patients according to their clinical characteristics.

Variable	ROC AUC (95% CI)	Sensitivity (%)	Specificity (%)	Survival (%, 95% CI)	*p*-value
Fold change in VR	0.8441 (0.7521–0.9361)	63.33	88.24		<0.0001
≥-0.0351				11.68 (1.09–36.03)	
<-0.0351				61.82 (36.03–79.72)	
Fold change in lymphocytes	0.8039 (0.6981–0-9098)	63.33	85.29		<0.0001
≥0.127				68.51 (48.44–82.09)	
<0.127				8.31 (0.58–29.97)	
AKIN	N/A	96.67	59.46		<0.0001
Yes				22.53 (7.84–41.79)	
No				95.00 (69.47–99.28)	
Uric acid (mg/dL)	0.6971 (0.5682–0.8260)	90	44.12		0.025
≥3.085				32.29 (16.25–49.49)	
<3.085				83.33 (56.76–94.29)	
LDH (U/L)	0.6245 (0.4822–0.7668)	60	73.53		0.0035
≥528.5				19.10 (4.30–41.85)	
<528.5				61.09 (35.88–78.90)	
PaO_2/FiO_2 (mmHg)	0.6569 (0.5232–0.7905)	76.67	50		0.0706
≥157.5				58.18 (27.79–79.53)	
<157.5				32.28 (13.51–52.78)	

95% CI, 95% confidence interval; AKIN, acute kidney injury; AUC, area under the curve; FiO_2, fraction of inspired oxygen; LDH, lactate dehydrogenase; N/A, not applicable; PaO_2, partial pressure of oxygen in arterial blood; ROC, receiver operating characteristic curve; VR, ventilatory ratio. Survival rates at 28 days of admission, and their 95% CI were estimated using the Kaplan-Meyer method and the log-rank test. Best ROC curve thresholds were calculated with the Youden index. Sensitivity and specificity for AKIN were calculated by the Wilson/Brown method. Fold changes in lymphocyte counts, and VR are defined as the ratio of the difference between values at discharge/death and values at admission divided by the initial values of these variables.

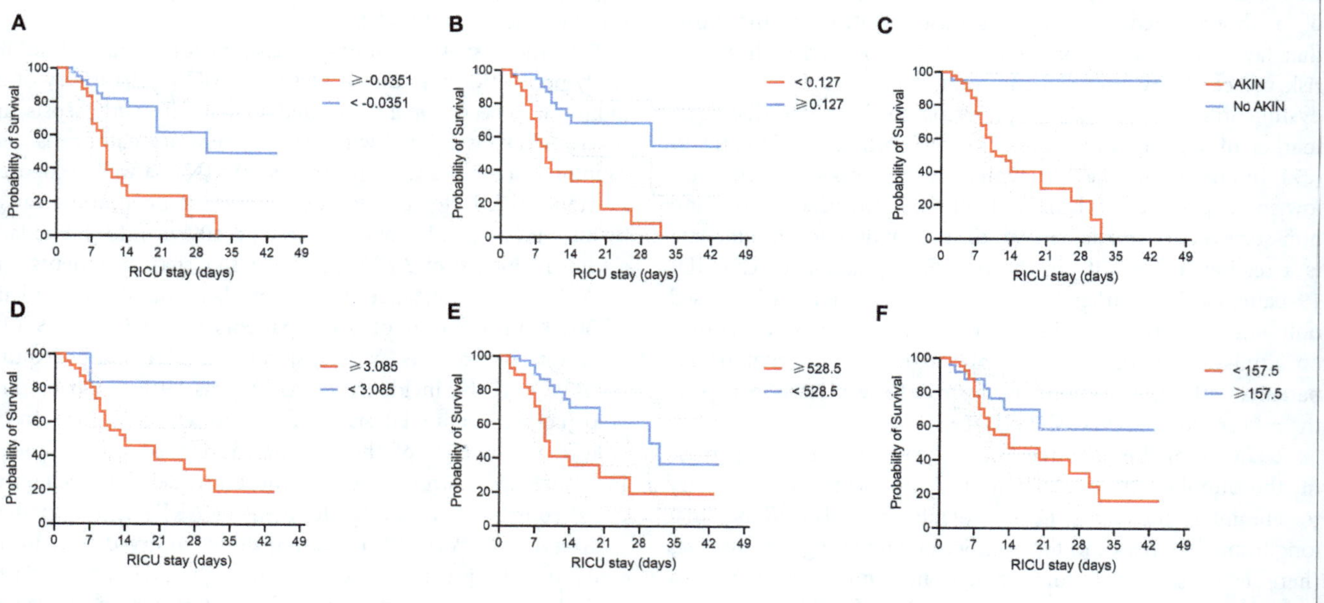

FIGURE 2 | Survival of COVID-19 patients admitted to the RICU according to their clinical characteristics. Critically ill COVID-19 patients were categorized according to different clinical risk factors for mortality identified by rancom forests and binomial logistic regression analyses. **(A)** Fold change in the ventilatory ratio (VR). **(B)** Fold change in lymphocytes. **(C)** Acute kidney injury (AKIN). **(D)** Uric acid levels. **(E)** Lactate dehydrogenase (LDH) levels. **(F)** PaO_2/FiO_2 index. Survival curves were compared using the Kaplan-Meyer method and the log-rank test. Continuous variables were dichotomized using the best ROC curve threshold determined using the Youden index. Fold changes in lymphocyte counts and VR are defined as the ratio of the difference between values at discharge/death and values at admission divided by the initial values of these variables.

the prognostic value of uric acid in COVID-19. Hence, ours is among the first studies that bring forward this marker for mortality prediction after SARS-CoV-2 infection. As uric acid levels primarily depend on the balance between its production and excretion through the urine, we speculate that the elevated uric acid levels observed among critically ill COVID-19 that died are related to the high incidence of renal dysfunction in these individuals. Notably, other biomarkers of renal function, such as Cr, were not associated with mortality. Collectively, these data indicate that uric acid may be a more useful readout of the renal function status than Cr and blood ureic nitrogen (BUN) among patients with COVID-19 in critical conditions. Regarding LDH, several studies have reported that this is a good marker to predict mortality in patients infected with SARS-CoV-2 (39, 40). Hence, our study reinforces the usage of LDH as a prognostic indicator of mortality that could be useful to guide therapeutic interventions.

Finally, the PaO2/FiO2 ratio showed a significant protective effect against mortality in our analyses. The PaO2/FiO2 ratio is a crucial determinant of the severity of ARDS, according to the Berlin definition (20). The majority of our patients showed ground-glass opacities on chest tomography, without extensive consolidation images. This explains the rapid response of many patients to oxygen administration and the poor response at this stage to recruitment maneuvers because there are no extensive recruitable consolidation areas. Therefore, the primary mechanism of hypoxemia in these patients in the initial phase is an abnormality in the distribution between ventilation and blood flow; the latter is assumed to be abnormal due to endothelial and vascular alterations documented among COVID-19 patients (41). Therefore, the PaO2/FiO2 ratio may be a good physiological biomarker of the amount of pulmonary shunt and lung parenchymal damage in the early phase of ARDS due to COVID-19, which explains why this parameter was a protective factor against mortality in our study. In contrast with our results, other investigations have shown that the PaO2/FiO2 ratio is not a strong predictor of mortality, which may be related to the clinical heterogeneity observed in studies involving patients with moderate-to-severe COVID-19.

One limitation of the study is the small size of the cohort, which originated from a single third-level center in Mexico City. Therefore, although our results are consistent with those reported in China, Europe, and North America, and despite the machine-learning approach used in our study may compensate for this caveat, the predictive value of the mortality risk factors identified here require further external validations in larger cohorts. In summary, we described the clinical characteristics of a cohort of critically ill Mexican patients with COVID-19 and identified independent factors associated with mortality. Based on our results, it is possible to suggest some management recommendations in patients with COVID-19 who require intensive care. These include respiratory management based on low tidal volumes and adjustment of parameters according to the VR. Measures to protect kidney function and adjustment of fluid balance according to volume responsiveness is also recommendable. Furthermore, the avoidance of immunosuppressants in patients who do not show lymphocyte recovery, strict measures to prevent nosocomial infections, early detection, and aggressive treatment of suspected coinfections are crucial interventions. These simple measures could reduce the risk of mortality until an effective therapy against SARS-CoV-2 infection is available.

AUTHOR CONTRIBUTIONS

CH-C, JC-P, JZ, and GL-G: designed the research study. CH-C, CT-S, FJ, HS-S, CA, JG-O, DH-G, and GL-G: recruited patients. CH-C, JC-P, CT-S, FJ, HS-S, CA, JG-O, DH-G, and GL-G: retrieved clinical data. JC-P and EC-P: performed statistical analyses of the data. JZ: discussed the manuscript. JC-P, JZ, CH-C, and GL-G: drafted the manuscript. All authors contributed to the article and approved the submitted version.

FUNDING

This work was supported by the Institutional research funds of INER, and also received funding from the National Council of Science and Technology of Mexico (CONACyT) under the research contracts: SECTEI/050/2020, Secretaría de Ciencia, Tecnología e Innovación de la Ciudad de México (SECTEI CDMX); FORDECYT/10SE/2020/05/14-06 and FORDECYT/10SE/2020/05/14-07 from the Fondo Institucional de Fomento Regional para el Desarrollo Científico y Tecnológico y de Innovación (FORDECYT). JC-P was supported by a scholarship (CVU 737347) from CONACyT to his Ph.D. degree. Funders did not play any role in the study design and conduction.

ACKNOWLEDGMENTS

To all study participants and their family members.

REFERENCES

1. Richardson S, Hirsch JS, Narasimhan M, Crawford JM, Mcginn T, Davidson KW, et al. Presenting characteristics, comorbidities, and outcomes among 5700 patients hospitalized with COVID-19 in the New York City Area. *Jama.* (2020) 323:2052–9. doi: 10.1001/jama.2020.6775
2. Wu Z, Mcgoogan JM. Characteristics of and important lessons from the coronavirus disease 2019 (COVID-19) outbreak in china: summary of a report of 72314 cases from the Chinese Center For Disease Control And Prevention. *JAMA.* (2020) 323:1239–42. doi: 10.1001/jama.2020.2648
3. Menter T, Haslbauer JD, Nienhold R, Savic S, Hopfer H, Deigendesch N, et al. Postmortem examination of COVID-19 patients reveals diffuse alveolar damage with severe capillary congestion and variegated findings in lungs and other organs suggesting vascular dysfunction. *Histopathology.* (2020) 77:198–209. doi: 10.1111/his.14134
4. Tian S, Xiong Y, Liu H, Niu L, Guo J, Liao M, et al. Pathological study of the 2019 novel coronavirus disease (COVID-19) through postmortem core biopsies. *Mod Pathol.* (2020) 33:1007–14. doi: 10.1038/s41379-020-0536-x

5. Varga Z, Flammer AJ, Steiger P, Haberecker M, Andermatt R, Zinkernagel AS, et al. Endothelial cell infection and endotheliitis in COVID-19. *Lancet.* (2020) 395:1417–8. doi: 10.1016/S0140-6736(20)30937-5
6. Spiezia L, Boscolo A, Poletto F, Cerruti L, Tiberio I, Campello E, et al. COVID-19-related severe hypercoagulability in patients admitted to intensive care unit for acute respiratory failure. *Thromb Haemost.* (2020) 120:998–1000. doi: 10.1055/s-0040-1714350
7. Behzad S, Aghaghazvini L, Radmard AR, Gholamrezanezhad A. Extrapulmonary manifestations of COVID-19: radiologic and clinical overview. *Clin Imaging.* (2020) 66:35–41. doi: 10.1016/j.clinimag.2020.05.013
8. Lazzerini M, Putoto G. COVID-19 in Italy: momentous decisions and many uncertainties. *Lancet Glob Health.* (2020) 8:e641–2. doi: 10.1016/S2214-109X(20)30110-8
9. Chen N, Zhou M, Dong X, Qu J, Gong F, Han Y, et al. Epidemiological and clinical characteristics of 99 cases of 2019 novel coronavirus pneumonia in Wuhan, China: a descriptive study. *Lancet.* (2020) 395:507–13. doi: 10.1016/S0140-6736(20)30211-7
10. Jin JM, Bai P, He W, Wu F, Liu XF, Han DM, et al. Gender differences in patients with covid-19: focus on severity and mortality. *Front Public Health.* (2020) 8:152. doi: 10.3389/fpubh.2020.00152
11. Li X, Xu S, Yu M, Wang K, Tao Y, Zhou Y, et al. Risk factors for severity and mortality in adult COVID-19 inpatients in Wuhan. *J Allergy Clin Immunol.* (2020) 146:110–18. doi: 10.1016/j.jaci.2020.04.006
12. Ruan Q, Yang K, Wang W, Jiang L, Song J. Clinical predictors of mortality due to COVID-19 based on an analysis of data of 150 patients from Wuhan, China. *Intensive Care Med.* (2020) 46:846–8. doi: 10.1007/s00134-020-05991-x
13. Weiss P, Murdoch DR. Clinical course and mortality risk of severe COVID-19. *Lancet.* (2020) 395:1014–5. doi: 10.1016/S0140-6736(20)30633-4
14. Wu C, Chen X, Cai Y, Xia J, Zhou X, Xu S, et al. Risk factors associated with acute respiratory distress syndrome and death in patients with Coronavirus Disease 2019 pneumonia in Wuhan, China. *JAMA Intern Med.* (2020) 180:934–43. doi: 10.1001/jamainternmed.2020.0994
15. Zhu Z, Cai T, Fan L, Lou K, Hua X, Huang Z, et al. Clinical value of immune-inflammatory parameters to assess the severity of coronavirus disease 2019. *Int J Infect Dis.* (2020) 95:332–9. doi: 10.1016/j.ijid.2020.04.041
16. Arentz M, Yim E, Klaff L, Lokhandwala S, Riedo FX, Chong M, et al. Characteristics and Outcomes of 21 Critically Ill Patients With COVID-19 in Washington State. *JAMA.* (2020) 323:1612–4. doi: 10.1001/jama.2020.4326
17. Grasselli G, Zangrillo A, Zanella A, Antonelli M, Cabrini L, Castelli A, et al. Baseline characteristics and outcomes of 1591 patients infected with SARS-CoV-2 admitted to ICUs of the Lombardy Region, Italy. *JAMA.* (2020) 323:1574–81. doi: 10.1001/jama.2020.5394
18. Yang X, Yu Y, Xu J, Shu H, Xia J, Liu H, et al. Clinical course and outcomes of critically ill patients with SARS-CoV-2 pneumonia in Wuhan, China: a single-centered, retrospective, observational study. *Lancet Respir Med.* (2020) 8:475–81. doi: 10.1016/S2213-2600(20)30079-5
19. Corman VM, Landt O, Kaiser M, Molenkamp R, Meijer A, Chu DK, et al. Detection of 2019 novel coronavirus (2019-nCoV) by real-time RT-PCR. *Euro Surveill.* (2020) 25:2000045. doi: 10.2807/1560-7917.ES.2020.25.3.2000045
20. Force ADT, Ranieri VM, Rubenfeld GD, Thompson BT, Ferguson ND, Caldwell E, et al. Acute respiratory distress syndrome: the Berlin Definition. *JAMA.* (2012) 307:2526–33. doi: 10.1001/jama.2012.5669
21. Khwaja A. KDIGO clinical practice guidelines for acute kidney injury. *Nephron Clin Pract.* (2012) 120:c179–84. doi: 10.1159/000339789
22. Rigatti SJ. Random forest. *J Insur Med.* (2017) 47:31–9. doi: 10.17849/insm-47-01-31-39.1
23. Diao B, Wang C, Tan Y, Chen X, Liu Y, Ning L, et al. Reduction and functional exhaustion of t cells in patients with coronavirus disease 2019 (COVID-19). *Front Immunol.* (2020) 11:827. doi: 10.3389/fimmu.2020.00827
24. Wang F, Nie J, Wang H, Zhao Q, Xiong Y, Deng L, et al. Characteristics of peripheral lymphocyte subset alteration in COVID-19 pneumonia. *J Infect Dis.* (2020) 221:1762–9. doi: 10.1093/infdis/jiaa150
25. Wang W, Su B, Pang L, Qiao L, Feng Y, Ouyang Y, et al. High-dimensional immune profiling by mass cytometry revealed immunosuppression and dysfunction of immunity in COVID-19 patients. *Cell Mol Immunol.* (2020) 17:650–2. doi: 10.1038/s41423-020-0447-2
26. Bermejo-Martin JF, Cilloniz C, Mendez R, Almansa R, Gabarrus A, Ceccato A, et al. Lymphopenic Community Acquired Pneumonia (L-CAP), an immunological phenotype associated with higher risk of mortality. *EBioMedicine.* (2017) 24:231–6. doi: 10.1016/j.ebiom.2017.09.023
27. Tan L, Wang Q, Zhang D, Ding J, Huang Q, Tang Y-Q, et al. Lymphopenia predicts disease severity of COVID-19: a descriptive and predictive study. *Signal Transduct Target Ther.* (2020) 5:33. doi: 10.1038/s41392-020-0148-4
28. Odak I, Barros-Martins J, Bošnjak B, Stahl K, David S, Wiesner O, et al. Reappearance of effector T cells is associated with recovery from COVID-19. *EBioMedicine.* (2020) 57:102885. doi: 10.1016/j.ebiom.2020.102885
29. Francois B, Jeannet R, Daix T, Walton AH, Shotwell MS, Unsinger J, et al. Interleukin-7 restores lymphocytes in septic shock: the IRIS-7 randomized clinical trial. *JCI Insight.* (2018) 3:98960. doi: 10.1172/jci.insight.98960
30. Nuckton TJ, Alonso JA, Kallet RH, Daniel BM, Pittet JF, Eisner MD, et al. Pulmonary dead-space fraction as a risk factor for death in the acute respiratory distress syndrome. *N Engl J Med.* (2002) 346:1281–6. doi: 10.1056/NEJMoa012835
31. Kallet RH, Alonso JA, Pittet JF, Matthay MA. Prognostic value of the pulmonary dead-space fraction during the first 6 days of acute respiratory distress syndrome. *Respir Care.* (2004) 49:1008–14.
32. Morales-Quinteros L, Schultz MJ, Bringué J, Calfee CS, Camprubí M, Cremer OL, et al. Estimated dead space fraction and the ventilatory ratio are associated with mortality in early ARDS. *Ann Intensive Care.* (2019) 9:128. doi: 10.1186/s13613-019-0601-0
33. Liu X, Liu X, Xu Y, Xu Z, Huang Y, Chen S, et al. Ventilatory ratio in hypercapnic mechanically ventilated patients with COVID-19-associated acute respiratory distress syndrome. *Am J Respir Crit Care Med.* (2020) 201:1297–9. doi: 10.1164/rccm.202002-0373LE
34. Demirjian SG, Raina R, Bhimraj A, Navaneethan SD, Gordon SM, Schreiber J, Jr., et al. 2009 influenza A infection and acute kidney injury: incidence, risk factors, and complications. *Am J Nephrol.* (2011) 34:1–8. doi: 10.1159/000328386
35. Martin-Loeches I, Papiol E, Rodríguez A, Diaz E, Zaragoza R, Granada RM, et al. Acute kidney injury in critical ill patients affected by influenza A (H1N1) virus infection. *Critical care (London, England).* (2011) 15:R66. doi: 10.1186/cc10046
36. Bautista E, Arcos M, Jimenez-Alvarez L, Garcia-Sancho MC, Vazquez ME, Pena E, et al. Angiogenic and inflammatory markers in acute respiratory distress syndrome and renal injury associated to A/H1N1 virus infection. *Exp Mol Pathol.* (2013) 94:486–92. doi: 10.1016/j.yexmp.2013.03.007
37. Dalbhi SA, Alshahrani HA, Almadi A, Busaleh H, Alotaibi M, Almutairi W, et al. Prevalence and mortality due to acute kidney injuries in patients with influenza A (H1N1) viral infection: a systemic narrative review. *Int J Health Sci.* (2019) 13:56–62.
38. Hirsch JS, Ng JH, Ross DW, Sharma P, Shah HH, Barnett RL, et al. Acute kidney injury in patients hospitalized with COVID-19. *Kidney Int.* (2020) 98:209–18. doi: 10.1016/j.kint.2020.05.006
39. Henry BM, Aggarwal G, Wong J, Benoit S, Vikse J, Plebani M, et al. Lactate dehydrogenase levels predict coronavirus disease 2019 (COVID-19) severity and mortality: A pooled analysis. *Am J Emerg Med.* (2020) 38:1722–6. doi: 10.1016/j.ajem.2020.05.073
40. Yan L, Zhang, H.-T., Goncalves J, Xiao Y, Wang M, et al. An interpretable mortality prediction model for COVID-19 patients. *Nat Mach Intell.* (2020) 2:283–8. doi: 10.1038/s42256-020-0180-7
41. Gattinoni L, Coppola S, Cressoni M, Busana M, Rossi S, Chiumello D. COVID-19 does not lead to a "typical" acute respiratory distress syndrome. *Am J Respir Crit Care Med.* (2020) 201:1299–300. doi: 10.1164/rccm.202003-0817LE

9

The Common Haplotype GATGACA in Surfactant-Protein B Gene is Protective for Respiratory Distress Syndrome in Preterm Neonates

Silvia Mikolajcikova [1], Zora Lasabova [2], Veronika Holubekova [3], Maria Skerenova [3], Jana Zibolenova [4], Katarina Matasova Sr. [1*], Mirko Zibolen [1] and Andrea Calkovska [5]*

[1] Clinic of Neonatology, Jessenius Faculty of Medicine, Comenius University and University Hospital, Martin, Slovakia,
[2] Department of Molecular Biology and Genomics, Jessenius Faculty of Medicine, Comenius University, Martin, Slovakia,
[3] Biomedical Centre Martin, Jessenius Faculty of Medicine, Comenius University, Martin, Slovakia, [4] Department of Public Health, Jessenius Faculty of Medicine, Comenius University, Martin, Slovakia, [5] Department of Physiology, Jessenius Faculty of Medicine, Comenius University, Martin, Slovakia

***Correspondence:**
Zora Lasabova
zora.lasabova@uniba.sk
Katarina Matasova Sr.
matasova.katarina@gmail.com

Background: Respiratory distress syndrome (RDS), a disorder of primary surfactant deficiency resulting in pulmonary insufficiency, remains a significant problem for preterm neonates. Associations between genetic variants of surfactant proteins and RDS have been reported, but haplotypes of the surfactant protein B gene (*SFTPB*) have not been studied. The aim of the study was to prove the hypothesis that certain haplotypes of *SFTPB* may be protective or risk factors for RDS.

Methods: The study was performed with 149 preterm infants, born <34 weeks of gestation, with 86 infants with mild RDS or without RDS (control group) and 63 infants with severe RDS (patient group). RDS was considered severe if multiple doses of exogenous surfactant and/or mechanical ventilation within the first 72 h of life were needed. The venous blood sample was used for the analysis of gene polymorphisms associated with RDS, genotyping, and haplotype estimation. Multivariate logistic regression analysis and the odds ratio were calculated to detect the contribution of the studied variables to the development of RDS.

Results: A new association of the common single nucleotide polymorphism (SNP) rs2304566 with RDS in premature infants was detected. Analysis of rs2304566 polymorphisms using a logistic regression model showed that there are two significant predictors inversely related to the occurrence of RDS (Apgar score of 5 min, CT and TT genotype in rs2304566 polymorphism). Gestational age, birth weight, and sex have border significance. Moreover, in the patient group, the frequency of the GATGACA haplotype in the *SFTPB* gene was lower ($p = 0.037$), and the GATGGCA haplotype was higher ($p = 0.059$) in comparison with the control group.

Conclusion: The common haplotype GATGACA of the *SFTPB* gene can be protective against RDS in preterm infants. The trend of a higher frequency of GATGGCA in the *SFTPB* gene in infants with severe RDS suggests that this haplotype may be a risk factor for RDS susceptibility.

Keywords: haplotype, *SFTPB*, surfactant, respiratory distress, neonate

INTRODUCTION

The successful fetal-neonatal pulmonary transition depends on the appropriate production of pulmonary surfactant *in utero* (1). Surfactant deficiency may result in respiratory distress syndrome (RDS), which is the most common form of respiratory failure in newborn infants. Although the incidence of RDS is inversely related to gestational age, preterm delivery alone does not determine the risk of developing the disorder. Several studies have suggested the possible involvement of surfactant protein (SP) SP-A2 and SP-B, SP-C, and SP-D common genetic polymorphisms in the genetic predisposition to RDS (2–8).

Surfactant protein B is encoded by the *SFTPB* gene located on human chromosome 2p11.2 that spans 9.7 kb and encodes mature SP-B of 79-amino acids (9). SP-B plays a critical role in the intracellular processing of surfactant components, and it is essential for low surface tension in the alveoli (10). Pathogenic recessive mutations in *SFTPB* are associated with SP-B deficiency (11), known as pulmonary surfactant metabolism dysfunction type 1 (OMIM #265120). Until now, more than 50 different disease-causing mutations, resulting in acute respiratory distress in full-term infants, have been identified enabling both prenatal and postnatal genetic diagnosis (12, 13). This very rare condition is progressive and usually fatal at 3–6 months of age.

However, common DNA polymorphisms of the *SFTPB* gene have been identified in neonatal RDS. A variable short tandem repeat (STR) region in intron 4 of SP-B was analyzed, and higher rates of variant alleles in populations of infants with RDS were found when compared with controls (14, 15). A functional study demonstrated the involvement of this STR in *SFTPB* mRNA splicing (15). In addition, it was also reported that a common non-synonymous single-nucleotide polymorphism (SNP) variant rs1130866 is associated with RDS in preterm newborns (6, 16). Therefore, *SFTPB* is considered a candidate gene for neonatal RDS, and the role of common variants has to be elucidated.

In our previous studies, we have identified a risk haplotype comprising common alleles that were associated with fetal loss in women with sticky platelet syndrome (17). Additionally, we have identified common missense variant haplotypes involved in this condition (18). Thus, it appears that certain haplotypes may be associated with a functional effect on gene expression. Since disease-causing variants in the *SFTPB* gene are loss-of-function variants, we assume in RDS that common variants may have minimal effect on protein function or gene expression that is not phenotypically manifested in the later life of the neonate. To confirm our assumption, we aimed to explore haplotypes of common tagged SNPs in order to evaluate the hypothesis that certain haplotypes of *SFTPB* may be protective or risk factors for RDS.

MATERIAL AND METHODS

Study Group

Preterm infants ($n = 149$) born at University Hospital Martin and admitted to the Clinic of Neonatology were enrolled in the study. The major inclusion criteria were as follows: (1) gestational age under 33rd + 6 weeks of gestation and (2) severity of respiratory distress. The newborns without or with mild respiratory distress were enrolled in the control group ($n = 86$); the infants with severe respiratory distress were included in the patient group ($n = 63$). Respiratory distress was considered severe if multiple doses of exogenous surfactant and/or mechanical ventilation within the first 72 h of life were needed. All the patients were Slovak and Caucasian. The exclusion criteria included severe perinatal asphyxia, early-onset sepsis, and congenital malformations.

The diagnosis of respiratory distress syndrome was based on the presence of clinical symptoms (tachypnea, dyspnea, retraction of jugulum, intercostal spaces and epigastrium, and cyanosis), X-ray findings with evidence of diffuse lung shading, and the need for ventilation support (19). All procedures related to postnatal stabilization and subsequent treatment were performed in accordance with the European consensus guidelines on the management of neonatal RDS in preterm infants (19, 20). The stabilization of the newborns was initiated in the delivery room by nasal continuous positive airway pressure (CPAP) applied through a face mask or short nasal prongs by T-resuscitator (Neopuff®) using a positive end-expiratory pressure (PEEP) of 6–8 cm H_2O. Oxygen administration was adjusted according to pre-ductal saturation obtained by pulse oximetry. When indicated, the exogenous porcine surfactant (Curosurf, Chiesi Farmaceutici SpA, Parma, Italy) in 100–200 mg/kg doses was administered by INSURE or LISA methods. Subsequently, neonates were managed by non-invasive respiratory support either by nasal continuous positive airway pressure (CPAP) or nasal biphasic positive airway pressure (nBiPAP) (InfantFlow®). Indications for mechanical ventilation were apnoeic episodes and respiratory insufficiency despite the appropriate non-invasive respiratory support. Mechanical ventilation was performed in the pressure support ventilation (PSV+VG) mode. A second dose and, rarely, a third dose of surfactant were given when there was ongoing evidence of RDS, hypercarbia, high oxygen requirement, and other causative problems have been excluded. Gestational age, birthweight, gender, Apgar score, antenatal steroids, and preterm rupture of membranes (PROM) were recorded and assessed.

DNA Isolation

The sample of venous blood (0.5 ml) was drawn into the EDTA tube. The DNA was extracted from blood samples at a volume of 0.2 ml by using the DNeasy Blood and Tissue DNA Isolation Kit (Qiagen, Germany) according to the manufacturer's instructions. DNA samples were diluted to 20 ng/μl and stored at −20°C before further processing.

Selection of Tagged SNPs in the *SFTPB* Gene

In total, seven tagged SNPs (tagSNPs), such as rs9752, rs762548, rs2304566, rs893159, rs1130866, rs3024791, and rs4616480, were chosen directly in or near of *SFTPB* gene (chromosome 2, position from 85659544 to 85670645 according GRCh38.p7) and

TABLE 1 | Characterization of tagged SNPs.

SNP	Chromosome	HGVS name
rs9752	2	NC_000002.12:g.85659544G>C
rs762548	2	NC_000002.12:g.85663630A>G
rs2304566	2	NC_000002.12:g.85663635T>C
rs893159	2	NC_000002.12:g.85663648T>G
rs1130866	2	NC_000002.12:g.85666618G>A
rs3024791	2	NC_000002.12:g.85668581C>T
rs4616480	2	NC_000002.12:g.85670645G>A

are characterized in **Table 1**. For the tag selection, we used Hap Map Data Rel 27/phase II + III on the NCBI B36 assembly, dbSNP b126 with minor allele frequency MAF > 0.1 in the Caucasian population, and Haploview software (Broad Institute, USA) applying the r^2 threshold of 0.8. The distribution of tagged SNPs is shown in **Figure 1**.

Genotyping by Allelic Discrimination

DNA genotyping of tagged SNPs was performed by allelic discrimination. We used the commercially available TaqMan Universal PCR Mastermix (Applied Biosystems, USA) and TaqMan SNP Genotyping Assays (Applied Biosystems, USA) C_8696006_10 for rs9752, C_8695999_20 for rs893159, C_15984495_10 for rs3024791, and C_30785447_10 for rs4616480. The PCR was performed with 20 ng of DNA in a 20 μl volume according to the protocol of the manufacturer. Briefly, 10 μl of the 2× concentrated TaqMan Universal Master Mix (Applied Biosystems, USA), 0.5 μl of the 40× concentrated, or 1 μl of the 20× concentrated appropriate TaqMan SNP Genotyping Assay (Applied Biosystems, USA), and 1 μl of the diluted DNA were amplified for 2 min at 50°C, 10 min at 95°C, and 40 times at 92°C for 15 s, and 60°C for 1 min. The genotypes were evaluated from the allelic discrimination plot using software version 2.0.1.

Genotyping by High Resolution Melting Analysis (HRMA) and Confirmation by Dideoxysequencing

For the rs762548, the HRMA was performed in a 15 μl reaction with forward primer 5′-GCGCTGGCCCAAGTGA-3′ and reverse primer 5′- CATGCAGTGGCAGGGTAGG-3′ using 7.5 μl LighCycler 480 High Resolution Melting Master (Roche, Switzerland), 3 mM final concentration of Mg^{2+}, 0.25 μM of each forward and reverse primer, and 15 ng of template DNA. The annealing temperature was 60°C, and the size of the amplified PCR products was 79 bp. In 10% of cases, the genotype was confirmed by dideoxysequencing using the forward primer as for HRMA and the reverse primer 5′-GCCACCCTACAGAGGTGTTT-3′. The PCR for sequencing was performed with 100 ng of extracted DNA in a final volume of 20 μl using FastStart Taq polymerase (Roche, Switzerland) with a 1.5 mM of Mg^{2+} concentration. The PCR conditions were 10 min at 95°C and 30 cycles at 95°C for 30 s, appropriate annealing temperature for 30 s, and 72°C for 30 s. The presence of PCR products was verified by using 1.75% agarose gel electrophoresis. Subsequently, PCR products were purified with the NucleoSpin Extract II kit (Machery-Nagel, UK), and the sequencing reaction was performed using the BigDye Terminator kit version 1.1 (Applied Biosystems, USA) at 95°C for 2 min and 35 times at 95°C for 15 min and 60°C for 4 min. The fragments were separated on the automatic genetic analyzer AB3500 and subsequently evaluated with DNA Sequencing Analysis Software version 5.4 (Applied Biosystems, USA) and ChromasPro version 2.4.4 (Technelysium, Australia).

Statistical Analysis

Hardy–Weinberg equilibrium (HWE), genotype, allele, haplotype frequencies, and linkage disequilibrium between the gene polymorphisms were analyzed by using SHEsis software (http://shesisplus.bio-x.cn/SHEsis.html). Haplotype analysis was done using SVS 8 software (SNP and Variation Suite version 8.1, Golden Helix, Bozeman, MT).

Pearson's chi-square test was used for univariate comparisons of allele and genotype frequencies between the patient group and control group and for checking for deviation from HWE. Odds ratios (OR) with 95% confidence intervals (95% CI) were calculated to identify the relationship between SNPs and RDS.

Epi Info 7 was used for the rest of the analysis. Continuous variables were expressed as mean ± SD and compared by *t*-test, while the binomial variables were tabulated and compared with the chi-square test using Yates's correction.

Multivariate logistic regression analysis and the odds ratio were calculated to detect the contribution of the studied variables to the development of RDS. The following variables were included in the logistic model: gestational age, Apgar score of 5 min, birth weight, sex, antenatal steroids, and rs2304566 (model 1) or rs9752 (model 2). The value of $p < 0.05$ was regarded as statistically significant.

RESULTS

Clinical Description of the Study Population

The main characteristics of both groups are summarized in **Table 2**. The patient and control groups differed significantly by gestational age, birthweight, and postnatal adaptation is expressed by Apgar scores.

Analysis of Individual Polymorphisms in *SFTPB* Gene

The comparison of individual polymorphisms localized in the *SFTPB* gene in patients ($n = 63$) and control ($n = 86$) groups is shown in **Table 3**. Based on a calculation of Hardy–Weinberg equilibrium, the distribution of genotypes is consistent with control and patient groups ($p > 0.05$). Using a general genetic model for the estimation of associations between genotypes and RDS, no significant correlation was found. However, when we

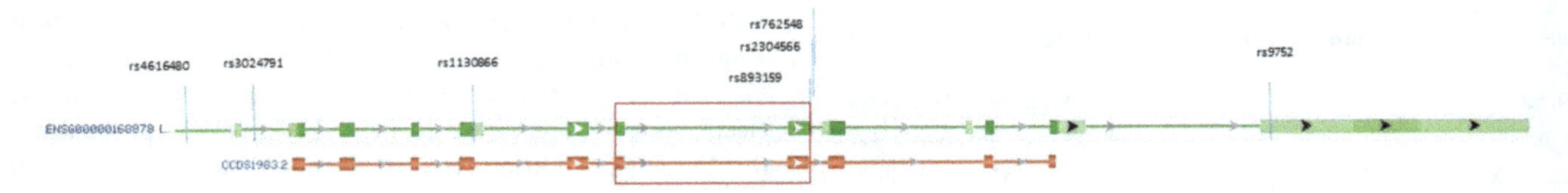

FIGURE 1 | The reference transcript for the *SFTPB* gene (green section) and the SP-B preprotein (red section). The *SFTPB* gene reference transcript ENSG00000168878 is composed of 11 exons, with dark green rectangles aligning the exons that encode the SP-B preprotein, which is composed of 381 amino acid residues (CCDS1983.2, red section below transcript). The mature SP-B protein contains amino acid residues at codons 201 to 279 (28, 29), and protein-encoding exons 6 and 7 are indicated by a large red rectangle. Three of the tagged SNPs (rs893159, rs2304566, and rs762548) are in the second exon encoding mature SP-B, and SNP rs9752 is at 3′UTR in the flanking arm of the preprotein (light green transcript rectangle). https://www.ncbi.nlm.nih.gov/gene/6439 (modified).

TABLE 2 | Characterization of enrolled subjects.

Variable	Patients ($n = 63$)	Control ($n = 86$)	*P*-value
Gestational age (weeks)	27.2 ± 2.7	30.6 ± 2.0	<0.001
Birth weight (g)	1001.8 ± 393.2	1526.7 ± 391.7	<0.001
1 min Apgar score	4 [0–9]	6 [3–9]	<0.001
5 min Apgar score	6 [2–8]	7 [5–10]	<0.001
Male gender	34 (54.0%)	44 (51.2%)	0.8628
Preterm rupture of membranes	13 (20.6%)	19 (22.1%)	0.9902
Antenatal steroids	36 (57.1%)	37 (43.0%)	0.1012

Gestational age and birth weight are displayed as mean ± SD; Apgar score is shown as median and the interval; and other variables are shown as number of subjects and percentage.

TABLE 3 | Comparison of gene polymorphisms (SNPs) in the *SFTPB* gene.

SNP	Group	Genotype a genotype frequency			*P*-value
rs9752		G/G	G/C	C/C	
	patient	27(0.428)	25(0.396)	11(0.174)	0.159
	control	49(0.569)	29(0.337)	8(0.093)	
rs762548		A/A	A/G	G/G	
	patient	54(0.857)	8(0.126)	1(0.015)	0.496
	control	75(0.882)	10(0.117)	0(0)	
rs2304566		T/T	T/C	C/C	
	patient	36(0.571)	20(0.317)	7(0.111)	0.16
	control	60(0.705)	21(0.247)	4(0.047)	
rs893159		T/T	T/G	G/G	
	patient	1(0.015)	10(0.158)	52(0.825)	0.725
	control	1(0.011)	18(0.209)	67(0.779)	
rs1130866		G/G	G/A	A/A	
	patient	12(0.19)	33(0.523)	18(0.285)	0.382
	control	14(0.162)	38(0.441)	34(0.395)	
rs3024791		C/C	C/T	T/T	
	patient	51(0.809)	11(0.174)	1(0.015)	0.355
	control	75(0.872)	11(0.127)	0(0)	
rs4616480		G/G	G/A	A/A	
	patient	17(0.269)	32(0.507)	14(0.222)	0.674
	control	29(0.337)	39(0.453)	18(0.209)	

analyzed the distribution of single alleles (**Table 4**), we could show that the frequency of the C (minor) allele for rs9752 was significantly higher in the patient group compared to the control group (0.373 vs. 0.261) ($p = 0.039$, OR 1.679, 95% CI: 1.022–2.757). Similarly, the C (minor) allele of rs2304566 was significantly more frequent in the patient group compared with controls (0.269 vs. 0.171) ($p = 0.039$; OR 1.796, 95% CI: 1.025–3.148). For the other SNPs, only insignificant differences in the allele frequencies between the two groups were present ($p > 0.05$). After the false discovery rate was controlled at a level of 0.05 (Benjamini–Hochberg method), none of the differences in allele frequencies remained significant.

Haplotype Estimation of Tagged SNPs in *SFTPB* Gene

Haplotype analysis was performed on seven tagged SNPs. The most frequent haplotypes are shown in **Table 5**. The frequency of haplotype GATGACA (in the following order: rs9752, rs762548, rs2304566, rs893159, rs1130866, rs3024791, and rs4616480) was lower in neonates with severe respiratory symptoms compared to neonates with no or only mild respiratory symptoms (0.126 vs. 0.223); the difference was statistically significant ($p = 0.037$; OR 0.512, 95% CI: 0.271–0.969). A similar trend close to statistical significance ($p = 0.073$; OR 0.427, 95% CI: 0.164–1.11) was present in the distribution of haplotype GATGACG. Its presence in the patient group was lower than in the control group (0.047 vs. 0.105). On the contrary, the frequency of haplotype GATGGCA was higher in the patient group than in the control group (0.15 vs. 0.082) ($p = 0.059$, OR 2.004, 95% CI: 0.963–4.169).

Multivariate Logistic Regression Analysis

Analysis of rs2304566 polymorphisms (model 1) using a logistic regression model showed that there are two significant predictors inversely related to the occurrence of RDS (Apgar score of 5 min, CT and TT genotype in rs2304566 polymorphism). Moreover, gestational age, birth weight, and sex have borderline significance (**Table 6**).

After including polymorphism rs9752 (model 2, results not shown) into the logistic regression model, it was found that this polymorphism is not associated with RDS.

TABLE 4 | Distribution of individual genotypes in gene *SFTPB*.

SNP	Group	Genotype frequency		P-value	OR (95% CI)	HWE (patient) *P*-value	HWE (control) *P*-value
rs9752		G	C				
	patient	79 (0.626)	47 (0.373)	0.039	1.679	0.484	0.498
	control	127 (0.738)	45 (0.261)		(1.022–2.757)		
rs762548		A	G				
	patient	116 (0.92)	10 (0.079)	0.486	1.379	0.582	0.847
	control	160 (0.941)	10 (0.058)		(0.556–3.421)		
rs2304566		T	C				
	patient	92 (0.73)	34(0.269)	0.039	1.796	0.304	0.504
	control	141 (0.829)	29 (0.17)		(1.025–3.148)		
rs893159		T	G				
	patient	12 (0.095)	114 (0.904)	0.562	0.8	0.821	0.985
	control	20 (0.116)	152 (0.883)		(0.375–1.703)		
rs1130866		G	A				
	patient	57 (0.452)	69 (0.547)	0.234	1.326	0.902	0.83
	control	66 (0.383)	106 (0.616)		(0.832–2.115)		
rs3024791		T	C				
	patient	13 (0.103)	113 (0.896)	0.219	1.683	0.904	0.818
	control	11 (0.063)	161 (0.936)		(0.728–3.893)		
rs4616480		G	A				
	patient	66 (0.523)	60 (0.476)	0.491	1.175	0.989	0.77
	control	97 (0.563)	75 (0.436)		(0.741–1.865)		

TABLE 5 | Comparison of haplotypes in gene *SFTPB*.

Haplotype	Patients (frequency)	Control (frequency)	Chi^2	Fisher p-value	Pearson p-value	OR [95% CI]
CACGACA	20 (0.158)	20 (0.117)	1.127	0.306	0.288	1.433 [0.735~2.795]
GATGACA	16 (0.126)	38 (0.223)	4.326	0.047	0.037	0.512 [0.271~0.969]
GATTACG	9 (0.071)	12 (0.07)	0.003	1	0.955	1.025 [0.418~2.514]
GATTGCG	3 (0.023)	6 (0.035)	0.304	0.738	0.581	0.674 [0.165~2.751]
GATGGCA	19 (0.15)	14 (0.082)	3.556	0.064	0.059	2.004 [0.963~4.169]
GATGGCG	20 (0.158)	32 (0.188)	0.376	0.643	0.539	0.825 [0.447~0.523]
GATGACG	6 (0.047)	18 (0.105)	3.194	0.086	0.073	0.427 [0.164~1.11]
CGTGACG	4 (0.031)	5 (0.029)	0.017	1	0.893	1.095 [0.288~4.162]
CATGACG	3 (0.023)	8 (0.047)	1.054	0.366	0.304	0.5 [0.129~1.923]

DISCUSSION

The etiology of RDS is multifactorial, and the phenotype of the RDS is likely influenced by several genetic factors, the proportion of which is estimated between 35 and 65% (21). The incidence and severity are inversely proportional to gestational age. Based on Vermont Oxford Network data in 2017, the incidence of RDS is about 80% in babies born at the 28th week of gestation increasing to 90% at the 24th week of gestation (19). The lower gestational age in the patient group in our study, where only infants with severe RDS were included, is consistent with this data. The differences between the patient and control groups in birth weight and postnatal adaptation expressed by the Apgar score can be attributed to lower gestational age. The literary data supports this assumption (22). Antenatal steroids as a protective factor and male gender as a risk factor can affect the course of RDS (23, 24), but the patient and control groups in our study did not differ in these variables.

The aim of our study was to explore the association of *SFTPB* gene haplotypes that were derived from a common SNP with a MAF > 0.1. We also analyzed all 7 tagged SNPs spanning the *SFTPB* gene separately in all enrolled subjects. The statistical evaluation of each SNP individually did not reveal any significant association with RDS in our cohort, and there were no differences observed between the patients and controls, as we expected. Nevertheless, we found an intronic TT genotype in the rs2304566 polymorphism to be protective of severe RDS, but its functional impact is not known yet. The second SNP

TABLE 6 | Logistic regression analysis (model 1).

Variable	Odds Ratio	Lower limit (95% CI)	Upper limit (95% CI)	Coefficient	S.E.	Z-Statistic	*P*-Value
Gestational age	0.7372	0.5422	1.0024	−0.3049	0.1568	−1.9445	0.0518
Apgar in 5th minute	0.4017	0.2485	0.6491	−0.9121	0.2449	−3.7246	0.0002
Birth weight	0.9982	0.9963	1.0001	−0.0018	0.001	−1.8248	0.068
Gender—male (ref. female)	2.6192	0.921	7.4484	0.9629	0.5332	1.8056	0.071
Antenatal steroids	2.0253	0.7477	5.4861	0.7057	0.5084	1.3881	0.1651
rs2304566 - C/T (ref C/C)	**0.1295**	**0.0184**	**0.9105**	**−2.0441**	**0.9951**	**−2.0541**	**0.04**
rs2304566 - T/T (ref C/C)	**0.0709**	**0.0107**	**0.4704**	**−2.6468**	**0.9656**	**−2.7411**	**0.0061**
CONSTANT				18.4075	4.3608	4.2211	<0.0001

SE, standard error; CI, confidence interval.

where we found a significant association with RDS is rs9752. SNP rs9752 is located at 3′UTR. Recently, the association of recessive homozygotes harboring the CC genotype and heterozygotes with the CT genotype has been demonstrated with reduced plasma pro-SFTPB in non-small cell lung cancer patients (25), which could also indicate some functional effects of this SNP on gene expression.

The missenses SNP rs1130866 (Thr131Ile) was one of the included SNPs in this analysis; however, the association with RDS was not confirmed. Contrary to our result, an association between the SP-B Ile131Thr polymorphism and RDS was found in the twin study. The authors conclude that the concordance difference between monozygotic and dizygotic twin pairs underestimates the genetic impact on the risk of RDS (16). In the Greek population, no association between the SP-B Ile131Thr polymorphism and RDS was found (6).

A very recent study used 17 well-studied SNPs of *SFTPA1*, *SFTPA2*, *SFTPB*, *SFTPC*, and *SFTPD* to investigate the impact of individual SNPs and their interactions among SNPs in the same gene or between two or among three different genes on RDS. The authors show not only the association of a single SNP but also of two and three SNP interactions associated with RDS susceptibility. In the *SFTPB* gene, there was one significant intragenic interaction (rs2077079, rs3024798, and rs7316). Each SNP exhibited a dominant effect, and this interaction was associated with a decreased risk of RDS (2).

In our study, genotyping followed by a comparison of the *SFTPB* polymorphisms by Hardy–Weinberg equilibrium revealed a consistent distribution of different genotypes in both groups, namely controls and patients. However, for rs230456 polymorphisms, the minor allele C frequency was significantly higher in patients than in the control group.

We found out that the haplotype GATGACA (in the following order: rs9752G, rs762548A, rs2304566T, rs893159G, rs1130866A, rs3024791C, and rs4616480A) in the *SFTPB* gene showed significantly lower frequency in preterm infants with severe RDS compared to controls. The rs2304566 minor allele C associated with RDS in preterm neonates, as mentioned above, is not present in this haplotype. A similar trend, close to statistical significance, was observed in haplotype GATGACG (rs in the above-mentioned order) distribution. Its frequency in the patient group was lower than in the control group. The rs2304566 is here also represented by major allele T. Taken together, these two haplotypes can be considered as protective factors against the development of RDS in preterm infants. To the best of our knowledge, only one study analyzing SP-B haplotypes based on common SNPs in association with RDS has been published. However, this study used the family-based association test (FBAT) and extended transmission disequilibrium test (ETDT) to test −18 A/C (rs2077079 g.85668215T>C), 1,013 A/C (rs3024798 g.85667185G>T), 1,580 C/T (rs1130866 g.85666618G>A; Thr131Ile), and 9,306 A/G (rs7316 g.85658890T>C). By FBAT, two protective haplotypes have been identified and, in both cases, the rs1130866 was present as the Ile allele (3). In protective haplotypes in our study, the rs1130866 is also present as the Ile allele.

On the contrary, the haplotype GATGGCA in the patient group tended to be higher than in the control group. It means that the probability of the occurrence of RDS in exposed individuals is higher, and thus this haplotype can be identified as a risk factor for the development of RDS. In this case, the rs1130866 is present as the Thr allele. For that reason, the role of rs1130866 in the development of RDS in preterm neonates remains to be elucidated.

We suggest that other genetic and epigenetic factors can play a modifying role, or in certain populations, the rs1130866 can be linked to the locus affecting the expression of the *SFTPB* gene, and therefore, the results for rs1130866 are still controversial. Glycosylation of pro-SP-B or genetic polymorphisms within the promoter region has a role in genetic susceptibility to RDS. In a mice model, SP-B levels were correlated with the Ile131Thr genotype, and the lowest SP-B levels were observed in Thr/Thr homozygotes. This rs1130866 variation-dependent N-glycosylation was associated with the decreased levels of SP-B, which was secreted from fetal lung to amniotic fluid (26). Lower levels of pro-SP-B were also confirmed in human amniotic fluid samples and were associated with rs1130866 (9).

The results of our study contribute to a better understanding of the genetic background of RDS in preterm infants. The main strength of this study was the ethnically homogenous study group. The other advantages were the strict inclusion and exclusion criteria and homogenous management of obstetrical and neonatal care. On the contrary, the study had some limitations. It was conducted as a single-center study, and the number of participants is limited. The results should be replicated in future larger studies.

CONCLUSION

At least one common haplotype GATGACA of the *SFTPB* gene can protect preterm newborns from RDS. The trend of higher frequency of GATGGCA in the *SFTPB* gene in preterm infants with severe respiratory distress suggests that this haplotype may be a risk factor for the occurrence of RDS. However, other genetic factors must be elucidated as candidate genes for the genetic susceptibility for RDS in preterm neonates. Further research is required to clarify the exact mechanism by which these genetic variants predispose to neonatal RDS.

Common SNPs tagged to a haplotype have been shown to have some protective and risk associated with RDS in premature newborns, emphasizing the genetic component of RDS. However, this association is weak and rather indicates a linkage disequilibrium of a certain haplotype or SNP with rare alleles in some patients. However, in the study design, we only concentrated on MAF > 0.1 and thus could not identify rare alleles. Sequencing analyses of whole genes in premature infants have identified novel rare variants associated with RDS. These are mostly in-frame deletions, missense synonyms, and variants in introns and 3′UTR, and according to the ACMG-AMP criteria, these are classified as variants of unknown significance (27). Therefore, it is necessary for the future to focus on the sequencing of whole genes and the identification of rare variants, which cannot be captured by haplotypes with common SNPs. Functional studies and patient follow-up can further identify the effect of these variants on the protein function and disease course, respectively.

Protection, US Department of Health and Human Services, and certified with the code IRB00005636 Jessenius Faculty of Medicine, Comenius University in Martin IRB # 1. Written informed consent to participate in this study was provided by the participants' legal guardian/next of kin.

AUTHOR CONTRIBUTIONS

SM conceptualized the study, wrote the study protocol, included the patients, collected the data, and wrote the paper. ZL conceptualized the study, wrote the study protocol, and performed the final interpretation of the results. VH performed processing and analysis of biological samples. MS was engaged in the analysis of haplotypes. JZ performed the statistical analyses. KM supervised the study and participated in the interpretation of the results. MZ and AC designed the study, oversaw the data analysis and interpretation, and critically reviewed and revised the manuscript drafts. All authors contributed substantially to the writing of the manuscript. All authors read and approved the final manuscript.

ACKNOWLEDGMENTS

The authors thank P. Lukac for the help and assistance. The graphics of gene and protein in **Figure 1** was modified according to the NCBI webpage (https://www.ncbi.nlm.nih.gov/gene/6439).

REFERENCES

1. Hallman M. The surfactant system protects both fetus and newborn. *Neonatology.* (2013) 103:320–6. doi: 10.1159/000349994
2. Amatya S, Ye M, Yang L, Gandhi CK, Wu R, Nagourney B, et al. Single nucleotide polymorphisms interactions of the surfactant protein genes associated with respiratory distress syndrome susceptibility in preterm infants. *Front Pediatr.* (2021) 9:682160. doi: 10.3389/fped.2021.682160
3. Floros J, Thomas NJ, Liu W, Papagaroufalis C, Xanthou M, Pereira S, et al. Family-based association tests suggest linkage between surfactant protein B (SP-B) (and flanking region) and respiratory distress syndrome (RDS): SP-B haplotypes and alleles from SP-B-linked loci are risk factors for RDS. *Pediatr Res.* (2006) 59:616–21. doi: 10.1203/01.pdr.0000203145.48585.2c
4. Lyra PP, Diniz EM, Abe-Sandes K, Angelo AL, Machado TM, Cardeal M. Surfactant protein B gene polymorphism in preterm babies with respiratory distress syndrome. *Braz J Med Biol Res.* (2011) 44:66–72. doi: 10.1590/S0100-879X2010007500147
5. Abuelhamed WA, Zeidan N, Shahin WA, Rizk HI, Rabie WA. Human surfactant proteins A2 (SP-A2) and B (SP-B) genes as determinants of respiratory distress syndrome. *Indian Pediatr.* (2015) 52:391–4. doi: 10.1007/s13312-015-0643-9
6. Tsitoura MI, Stavrou EF, Maraziotis IA, Sarafidis K, Athanassiadou A, Dimitriou G. Surfactant protein A and B gene polymorphisms and risk of respiratory distress syndrome in late-preterm neonates. *PLoS ONE.* (2016) 11:e0166516. doi: 10.1371/journal.pone.0166516
7. Lahti M, Marttila R, Hallman M. Surfactant protein C gene variation in the Finnish population - association with perinatal respiratory disease. *Eur J Hum Genet.* (2004) 12:312–20. doi: 10.1038/sj.ejhg.5201137
8. Sorensen GL, Dahl M, Tan Q, Bendixen C, Holmskov U, Husby S. Surfactant protein-D-encoding gene variant polymorphisms are linked to respiratory outcome in premature infants. *J Pediatr.* (2014) 165:683–9. doi: 10.1016/j.jpeds.2014.05.042
9. Hamvas A, Wegner DJ, Carlson CS, Bergmann KR, Trusgnich MA, Fulton L, et al. Comprehensive genetic variant discovery in the surfactant protein B gene. *Pediatr Res.* (2007) 62:170–5. doi: 10.1203/PDR.0b013e3180a03232
10. Whitsett JA, Weaver TE. Hydrophobic surfactant proteins in lung function and disease. *N Engl J Med.* (2002) 347:2141–8. doi: 10.1056/NEJMra022387
11. Nogee LM, Wert SE, Proffit SA, Hull WM, Whitsett JA. Allelic heterogeneity in hereditary surfactant protein B (SP-B) deficiency. *Am J Respir Crit Care Med.* (2000) 161:973–81. doi: 10.1164/ajrccm.161.3.9903153
12. Nogee LM. Genetic causes of surfactant protein abnormalities. *Curr Opin Pediatr.* (2019) 31:330–9. doi: 10.1097/MOP.0000000000000751
13. Kurath-Koller S, Resch B, Kraschl R, Windpassinger C, Eber E. Surfactant protein B deficiency caused by homozygous C248X mutation-A case report and review of the literature. *AJP Rep.* (2015) 5:e53–59. doi: 10.1055/s-0035-1545668
14. Floros J, Veletza SV, Kotikalapudi P, Krizkova L, Karinch AM, Friedman C, et al. Dinucleotide repeats in the human surfactant

protein-B gene and respiratory-distress syndrome. *Biochem J.* (1995) 305:583–90. doi: 10.1042/bj3050583

15. Yang W, Ni L, Silveyra P, Wang G, Noutsios GT, Singh A, et al. Motifs within the CA-repeat-rich region of Surfactant Protein B (SFTPB) intron 4 differentially affect mRNA splicing. *J Mol Biochem.* (2013) 2:40–55.
16. Marttila R, Haataja R, Rämet M, Löfgren J, Hallman M. Surfactant protein B polymorphism and respiratory distress syndrome in premature twins. *Hum Genet.* (2003) 112:18–23. doi: 10.1007/s00439-002-0835-y
17. Sokol J, Biringer K, Skerenova M, Hasko M, Bartosova L, Stasko J, et al. Platelet aggregation abnormalities in patients with fetal losses: the GP6 gene polymorphism. *Fertil Steril.* (2012) 98:1170–4. doi: 10.1016/j.fertnstert.2012.07.1108
18. Škerenová M, Sokol J, Biringer K, Ivanková J, Staško J, Kubisz P, et al. GP6 haplotype of missense variants is associated with sticky platelet syndrome manifested by fetal loss. *Clin Appl Thromb Hemost.* (2018) 24:63–9. doi: 10.1177/1076029616685428
19. Sweet DG, Carnielli V, Greisen G, Hallman M, Ozek E, Te Pas A, et al. European consensus guidelines on the management of respiratory distress syndrome - 2019 update. *Neonatology.* (2019) 115:432–50. doi: 10.1159/000499361
20. Sweet DG, Carnielli V, Greisen G, Hallman M, Ozek E, Plavka R, et al. European consensus guidelines on the management of respiratory distress syndrome - 2016 update. *Neonatology.* (2017) 111:107–25. doi: 10.1159/000448985
21. Hallman M, Marttila R, Pertile R, Ojaniemi M, Haataja R. Genes and environment in common neonatal lung disease. *Neonatology.* (2007) 91:298–302. doi: 10.1159/000101345
22. Numerato D, Fattore G, Tediosi F, Zanini R, Peltola M, Banks H, et al. Mortality and length of stay of very low birth weight and very preterm infants: a EuroHOPE study. *PLoS ONE.* (2015) 10:e0131685. doi: 10.1371/journal.pone.0131685
23. O'Driscoll DN, McGovern M, Greene CM, Molloy EJ. Gender disparities in preterm neonatal outcomes. *Acta Paediatr.* (2018) 107:1494–9. doi: 10.1111/apa.14390
24. Roberts D, Brown J, Medley N, Dalziel SR. Antenatal corticosteroids for accelerating fetal lung maturation for women at risk of preterm birth. *Cochrane Database Syst Rev.* (2017) 3:CD004454. doi: 10.1002/14651858.CD004454.pub3
25. Wang K, Huang Q, Zhao G, Yang J, Huang Y. Gene polymorphisms of *SFTPB* rs7316, rs9752 and PAOX rs1046175 affect the diagnostic value of plasma Pro-SFTPB and DAS in Chinese Han non-small-cell lung cancer patients. *J Cell Biochem.* (2019) 120:14804–12. doi: 10.1002/jcb.28741
26. Taponen S, Huusko J, Petäjä-Repo U, Paananen R, Guttentag SH, Hallman M, et al. Allele-Specific N-glycosylation delays human surfactant protein B secretion in vitro and associates with decreased protein levels *in vivo*. *Pediatr Res.* (2013) 74:646–51. doi: 10.1038/pr.2013.151
27. Somaschini M, Presi S, Ferrari M, Vergani B, Carrera P. Surfactant proteins gene variants in premature newborn infants with severe respiratory distress syndrome. *J Perinatol.* (2018) 38:337–44. doi: 10.1038/s41372-017-0018-2
28. Hawgood S, Derrick M, Poulain F. Structure and properties of surfactant protein B. *Biochim Biophys Acta.* (1998) 1408:150–60. doi: 10.1016/S0925-4439(98)00064-7
29. Gargiulo P, Banfi C, Ghilardi S, Magri D, Giovannardi M, et al. Surfactant-derived proteins as markers of alveolar membrane damage in heart failure. *PLos ONE.* (2014) 9:e115030. doi: 10.1371/journal.pone.0115030

10

Positive End-Expiratory Pressure Setting in COVID-19-Related Acute Respiratory Distress Syndrome: Comparison Between Electrical Impedance Tomography, PEEP/FiO_2 Tables and Transpulmonary Pressure

Sébastien Gibot, Marie Conrad, Guilhem Courte and Aurélie Cravoisy*

Service de Réanimation Médicale, Hôpital Central, CHRU, Nancy, France

***Correspondence:**
Sébastien Gibot
s.gibot@chru-nancy.fr*

Introduction: The best way to titrate the positive end-expiratory pressure (PEEP) in patients suffering from acute respiratory distress syndrome is still matter of debate. Electrical impedance tomography (EIT) is a non-invasive technique that could guide PEEP setting based on an optimized ventilation homogeneity.

Methods: For this study, we enrolled the patients with 2019 coronavirus disease (COVID-19)-related acute respiratory distress syndrome (ARDS), who required mechanical ventilation and were admitted to the ICU in March 2021. Patients were monitored by an esophageal catheter and a 32-electrode EIT device. Within 48 h after the start of mechanical ventilation, different levels of PEEP were applied based upon PEEP/FiO_2 tables, positive end-expiratory transpulmonary (P_L)/ FiO2 table, and EIT. Respiratory mechanics variables were recorded.

Results: Seventeen patients were enrolled. PEEP values derived from EIT ($PEEP_{EIT}$) were different from those based upon other techniques and has poor in-between agreement. The $PEEP_{EIT}$ was associated with lower plateau pressure, mechanical power, transpulmonary pressures, and with a higher static compliance (Crs) and homogeneity of ventilation.

Conclusion: Personalized PEEP setting derived from EIT may help to achieve a more homogenous distribution of ventilation. Whether this approach may translate in outcome improvement remains to be investigated.

Keywords: ARDS, COVID-19, PEEP, electrical tomography impedance, mechanical ventilation

INTRODUCTION

Despite progresses in acute respiratory distress syndrome (ARDS) management, the best way to titrate a positive end-expiratory pressure (PEEP) is not straightforward (1). The "right" PEEP should allow for optimized lung recruitment while minimizing over-distention. To this aim, clinicians can use PEEP-FiO_2 tables (2), transpulmonary pressure (P_L) (3), or electrical impedance tomography (EIT).

The transpulmonary pressure is measured using an esophageal balloon catheter that approximates the pleural pressure. Using this technique, PEEP has to be set to maintain the end-expiratory P_L above zero to avoid collapse of dependent dorsal lung regions, and the end-inspiratory P_L below 20–25 cmH_2O to decrease the risk of overdistension of non-dependent regions.

Electrical impedance tomography (EIT) is a non-invasive technique giving dynamic information on regional ventilation that can be embarked in modern ventilators. Regional hypoventilated lung units ("Silent spaces") correspond to both collapsed areas in the dependent territories, and distended areas in the non-dependent regions. Using this technique, PEEP is set to minimize the percentage of total silent spaces.

We describe a case series of patients suffering from 2019 coronavirus disease (COVID-19)-related ARDS in whom we compared PEEP settings based on PEEP/FiO_2 tables, P_L/ FiO2 table, and EIT.

METHODS

In March 2021, we enrolled some mechanically ventilated patients who were admitted to our Intensive Care Unit (ICU) because of a COVID-19-related moderate-to-severe ARDS. The diagnosis of COVID-19 relied upon positive result on polymerase chain reaction of sputum or nasal swab. The Ethic Committee of our University Hospital approved this study with a waiver of informed consent because of the use of routine procedures, as well as the use of de-identified data.

All patients were ventilated in volume control mode [tidal volume (Vt): 6–7 ml/kg ideal body weight (IBW)], with FiO_2 set to achieve peripheral oxygen saturation (SpO_2) between 92 and 95%, and respiratory rate (RR) set to reach $PaCO_2$ between 38 and 45 mmHg. Transpulmonary pressures were measured with the use of an esophageal balloon catheter (Nutrivent; Sidam, Mirandola, Italy) after its correct positioning has been verified through passive chest compression during occlusion. As part of our routine monitoring, patients were also equipped with a 32-electrode soft-textile EIT belt (Sentec; Therwil, Switzerland), which was directly connected to the ventilator (ELISA 800 VIT, Lowenstein Medical; Kronberg, Germany). Some maneuvers were performed in supine position after 24–48 h of mechanical ventilation while the patients were still sedated (midazolam and sufentanyl) and paralyzed (cisatracurium or atracurium). Respiratory mechanics variables were recorded after 10 min at different PEEP levels while all the other parameters (FiO_2, Vt, RR, flow rates, etc.) remained unchanged.

Positive end-expiratory pressure (PEEP) was first set according to the lower, then, to the higher PEEP/FiO_2 ALVEOLI table (2). Next, PEEP as based upon end-expiratory P_L/FiO_2 table, was applied (3). Finally, an automated decremental PEEP trial was performed under EIT monitoring (Best-PEEP-Tool, Lowenstein Medical): PEEP was set at 24 cmH_2O (corresponding to the maximum PEEP in the PEEP/FiO_2 table) and was reduced by 2 cmH_2O every 10 inspirations until 6 cm H_2O, with a 3-s end-expiratory hold between decremental steps. For each PEEP values, percentages of relatively collapsed and overdistended lung regions were given by the EIT, and the "best" PEEP ($PEEP_{EIT}$) was considered as the lowest level associated with the lowest total percentage of the lung silent spaces (collapsed + distended).

Data are presented as median (interquartile range) and are compared using Wilcoxon signed-rank test. Bias and limits of agreement between different approaches were calculated with the Bland-Altman approach. Statistical analyses were performed by GraphPad software (La Jolla, CA, USA) with two-tailed $p < 0.05$ deemed as significant.

RESULTS

Seventeen patients (15 men, 2 women) were enrolled. Median age was 65 (62–71) years, and body mass index was 31.1 (28.5–33.0). The ARDS was severe in 6 and moderate in 11 patients, while the PaO_2/FiO_2 was 136 (103–155), Vt 6.6 (6.2–7.0) mL/kg IBW, and RR 24 (22–27), respectively. Twelve patients were under high-flow oxygen therapy for a median of 1 (1, 2) day before intubation. All patients, except for one, were discharged alive.

Positive end-expiratory pressure derived from EIT ($PEEP_{EIT}$), corresponding to the lowest level of PEEP achieving the lowest percentage of total silent spaces (distended + collapsed), was significantly different from the other PEEP values. It was higher than the lower PEEP/FiO_2 table, and lower than the higher PEEP/FiO_2 or P_L/FiO_2 tables (**Table 1**). The Bland-Altman analysis showed that $PEEP_{EIT}$ was 1.3 cm H_2O higher than the lower PEEP/FiO_2 table with limits of agreement from −8.5 to 11.2 cm H_2O. By contrast, $PEEP_{EIT}$ was 5 and 4 cm H_2O lower, respectively, than higher PEEP/FiO_2 and P_L/FiO_2 tables, with again wide limits of agreement (**Figure 1**).

In terms of respiratory mechanics, $PEEP_{EIT}$ was associated with lower plateau pressure, mechanical power, transpulmonary pressures, and with a higher static compliance (Crs) than higher PEEP/FiO_2 or P_L/FiO_2 tables (**Table 1**). Driving pressures were not significantly different.

A better distribution of ventilation was achieved with $PEEP_{EIT}$: lung collapse was lower with $PEEP_{EIT}$ than with lower PEEP/FiO_2 table (9 vs. 13%; $p = 0.04$), while lung distension was reduced as compared to higher PEEP/FiO_2 and P_L/FiO_2 tables (6 vs. 20 and 13%, respectively; $p < 0.01$) (**Figure 1**).

DISCUSSION

Personalized PEEP guided by EIT, with the aim to minimize relative alveolar distention and collapse, was different than PEEP based upon PEEP/FiO_2 or P_L/FiO_2 tables. Although in terms of respiratory mechanics, $PEEP_{EIT}$ did not differ from lower PEEP/FiO_2 table. There were very important individual variations as witnessed by the wide range of limit agreement in Bland-Altman analyses. Therefore, each patient exhibited different lung properties that cannot be ascertained by using global mechanics parameter such as driving or transpulmonary pressures, compliance, or pressure-volume curves. This may explain the negative results of important clinical trials, which compared low vs. high PEEP in ARDS patients (2, 4).

TABLE 1 | Effect of positive end-expiratory pressure (PEEP) settings on respiratory mechanics.

Variable	Lower PaO_2/FiO_2 table	Higher PaO_2/FiO_2 table	P_L/FiO_2 table	$PEEP_{EIT}$
PEEP (cm H_2O)	10 (10 to 14)	17 (16 to 20)	15 (14 to 20)	13 (12 to 14)*#
P_{PLAT} (cm H_2O)	23 (20 to 26)	33 (28 to 38)	29 (24 to 37)	25 (22 to 27)#
Driving Pressure (cm H_2O)	12 (10 to 14)	14 (12 to 18)	13 (11 to 16)	12 (11 to 13)
C_{RS} (mL/cm H_2O)	39 (34 to 48)	30 (24 to 37)	35 (26 to 43)	38 (34 to 45)#
Mechanical Power (J/min)	25.1 (22.7 to 34.3)	34.4 (28.0 to 43.6)	34.1 (26.0 to 40.7)	28.4 (24.4 to 32.0)#
Inspiratory Transpulmonary pressure (cm H_2O)	6.6 (4.3 to 13.5)	17.5 (9.9 to 21.6)	14.7 (9.4 to 18.7)	11.5 (6.4 to 14.3)#
Expiratory Transpulmonary pressure (cm H_2O)	−0.3 (−2.8 to 3.6)	5.0 (2.0 to 8.0)	4.0 (1.5 to 6.5)	1.3 (0.1 to 2.0)#
Silent spaces (%)	18 (10 to 26)	30 (13 to 48)	23 (17 to 35)	16 (9 to 23)#

*$p < 0.05$ $PEEP_{EIT}$ vs. Lower PaO_2/FiO_2 table.
#$p < 0.05$ $PEEP_{EIT}$ vs. Higher PaO_2/FiO_2 and P_L/FiO_2 tables.

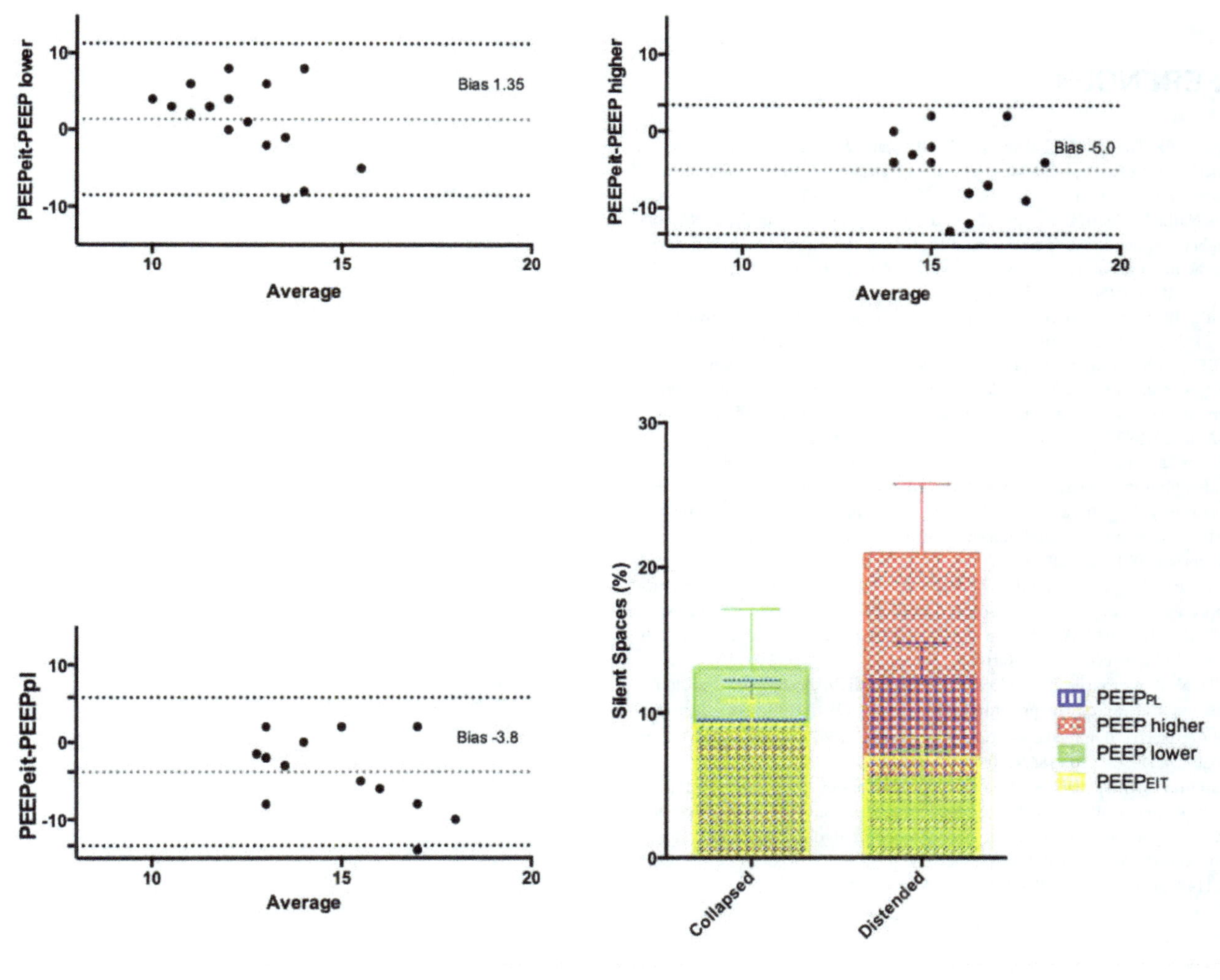

FIGURE 1 | Bland-Altman plots evaluating agreement between PEEP derived from EIT ($PEEP_{EIT}$) and positive end-expiratory pressure (PEEP) values derived from lower and higher $PEEP/FiO_2$ tables and P_L/FiO_2 table. Dotted lines: bias and its 95% confidence interval. Lower right panel: percentages of collapsed and distended lung regions measured by electrical impedance tomography (EIT) under different PEEP settings. Percentage of collapse was lower with $PEEP_{EIT}$ than with lower $PEEP/FiO_2$ table ($p = 0.04$), while percentage cf distended areas was reduced as compared to higher $PEEP/FiO_2$ and P_L/FiO_2 tables ($p < 0.01$).

Several other recent studies evaluated EIT-guided PEEP titration. Van der Zee et al. (5) and Sella et al. (6) have compared $PEEP_{EIT}$ vs. $PEEP/FiO_2$ tables in each of the 15 cases of COVID-19-related ARDS patients. In both studies, PEEP values differed with important individual variations. Interestingly, $PEEP_{EIT}$ was lower (12 cmH_2O) in the Sella study than in the

Van der Zee's (21 cm H_2O). This highlights the huge variability between patients with ARDS, depending on weight, age, sex, or duration of mechanical ventilation.

When comparing $PEEP_{EIT}$ and P_L/FiO_2 table, Scaramuzzo et al. (7), in 20 patients under non-COVID-19 ARDS, found no correlation between the values given by the 2 techniques. As in our study, $PEEP_{EIT}$ achieved a more homogenous distribution of ventilation.

Our work has several limitations. First, we only included patients with COVID-19. Whether these patients behaved similarly to those suffering from non-COVID-19 ARDS in terms of respiratory mechanics is still matter of debate. Second, most of our patients were over-weighted. Hence, this may have contributed to the low agreement between techniques. Finally, only 17 patients have been enrolled, precluding any generalization. However, each patient was its own control, and we just wanted to underline the poor agreement between routinely used techniques at the patient level.

The use of EIT allows for a personalized PEEP titration with the aim to minimize the total amount of pulmonary silent spaces. Whether this approach could translate in outcome improvement remains to be investigated.

AUTHOR CONTRIBUTIONS

SG designed the study, collected and analyzed data, and wrote the manuscript. MC, GC, and AC collected and analyzed data. All authors read and approved the manuscript.

REFERENCES

1. Sahetya SK, Golagher EC, Brower RG. Fifty years of research inn ARDS. Setting positive end-expiratory pressure in acute respiratory distress syndrome. *Am J Respir Crit Care Med.* (2017) 195:1429–38. doi: 10.1164/rccm.201610-2035CI
2. The National Heart, Lung, and Blood Institute ARDS Clinical Trials Network. Higher versus lower positive end-expiratory pressures in patients with the acute respiratory distress syndrome. *N Engl J Med.* (2004). 351:327–36. doi: 10.1056/NEJMoa032193
3. Beitler JR, Sarge T, Banner-Goodspeed VM, Gong MN, Cook D, Novack V, et al. EPVent-2 study group: effect of titrating positive end-expiratory pressure (PEEP) with an esophageal pressure-guided strategy vs an empirical high PEEP-FiO_2 strategy on death and days free from mechanical ventilation among patients with acute respiratory distress syndrome: a randomized clinical trial. *JAMA.* (2019) 321:846–57. doi: 10.1001/jama.2019.0555
4. Mercat A, Richard JC, Vielle B, Jaber S, Osman D, Diehl JL, et al. End-expiratory pressure (Express) study group. Positive end-expiratory pressure setting in adults with acute lung injury and acute respiratory distress syndrome: a randomized controlled trial. *JAMA.* (2008) 299:646–55. doi: 10.1001/jama.299.6.646
5. van der Zee P, Somhorst P, Endemann H, Gommers D. Electrical impedance tomography for positive end-expiratory pressure titration in COVID-19 related ARDS. *Am J Respir Crit Care Med.* (2020) 202:280–4. doi: 10.1164/rccm.202003-0816LE
6. Sella N, Zarantonello F, Andreatta G, Gagliardi V, Boscolo A, Navalesi P. Positive end-expiratory pressure titration in COVID-19 acute respiratory failure: electrical impedance tomography vs. PEEP/FiO_2 tables. *Crit Care.* (2020) 24:540. doi: 10.1186/s13054-020-03242-5
7. Scaramuzzo G, Spadaro S, Dalla Corte F, Waldmann AD, Böhm SH, Ragazzi R, et al. Personalized positive end-expiratory pressure in acute respiratory distress syndrome: Comparison between optimal distribution of regional ventilation and positive transpulmonary pressure. *Crit Care Med.* (2020) 48:1148–56. doi: 10.1097/CCM.0000000000004439

11

Methods of Weaning from Mechanical Ventilation in Adult

Hong-Jie Jhou [1,2†], *Po-Huang Chen* [3,4†], *Liang-Jun Ou-Yang* [5], *Chin Lin* [6,7], *Shih-En Tang* [8,9*] *and Cho-Hao Lee* [10*]

[1] Department of Neurology, Changhua Christian Hospital, Changhua, Taiwan, [2] School of Medicine, Kaohsiung Medical University, Kaohsiung, Taiwan, [3] Department of General Medicine, National Defense Medical Center, Tri-Service General Hospital, Taipei, Taiwan, [4] Department of Internal Medicine, National Defense Medical Center, Tri-Service General Hospital, Taipei, Taiwan, [5] Department of Physical Medicine and Rehabilitation, Chang Gung Memorial Hospital, Taoyuan, Taiwan, [6] School of Public Health, National Defense Medical Center, Taipei, Taiwan, [7] Department of Research and Development, National Defense Medical Center, Taipei, Taiwan, [8] Division of Pulmonary and Critical Care Medicine, Department of Internal Medicine, National Defense Medical Center, Tri-Service General Hospital, Taipei, Taiwan, [9] National Defense Medical Center, Graduate Institute of Aerospace and Undersea Medicine, Taipei, Taiwan, [10] Division of Hematology and Oncology Medicine, Department of Internal Medicine, National Defense Medical Center, Tri-Service General Hospital, Taipei, Taiwan

***Correspondence:**
Shih-En Tang
msetang@gmail.com
Cho-Hao Lee
drleechohao@gmail.com

† These authors have contributed equally to this work and share first authorship

Background/Objective: The aim of study is to assess the efficacy of each ventilator weaning method for ventilated patients in intensive care units (ICUs).

Methods: A systematic search was conducted using PubMed, Embase, and China National Knowledge Infrastructure to identify randomized control studies on ventilated patients regarding extubation associated outcomes (weaning success or failure, proportion requiring re-intubation, or mortality) from inception until April 01, 2020. Commonly used ventilation modes involved pressure support ventilation, synchronized intermittent mandatory ventilation, automatic tube compensation, continuous positive airway pressure, adaptive support ventilation, neurally adjusted ventilatory assist, proportional assisted ventilation, and SmartCare. Pooled estimates regarding extubation associated outcomes were calculated using network meta-analysis.

Results: Thirty-nine randomized controlled trials including 5,953 patients met inclusion criteria. SmartCare and proportional assist ventilation were found to be effective methods in increasing weaning success (odds ratio, 2.72, 95% confidence interval (CI), 1.33–5.58, *P*-score: 0.84; odds ratio, 2.56, 95% CI, 1.60–4.11, *P*-score: 0.83; respectively). Besides, proportional assist ventilation had superior in reducing proportion requiring re-intubation rate (odds ratio, 0.48, 95% CI, 0.25–0.92, *P*-score: 0.89) and mortality (odds ratio, 0.48, 95% CI, 0.26–0.92, *P*-score: 0.91) than others.

Conclusion: In general consideration, our study provided evidence that weaning with proportional assist ventilation has a high probability of being the most effective ventilation mode for patients with mechanical ventilation regarding a higher rate of weaning success, a lower proportion requiring reintubation, and a lower mortality rate than other ventilation modes.

Keywords: systemic review, network meta-analysis, weaning, T-piece, proportional assist ventilation, SmartCare

INTRODUCTION

The most common cause of vital organ failure was acute respiratory failure in critically ill patients. It was estimated that 40–65% of patients in intensive care units (ICUs) needed mechanical ventilation (1), which provided adequate oxygen and reduced the work of breathing for patients with respiratory failure of different etiologies (2). However, there were several complications associated with mechanical ventilation, such as initiating lung injury, ventilator-associated pneumonia (3), and respiratory muscle weakness (4).

Successful and timely weaning of patients from mechanical ventilation could shorten the duration of the ventilation and reduce infection risk, medical costs, and mortality. Some evidence showed that delay weaning might cause unnecessary discomfort, increase complication rates, and result to higher medical costs (5, 6). Even in scheduled extubated patients, up to one-third of patients needed reintubation because of extubation failure (7, 8). Reintubation was associated with high mortality due to new complications (9).

A spontaneous breathing trial (SBT) was the most common method to evaluate the ability of a patient to self-breathing and provided important clinical information for weaning. According to the American Thoracic Society Clinical Practice Guidelines on weaning and extubation (10, 11), an initial SBT was weakly recommended for weaning. PSV and T-piece for SBT in adults were commonly used modes for the liberation process. In a Cochrane review (12), Ladeira et al. found non-significant differences between the pressure support and T-piece modes regarding weaning success, pneumonia, reintubation, ICU mortality, and length of hospital stay.

Closed-loop weaning systems, an automatic system using physiological feedback signal to adjust the process of weaning, may facilitate systematic and early identification of spontaneous breathing ability and the potential for ventilation discontinuation through continuous monitoring and real-time interventions. The concept of closed-loop weaning systems is not new; however, with advanced technology from academia and industry, SmartCare is the first commercial closed-loop systems with intelligent modes in clinical use, and adaptive support ventilation, neurally adjusted ventilatory assist, and proportional assisted ventilation (PAV) have been further developed in recent decades (13). In current studies, closed-loop weaning systems show clinical benefit regarding a reduction of duration of weaning, mechanical ventilation, and length of ICU stay (13, 14).

PAV was first introduced by Younes in 1992 and adjusted the inspiratory pressure in proportion to the flow and volume generated by the patient. New software (PAV+) has been developed based on PAV to adapt to clinical needs through semi-continuous measurements and delivering pressure proportional to the instantaneous inspiratory flow and volume (13, 14). In a meta-analysis (15), PAV+ had benefits of decreasing the rate of weaning failure and the duration of mechanical ventilation in comparison with pressure support ventilation. Another meta-analysis provided the evidence that PAV increases the rate of weaning success, decreases proportion of patients requiring reintubation and the length of ICU stay, but does not reduce the mortality in comparison with pressure support ventilation (16).

Several meta-analyses have evaluated different ventilation modes for weaning; however, no study has presented a head-to-head comparison of the efficacy of different modes for liberation from mechanical ventilation. Therefore, we conducted this network meta-analysis to assess the relative efficacy of each technique with the aim of providing treatment recommendations to physicians in daily clinical practice.

METHODS

We performed this systematic review and network meta-analysis using established guidelines from the Preferred Reporting Items for Systematic Reviews and Meta-Analyses for Network Meta-Analyses (PRISMA-NMA) (17, 18) (**Supplementary Table 1**). The review protocol was registered in the Open Science Framework (OSF, protocol available at https://osf.io/fs8ze).

Data Sources and Search Strategy

We performed a comprehensive search without language restrictions using PubMed, Embase, and China National Knowledge Infrastructure (https://www.cnki.net) from inception until April 01, 2020. The goal was to identify all relevant trials while screening the titles and reviewing the abstracts. To ensure that no randomized controlled trials were missing, gray literature (conference abstracts and doctoral theses) were searched, and the reference lists of included articles were reviewed. Further ongoing trials were searched using Google Scholar, and the US Government Clinical Trials Database (www.ClinicalTrials.gov). The search terms comprised "Ventilation Weaning," "T-piece," "Pressure Support Ventilation," "Synchronized Intermittent Mandatory Ventilation," "Automatic Tube Compensation," "Continuous Positive Airway Pressure," "Adaptive Support Ventilation," "Neurally Adjusted Ventilatory Assist," "Proportional Assisted Ventilation," and "SmartCare," along with a list of all interventions and possibly relevant key words (**Supplementary Table 2**).

Study Selection

We included randomized control studies on mechanically ventilated adults (at least 18 years of age) that reported at least one of extubation associated outcomes (weaning success or failure, proportion requiring re-intubation, or mortality) with respiratory failure of various etiologies and received invasive mechanical ventilation (MV) for at least 24 h. The comparison included two or more ventilation modes for weaning. We excluded trials that evaluated neonatal or pediatrics subjects, enrolled extubated patients directly to non-invasive ventilation for weaning, compared without controls or same ventilation mode but different parameters.

Two authors (HJJ, LJOY) independently selected trials that met the inclusion criteria, and another author (PHC) adjudicated differences. In the case of disagreement, the same authors consulted with another author (CHL) to obtain decisions after group discussion.

Data Extraction and Bias Assessment

Two reviewers (HJJ and PHC) independently assessed the eligibility of identified citations and extracted data. Data extraction was performed with a form to capture information regarding study, participants, and treatment characteristics. We contacted the corresponding authors for missing data (**Supplementary Table 3**).

The same authors independently appraised each study using the Cochrane Risk of Bias (RoB) tool (**Supplementary Figure 1**) (19). We produced RoB graphs using the software Review Manager 5.3 (20). Discrepancies were resolved by consensus in consultation with a third reviewer (CHL) or deliberation through group discussion.

Outcome Measures

1. Weaning success: the absence of the requirement for invasive mechanical ventilation support, without cardiac arrest events, or mortality for 48 h after the extubation (translaryngeal tube) or withdrawal (tracheostomy tube), or as defined by the study authors (**Supplementary Table 4**).
2. The proportion requiring reintubation: the patient requiring reintubation in 48 h after extubation or as defined by the study authors.
3. All-cause mortality: hospital mortality or as defined by the study authors.

Data Synthesis and Statistical Analysis

We performed the network meta-analysis using a frequentist approach and provided a point estimated using a 95% confidence interval (CI) with the frequency distribution. All network meta-analyses were done with the statistical package "netmeta" in R 3.4.2 (R Core Team, Vienna, Austria) and Stata version 16 (Stata Corp, College Station, Texas, USA). We examined the symmetry and geometry of the evidence by producing a network plot with nodes for the number of study subjects and connection size corresponding to the number of studies. The estimation of mixed estimate of the network summary effects was calculated using the combination of the direct and indirect treatment effect and comprised network structure (**Supplementary Figure 2**) (21). For the dichotomous variables, we produced the pooled odds ratio (OR) with 95% CIs to summarize the effects of each comparison tested using a random-effects model (22), allowed for across studies variation.

The probability of a mode being ranked was calculated as its surface under the cumulative ranking curve (SUCRA) in frequentist framework, which is the percentage of efficacy achieved by an approach compared with an imaginary approach that is always the best without uncertainty (i.e., SUCRA = 100%). SUCRA provides a hierarchy of treatments and accounts for the variance of all relative intervention effects (23–25). In the frequentist model, *P*-score is an interpretation analogous to the SUCRA and measures certainty of whether a treatment is better than another treatment. Higher *P*-score scores correspond to a greater weaning success rate, lower proportion requiring reintubation and lower mortality (26).

Forest plots summarized relative mean effects, 95% CIs, and *P*-score for all comparisons together (27). The *P*-score results were summarized in a rank-heat plot (28). We used a multivariate random-effects meta-regression with a consistency model by White et al. (29). We assessed potential inconsistencies by comparing deviance and deviance estimates for each comparison between consistency and inconsistency using a random-effects design-by-treatment interaction model (30, 31) and the node-splitting technique (32, 33). Statistical significance was set at 5% for both analyses.

Network transitivity was examined by visually inspecting tables with study-related characteristics that may modify treatment effects, including differences in patient characteristics, study designs, details of the intervention, and differences in measurements of the outcome. Sensitivity analyses were performed to examine the validity of study findings (34). Subgroup analyses were conducted based on the following effect modifiers: endotracheal prosthesis defined as the methods for attaching to a ventilator such as ventilation through endotracheal tube or tracheostomy, publication year before and after 2008 which was the first published randomized control trial of PAV for weaning, and patients with COPD.

We evaluated whether treatment effects for the outcomes were robust and examined the relationship using random-effect network meta-regression with study characteristics. Comparison-adjusted funnel plots and Egger's test were also used to assess publication bias or other small study effects for available interventions (23). The quality of evidence derived from the GRADE framework. (35, 36) (**Supplementary Table 5**).

RESULTS

Systematic Literature Review

Totally, 39 articles met our inclusion criteria in our study. The studies regarding neurally adjusted ventilatory assist were excluded because of no adequate information. **Figure 1** showed the flowchart. The 39 trials (37–75) investigated a total of 5,953 participants who were randomized into the following interventions: adaptive support ventilation (ASV), automatic tube compensation (ATC), continuous positive airway pressure (CPAP), PAV (including PAV plus mode), pressure support ventilation (PSV), SmartCare, synchronized intermittent mandatory ventilation (SIMV), and the T-piece.

Study characteristics was summarized in **Supplementary Table 3**. The studies were with sample sizes ranging from 23 to 1,153 patients. There were 62.8% males. The mean age of subjects was 62.1 years old (standard deviation (SD): 8.0 years old), and the mean mechanical ventilation duration prior to randomization was 5.4 days (SD: 3.2 days). The mean Acute Physiology and Chronic Health Evaluation II score was 19.8 (SD: 5.6).

Result of Weaning Success

There were 36 studies (5,008 patients; 8 treatment nodes) regarding the weaning success with maintained transitivity (**Figure 2A**). **Figure 3A** presented the results of weaning success, in which the T-piece was used as a comparator. PAV and SmartCare had a significantly better weaning success

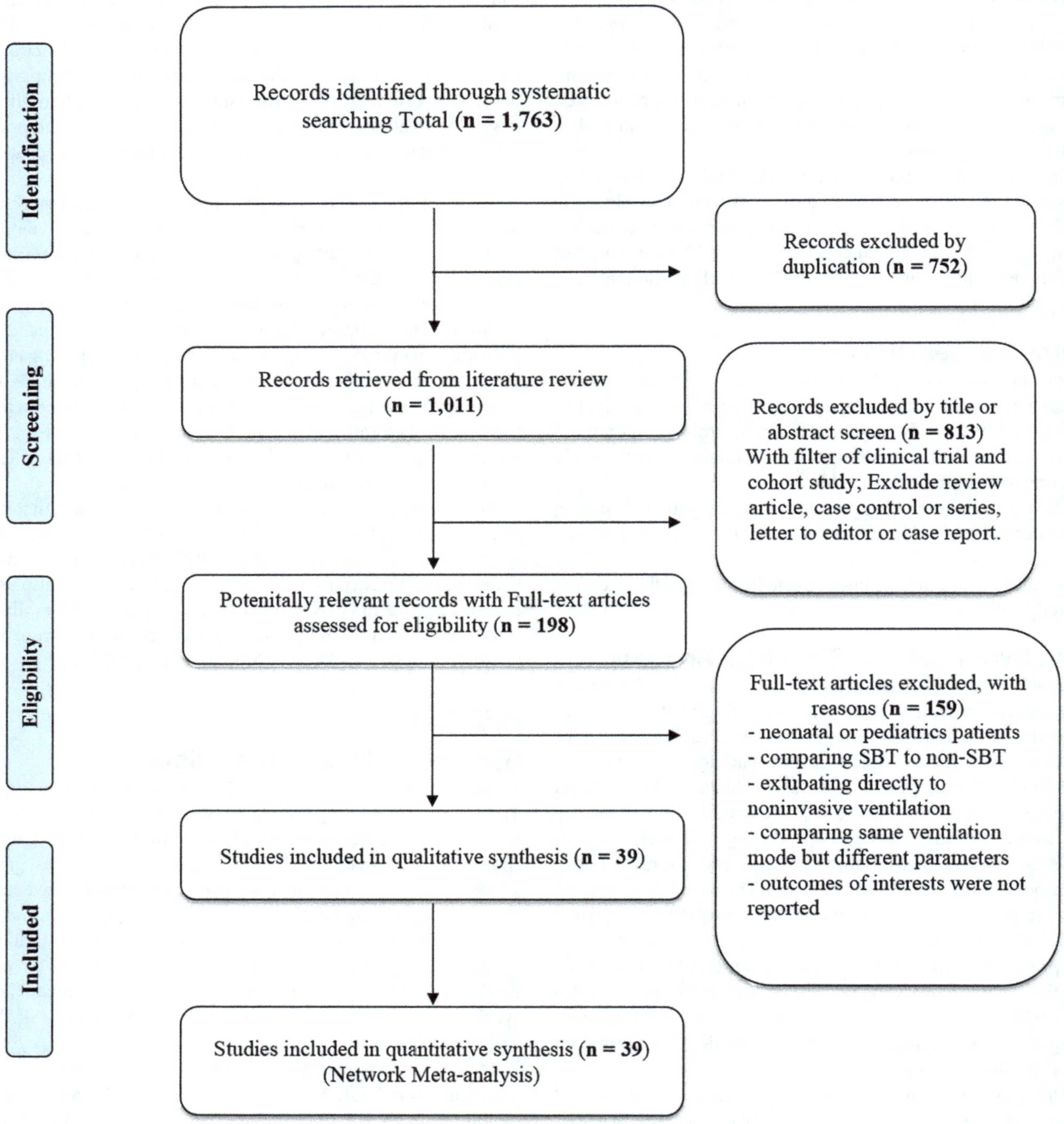

FIGURE 1 | PRISMA flow diagram of included studies.

rate (PAV: OR, 2.56; 95% CI, 1.60–4.11, P-score: 0.83; SmartCare: OR, 2.72; 95% CI, 1.33–5.58, P-score: 0.84; **Figure 4**). **Supplementary Table 6** shows details of the head-to-head comparison of outcomes.

In the sensitivity analyses of, the *P*-score rankings were changed. PAV became the first ranking in weaning success after omitting the small trials (<25th percentiles) or excluding the high risk-of-bias studies (**Supplementary Figure 4**). All the subgroup analyses revealed similar results, favoring PAV, including patients with an endotracheal prosthesis type of translaryngeal tube (PAV: OR, 3.12; 95% CI, 1.67–5.82; *P*-score: 0.91) and patients with COPD (PAV: OR, 5.89; 95% CI, 1.31–26.43; P-score: 0.88). In the subgroup of publication years after 2008, PAV and SmartCare had similar efficacy for weaning success (PAV: OR, 2.69; 95% CI, 1.66–4.37, P-score: 0.84; SmartCare: OR, 2.91; 95% CI, 1.29–6.54, P-score: 0.85; **Supplementary Figure 4**).

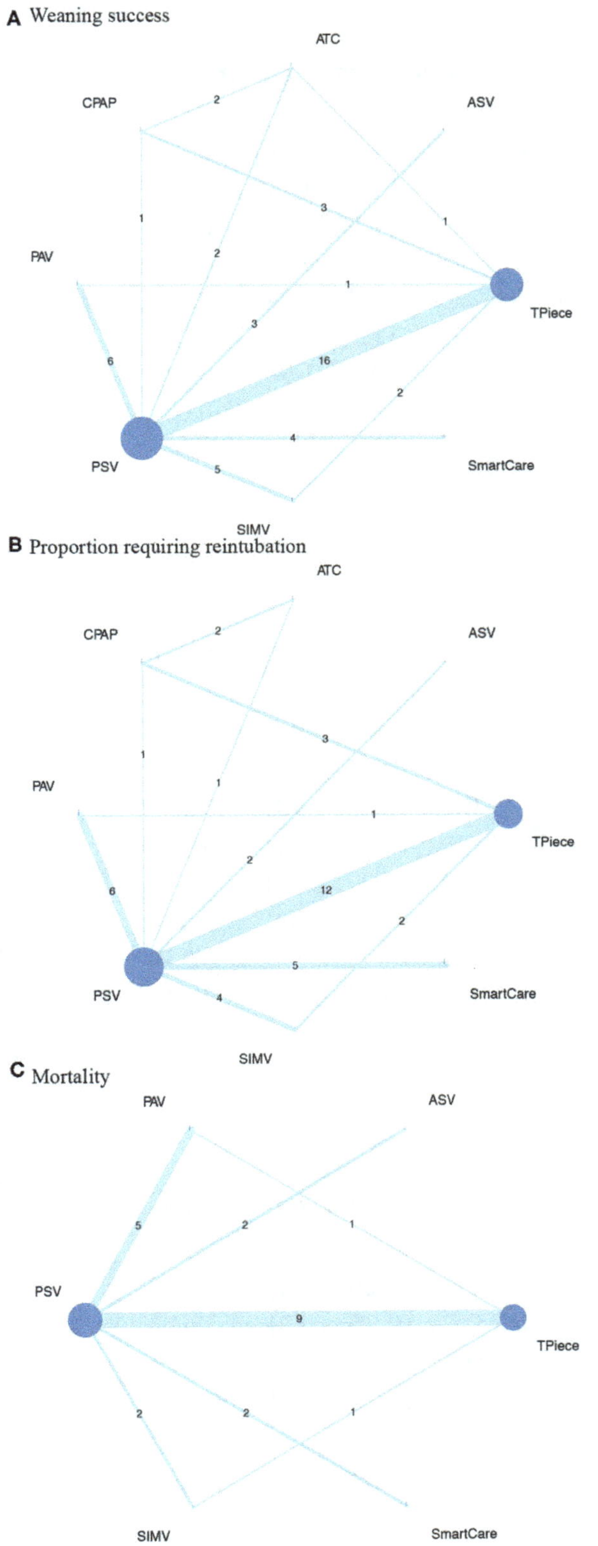

FIGURE 2 | Network plot of comparisons in **(A)**, weaning success **(B)**, proportion requiring reintubation, and mortality among different ventilator modes **(C)**. ASV, Adaptive support ventilation; ATC, Automatic tube compensation; CPAP, Continuous positive airway pressure; PAV, Proportional assist ventilation; PSV, Pressure support ventilation; SIMV, Synchronized intermittent mandatory ventilation.

Result of Proportion Requiring Reintubation

There were 31 studies (4,644 patients; 8 treatment nodes) regarding the proportion requiring reintubation with maintained transitivity (**Figure 2B**). **Figure 3B** presented the results of the proportion requiring reintubation, in which the T-piece was used as a comparator. PAV had a significantly lower proportion of re-intubation (PAV: OR, 0.48; 95% CI, 0.25–0.92; *P*-score: 0.90) (**Figure 4**). The first ranking of PAV was unchanged in sensitivity analyses. Moreover, PAV was the most highly ranked intervention in all subgroups (**Supplementary Figure 4**).

Result of Mortality

There were 18 studies (3,727 patients; 6 treatment nodes) regarding mortality with maintained transitivity (**Figure 2C**). **Figure 3C** presented the results of mortality rate, in which the T-piece was used as a comparator. PAV was significantly beneficial for mortality (PAV: OR, 0.48; 95% CI, 0.26–0.92; P-score: 0.91) (**Figure 4**). The top ranking of PAV was unchanged in sensitivity analyses. Moreover, PAV was the most highly ranked intervention in all subgroups, but no statistical significance (**Supplementary Figure 4**).

Inconsistency, Meta-Regression Analysis, and Publication Bias

In the design-by-treatment interaction model, there was no evidence of global inconsistency in any outcomes (**Supplementary Table 7**). In the node-splitting model, there was no evidence of substantial statistical inconsistency between direct and indirect evidence except for the proportion requiring reintubation. There was local inconsistency between the comparisons of ATC vs. CPAP, ATC vs. PSV, and CPAP vs. the T-piece.

In the meta-regression analysis, there was no relationship between the intervention outcomes and the study characteristics (**Supplementary Table 8**). In all the outcomes, there was no evidence of potential small-study effects or publication bias according to Egger's test and the comparison-adjusted funnel plots, respectively (**Supplementary Figure 5**).

DISCUSSION

We conducted a systematic review and network meta-analysis to compare the efficacy of different modes for weaning in patients with mechanical ventilation. PAV and SmartCare had a higher ratio for weaning success. Furthermore, PAV ranked as the best intervention for the lowest proportion requiring reintubation and mortality rate comparing mechanical ventilator with any other modes for weaning. Therefore, PAV seemed to be the best weaning mode in our analysis.

The difficulty of weaning was associated with two major parameters: the duration of the weaning and the level of support pressure (76–78). In concerned with latest study (65), patients in the 30-min PSV had a higher rate of weaning success and lower hospital mortality than patients in the 2-h T-piece SBT. There was no difference of the proportion

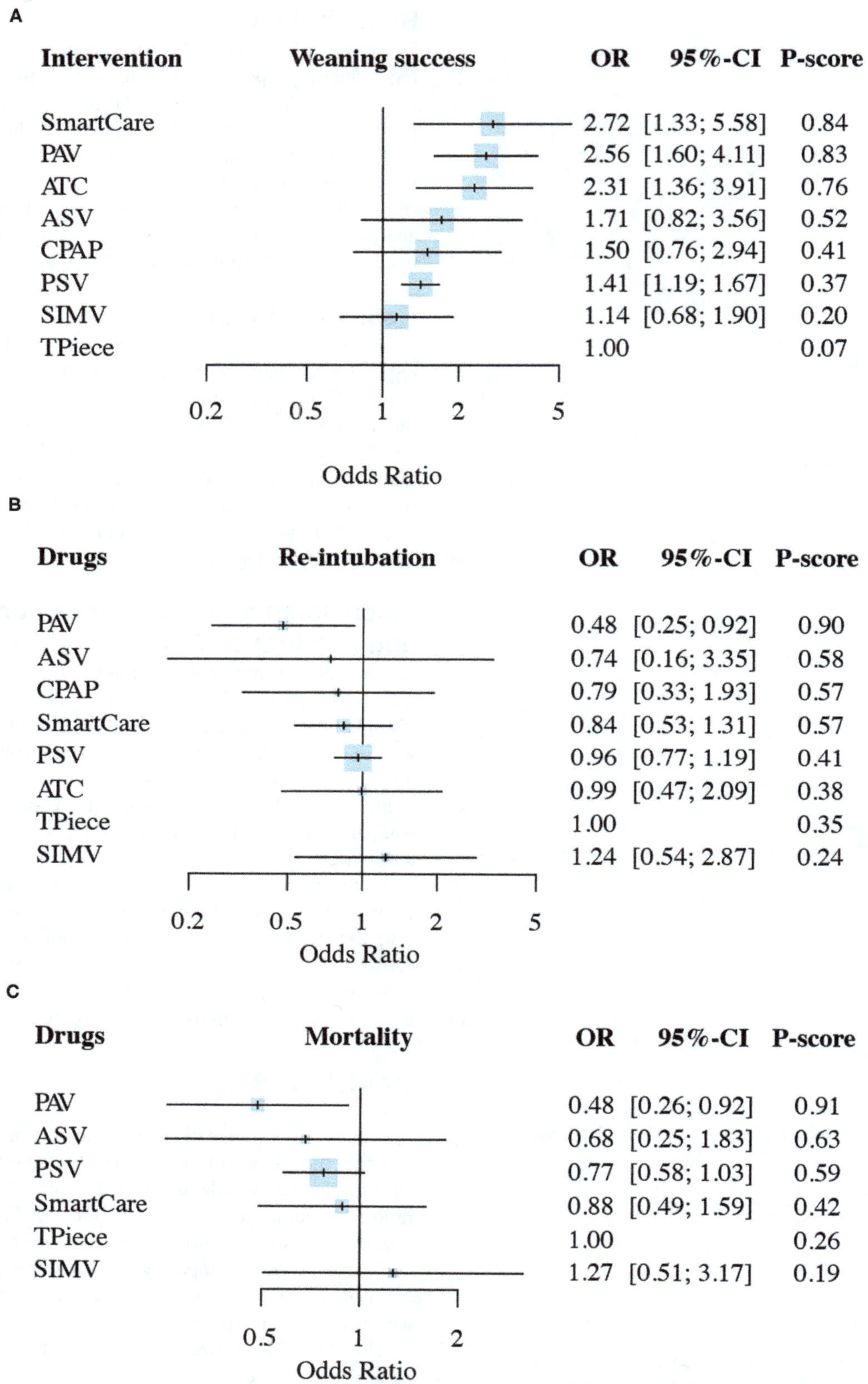

FIGURE 3 | Network meta-analysis results of **(A)**, weaning success **(B)** proportion requiring reintubation, and mortality **(C)**. ASV, Adaptive support ventilation; ATC, Automatic tube compensation; CPAP, Continuous positive airway pressure; PAV, Proportional assist ventilation; PSV, Pressure support ventilation; SIMV, Synchronized intermittent mandatory ventilation; OR, odds ratio; CI, confidence interval.

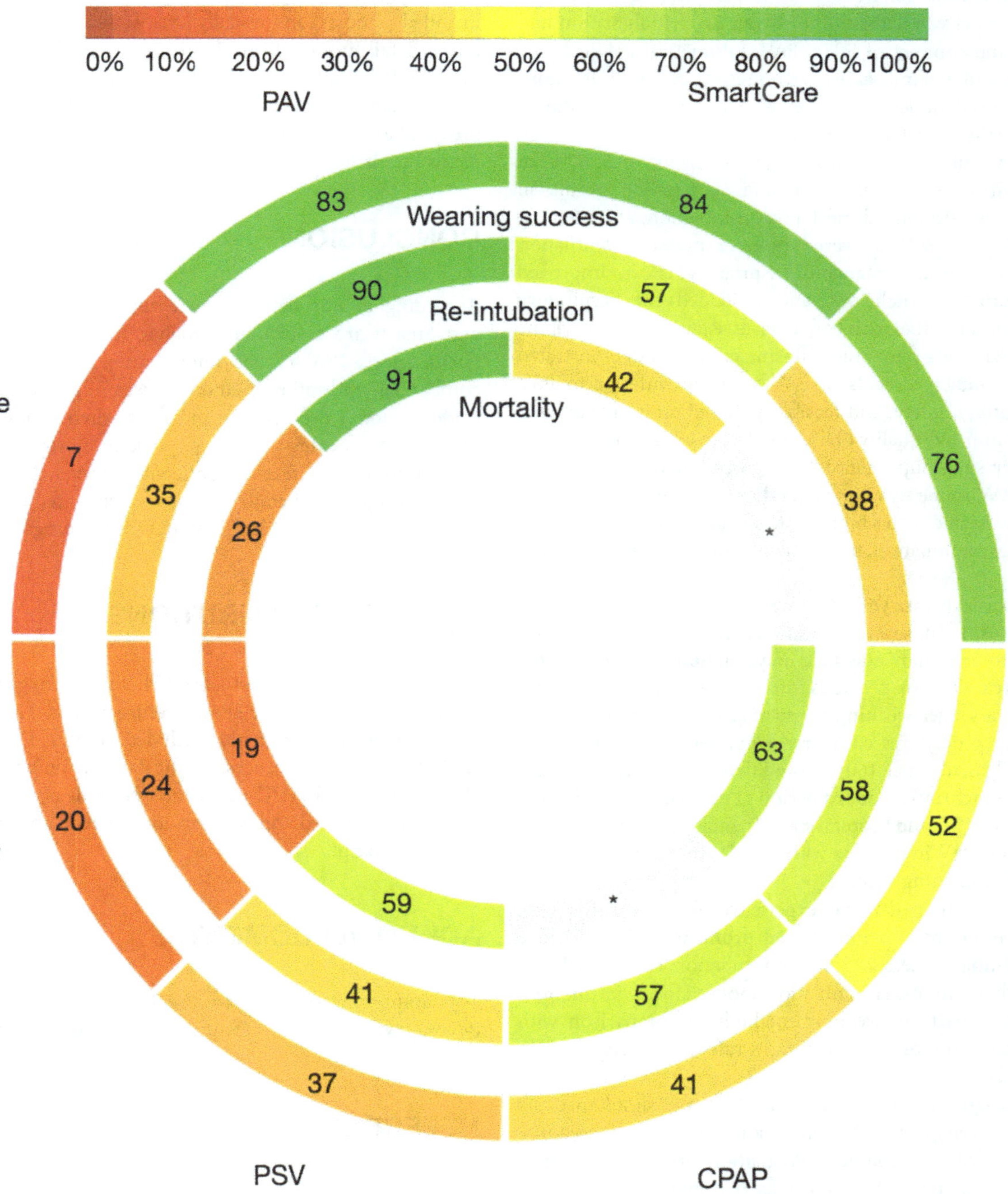

FIGURE 4 | Rank-heat plot of *P*-score values among different ventilator modes targeting outcomes of weaning success, proportion requiring reintubation and mortality. ASV, Adaptive support ventilation; ATC, Automatic tube compensation; CPAP, Continuous positive airway pressure; PAV, Proportional assist ventilation; PSV, Pressure support ventilation; SIMV, Synchronized intermittent mandatory ventilation; OR, odds ratio; CI, confidence interval.

requiring reintubation and tracheotomy rate between these two groups. Similarly, the comparison between PSV and T-piece in our study, PSV increased the rate of weaning success but did not reduce the rates of reintubation and mortality. The T-piece seemed to be more difficult than the PSV because there was no ventilation support for the T-piece.

Weaning can be accomplished by several methods. PSV or T-piece as a period of SBTs remain common methods for weaning. Automated modes of mechanical ventilation achieve synchrony of interaction between patient and ventilator, thereby improving the patient-ventilator relationship with closed-loop control system. ASV is an automated system that adapts inspiratory pressure to achieve a target tidal volume and a desired minimum minute ventilation. SmartCare measures selected respiratory variables, adapts ventilator output by an explicit algorithm and automates the conduct of SBTs. PAV automatically adjusts the flow assist and volume assist to represent constant fractions of the measured values resistance and elasticity of the patient's respiratory system instantaneously (13, 14).

Patient–ventilator asynchrony was seen in ~25–80% of patients with mechanical ventilation and might result in patient distress, prolonged mechanical ventilation, and weaning failure (79, 80). PAV delivered positive pressure ventilation in proportion to instantaneous inspiratory effort, improved patient–ventilator synchrony, and unloaded the respiratory muscles without the risk of over-assistance and periodic breathing (81). In a pilot study, Bosma et al. (55) demonstrated that the weaning protocols of PAV were not inferior to PSV regarding utility, safety, and feasibility. Based on its advantages, PAV might improve quality of life and decreased health care costs (82). In our subgroup analysis of publication years after 2008 when the PAV mode was first applied to weaning, we found that PAV was associated with a higher rate of successful weaning and a lower rate of reintubation, but there was no significant difference in mortality.

COPD was a disease with increasing prevalence and mortality worldwide (83). In severe conditions, mechanical ventilation was used to maintain adequate oxygenation and reduce the work of breathing. In previous studies (84, 85), patients with COPD had a longer weaning phase and a lower success rate of the weaning procedures compared to patients without COPD. However, Elganady et al. (60) showed that PAV was less patient–ventilator asynchrony, reduced period of mechanical ventilation, and shortened ICU and hospital stays. In our study, we found that weaning with PAV in patients with COPD was associated with a higher rate of weaning success.

Despite limited real-world experience about weaning with PAV, our results have demonstrated promising efficacy and a higher weaning success, a lower reintubation rate, and lower mortality than any other ventilation mode. However, due to a paucity of a variety of weaning methods in comparison with PAV, optimization of the weaning strategy was required in further studies.

The strength of this review was that we simultaneously compared seven different ventilation modes for weaning in patients with mechanical ventilation in ICUs using a network meta-analysis. To avoid bias, a comprehensive search, study selection, data extraction, and bias assessment by two reviewers were performed. We produced a rank-heat plot to summarize the results and allowed readers to quickly visualize the highest ranked choice. Besides, inconsistency was properly identified by the node-splitting and design-by-treatment model. Finally, the certainty of evidence was rated by the GRADE approach.

There were several limitations in our study. Firstly, patient population were various cross the studies and it was difficult to separate the individual studies into subgroup analysis to conduct network meta-analysis with more specific aspect. Secondly, the variety of ventilation setting prior to or during weaning might flaw the clinical efficacy; therefore, we summarized the characteristics of included studies in visually inspecting tables to provide more detail information. Lastly, due to the small number of included studies, the results should be interpreted with caution. Despite these limitations, we still hoped our findings provided a rationale for designing future large-scale randomized control trials.

CONCLUSION

According to our network meta-analysis, weaning with PAV and SmartCare results in a higher rate of weaning success. Furthermore, PAV reduce reintubation rate and mortality in comparison with other methods of weaning. We hope that this evidence about the benefits and risks when choosing weaning methods for weaning will help physicians to properly provide the optimal course of actions for patients. However, the further head-to-head randomized control trials are warranted to examine the effects of different ventilation modes for weaning.

AUTHOR CONTRIBUTIONS

H-JJ and L-JO-Y conceptualized the research goals, planned the analyses, and guided the literature review. H-JJ and P-HC extracted the data from the included studies. P-HC, CL, and C-HL participated in processing the data and doing the statistical analysis. H-JJ and P-HC wrote the first draft of the paper. S-ET and C-HL reviewed and edit. All authors read and approved the final manuscript.

ACKNOWLEDGMENTS

The authors would like to thank UNIVERSAL LINK CO. (www.service-top1.com) for the English language review.

REFERENCES

1. Linko R, Okkonen M, Pettila V, Perttila J, Parviainen I, Ruokonen E, et al. Acute respiratory failure in intensive care units. FINNALI: a prospective cohort study. *Intensive Care Med.* (2009) 35:1352–61. doi: 10.1007/s00134-009-1519-z
2. Coursin Douglas B. Physiological basis of ventilatory support. *Anesthesiology.* (1999) 90:1495–6. doi: 10.1097/00000542-199905000-00049
3. Eggimann P, Pittet D. Infection control in the ICU. *Chest.* (2001) 120:2059–93. doi: 10.1378/chest.120.6.2059
4. Powers SK, Shanely RA, Coombes JS, Koesterer TJ, McKenzie M, Van Gammeren D, et al. Mechanical ventilation results in progressive contractile dysfunction in the diaphragm. *J Appl Physiol.* (1985) 92:1851–8. doi: 10.1152/japplphysiol.00881.2001
5. Esteban A, Anzueto A, Frutos F, Alia I, Brochard L, Stewart TE, et al. Characteristics and outcomes in adult patients receiving mechanical ventilation: a 28-day international study. *JAMA.* (2002) 287:345–55. doi: 10.1001/jama.287.3.345

6. Cooper LM, Linde-Zwirble WT. Medicare intensive care unit use: analysis of incidence, cost, and payment. *Crit Care Med.* (2004) 32:2247–53. doi: 10.1097/01.CCM.0000146301.47334.BD
7. Frutos-Vivar F, Esteban A, Apezteguia C, Gonzalez M, Arabi Y, Restrepo MI, et al. Outcome of reintubated patients after scheduled extubation. *J Crit Care.* (2011) 26:502–9. doi: 10.1016/j.jcrc.2010.12.015
8. Jaber S, Quintard H, Cinotti R, Asehnoune K, Arnal JM, Guitton C, et al. Risk factors and outcomes for airway failure versus non-airway failure in the intensive care unit: a multicenter observational study of 1514 extubation procedures. *Crit Care.* (2018) 22:236. doi: 10.1186/s13054-018-2150-6
9. Bittner EA, Schmidt UH. Tracheal reintubation: caused by "too much of a good thing"? *Respir Care.* (2012) 57:1687–91. doi: 10.4187/respcare.02082
10. Schmidt GA, Girard TD, Kress JP, Morris PE, Ouellette DR, Alhazzani W, et al. Liberation from mechanical ventilation in critically ill adults: executive summary of an Official American College of Chest Physicians/American Thoracic Society Clinical Practice Guideline. *Chest.* (2017) 151:160–5. doi: 10.1016/j.chest.2016.10.036
11. Girard TD, Alhazzani W, Kress JP, Ouellette DR, Schmidt GA, Truwit JD, et al. An Official American Thoracic Society/American College of Chest Physicians clinical practice guideline: liberation from mechanical ventilation in critically ill adults. Rehabilitation protocols, ventilator liberation protocols, and cuff leak tests. *Am J Respir Crit Care Med.* (2017) 195:120–33. doi: 10.1164/rccm.201610-2075ST
12. Ladeira MT, Vital FM, Andriolo RB, Andriolo BN, Atallah AN, Peccin MS. Pressure support versus T-tube for weaning from mechanical ventilation in adults. *Cochrane Database Syst Rev.* (2014) 2014:Cd006056. doi: 10.1002/14651858.CD006056.pub2
13. Delgado M, Zavala E, Tomas R, Fernandez R. Clinical factors associated with success of proportional assist ventilation in the acute phase of critical illness: pilot study. *Med Intensiva.* (2014) 38:65–72. doi: 10.1016/j.medine.2013.07.003
14. Younes M. Proportional assist ventilation, a new approach to ventilatory support. *Theory Am Rev Respir Dis.* (1992) 145:114–20. doi: 10.1164/ajrccm/145.1.114
15. Kataoka J, Kuriyama A, Norisue Y, Fujitani S. Proportional modes versus pressure support ventilation: a systematic review and meta-analysis. *Ann Intensive Care.* (2018) 8:123. doi: 10.1186/s13613-018-0470-y
16. Ou-Yang LJ, Chen PH, Jhou HJ, Su VY, Lee CH. Proportional assist ventilation versus pressure support ventilation for weaning from mechanical ventilation in adults: a meta-analysis and trial sequential analysis. *Crit Care.* (2020) 24:556. doi: 10.1186/s13054-020-03251-4
17. Hutton B, Salanti G, Caldwell DM, Chaimani A, Schmid CH, Cameron C, et al. The PRISMA extension statement for reporting of systematic reviews incorporating network meta-analyses of health care interventions: checklist and explanations. *Ann Intern Med.* (2015) 162:777–84. doi: 10.7326/M14-2385
18. Shamseer L, Moher D, Clarke M, Ghersi D, Liberati A, Petticrew M, et al. Preferred reporting items for systematic review and meta-analysis protocols (PRISMA-P) 2015: elaboration and explanation. *BMJ.* (2015) 349:g7647. doi: 10.1136/bmj.g7647
19. Higgins JPT TJ, Chandler J, Cumpston M, Li T, Page MJ, Welch VA (editors). *Cochrane Handbook for Systematic Reviews of Interventions version 6.0 (updated July 2019).* Cochrane (2019). Available online at: www.training.cochrane.org/handbook. doi: 10.1002/9781119536604
20. Review Manager (RevMan). *Version 5.3.* Copenhagen: The Nordic Cochrane Centre; The Cochrane Collaboration (2014).
21. Krahn U, Binder H, Konig J, A. graphical tool for locating inconsistency in network meta-analyses. *BMC Med Res Methodol.* (2013) 13:35. doi: 10.1186/1471-2288-13-35
22. DerSimonian R, Laird N. Meta-analysis in clinical trials. *Control Clin Trials.* (1986) 7:177–88. doi: 10.1016/0197-2456(86)90046-2
23. Chaimani A, Higgins JPT, Mavridis D, Spyridonos P, Salanti G. Graphical tools for network meta-analysis in STATA. *PLoS ONE.* (2013) 8:e76654. doi: 10.1371/journal.pone.0076654
24. Jansen JP, Trikalinos T, Cappelleri JC, Daw J, Andes S, Eldessouki R, et al. Indirect treatment comparison/network meta-analysis study questionnaire to assess relevance and credibility to inform health care decision making: an ISPOR-AMCP-NPC Good Practice Task Force report. *Value Health.* (2014) 17:157–73. doi: 10.1016/j.jval.2014.01.004
25. Salanti G, Del Giovane C, Chaimani A, Caldwell DM, Higgins JP. Evaluating the quality of evidence from a network meta-analysis. *PLoS One.* (2014) 9:e99682. doi: 10.1371/journal.pone.0099682
26. Rücker G, Schwarzer G. Ranking treatments in frequentist network meta-analysis works without resampling methods. *BMC Med Res Methodol.* (2015) 15:58. doi: 10.1186/s12874-015-0060-8
27. Jackson D, White IR, Riley RD. Quantifying the impact of between-study heterogeneity in multivariate meta-analyses. *Stat Med.* (2012) 31:3805–20. doi: 10.1002/sim.5453
28. Veroniki AA, Straus SE, Fyraridis A, Tricco AC. The rank-heat plot is a novel way to present the results from a network meta-analysis including multiple outcomes. *J Clin Epidemiol.* (2016) 76:193–9. doi: 10.1016/j.jclinepi.2016.02.016
29. White IR, Barrett JK, Jackson D, Higgins JP. Consistency and inconsistency in network meta-anlysis: model estimation using multivariate meta-regression. *Res Synth Methods.* (2012) 3:111–25. doi: 10.1002/jrsm.1045
30. Dias S, Welton NJ, Sutton AJ, Caldwell DM, Lu G, Ades AE. Evidence synthesis for decision making 4: inconsistency in networks of evidence based on randomized controlled trials. *Med Decis Making.* (2013) 33:641–56. doi: 10.1177/0272989X12455847
31. Higgins JPT, Jackson D, Barrett JK, Lu G, Ades AE, White IR. Consistency and inconsistency in network meta-analysis: concepts and models for multi-arm studies. *Res Synth Methods.* (2012) 3:98–110. doi: 10.1002/jrsm.1044
32. Yu-Kang T. Node-splitting generalized linear mixed models for evaluation of inconsistency in network meta-analysis. *Value Health.* (2016) 19:957–63. doi: 10.1016/j.jval.2016.07.005
33. Dias S, Welton NJ, Caldwell DM, Ades AE. Checking consistency in mixed treatment comparison meta-analysis. *Stat Med.* (2010) 29:932–44. doi: 10.1002/sim.3767
34. Dechartres A, Altman DG, Trinquart L, Boutron I, Ravaud P. Association between analytic strategy and estimates of treatment outcomes in meta-analyses. *JAMA.* (2014) 312:623–30. doi: 10.1001/jama.2014.8166
35. Guyatt G, Oxman AD, Akl EA, Kunz R, Vist G, Brozek J, et al. GRADE guidelines: 1. Introduction-GRADE evidence profiles and summary of findings tables. *J Clin Epidemiol.* (2011) 64:383–94. doi: 10.1016/j.jclinepi.2010.04.026
36. Puhan MA, Schünemann HJ, Murad MH Li T, Brignardello-Petersen R, Singh JA, et al. A GRADE Working Group approach for rating the quality of treatment effect estimates from network meta-analysis. *BMJ.* (2014) 349:g5630. doi: 10.1136/bmj.g5630
37. Brochard L, Rauss A, Benito S, Conti G, Mancebo J, Rekik N, et al. Comparison of three methods of gradual withdrawal from ventilatory support during weaning from mechanical ventilation. *Am J Respir Crit Care Med.* (1994) 150:896–903. doi: 10.1164/ajrccm.150.4.7921460
38. Esteban A, Alia I, Gordo F, Fernandez R, Solsona JF, Vallverdu I, et al. Extubation outcome after spontaneous breathing trials with T-tube or pressure support ventilation. The Spanish Lung Failure Collaborative Group. *Am J Respir Crit Care Med.* (1997) 156:459–65. doi: 10.1164/ajrccm.156.2.9610109
39. Esteban A, Frutos F, Tobin MJ, Alía I, Solsona JF, Valverdu V, et al. A Comparison of Four Methods of Weaning Patients from Mechanical Ventilation. *N Engl J Med.* (1995) 332:345–50. doi: 10.1056/NEJM199502093320601
40. Haberthur C, Mols G, Elsasser S, Bingisser R, Stocker R, Guttmann J. Extubation after breathing trials with automatic tube compensation, T-tube, or pressure support ventilation. *Acta Anaesthesiol Scand.* (2002) 46:973–9. doi: 10.1034/j.1399-6576.2002.460808.x
41. Koh Y, Hong SB, Lim CM, Lee SD, Kim WS, Kim DS, et al. Effect of an additional 1-hour T-piece trial on weaning outcome at minimal pressure support. *J Crit Care.* (2000) 15:41–5. doi: 10.1053/jcrc.2000.7898
42. Koksal GM, Sayilgan C, Sen O, Oz H. The effects of different weaning modes on the endocrine stress response. *Crit Care.* (2004) 8:R31–R4. doi: 10.1186/cc2413
43. Vitacca M, Vianello A, Colombo D, Clini E, Porta R, Bianchi L, et al. Comparison of two methods for weaning patients with chronic obstructive pulmonary disease requiring mechanical ventilation for more than 15 days. *Am J Respir Crit Care Med.* (2001) 164:225–30. doi: 10.1164/ajrccm.164.2.2008160

44. Matic I, Majeric-Kogler V. Comparison of pressure support and T-tube weaning from mechanical ventilation: randomized prospective study. *Croat Med J.* (2004) 45:162–6.
45. Ma YM, Pan L, Liu YN. A comparison of T-tube and pressure support ventilation for programatic extubation. *Biomed Eng Clin Med.* (2005) 5:277–80. Available online at: http://caod.oriprobe.com/articles/9226886/A_comparison_of_T_tube_and_pressure_support_ventilation_for_programati.htm
46. Cohen J, Shapiro M, Grozovski E, Fox B, Lev S, Singer P. Prediction of extubation outcome: a randomised, controlled trial with automatic tube compensation vs. pressure support ventilation. *Crit Care.* (2009) 13:R21. doi: 10.1186/cc7724
47. Cohen JD, Shapiro M, Grozovski E, Lev S, Fisher H, Singer P. Extubation outcome following a spontaneous breathing trial with automatic tube compensation versus continuous positive airway pressure. *Crit Care Med.* (2006) 34:682–6. doi: 10.1097/01.CCM.0000201888.32663.6A
48. Matic I, Danic D, Majeric-Kogler V, Jurjevic M, Mirkovic I, Mrzljak Vucinic N. Chronic obstructive pulmonary disease and weaning of difficult-to-wean patients from mechanical ventilation: randomized prospective study. *Croat Med J.* (2007) 48:51–8.
49. Xirouchaki N, Kondili E, Vaporidi K, Xirouchakis G, Klimathianaki M, Gavriilidis G, et al. Proportional assist ventilation with load-adjustable gain factors in critically ill patients: comparison with pressure support. *Intensive Care Med.* (2008) 34:2026–34. doi: 10.1007/s00134-008-1209-2
50. Deng J-J, Wang Q-L. The comparison of two method to liberation from mechenical ventilation in ICU (ICU zhong liang zhong ji xie tong qi che li mo shi de bi jiao). In: *The Medical Forum.* (Shanxi) (2009).
51. Figueroa-Casas JB, Montoya R, Arzabala A, Connery SM. Comparison between automatic tube compensation and continuous positive airway pressure during spontaneous breathing trials. *Respir Care.* (2010) 55:549–54.
52. He H, Chen Z, Yang C. Comparison of two modes of spontaneous breathing trial for weaning from mechanical ventilation. *JiangXi Med J.* (2010) 45:1167–9. Available online at: https://caod.oriprobe.com/articles/25726429/Comparison_of_two_modes_of_spontanenous_breathing_.htm
53. Li C, Yan C-Z, Wang Z-Y. Comparison of two weaning methods for patients with chronic obstructive pulmonary disease. *J Xinj Med Univ.* (2010) 33. Available online at: http://caod.oriprobe.com/articles/24135407/Comparison_of_two_weaning_methods_for_patients_with_chronic_obstructiv.htm
54. Molina-Saldarriaga FJ, Fonseca-Ruiz NJ, Cuesta-Castro DP, Esteban A, Frutos-Vivar F. Ensayo de respiración espontánea en pacientes con enfermedad pulmonar obstructiva crónica: presión positiva continua de la vía aérea (CPAP) versus Tubo en T. *Med Intens.* (2010) 34:453–8. doi: 10.1016/j.medin.2010.03.007
55. Bosma KJ, Read BA, Bahrgard Nikoo MJ, Jones PM, Priestap FA, Lewis JF, et al. Pilot randomized trial comparing weaning from mechanical ventilation on pressure support versus proportional assist ventilation. *Crit Care Med.* (2016) 44:1098–108. doi: 10.1097/CCM.0000000000001600
56. Botha J, Green C, Carney I, Haji K, Gupta S, Tiruvoipati R. Proportional assist ventilation versus pressure support ventilation in weaning ventilation: a pilot randomised controlled trial. *Crit Care Resusc.* (2018) 20:33–40.
57. Cekmen N, Erdemli O. The comparison of the effects of T-piece and CPAP on hemodynamic parameters, arterial blood gases and success of weaning. *Bratisl Lek Listy.* (2011) 112:512–6.
58. Chen F. COPD huan zhe ji xie tong qi che ji fang fa de lin chuang dui zhao yan jiu. *Med Innov China.* (2012) 28:28–9. Available online at: https://caod.oriprobe.com/articles/45031969/copd_huan_zhe_ji_xie_tong_qi_che_ji_fang_fa_de_lin.htm
59. Chittawatanarat K, Orrapin S, Jitkaroon K, Mueakwan S, Sroison U. An open label randomized controlled trial to compare low level pressure support and t-piece as strategies for discontinuation of mechanical ventilation in a general surgical intensive care unit. *Med Arch.* (2018) 72:51–7. doi: 10.5455/medarh.2018.72.51-57
60. Elganady AA, Beshey BN, Abdelaziz AAH. Proportional assist ventilation versus pressure support ventilation in the weaning of patients with acute exacerbation of chronic obstructive pulmonary disease. *Egypt J Chest Dis Tuber.* (2014) 63:643–50. doi: 10.1016/j.ejcdt.2014.04.001
61. Kirakli C, Ozdemir I, Ucar ZZ, Cimen P, Kepil S, Ozkan SA. Adaptive support ventilation for faster weaning in COPD: a randomised controlled trial. *Eur Respir J.* (2011) 38:774–80. doi: 10.1183/09031936.00081510
62. Mohamed KAE. El Maraghi Sk. Role of adaptive support ventilation in weaning of COPD patients. *Egypt J Chest Dis Tuber.* (2014) 63:449–54. doi: 10.1016/j.ejcdt.2013.12.017
63. Santos Pellegrini JA, Boniatti MM, Boniatti VC, Zigiotto C, Viana MV, Nedel WL, et al. Pressure-support ventilation or T-piece spontaneous breathing trials for patients with chronic obstructive pulmonary disease - A randomized controlled trial. *PLoS ONE.* (2018) 13:e0202404. doi: 10.1371/journal.pone.0202404
64. Sasikumar S, Shanbhag V, Shenoy A, Unnikrishnan R. Comparison of pressure support and proportional assist ventilation with load-adjustable gain factors for weaning from mechanical ventilation in critically ill patients. *Euro Respir J.* (2013) 42:P4926. Available online at: https://www.ers-education.org/lr/show-details/?idP=130196
65. Subira C, Hernandez G, Vazquez A, Rodriguez-Garcia R, Gonzalez-Castro A, Garcia C, et al. Effect of pressure support vs t-piece ventilation strategies during spontaneous breathing trials on successful extubation among patients receiving mechanical ventilation: a randomized clinical trial. *JAMA.* (2019) 321:2175–82. doi: 10.1001/jama.2019.7234
66. Teixeira SN, Osaku EF, Costa CR, Toccolini BF, Costa NL, Candia MF, et al. Comparison of proportional assist ventilation plus, T-tube ventilation, and pressure support ventilation as spontaneous breathing trials for extubation: a randomized study. *Respir Care.* (2015) 60:1527–35. doi: 10.4187/respcare.03915
67. Zhang B, Qin YZ. Comparison of pressure support ventilation and T-piece in determining rapid shallow breathing index in spontaneous breathing trials. *Am J Med Sci.* (2014) 348:300–5. doi: 10.1097/MAJ.0000000000000286
68. Burns KE, Meade MO, Lessard MR, Keenan SP, Lellouche F. Wean Earlier and Automatically with New technology (the WEAN study): a protocol of a multicentre, pilot randomized controlled trial. *Trials.* (2009) 10:81. doi: 10.1186/1745-6215-10-81
69. Jiang H, Yu S, Wang L. Comparison of SmartCare and spontaneous breathing trials for weaning old patients with chronic obstructive pulmonary diseases. *Zhonghua Jie He He Hu Xi Za Zhi.* (2006) 29:545–8.
70. Ma Y, Yang X, Cao X, Ma X. Comparison of computer-driven weaning and physician-directed weaning from mechanical ventilation: a randomized prospective study. *Zhonghua Jie He He Hu Xi Za Zhi.* (2010) 33:174–8.
71. Rose L, Presneill JJ, Johnston L, Cade JF, A. randomised, controlled trial of conventional versus automated weaning from mechanical ventilation using SmartCare/PS. *Intensive Care Med.* (2008) 34:1788–95. doi: 10.1007/s00134-008-1179-4
72. Schadler D, Engel C, Elke G, Pulletz S, Haake N, Frerichs I, et al. Automatic control of pressure support for ventilator weaning in surgical intensive care patients. *Am J Respir Crit Care Med.* (2012) 185:637–44. doi: 10.1164/rccm.201106-1127OC
73. Sulzer CF, Chiolero R, Chassot PG, Mueller XM, Revelly JP. Adaptive support ventilation for fast tracheal extubation after cardiac surgery: a randomized controlled study. *Anesthesiology.* (2001) 95:1339–45. doi: 10.1097/00000542-200112000-00010
74. Taniguchi C, Victor ES, Pieri T, Henn R, Santana C, Giovanetti E, et al. Smart Care versus respiratory physiotherapy-driven manual weaning for critically ill adult patients: a randomized controlled trial. *Crit Care.* (2015) 19:246. doi: 10.1186/s13054-015-0978-6
75. Tong L, Liu Y. Research on measures of weaning from mechanical Ventilation-dependency patients with chronic obstructive pulmonary diseases. *Chin Modern Med.* (2014) 21. Available online at: https://kns.cnki.net/kcms/detail/detail.aspx?dbcode=CJFD&dbname=CJFDLAST2015&filename=ZGUD201433066&uniplatform=NZKPT&v=fBVGTqy8WBKcDVhZPtU7%25mmd2BTIVz3HxsD%25mmd2BjDbygal4PDgZROtMFYP7HWeLsJlB9YAnh
76. Dasta JF, McLaughlin TP, Mody SH, Piech CT. Daily cost of an intensive care unit day: the contribution of mechanical ventilation. *Crit Care Med.* (2005) 33:1266–71. doi: 10.1097/01.CCM.0000164543.14619.00
77. Esteban A, Alia I, Tobin MJ, Gil A, Gordo F, Vallverdu I, et al. Effect of spontaneous breathing trial duration on outcome of attempts to discontinue

mechanical ventilation. Spanish Lung Failure Collaborative Group. *Am J Respir Crit Care Med.* (1999) 159:512–8. doi: 10.1164/ajrccm.159.2.9803106

78. Godard S, Herry C, Westergaard P, Scales N, Brown SM, Burns K, et al. Practice variation in spontaneous breathing trial performance and reporting. *Can Respir J.* (2016) 2016:9848942. doi: 10.1155/2016/9848942
79. Thille AW, Rodriguez P, Cabello B, Lellouche F, Brochard L. Patient-ventilator asynchrony during assisted mechanical ventilation. *Intensive Care Med.* (2006) 32:1515–22. doi: 10.1007/s00134-006-0301-8
80. Purro A, Appendini L, De Gaetano A, Gudjonsdottir M, Donner CF, Rossi A. Physiologic determinants of ventilator dependence in long-term mechanically ventilated patients. *Am J Respir Crit Care Med.* (2000) 161:1115–23. doi: 10.1164/ajrccm.161.4.9812160
81. Alexopoulou C, Kondili E, Plataki M, Georgopoulos D. Patient-ventilator synchrony and sleep quality with proportional assist and pressure support ventilation. *Intensive Care Med.* (2013) 39:1040–7. doi: 10.1007/s00134-013-2850-y
82. Saunders R, Geogopoulos D. Evaluating the cost-effectiveness of proportional-assist ventilation plus vs. Pressure support ventilation in the intensive care unit in two countries. *Front Public Health.* (2018) 6:168. doi: 10.3389/fpubh.2018.00168
83. Vestbo J, Hurd SS, Agusti AG, Jones PW, Vogelmeier C, Anzueto A, et al. Global strategy for the diagnosis, management, and prevention of chronic obstructive pulmonary disease: GOLD executive summary. *Am J Respir Crit Care Med.* (2013) 187:347–65. doi: 10.1164/rccm.201204-0596PP
84. Lemaire F. Difficult weaning. *Intensive Care Med.* (1993) 19:S69–73. doi: 10.1007/BF01708804
85. Esteban A, Alia I, Ibanez J, Benito S, Tobin MJ. Modes of mechanical ventilation and weaning. A national survey of Spanish hospitals. The Spanish Lung Failure Collaborative Group. *Chest.* (1994) 106:1188–93. doi: 10.1378/chest.106.4.1188

12

Surfactant Therapy for Respiratory Distress Syndrome in High- and Ultra-High-Altitude Settings

Xudong Duan[1,2], Jiujun Li[1,2], Long Chen[3], Yuan Shi[3], Xianyang Chen[4,5], Teng Xue[5,6], Chongde Liu[7], Xiaorong Wang[7], Quanfang Qiu[8], Zhen Yu[8], Bacuozhen Qiang[8], Hong Wu[9], Tianqi Wu[9], Lihong Zhang[10], Zhangsheng Chen[11], Dobje Jigme[12], Aili Xu[13], Zhuoga Mima[13], Zhen Da[14], Min Ren[14], Deji Gesang[15], Zhaxi Pubu[15], Chun Li[16], Yanchao Lv[16], Haoquan Zhou[17,18], Xue Zhang[17,18], Zhuoma Dawa[19], Wujin Gongjue[19], Li Wang[20], Li Wu[20] and Xuelian Li[20]*

[1] Department of Pediatrics, Shengjing Hospital of China Medical University, Shenyang, China, [2] Plateau Medical Research Center of China Medical University, Shenyang, China, [3] Department of Neonatology, Children's Hospital Affiliated Chongqing Medical University, Chongqing, China, [4] BaoFeng Key Laboratory of Genetics and Metabolism, Beijing, China, [5] Zhongguancun Biological and Medical Big Data Center, Beijing, China, [6] Zhongyuanborui (Hengqin, Zhuhai) Key Laboratory of Genetics and Metabolism, Zhuhai, China, [7] Department of Neonatology, Qinghai Women and Children's Hospital, Xining, China, [8] Department of Pediatrics, Lhasa People's Hospital, Lhasa, China, [9] Department of Pediatrics, People's Hospital of Tibet, Tibet, China, [10] Department of Pediatrics, Linzhi People's Hospital, Tibet, China, [11] Center of Pediatrics, Zhujiang Hospital, Southern Medical University, Guangzhou, China, [12] Department of Pediatrics, Naqu People's Hospital, Tibet, China, [13] Department of Pediatrics, Shigatse People's Hospital, Tibet, China, [14] Department of Pediatrics, Second People's Hospital of Tibet, Tibet, China, [15] Department of Pediatrics, Shannan People's Hospital, Tibet, China, [16] Department of Pediatrics, Changdu People's Hospital, Tibet, China, [17] Department of Pediatrics, The First Affiliated Hospital of University of Science and Technology of China, Hefei, China, [18] Division of Life Science and Medicine, University of Science and Technology of China, Hefei, China, [19] Department of Pediatrics, People's Hospital of Ali District, Tibet, China, [20] Department of Pediatrics, Daping Hospital, Third Military Medical University, Chongqing, China

***Correspondence:**
Jiujun Li
lijj@sj-hospital.org

Objective: The objective of this study is to investigate the therapeutic effect of surfactant replacement therapy (SRT) on respiratory distress syndrome (RDS) in premature infants in the Qinghai-Tibet Plateau.

Materials and Methods: This multi-center retrospective cohort study collected and screened reasonable clinical data of 337 premature infants with RDS from 10 hospitals in the Qinghai-Tibet Plateau from 2015 to 2017. We grouped the cases by rationally analyzing their baseline characteristics, using logistic analysis to evaluate each factor's effect on the prognosis of the infants, and comparing the short-term improvement in blood gas and mortality after SRT treatment at different altitudes, in high-altitude (1,500–3,500 m) and ultra-high-altitude (3,500–5,500 m) groups.

Results: Independent of altitude, the mortality rate of children with RDS in the SRT group was significantly lower than that of children in the non-SRT group (both $P < 0.05$). The effect of SRT on preterm infants with RDS in the high-altitude group [odds ratio (OR) = 0.44, 95% confidence interval (CI) = 0.22–0.87, $P = 0.02$] was better than that in the infants in the ultra-high-altitude group (OR = 0.26, 95% CI = 0.13–0.58, $P < 0.01$), with death rates of 34.34 and 49.71%, respectively.

Similarly, after SRT, the improvement of PaO_2/FiO_2 and pH of children at high altitude was significantly better than those of children at ultra-high altitude (all $P < 0.01$).

Conclusions: SRT plays a prominent role in curing infants with RDS in both high- and ultra-high-altitude regions, although with better effects at high rather than ultra-high altitude. This study provides a basis for further large-scale studies on SRT for RDS treatment at high altitudes.

Keywords: high-altitude, ultra-high-altitude, surfactant replacement therapy, respiratory distress syndrome, premature infants, logistic regression

INTRODUCTION

Respiratory distress syndrome (RDS) due to surfactant deficiency is a major cause of morbidity and mortality due to respiratory failure in newborn infants, especially those born prematurely (1, 2). Since the 1990s, surfactant replacement therapy (SRT) has been effective in treating RDS (3) and has been confirmed to effectively reduce RDS-related mortality, pneumothorax incidence, and the risk of chronic lung disease (4–8). Nowadays, SRT is part of the core treatment strategy for RDS, which can prevent the collapse of alveoli and increase lung compliance, thereby improving survival and reducing respiratory morbidities (9). Additionally, the development of neonatal care and less-invasive methods of surfactant delivery has further promoted the widespread clinical use of SRT (10, 11).

High-altitude regions are regions at an altitude >1,500 m; globally, about 2% of the population lives in these regions (12). Additionally, three altitude regions can be defined according to the Society of Mountain Medicine: high altitude (1,500–3,500 m above sea level), ultra-high altitude (3,500–5,500 m above sea level), and extreme altitude (above 5,500 m above sea level) (13). In high-altitude regions, due to gravity, with increasing altitude, the atmospheric pressure decreases. While the proportion of oxygen in the atmosphere remains unchanged, the oxygen partial pressure and, hence, the driving pressure for gas exchange in the lungs decrease, and a hypoxic environment is formed (14). This determines the uniqueness of various pulmonary diseases and their therapy in high-altitude regions.

Since the 20th century, in the Qinghai-Tibet Plateau, SRT has been used in the therapy of neonatal RDS. Recently, as medical technology gradually developed in high-altitude regions, the use of technologies such as ventilation support has increased as well. Additionally, in high-altitude areas, mechanical ventilation has been shown to effectively improve the arterial partial oxygen pressure in newborns with RDS and reduce their mortality (15). However, most clinical research data on SRT treatment for RDS so far comes from plain or hilly areas, and relevant research in high-altitude regions is non-existent.

Due to various reasons, such as lagging medical and economic progress and differences in language and customs, collecting data of clinical cases in high-altitude regions is very difficult. Although SRT is now more commonly used in RDS treatment in high-altitude regions, there is no specific study to confirm the efficacy of this therapy in such conditions or the effects of SRT at different altitudes. Therefore, clarifying the effect of SRT on RDS in premature infants in high-altitude regions is important to improve the prenatal healthcare quality in high-altitude regions. This study aimed to investigate the important role of SRT therapy in premature infants with RDS in the Qinghai-Tibet Plateau.

MATERIALS AND METHODS

Subjects

This was a multi-center retrospective cohort study conducted in 10 hospitals (Lhasa People's Hospital; People's Hospital of Tibet; Second People's Hospital of Tibet; Naqu People's Hospital, Tibet; Shannan People's Hospital, Tibet; Linzhi People's Hospital, Tibet; Changdu People's Hospital, Tibet; People's Hospital of Ali District, Tibet; Shigatse People's Hospital, Tibet; and Qinghai Women and Children's Hospital) in the Tibetan Plateau from January 2015 to December 2017. We reviewed 632 cases of preterm infants with RDS and finally included 337 cases according to the inclusion criteria (**Figure 1**). The study was approved by the Ethics Committee of Shengjing Hospital Affiliated to China Medical University and registered in ClinicalTrials.gov (NCT03440333). Written informed consent from the participants' legal guardian/next of kin was not required to participate in this study in accordance with the national legislation and the institutional requirements.

Sample Collection

A total of 337 clinical cases were grouped and evaluated based on the use of SRT and the altitude of the infants' birth area. We collected other basic information, which may affect the children's outcomes. In addition, we included SRT use, the altitude of the infant's birthplace, and indicators of treatment effect, such as mortality, blood gas results, etc. Then, we compared the various indicators under different treatment methods and at different altitudes to determine whether there was any difference in the therapeutic effect.

Patient Identification

The diagnosis of RDS was based on clinical manifestations (dyspnea, nasal flaring, groaning, and cyanosis after birth) and chest X-ray (CR) findings. Based on the characteristics of the infants' CR, RDS can be classified into four degrees: grade 1 (ground glass shadowing), grade 2 (ground glass shadowing with air bronchograms), grade 3 (confluent alveolar shadowing), and grade 4 (complete white lungs obscuring the cardiac border) (16).

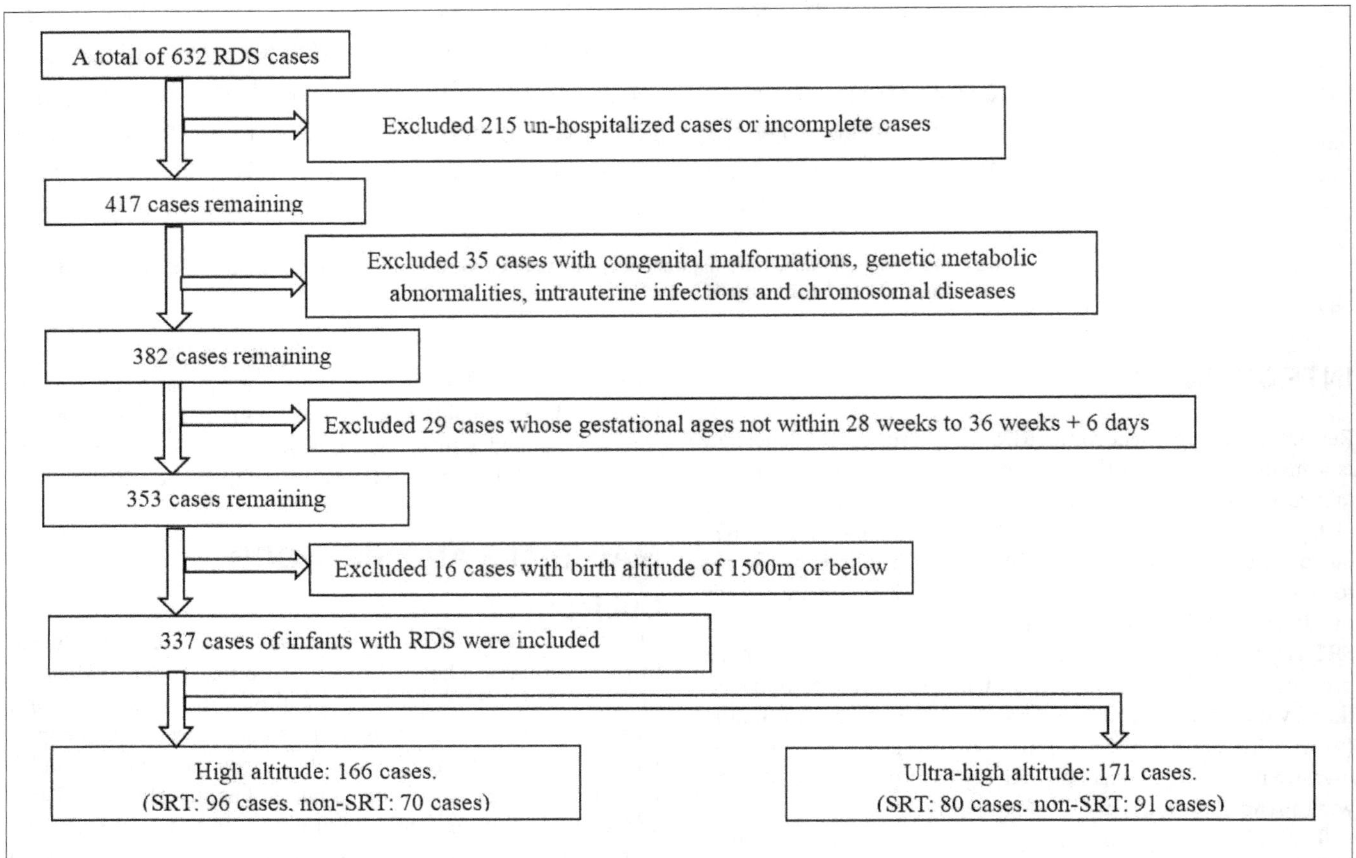

FIGURE 1 | Qualitative and basic sample exclusion (RDS, respiratory distress syndrome; SRT, surfactant replacement therapy).

In this study, we set grades 1 and 2 as mild RDS and grades 3 and 4 as severe RDS.

There were no obvious differences in the methods and technology used for RDS therapy among the neonatal intensive care unit (NICU) of the 10 hospitals. Furthermore, all infants were intubated to receive a surfactant (Curosurf, Chiesi Pharmaceuticals, Parma, Italy), which was used only once at a dose of 200 mg/kg.

Data Analysis

The Wilcoxon test (Mann–Whitney *U* test) was used to compare categorical indicators between the subgroups. The Fisher exact test was adopted to analyze the relationships between the characteristics. Multivariate analysis *via* logistic regression was performed for quantizing the factors' effects. For detailed comparisons, each altitude category was modeled twice, including a model of patients without SRT treatment at high altitude (Model I), a model of the whole population at high altitude (Model II), a model of the population without SRT at ultra-high altitude (Model III), and a multiple regression model of the whole sample (Model IV). Redundancy analysis (RDA) was performed to remove redundant information in blood gas targets. The significance levels (type I error, α) were unified to 0.05 in this study. All analyses were performed on R (version 3.6.3, 64-bit, 2020-02-29).

RESULTS

General Information

We identified 632 infants in the Tibetan Plateau diagnosed with RDS during the study period. Of these, we excluded 215 patients as they were not hospitalized after diagnosis or had incomplete clinical data; 35 for having congenital malformations, genetic metabolic abnormalities, intrauterine infections, and chromosomal diseases; 29 whose gestational ages were outside the study range; and 16 infants whose birthplace altitudes were <1,500 m, leaving 337 patients for analysis (**Figure 1**).

The study population characteristics are shown in **Table 1**. Most subjects were male (209, 60.2%), and the median birth weight was 1.7 kg. The Apgar score at 5 min varied between 7 and 8 points. Over 80% of subjects had a gestational age in 28–33 weeks + 6 days. Overall, 174 (51.6%) were judged as having severe RDS. SRT was used in 150 patients (44.5%), and the rest were treated without SRT. Only the Apgar score at 5 min and RDS severity were significantly different at baseline between the high- and ultra-high-altitude groups. Particularly, the change in health status of patients showed a significant difference between the high-altitude and ultra-high-altitude groups, and the death rates were 34.34% and 49.71%, respectively ($P = 0.006$; **Figure 2A**). At the same time, SRT impacted significantly on the improvements of death at both high-altitude and ultra-high-altitude groups ($P = 0.013, 0.047$; **Figures 2B,C**).

TABLE 1 | Baseline characteristics in high-altitude and ultra-high-altitude groups.

Characteristic	High altitude	Ultra-high altitude	W/χ^{2-} value	p
Sex, *n* (%)				
Male	104 (62.65)	105 (61.40)	0.015	0.902
Female	62 (37.35)	66 (38.60)		
Birth weight (kg), median (IQR)	1.7 (1.35–2)	1.7 (1.5–2)	13,590	0.259
Gestational age, *n* (%)				
28–33 weeks + 6	139 (83.73)	136 (79.53)	0.731	0.393
34–36 weeks + 6	27 (16.27)	35 (20.47)		
Apgar score at 5 min, median (IQR)	7 (7,8)	8 (7,8)	12,669	0.028
RDS severity, *n* (%)				
Mild	68 (40.96)	106 (61.99)	14.079	0.000
Severe	98 (59.04)	65 (38.01)		
Clinical intervention, *n* (%)				
SRT	96 (57.83)	80 (46.78)	0.552	0.458
Without SRT	70 (42.17)	91 (53.22)		

RDS, respiratory distress syndrome; SRT, surfactant replacement therapy; IQR, inter-quartile range.

Correlation of Diverse Indicators in High and Ultra-High Altitude

In the high-altitude group, the change in health status was positively correlated with RDS severity ($r = 0.22$, $P < 0.05$) and inversely correlated with SRT ($r = -0.2$, $P < 0.05$). Birth weight correlated with the Apgar score at 5 min and gestational age ($r =$ 0.17 and 0.47, respectively, $P < 0.05$ for both; **Figure 3A**).

Similarly, in the ultra-high-altitude group, the change in health status was negatively correlated with sex ($r = -0.2$, $P <$ 0.05), birth weight ($r = -0.28$, $P < 0.05$), gestational age ($r = -0.27$, $P < 0.05$), and SRT ($r = -0.16$, $P < 0.05$) and positively correlated with RDS severity ($r = 0.26$, $P < 0.05$); birth weight was positively correlated with gestational age ($r = 0.52$, $P < 0.05$). Specifically, gestational age was negatively correlated with SRT ($r = -0.27$, $P < 0.05$), and sex was correlated with birth weight and gestational age ($r = 0.26$ and 0.16, respectively, $P < 0.05$ for both; **Figure 3B**).

Multivariate Analysis of Factor Contributions to RDS Treatment

Binary logistic regression analysis based on altitude and therapeutic intervention was used to analyze the risk factors related to change in status. The result showed that RDS severity [odds ratio (OR) = 3.76, $P = 0.03$) was a risk factor and birth weight (OR = 0.22, $P = 0.03$) was a protective factor in the non-SRT subset of the high-altitude group (**Figure 4A**). Nevertheless, SRT (OR = 0.44, $P = 0.02$) became a new protective factor in the model of overall high-altitude samples (**Figure 4B**).

Further correlation analysis in the ultra-high-altitude group showed that RDS severity (OR = 6.42, $P = 0.00$) was still a risk factor, while gestational age (OR = 0.16, $P = 0.01$) was a protective factor in the non-SRT subset (**Figure 4C**). Similar to the model of overall high-altitude samples, SRT (OR = 0.28, $P <$ 0.01) still appeared protective in the model of overall ultra-high-altitude samples (**Figure 4D**). Notably, the OR of risk factors decreased and that of protective factors increased after importing SRT at two altitude levels.

To compare the role of indicators in the model, we calculated each hotspot coding feature and summarized the importance of variables. On this occasion, the scores represented the similarity between the model and the variables. Interestingly, by leading in SRT, although the SRT score in the overall high-altitude group model (score = 0.4) was slightly lower than in the overall ultra-high-altitude group model (score = 0.64), there was a greater decrease in protective factors' scores (birth weight: 0.65–0.38; gestational age: 0.86–0.55) (**Table 2**).

Synthesis Evaluation by Blood Gas Targets

Blood gas analyses were used to demonstrate diverse improvements in patients at various altitudes. To avoid amplifying redundant information from various times, pH, $PaCO_2$, and PaO_2/FiO_2(p/f) were tested; RDA was conducted to reveal the comprehensive effect of variables in the high-altitude and ultra-high-altitude group, and prognostic pH, $PaCO_2$, and p/f at 6, 12, and 24 h after SRT were regarded as "outcome variables" and sex, Apgar score at 5 min, RDS severity, birth weight, and gestational age as "environmental variables". The results showed that the highest value of RDA1 axis in variables is 0.9188 in the severity of RDS, indicating that RDS severity was the most influential factor in the high-altitude group, while it was the Apgar score at 5 min ($|RDA1| = 0.6581$) in the ultra-high-altitude group. Additionally, other results showed that the lowest value of RDA1 in variables is 0.1703 in gestational age (GA), indicating GA was the least influential factor in the high-altitude group, while it was sex ($|RDA1| = 0.1093$) in the ultra-high-altitude group (**Figures 5A,B**).

We chose pH, $PaCO_2$, and p/f and examined the changes with SRT at different altitudes. The temporal dynamics curves showed clear differences in pH and p/f at various altitudes over time. In summary, compared with patients at ultra-high altitude, patients who were at high altitude do faster entry or almost normal entry ranges after SRT (**Figures 5C–E**).

DISCUSSION

To our knowledge, this multi-center retrospective study is the first study focusing on the efficacy of SRT in the treatment for RDS in premature infants in high-altitude regions. In this study, we provide a theoretical basis to continue to use exogenous pulmonary surfactant to treat RDS in premature infants in high-altitude regions. There were significant differences in patients who were and were not treated using SRT in both high- and ultra-high-altitude regions. In fact, other indicators did not differ after strictly controlled grouping, considered unmatched patients and therefore were not excluded outside subgroup classification. This shows that SRT can effectively reduce alveolar surface tension and increase lung compliance in preterm infants with RDS in

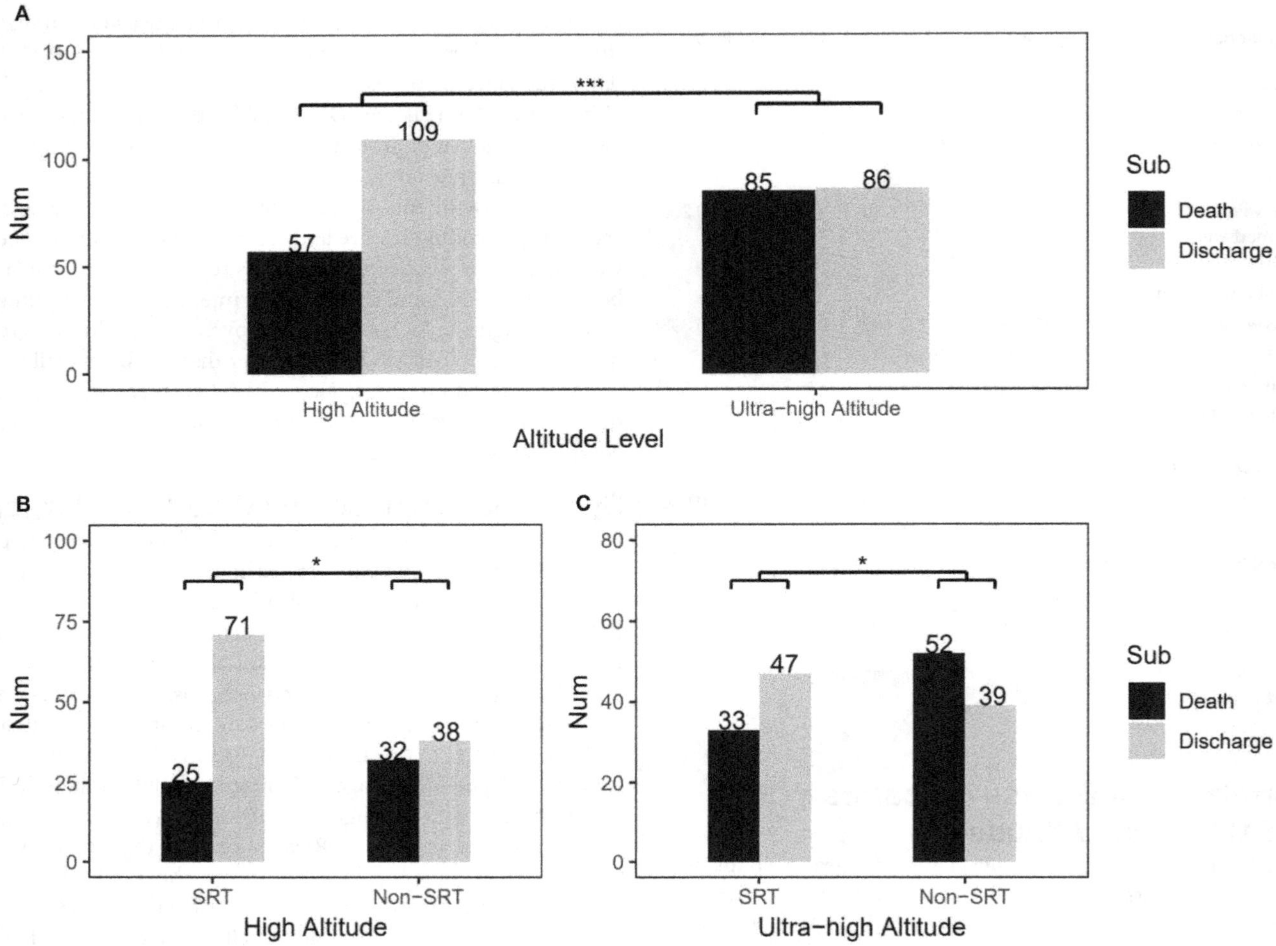

FIGURE 2 | Change in patients' health status and comparisons of therapeutic effects of surfactant replacement therapy between the high-altitude and ultra-high-altitude groups. **(A)** Overall health status'changes at different altitudes, **(B)** Comparison of therapeutic effects of surfactant replacement therapy in the high-altitude group, and **(C)** Comparison of therapeutic effects of surfactant replacement therapy in the ultra-high-altitude group. The numbers on the graph represent frequency in the different subgroups. Sub, subgroups of various outcomes; SRT, surfactant replacement therapy; non-SRT, without using surfactant replacement therapy. ***$P < 0.001$ and *$0.01 < P < 0.05$ (chi-square test).

high-altitude regions. SRT can achieve better lung dynamics and oxygenation, reduce hypoxic damage in various organs and systems, and improve the prognosis.

Based on the early improvement in the infants' blood gas analysis results and the improved final prognosis, the efficacy of SRT is better in high-altitude regions than in ultra-high-altitude regions. This result may be related to the unique natural environmental characteristics of high-altitude areas, mainly the low atmospheric pressure. Preterm infants fail to fully expand the lungs after birth due to RDS, and a vicious cycle of worsening hypoxemia can result from pulmonary vasoconstriction, pulmonary hypoperfusion, increased right heart pressure, and right to left shunting across the foramen ovale and the ductus arteriosus (17). As a result of the worsening oxygenation, preterm infants with RDS born at high altitude might have a greater demand for SRT after early mechanical or non-invasive ventilation than those born at lower altitudes (18). Under hypoxia, pulmonary capillary damage and changes in membrane permeability function occur (19, 20); aquaporin expression in lung tissue is inhibited (21), and the activity of $Na+$-$K+$-ATPase on the lung base membrane is inhibited (22). All these conditions could cause severe pulmonary edema in infants, in turn influencing the effect of SRT on RDS in preterm infants. In addition, the exposure of the lung surfactant to high-altitude-induced oxidative stress may result in the peroxidation of unsaturated phospholipids, surfactant inactivation, airspace collapse, and impaired gas exchange, which would reduce SRT's curative effects (23). Furthermore, the hypoxic environment in high-altitude regions appears to increase the incidence of intrauterine growth retardation (24). Compared to areas at sea level, the development of various organs of the same gestational age fetuses in high-altitude regions is slower. Usually, when the fetus reaches 35 weeks of gestation, the synthesis and secretion of pulmonary surfactant by alveolar type II

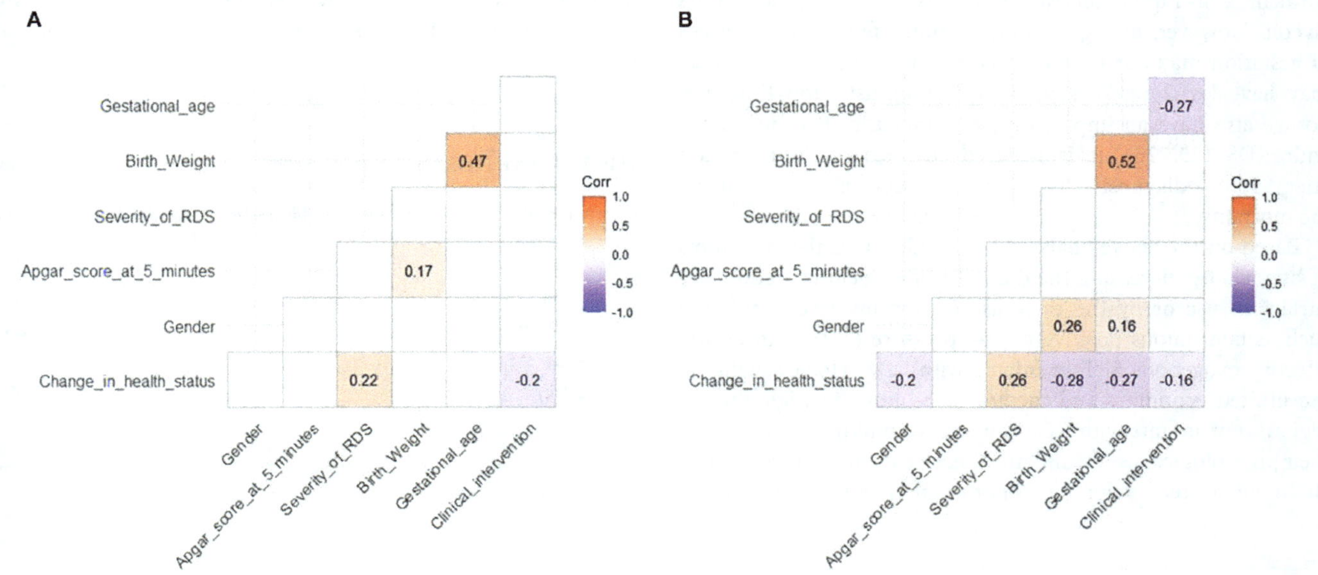

FIGURE 3 | Correlation between various indicators. **(A)** High altitude and **(B)** ultra-high altitude. Correlation coefficients were calculated before correlation tests. Blue indicates significant negative correlations and rec significant positive correlations. The darker the color, the more significant. Unrelated situations are not shown. The level of significance is 0.05.

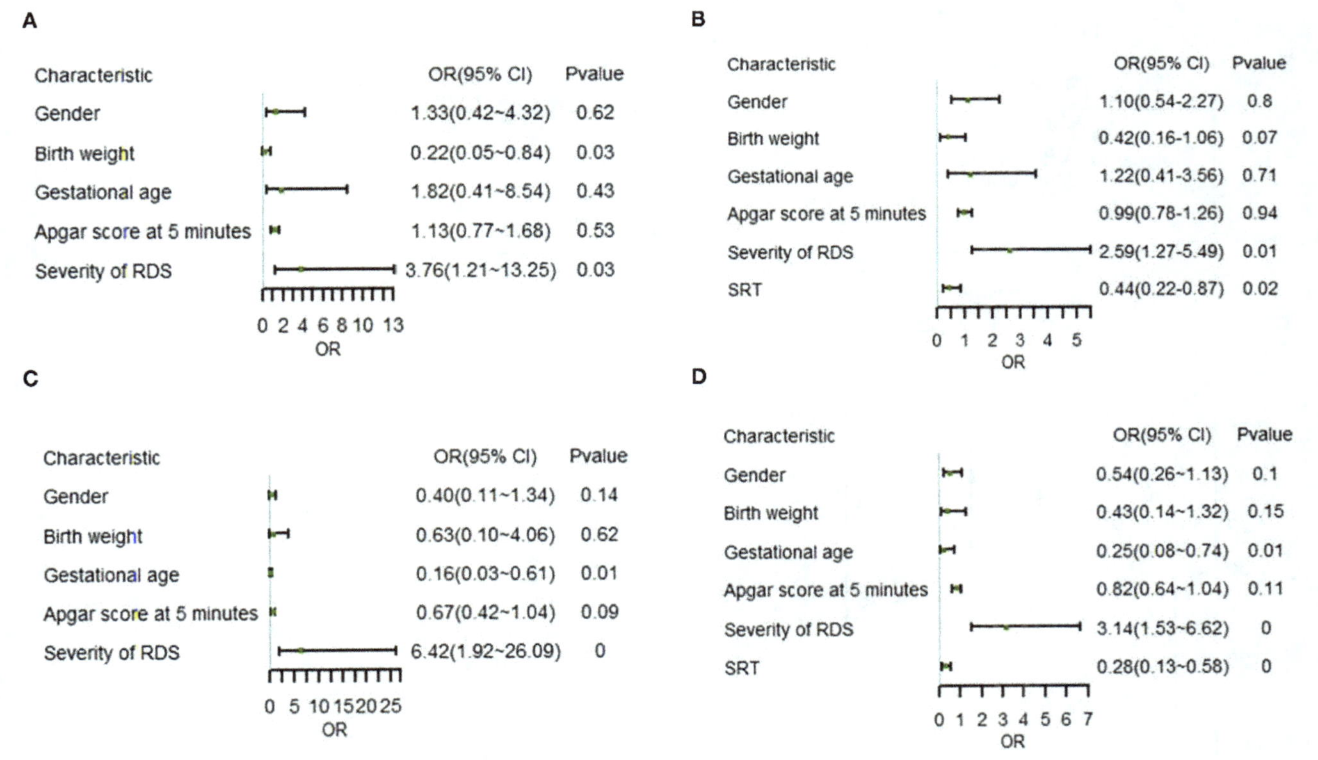

FIGURE 4 | Correlation between various indicators and outcomes in multivariate logistic regression. **(A)** Model I for non-SRT samples in the high-altitude group, **(B)** Model II for whole samples in the high-altitude group, **(C)** Model III for non-SRT samples in the ultra-high-altitude group, and **(D)** Model IV for whole samples in the ultra-high-altitude group. OR, odds ratio; 95% CI, 95% confidence interval; RDS, respiratory distress syndrome; SRT, surfactant replacement therapy. 0 represents $P < 0.01$.

epithelial cells rapidly increase and transfer to the surface of the alveoli. However, in high-altitude regions, fetuses at 35 weeks of gestation may not have reached this peak period; thus, they may have less lung surfactant. SRT administration time and dosage also have an impact on its therapeutic effect in infants with RDS (25, 26). It is believed that early administration after RDS diagnosis is more conducive to reducing the mortality.

Based on the above analysis, we could reduce the symptoms of hypoxia by increasing the duration of exogenous pulmonary surfactant use or by the early use of non-invasive ventilation such as continuous positive airway pressure (CPAP) to ensure effective exogenous SRT in infants with RDS. However, due to the limited economic and medical conditions in high-altitude regions, few infants with RDS can receive multiple SRT to meet their physiological needs, and most receive it either once or not at all. In the future, developing economic and medical conditions in high-altitude regions may allow the comparison of the efficacy of SRT with different drug dosages for neonatal or preterm infants with RDS.

TABLE 2 | Relative importance score of variables in multivariate logistic regression.

Characteristic	Model I	Model II	Model III	Model IV
Sex	0.14	0.05	0.45	0.3
Birth weight	0.65	0.38	0.17	0.33
Gestational age	0.23	0.07	0.86	0.55
Apgar score at 5 min	0.17	0.01	0.55	0.3
RDS severity	0.63	0.47	0.89	0.56
SRT	–	0.4	–	0.64

*Model I to Model IV are consistent with **Figure 4**. RDS, respiratory distress syndrome; SRT, surfactant replacement therapy.*

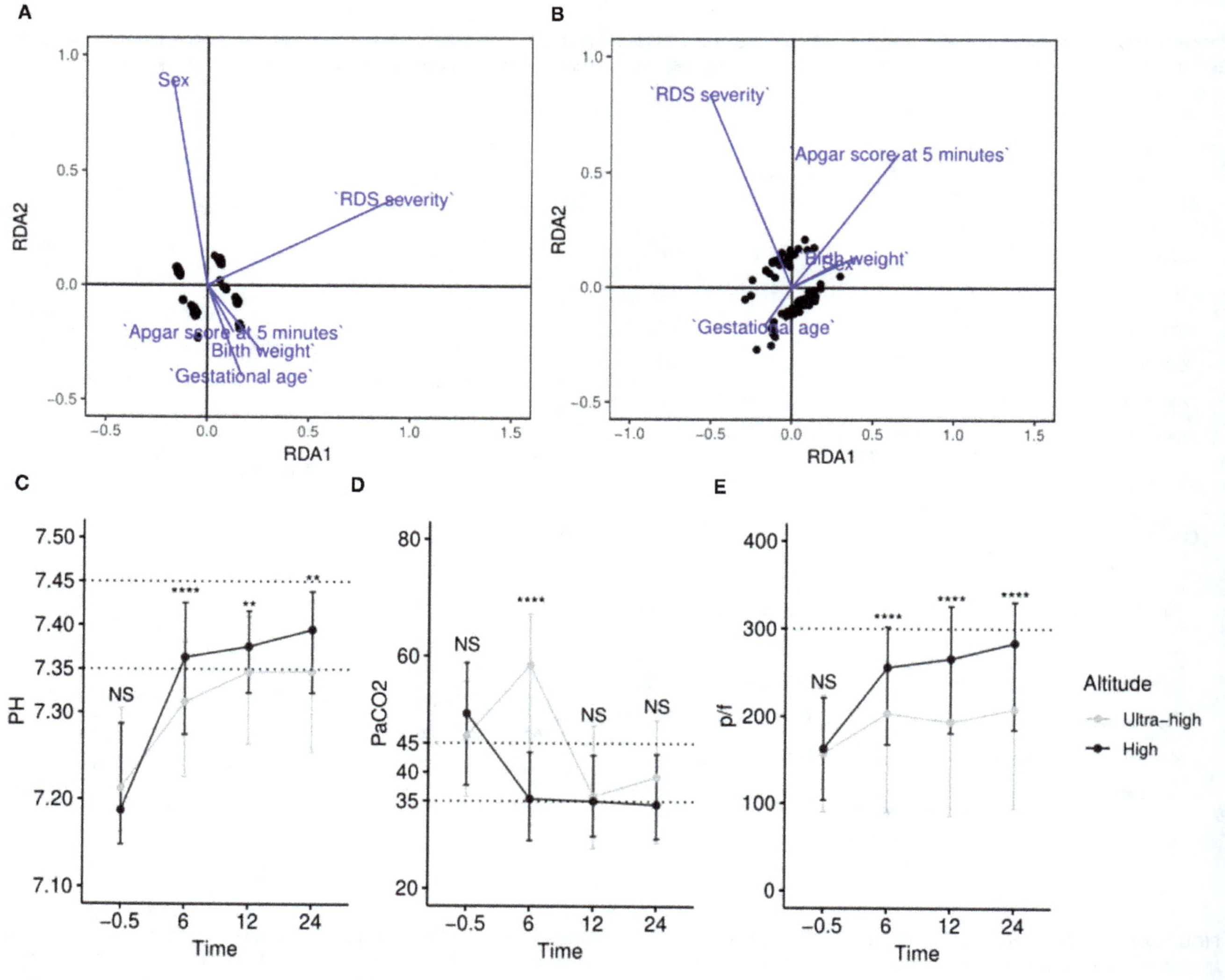

FIGURE 5 | Comprehensive evaluation by redundancy analysis and comparison of blood gas targets at various time points in different altitudes. **(A)** RDA model of samples in high altitude; **(B)** RDA model of samples in ultra-high altitude; **(C–E)** changes of pH, $PaCO_2$, and p/f at various time points at different altitudes. $^{NS}P > 0.05$; $^{**}0.001 < P < 0.01$; $^{****}P < 0.0001$.

Factors such as sex, gestational age, RDS severity, and birth weight affect SRT efficacy. Therefore, we conducted a multi-factor analysis to compare their effects on SRT efficacy in high-altitude regions. RDS severity was a risk factor in all groups. Even with SRT, the prognosis of preterm infants with RDS was largely affected by RDS severity in both high-altitude and ultra-high-altitude groups. This means that in high-altitude regions, for infants with severe RDS, exogenous SRT may not achieve the expected results, which needs to be considered in advance.

Some maternal conditions during pregnancy, such as hypertension, diabetes, etc., will also affect the maturity of the lungs of the infant, which may affect the efficacy of SRT.

Various studies on SRT have shown that the effect of a first dose of pulmonary surfactant of 200 mg/kg is better than 100 mg/kg (10) and that early initiation of CPAP with subsequent selective surfactant replacement is superior to prophylactic surfactant therapy (27, 28). However, these studies only included infants at sea level or in non-high-altitude areas. In high-altitude areas, due to factors such as hypoxia, the response of infants with RDS to various treatments might differ, and this requires further study. Our research proves the value of SRT for RDS in high-altitude regions. In addition, on the basis of this research, more in-depth research can be carried out, for example, studies on immature or ultra-low birth weight infants.

Our study had some limitations. First, some objective conditions in the high-altitude regions had great impact on our data collection. However, this also confirms the importance of the data collected for this study. Second, due to medical conditions, economic conditions, and other restrictions, many mothers did not undergo systematic examinations during pregnancy, which has led to a regrettable lack of some baseline characteristics in our data collection. With the continued development of high-altitude areas, we will further expand the sample size and add to the various indicators for children and pregnant women in future studies. Third, other complications of preterm infants, such as patent ductus arteriosus (PDA), will also affect the treatment of RDS. However, due to objective medical conditions, we have not successfully collected data related to PDA in the hospitals of Qinghai-Tibet Plateau, which is quite regrettable. In the future, we will try our best to promote the application of new medical technologies (such as bedside ultrasound technology), continue to work on neonatal diseases and treatment-related research in high altitude areas, and further improve these contents.

Our research was limited to the Qinghai-Tibet Plateau, and the characteristics of other high-altitude areas worldwide might differ; therefore, our results need to be validated by studies in other high-altitude areas. We hope that our findings can provide insights for the treatment of RDS in other regions. We also look forward to cooperating with other regions to conduct a comprehensive large-scale multi-center research.

CONCLUSION

In conclusion, this multi-center retrospective study confirms that SRT is effective for the treatment of RDS in premature infants in high-altitude regions, but its therapeutic effect was affected by the plateau environment. In high-altitude regions, SRT efficacy decreases with increasing altitude. The present results serve as initial evidence of SRT use in high-altitude and reflect the need for standardized guidelines for SRT in high-altitude regions.

AUTHOR CONTRIBUTIONS

All authors listed have made a substantial, direct, and intellectual contribution to the work and approved it for publication.

ACKNOWLEDGMENTS

The authors are grateful to each participant from the 10 hospitals in the Tibetan Plateau and the Plateau Medical Research Center of China Medical University.

REFERENCES

1. Reuter S, Moser C, Baack M. Respiratory distress in the newborn. *Pediatr Revl* (2014) 35:417–29. doi: 10.1542/pir.35.10.417
2. Sardesai S, Biniwale M, Wertheimer F, Garingo A, Ramanathan R. Evolution of surfactant therapy for respiratory distress syndrome: past, present, and future. *Pediatr Res.* (2017) 81:240–8. doi: 10.1038/pr.2016.203
3. Fujiwara T, Chida S, Watabe Y, Maeta H, Morita T, Abe T. Artificia surfactant therapy in hyaline-membrane disease. *Lancet.* (1980) 1:55–9. doi: 10.1016/S0140-6736(80)90489-4
4. Bae CW, Kim CY, Chung SH, Choi YS. History of pulmonary surfactant replacement therapy for neonatal respiratory distress syndrome in Korea. *J Korean Med Sci.* (2019) 34 e175. doi: 10.3346/jkms.2019.34.e175
5. Seger N, Soll R. Animal derived surfactant extract for treatment of respiratory distress syndrome. *Cochrane Database Syst Rev.* (2009) 2:CD007836. doi: 10.1002/14651858.CD007836
6. Iyer NP, Mhanna MJ. The role of surfactant and non-invasive mechanical ventilation in early management of respiratory distress syndrome in premature infants. *World J Pediatr.* (2014) 10:204–10. doi: 10.1007/s12519-014-0494-9
7. Rojas-Reyes MX, Morley CJ, Soll R. Prophylactic versus selective use of surfactant in preventing morbidity and mortality in preterm infants. *Cochrane Database Syst Rev.* (2012) 3:CD000510. doi: 10.1002/14651858.CD000510.pub2
8. Bahadue FL, Soll R. Early versus delayed selective surfactant treatment for neonatal respiratory distress syndrome. *Cochrane Database Syst Rev.* (2012) 11:CD001456. doi: 10.1002/14651858.CD001456.pub2
9. Ng EH, Shah V. Guidelines for surfactant replacement therapy in neonates. *Paediatr Child Health.* (2021) 26:35–49. doi: 10.1093/pch/pxaa116
10. Sweet DG, Carnielli V, Greisen G, Hallman M, Ozek E, Plavka R, et al. European consensus guidelines on the management of respiratory distress syndrome-2016 update. *Neonatology.* (2017) 111:107–25. doi: 10.1159/000448985
11. Shin JE, Yoon SJ, Lim J, Han J, Eun HS, Park MS, et al. Pulmonary surfactant replacement therapy for respiratory distress syndrome in neonates:

a nationwide epidemiological study in Korea. *J Korean Med Sci.* (2020) 35:e253. doi: 10.3346/jkms.2020.35.e253

12. Beall CM. Andean, Tibetan, and Ethiopian patterns of adaptation to high-altitude hypoxia. *Integr Comp Biol.* (2006) 46:18–24. doi: 10.1093/icb/icj004
13. Mathew TM, Sharma S. *High Altitude Oxygenation.* Treasure Island, FL: StatPearls Publishing (2021).
14. Coşkun Yavuz Y, Altun E, Sevinc C, Guney I, Korez MK, Biyik Z, et al. Does altitude affect blood gases in hemodialysis patients? *Hemodial Int.* (2020) 24:323–9. doi: 10.1111/hdi.12844
15. Chen D, Liu X, Li J. Mechanical ventilation in neonatal respiratory distress syndrome at high altitude: a retrospective study from Tibet. *Front Pediatr.* (2019) 7:476. doi: 10.3389/fped.2019.00476
16. Bae CW, Hahn WH. Surfactant therapy for neonatal respiratory distress syndrome: a review of Korean experiences over 17 years. *J Korean Med Sci.* (2009) 24:1110–8. doi: 10.3346/jkms.2009.24.6.1110
17. Niermeyer S. Going to high altitude with a newborn infant. *High Alt Med Biol.* (2007) 8:117–23. doi: 10.1089/ham.2007.1068
18. Alshehri MA. Are preterm infants at high altitude at greater risk for the development of bronchopulmonary dysplasia? *J Trop Pediatr.* (2014) 60:68–73. doi: 10.1093/tropej/fmt079
19. Madonna R, Cocco N, De Caterina R. Pathways and drugs in pulmonary arterial hypertension - focus on the role of endothelin receptor antagonists. *Cardiovasc Drugs Ther.* (2015) 29:469–79. doi: 10.1007/s10557-015-6605-6
20. Lee SJ, Zhang M, Hu K, Lin L, Zhang D, Jin Y. CCN1 suppresses pulmonary vascular smooth muscle contraction in response to hypoxia. *Pulm Circ.* (2015) 5:716–22. doi: 10.1086/683812
21. Jiao GY, Li ER, Yu RJ. Decreased expression of AQP- 1 and AQP-5 in acute injured lungs in rats. *Chin Med J.* (2002) 115:963–7. doi: 10.1097/00000441-200207000-00008
22. Dada LA, Sznajder JL. Hypoxic inhibition of alveolar fluid reabsorption. *Adv Exp Med Biol.* (2007) 618:159–68. doi: 10.1007/978-0-387-75434-5_12
23. Saxena S, Kumar R, Madan T, Gupta V, Muralidhar K, Sarma PU. Association of polymorphisms in pulmonary surfactant protein A1 and A2 genes with high-altitude pulmonary edema. *Chest.* (2005) 128:1611–9. doi: 10.1378/chest.128.3.1611
24. Yangzom Y, Qian L, Shan M, La Y, Meiduo D, Hu X, et al. Outcome of hospital deliveries of women living at high altitude: a study from Lhasa in Tibet. *Acta Paediatr.* (2008) 97:317–21. doi: 10.1111/j.1651-2227.2008.00628.x
25. Jourdain G, Zacaria F, Ammar F, De Luca D. Appropriateness of surfactant dosing for preterm babies with respiratory distress syndrome: retrospective cohort study. *Arch Dis Child Fetal Neonatal Ed.* (2016) 101:182–3. doi: 10.1136/archdischild-2015-310195
26. Challis P, Nydert P, Håkansson S, Norman M. Association of adherence to surfactant best practice uses with clinical outcomes among neonates in Sweden. *JAMA Netw Open.* (2021) 4:e217269. doi: 10.1001/jamanetworkopen.2021.7269
27. Murki S, Deorari A, Vidyasagar D. Use of CPAP and surfactant therapy in newborns with respiratory distress syndrome. *Indian J Pediatr.* (2014) 81:481–8. doi: 10.1007/s12098-014-1405-8
28. Shim GH. Update of minimally invasive surfactant therapy. *Korean J Pediatr.* (2017) 60:273–81. doi: 10.3345/kjp.2017.60.9.273

13

Optimal Positive End Expiratory Pressure Levels in Ventilated Patients without Acute Respiratory Distress Syndrome

Jing Zhou[1†], Zhimin Lin[1†], Xiumei Deng[1†], Baiyun Liu[1†], Yu Zhang[1], Yongxin Zheng[1], Haichong Zheng[1], Yingzhi Wang[1], Yan Lai[1], Weixiang Huang[1], Xiaoqing Liu[1], Weiqun He[1], Yuanda Xu[1], Yimin Li[1], Yongbo Huang[1] and Ling Sang[1,2*]*

[1] State Key Laboratory of Respiratory Disease, National Clinical Research Center for Respiratory Disease, Guangzhou Institute of Respiratory Health, The First Affiliated Hospital of Guangzhou Medical University, Guangzhou, China, [2] Guangzhou Laboratory, Guangdong, China

Correspondence:
Yongbo Huang
yongbo2046@163.com
Ling Sang
sonysang999@vip.163.com

†These authors contribute equally to this work and share first authorship

Background: To find the optimal positive end expiratory pressure (PEEP) in mechanical ventilated patients without Acute Respiratory Distress Syndrome (ARDS), we conducted a Bayesian network meta-analysis and systematic review of randomized controlled trials (RCTs) comparing different level of PEEP based on a novel classification of PEEP level: ZEEP group (PEEP = 0 cm H2O); lower PEEP group (PEEP = 1–6 cm H2O); intermediate PEEP group (PEEP = 7–10 cm H2O); higher PEEP group (PEEP > 10 cm H2O).

Result: Twenty eight eligible studies with 2,712 patients were included. There were no significant differences in the duration of mechanical ventilation between higher and intermediate PEEP (MD: 0.020, 95% CI: −0.14, 0.28), higher and lower PEEP (MD: −0.010, 95% CI: −0.23, 0.22), higher PEEP and ZEEP (MD: 0.010, 95% CI: −0.40, 0.22), intermediate and lower PEEP (MD: −0.040, 95% CI: −0.18, 0.040), intermediate PEEP and ZEEP (MD: −0.010, 95% CI: −0.42, 0.10), lower PEEP and ZEEP (MD: 0.020, 95% CI: −0.32, 0.13), respectively. Higher PEEP was associated with significantly higher PaO2/FiO2 ratio(PFR) when compared to ZEEP (MD: 73.24, 95% CI: 11.03, 130.7), and higher incidence of pneumothorax when compared to intermediate PEEP, lower PEEP and ZEEP (OR: 2.91e + 12, 95% CI: 40.3, 1.76e + 39; OR: 1.85e + 12, 95% CI: 29.2, 1.18e + 39; and OR: 1.44e + 12, 95% CI: 16.9, 8.70e + 38, respectively). There was no association between PEEP levels and other secondary outcomes.

Conclusion: We identified higher PEEP was associated with significantly higher PFR and higher incidence of pneumothorax. Nonetheless, in terms of other outcomes, no significant differences were detected among four levels of PEEP.

Systematic Review Registration: The study had registered on an international prospective register of systematic reviews, PROSPERO, on 09 April 2021, identifier: [CRD42021241745].

Keywords: Acute respiratory distress syndrome, Mechanical ventilation, Positive end expiratory pressure, Pneumothorax, Mortality

INTRODUCTION

Although invasive mechanical ventilation is a lifesaving strategy for critically ill patients, previous studies have considered it a potentially harmful intervention (1, 2). Positive end expiratory pressure (PEEP) has shown efficacy in maintaining alveoli opening, improvement of gas exchange and reduction of injurious shear forces in acute respiratory distress syndrome (ARDS) patients since 1960 s (3). To date, however, the optimal PEEP levels remain unclear, owing to occurrence of potential negative effects that cause overdistention of the lungs, exacerbate lung stress as well as strain and impair hemodynamics by reducing venous return and increasing pulmonary vascular resistance. Therefore, PEEP's net benefits or harm are depended on the balance between alveolar recruitment and overdistension, and should be particularly beneficial in disease states with substantial alveolar collapse (4). Nevertheless, this trade-off is often difficult to achieve clinically.

Similarly, the optimal PEEP level for mechanical ventilated patients without ARDS remains unclear. Several studies have demonstrated that higher PEEP levels could improve oxygenation, reduce occurrence of ventilator-associated pneumonia (VAP), prevent ARDS in this population (5). In fact, application of PEEP has increased in clinical practice (6). However, PEEP level in a relatively healthy lung is expected to be lower because of less lung collapse which requires less pressure to open the collapsed lung. In addition, previous research evidences from animal studies have shown that ventilation with higher PEEP levels might worsen existing lung injuries or cause development of new ones (7–9). A recent RELAx trial demonstrated that a higher PEEP strategy generated clinically superior outcomes than lower levels with regards to the number of ventilator-free days (VFD) at day 28 in ventilated patients without ARDS, although there was a possibility of elevated hypoxemia in the lower PEEP group (10).

A previous systematic review and meta-analysis compared efficacy of different PEEP levels in patients without ARDS (11). However, the findings therein should be interpreted with caution, owing to a moderate to high heterogeneity, a low to very low quality of evidences (QoE), and the fact that the included studies could not allow the authors to comprehensively address the effects of moderate PEEP levels. In the present study, we conducted a Bayesian network meta-analysis and systematic review of RCTs to compare efficacy of different PEEP levels in ventilated patients without ARDS, and identify the optimal level for this population. Specifically, we divided the patients into four groups according to their PEEP levels. We chose a novel classification, based on patients' PEEP levels, which is closer to clinical practice, and can allow for reduction of heterogeneity in the analysis as well as precise evaluation of the effects of different PEEP levels.

MATERIALS AND METHODS

This meta-analysis was performed in accordance with the guidelines of the Preferred Reporting Items for Systematic Reviews and Meta-analyses extension statement for reporting network meta-analyses (PRISMA- NMA) (12). The study was also prospectively registered on PROSPERO database (Registration number: CRD42021241745).

Data Sources and Study Search

We searched PubMed, Web of Science, Embase, Cochrane Library, Embase up to January 2021. Reference lists of relevant articles were also reviewed. The inclusion criteria were as follows: (i) studies were RCTs; (ii) the study population comprised ventilated patients without ARDS; (iii) intervention included higher *vs.* lower PEEP; and (iv) studies were published in English. The exclusion criteria were as follows: (i) studies that analyzed pediatric patients; (ii) patients were not in ICU; (iii) data were unavailable; and (iv) duplicate publications.

Study Selection and Data Extraction

Meta-analysis was performed by two researchers (JZ and ZML), who independently screened the citations and abstracts in duplicate and extracted the data. All references that were judged potentially relevant were evaluated for full-text eligibility. Discrepancies were resolved by consensus with a third author (YBH). In cases where relevant data or information was missing, we attempted to contact the authors of the studies.

Outcome Measures

Primary outcome was the duration of mechanical ventilation, whereas secondary outcomes included PaO_2/FiO_2 ratio (PFR), length of stay (LOS) in ICU, LOS in hospital, hospital mortality, 28-day mortality, ICU mortality, occurrence of ARDS, pneumothorax, atelectasis and hypoxemia.

Assessment of Risk of Bias

Two authors (JZ and ZML) independently assessed the risk of bias (RoB) in individual studies, using the revised Cochrane risk-of-bias tool for randomized trials (13), and classified them as either low or high. Any disagreements between them were resolved by discussion and consensus with a third author (YBH). Low-biased studies were defined as those with no <4 low-risk items, based on the Cochrane risk-of-bias tool.

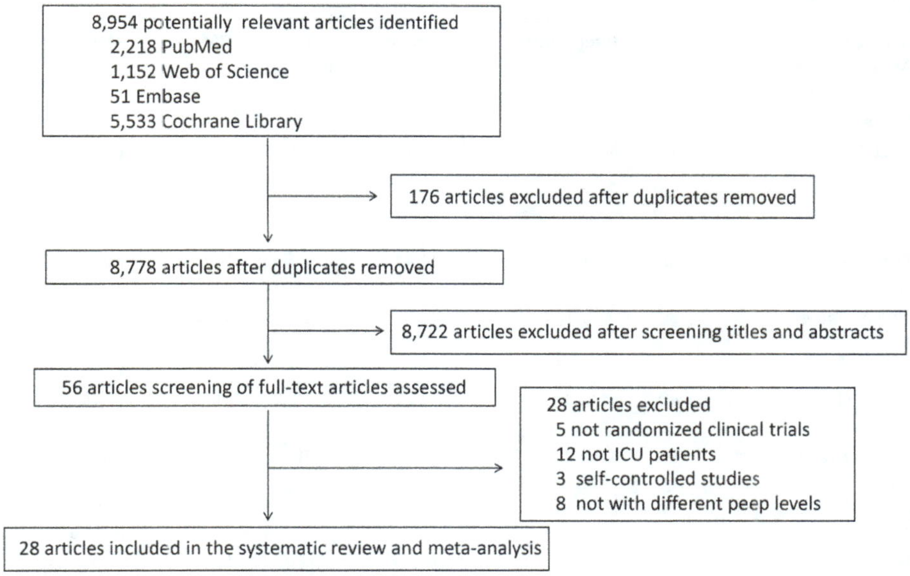

FIGURE 1 | PRISMA Flowchart.

Statistical Analysis

A random effects network meta-analysis was performed using a Bayesian framework. We also calculated mean differences for continuous outcomes and odds ratios (ORs) for dichotomous outcomes, then converted medians and interquartile ranges to means and standard deviations as previously described (14). Network meta-analysis was performed using the "gemtc" package (version 0.8–2) implemented in R version 3.4.4 (https://www.r-project.org/). This package is based on an approach that follows the graph-theoretical methodology. We ranked the treatments using the P-score to reveal the degree of certainty that a specific treatment was better than the others. Based on this, P-scores close to 1 and 0 denoted the best and worst treatments, respectively. Moreover, studies followed by a value of $I^2 \geq 50\%$ were considered to have substantial heterogeneity. To limit the possibility of type I error, we performed a Trial sequential analysis (TSA) using TSA version 0.9.5.10.

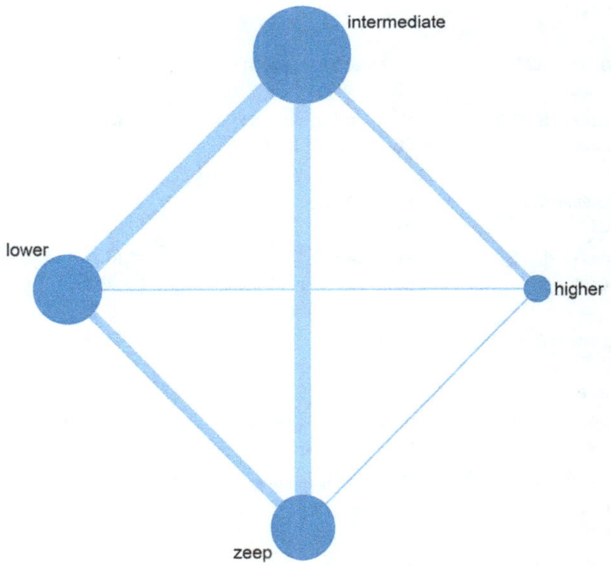

FIGURE 2 | Network geometry of included studies. The size of the nodes is proportional to the number of patients randomized to receive the intervention. The width of the lines is proportional to the number of trials comparing the connected intervention.

RESULTS

Eligible Studies

A total of 8,954 articles were retrieved from the aforementioned databases, of which 56 were considered potentially eligible after reviewing their full texts. Finally, 28 studies (5, 10, 15–40), comprising 2,712 patients, met all our inclusion criteria and were included in the meta-analysis (**Figure 1**).

Among the 28 eligible trials, 1 compared higher PEEP levels with ZEEP, 7 compared intermediate PEEP with ZEEP, 4 compared lower PEEP with ZEEP, 1 compared higher with lower PEEP, 4 compared higher with intermediate PEEP, 8 compared intermediate with lower PEEP, while 3 compared intermediate with lower PEEP and ZEEP. Sample sizes in these trials ranged from 15 to 969 patients. The network geometry is shown in **Figure 2**. With regards to regions, the eligible RCTs were conducted across different countries in the world, with 16 of them focusing on post-cardiac patients. Meanwhile, the year of publication widely varied across the studies, with 12 of them published before 2000 (**Table 1**). RoB was high in 18 (15–17, 20, 23, 24, 27, 28, 30–32, 34–38, 40, 41) and low in 10 (5, 10, 18, 19, 21, 22, 25, 26, 29, 33) trials. The high RoB was

TABLE 1 | Characteristics of included studies.

Study; country	Type of patients; Mean age (years)	N	Interventions	Sample Size	TV (ml/kg)	RM	Main findings
Post-Cardiac Surgery Patients							
Borges et al. (15); Brazil	Post-CABG; 60	136	M vs. L	92/44	6~8	NO	Better pulmonary compliance values, oxygenation indexes, and lower frequency of hypoxemia were found in higher PEEP group
Lago Borges et al. (16); Brazil	Post-CABG; 60	136	M vs. L	92/44	6~8	NO	Patients in higher PEEP group had shorter duration of mechanical ventilation.
Carroll et al. (17); America	Postoperative; 63	50	H vs. L	22/28	12	YES	Higher incidence of barotrauma and hypotension and death and higher duration of ventilation with higher PEEP.
Celebi et al. (18); Turkey	Post-CABG; 56	40	M vs. L	20/20	7	YES	Higher P/F ratio in the first 4h and less atelectasis in higher PEEP group.
Collier et al. (19); America	Post-cardiac surgery; 66	84	M vs. L	40/44	10	NO	Higher PEEP does not decrease chest-tube output or transfusion requirements but it may increase the fluid requirements.
Cordeiro et al. (20); Brazil	Post-CABG; 61	30	H vs. M	20/10	6~8	NO	Non-invasive ventilation with PEEP 15cm H2O represented an improvement in oxygenation levels.
Cordeiro et al. (21); Brazil	Post-cardiac surgery; 64	60	H vs. M	41/19	6	NO	Significant improvement in the oxygenation rate with higher peep.
Dyhr et al. (22); Denmark	Post-CABG; 60	15	H vs. Z	7/8	6	YES	Improvement in P/F ratio and end-expiratory lung volume in PEEP group.
Good et al. (23); America	Post-cardiac surgery; 55	24	M vs. Z	10/14	10~12	NO	Routine PEEP did not prevent atelectasis or improve pulmonary oxygen transport.
Holland et al. (24); Germany	Post-cardiac surgery; 66	28	M vs. L	14/14	6~8	NO	A PEEP of 10 mbar over 2 h did not compromise liver function and gastric mucosal perfusion
Lima et al. (25); Brazil	Post-CABG; 62	78	M vs. L	46/32	6~8	NO	No difference in gas exchange in the first 6 h after extubation between groups.
Marvel et al. (26); America	Post-CABG; 59	44	M vs. L vs. Z	12/15/17	NA	NO	No difference in the incidence of atelectasis or duration of hospitalization among groups.
Michalopoulos et al. (27); Greece	Post-CABG; 61	67	M vs. L vs. Z	21/24/22	NA	No	No differences in PaO_2/FiO_2, SvO_2, PvO_2 and in cardiac index among the three groups
Murphy et al. (28); America	Post-cardiac surgery; NA	139	M vs. Z	NA	NA	NO	PEEP reduced mediastinal bleeding after cardiac operations
Setak-Berenjestanaki et al. (29); Iran	Post-cardiac surgery; 56	180	M vs. L	120/60	NA	NO	Higher peep resulted in lower incidence of atelectasis and shorter duration of intubation
Zurick et al. (30); America	Post-cardiac surgery; 57	83	M vs. Z	41/42	NA	NO	PEEP did not reduce the amount of blood loss, the need for reexploration for bleeding, or the blood requirements
Non-Post-Cardiac Surgery Patients							
Cujec et al. (31); Canada	ARF: 59	46	M vs. Z	NA	NA	NO	Higher PEEP reduced alveolar–arterial oxygen difference and shunt fraction
Koutsoukou et al. (32); Greece	Severe brain damage; 41	21	M vs. Z	11/10	8~10	NO	Five days of mechanical ventilation on ZEEP resulted in higher static elastance and minimal resistance
Lesur et al. (33); Canada	ARF; 64	63	L vs. Z	30/33	6~9	NO	No difference in the occurrence of hypotension and duration of ventilation and mortality
Ma et al. (31); China	NPE; 64	120	H vs. M	60/60	6~8	NO	Higher PEEP resulted in lower 28-day morality rate and higher P/F ratio

(Continued)

TABLE 1 | Continued

Study; country	Type of patients; Mean age (years)	N	Interventions	Sample Size	TV (ml/kg)	RM	Main findings
Nelson et al. (35); America	At risk of ARF; 54	38	H vs. M	20/18	NA	NO	No difference in entry PaO2, intubated/ICU/hospitalization days, incidence of barotrauma, ICU/overall mortality between groups.
Pepe et al. (36) America	At risk of ARDS; 44	92	M vs. Z	44/48	12	NO	No difference in the incidence of the ARDS or other associated complications between groups.
Vigil et al. (37); America	Trauma; 34	44	L vs. Z	23/21	12~15	NO	Significantly less hospitalization days in zeep group whereas higher P/F ratio in the peep group.
Weijelt et al. (38); America	At risk of ARDS; 45	79	L vs. Z	45/34	15	NO	Peep altered the degree of deterioration and incidence of ARDS rather than preventing its occurrence
Miscellaneous Patients							
Algera et al. (10) Netherlands	Receiving IMV; 66	969	M vs. L	493/476	6~8	NO	With regard to the number of ventilator-free days at day 28, no difference was found between the two groups
Cao et al. (39); China	Hypovolemic patients; 44	30	M vs. L vs. Z	10/10/10	6~8	NO	Higher levels of PEEP increased CVP and CIVP
Manzano et al. (5); Spain	Without hypoxemia; 45	127	M vs. Z	64/63	8~9	NO	Application of prophylactic PEEP reduced the number of hypoxemia episodes and the incidence of ventilator-associated pneumonia
Feeley et al. (40); America	ARF; 61	25	L vs. Z	12/13	10	NO	PEEP may be useful in weaning patients who have a low vital capacity and inspiratory force

N means total number of participants in each study; Sample Size means number of participants in each group in study; NA, not available; TV, tidal volume; RM, recruitment maneuvers; PEEP, positive end-expiratory pressure (in cmH2O); P/F ratio: PaO2/FiO2; IMV, invasive mechanical ventilation; CABG, coronary artery bypass grafting; ARF, acute respiratory failure; ARDS, acute respiratory distress syndrome; NPE, neurological pulmonary edema.

H, higher peep (peep level >10 cmH_2O); M, intermediate peep (5 < peep level ≤ 10 cmH_2O); L, lower peep (0 < peep level ≤ 5 cmH_2O); Z, zeep means peep level of zero.

attributed to blinding of participants, personnel and outcome assessors (**Figure 3**).

Primary Outcomes

A total of 11 eligible articles (5, 10, 16, 19, 21, 23, 25, 29, 33, 35, 38), with 1,848 participants, reported duration of mechanical ventilation. Among them, 6 studies (16, 19, 21, 23, 25, 29), with 572 patients (16, 19, 21, 23, 25, 29). A summary of the RoBs is shown in **Figure 3** while the resulting funnel plot is illustrated in **Figure 4**. A direct comparison revealed no significant differences in the duration of mechanical ventilation, between higher and intermediate PEEP levels (MD: 0.024, 95% CI: −0.14, 0.28), intermediate and lower PEEP (MD: −0.034, 95% CI: −0.17, 0.050), intermediate PEEP and ZEEP (MD: −0.62, 95% CI: −1.6, 0.35), as well as lower PEEP and ZEEP (MD: −0.028, 95% CI: −0.26, 0.16). Similarly, a direct comparison among a subpopulation of post-cardiac surgery patients revealed no significant differences in the duration of mechanical ventilation among different PEEP strategies (higher vs. intermediate: MD: 0.02, 95% CI: −0.034, 0.073; intermediate vs. lower: MD: −0.03, 95% CI: −0.078, 0.017; and lower PEEP *vs.* ZEEP: MD: 0.03, 95% CI: 0.015, 0.046) (**Figure 5A**). Results from Network Meta-Analysis, which combined direct and indirect comparison approaches, revealed no significant differences in the duration of mechanical ventilation between higher and intermediate PEEP (MD: 0.020, 95% CI: −0.14, 0.28), higher and lower PEEP (MD: −0.010, 95% CI: −0.23, 0.22), higher PEEP and ZEEP (MD: 0.010, 95% CI: −0.40, 0.22), intermediate and lower PEEP (MD: −0.040, 95% CI: −0.18, 0.040), intermediate PEEP and ZEEP (MD: −0.010, 95% CI: −0.42, 0.10), as well as lower PEEP and ZEEP (MD: 0.020, 95% CI: −0.32, 0.13) groups. Pooled estimates from the network meta-analysis were shown in **Table 2**. Network Meta-Analysis of the subpopulation of post-cardiac surgery patients also revealed no significant differences in their duration of mechanical ventilation among different PEEP strategies (higher vs. intermediate PEEP: MD: 0.02, 95% CI: −0.060, 0.090; higher vs. lower PEEP: MD: −0.010, 95% CI: −0.10, 0.080; higher PEEP vs. ZEEP: MD: 0.02, 95% CI: −0.090, 0.12; intermediate *vs.* lower PEEP: MD: −0.03, 95% CI: −0.080, 0.020; intermediate PEEP vs. ZEEP: MD: 0, 95% CI: −0.070, 0.070; lower PEEP vs. ZEEP: MD: 0.03, 95% CI: −0.030, 0.090) (**Figure 5B**). We also performed node-splitting analysis to assess inconsistency in network meta-analysis, and found no significant differences between intermediate *vs.* lower PEEP ($p = 0.22$), intermediate PEEP vs. ZEEP ($p = 0.26$), and lower PEEP vs. ZEEP ($p = 0.22$), indicating that the results

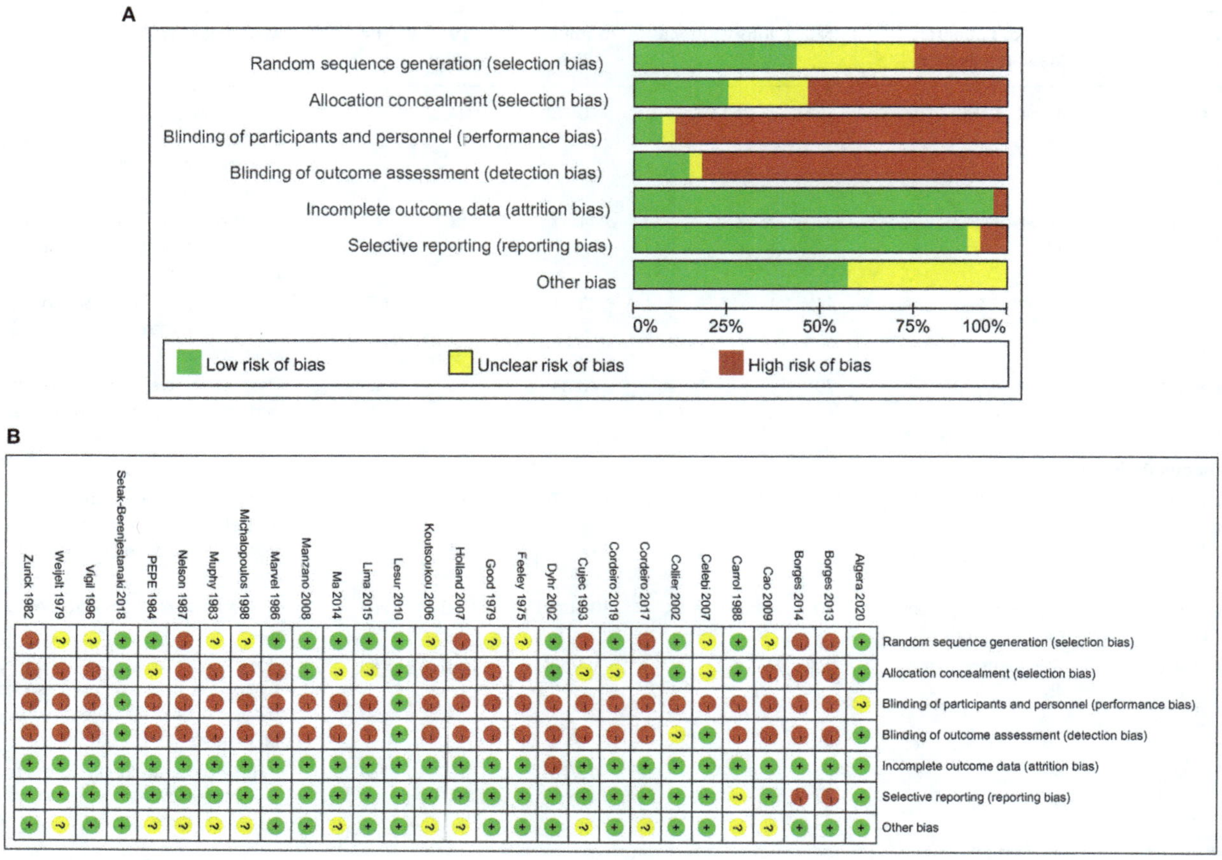

FIGURE 3 | Risk of bias of included studies. **(A)** Risk of bias graph based on the Cochrane Risk of Bias Tool. **(B)** Risk of bias summary based on the Cochrane Risk of Bias Tool.

from both direct and indirect comparisons across the three groups were highly consistent (**Figure 5C**). However, results from ranking analysis showed that intermediate PEEP levels could shorten the duration of mechanical ventilation, followed by ZEEP, higher PEEP and lower PEEP (**Figure 6**). Furthermore, TSA showed that conventional and O'Brien-Fleming significance boundaries were not crossed by the cumulative Z-curve, indicating that the evidence was not sufficient and conclusive. Therefore, further trials are needed to validate these findings. A graphical representation of this analysis is shown in **Figure 7**.

Secondary Outcomes

Eleven eligible studies, with 1,648 patients, reported on PFR (5, 10, 15, 20–22, 24, 25, 32–34), with 6 of them (comprising 347 patients) focusing on post-cardiac surgery patients (5, 10, 21, 22, 24, 33). Results of RoB are shown in **Figure 3** and **Supplementary Figure 1A**. Direct comparison revealed no significant differences in PFR among PEEP levels, in both general or post cardiac surgical patients (**Supplementary Figure 1B**). However, results from Network Meta-Analysis demonstrated that higher PEEP was associated with significantly higher PFR compared to ZEEP in the general population (MD: 73.24, 95% CI: 11.03, 130.7). Meawhile, there were no sigificant differences based on the other comparisons (**Figure 8**). Moreover, node-splitting analysis, based on both direct and indirect comparisons in these groups, revealed consistent results

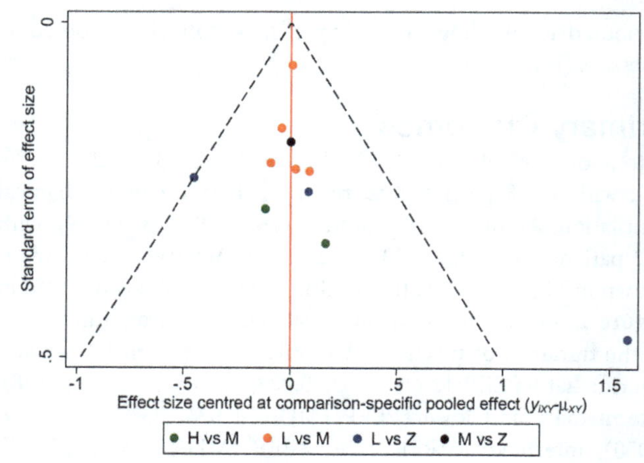

FIGURE 4 | Funnel plot for duration of mechanical ventilation. Funnel plot of association between estimated effect size for each study in terms of duration of mechanical ventilation.

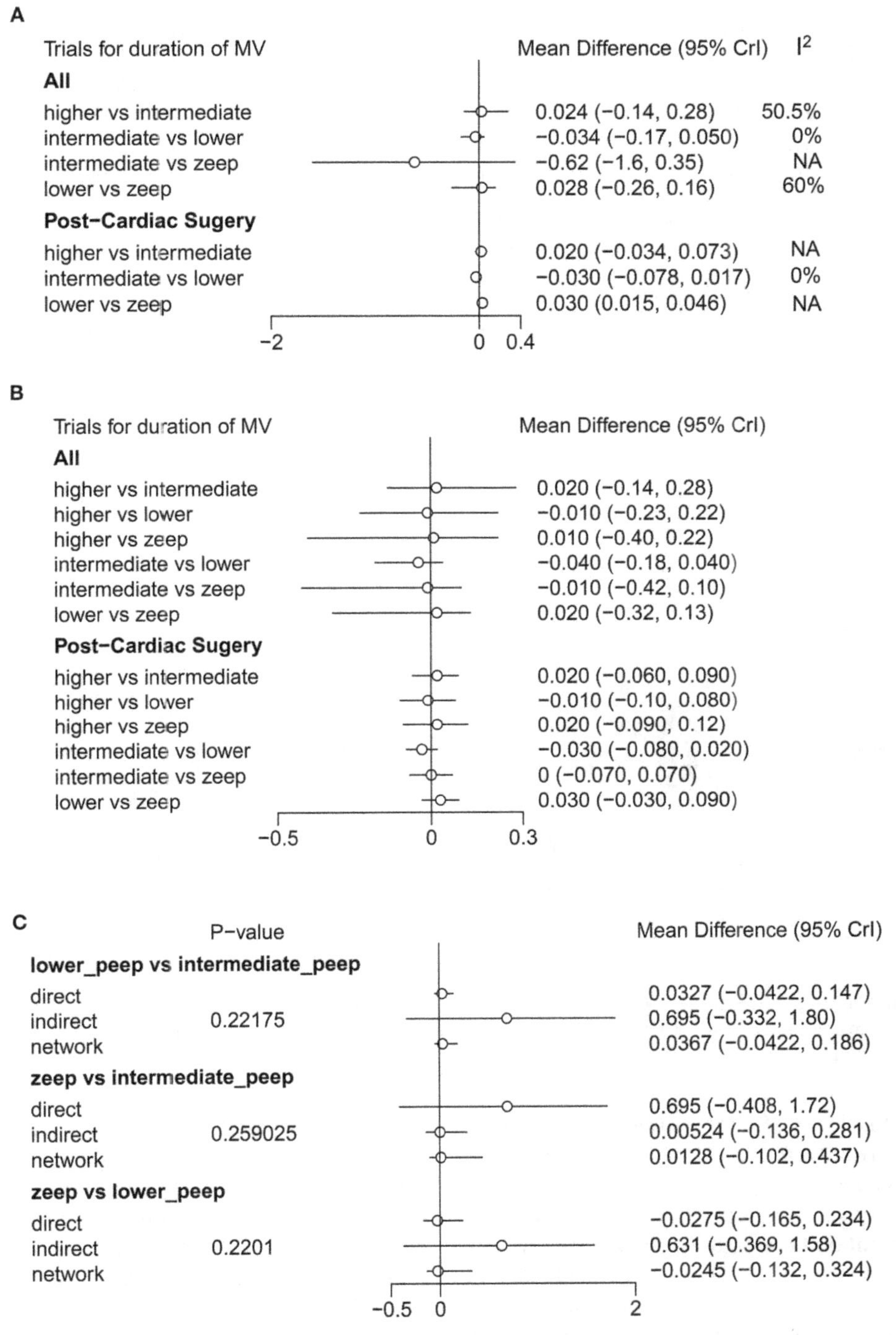

FIGURE 5 | Forest plot of duration of mechanical ventilation. **(A)** Results of direct comparison and heterogeneity test. **(B)** Results of Network Meta-Analysis. **(C)** Node-splitting analysis to assess inconsistency in network meta-analysis. In addition to general population (No statistic difference in inconsistency between direct result and indirect result when *P*-value > 0.05), **(A,B)** also show the results of analysis among post-cardiac surgery patients.

(all $p > 0.05$) (**Supplementary Figure 1C**). Ranking analysis showed that higher PEEP was associated with the best PFR, followed by intermediate and lower PEEP, and lastly ZEEP (**Supplementary Figure 1D**).

A total of 7 studies (5, 10, 18, 19, 26, 29, 35), comprising 1,482 patients, reported LOS of hospital, with 4 (18, 19, 26, 29) of them (that analyzed 348 patients) focusing on post-cardiac surgery patients. Direct comparisons and Network Meta-Analysis revealed no significant differences among all PEEP levels in either the general or post cardiac surgical patients (**Supplementary Figure 2**). Additionally, 6 studies (5, 10, 18, 29, 35, 38) (with 1,433 patients) reported LOS of ICU, with direct

TABLE 2 | Pooled estimates of the network meta-analysis for "duration of MV."

Relative effects	Higher	Intermediate	Lower	Zeep
Higher	–	−0.02 (−0.28, 0.14)	0.01 (−0.22, 0.23)	−0.01 (−0.22, 0.40)
Intermediate	0.02 (−0.14, 0.28)	–	0.04 (−0.04, 0.18)	0.01 (−0.10, 0.43)
Lower	−0.01 (−0.23, 0.22)	−0.04 (−0.18, 0.04)	–	−0.02 (−0.13, 0.32)
Zeep	0.01 (−0.40, 0.22)	−0.01 (−0.43, 0.10)	0.02 (−0.32, 0.13)	–

Results are MDs in the column-defining treatment compared with MDs in the row-defining treatment. Given that "duration of MV" is a negative outcome, MD < 0 favored the column-defining treatment. MD, mean difference; MV, mechanical ventilation.

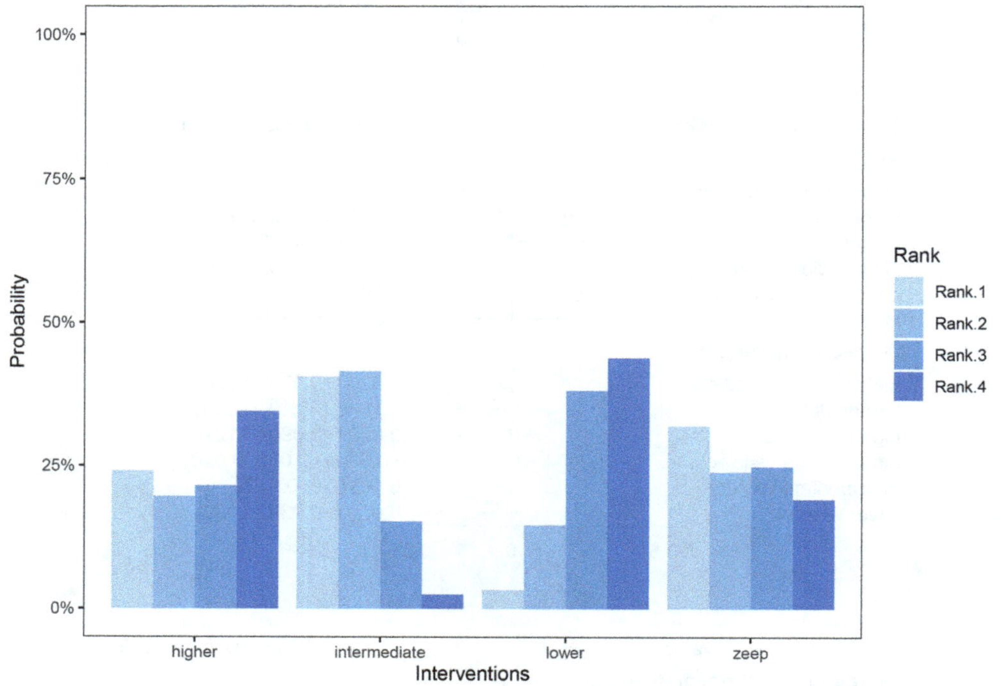

FIGURE 6 | Cumulative ranking bar graph for duration of mechanical ventilation. Ranks represent priority. For each intervention, cumulative ranking bar graph shows the probabilities when they are at Rank1/2/3/4 respectively. To sum up, the probabilities of every 4 columns in each intervention are 100%.

comparison showing that lower PEEP levels were associated with shorter LOS of ICU relative to ZEEP (MD: −6.00, 95% CI: −9.80, −2.20) (**Supplementary Figure 3A**). However, Network Meta-Analysis revealed no significant differences among all PEEP levels (**Supplementary Figure 3B**). Hospital mortality was reported in 9 eligible studies (5, 10, 17, 19, 27, 33, 35, 36, 38), comprising 1,561 patients, 28-days mortality was reported in 3 eligible studies (10, 33, 34), that analyzed 1,152 patients, while ICU mortality was reported in 3 eligible studies (10, 17, 35) (with 1,056 patients). Notably, only direct comparison showed that higher PEEP levels were associated with increased ICU mortality when compared to lower PEEP (OR: 10.1, 95% CI: 1.21, 91.9) (**Supplementary Figure 4A**). Results from Network Meta-Analysis revealed no significant differences among the PEEP levels with regards to hospital, 28 days and ICU mortality (**Supplementary Figure 4B**).

Four eligible studies (5, 10, 36, 38), comprising 1,267 patients, reported incidence of ARDS, 7 (5, 10, 17, 18, 27, 35, 36) (with 1,383 patients) described incidence of pneumothorax, 4 (5, 10, 29, 36) with a total of 1,368 patients reported incidence of atelectasis, while 4 (5, 10, 36) with 1,255 patients described incidence of hypoxemia. Direct comparison revealed no significant differences among PEEP levels in the various complications (**Supplementary Figure 5A**). Similarly, Network Meta-Analysis showed that there were no significant differences among the PEEP levels with regards to occurrence of ARDS,atelectasis and hypoxemia (**Supplementary Figure 5B**), although higher PEEP levels were associated with significantly higher incidence of pneumothorax relative to intermediate and lower PEEP, as well as ZEEP (OR: 2.91e + 12, 95% CI: 40.3, 1.76e + 39; OR: 1.85e + 12, 95% CI: 29.2, 1.18e + 39; and OR: 1.44e + 12, 95% CI: 16.9, 8.70e + 38, respectively) and there was no significant difference among intermediate PEEP, lower PEEP and ZEEP (**Figure 9**). Node-splitting analysis, based on both direct and indirect comparisons among groups, revealed consistent results (all $p > 0.05$) (**Supplementary Figure 6A**).

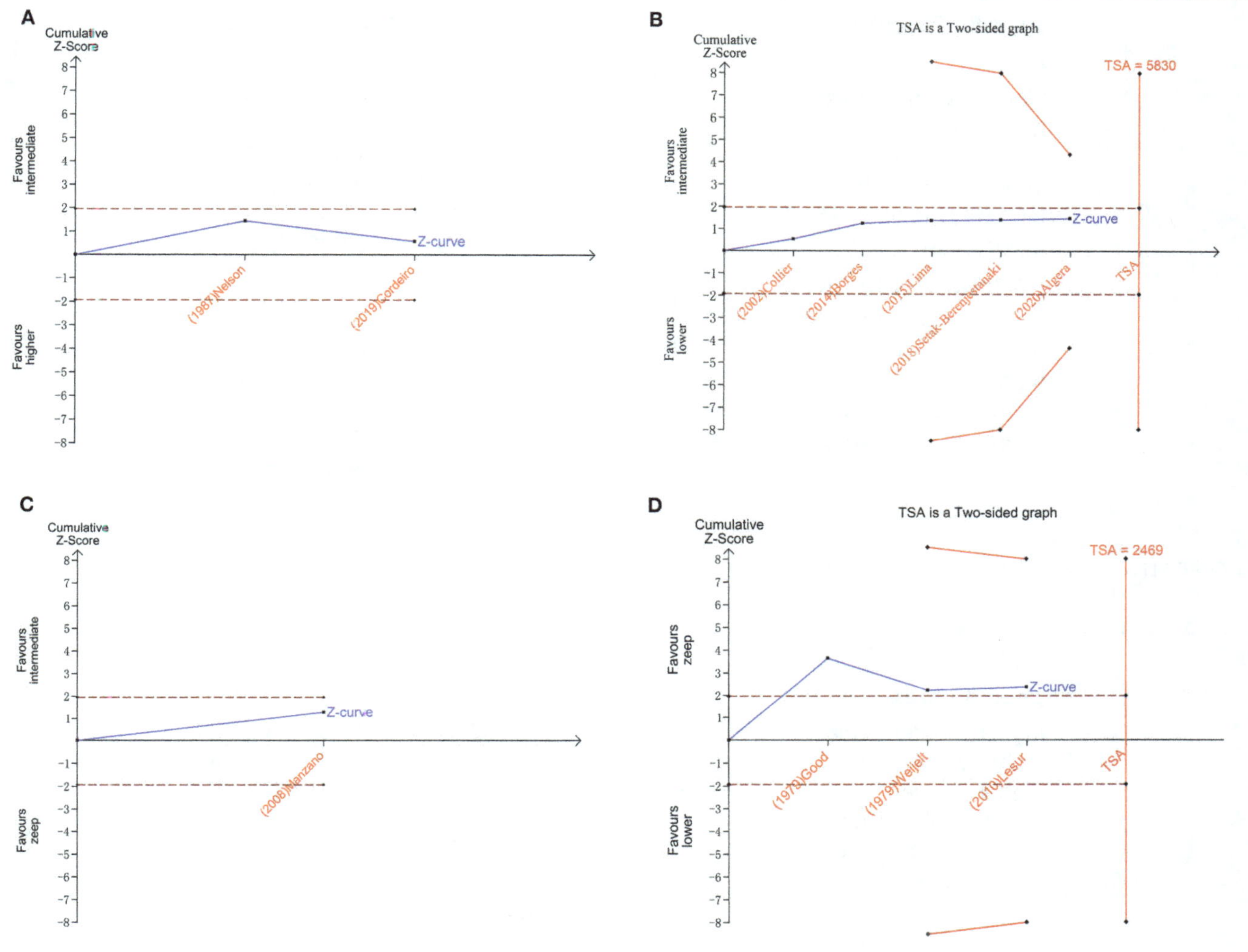

FIGURE 7 | Plots of trial sequential analysis (TSA) for duration of mechanical ventilation. **(A)** TSA for higher peep *vs.* intermediate peep; **(B)** TSA for intermediate peep vs. lower peep; **(C)** TSA for intermediate peep vs. Zeep; **(D)** TSA for lower peep vs. Zeep. TSA boundary is ignored due to too little information use in **A,C**.

Results from ranking analysis showed that high PEEP levels were associated with the highest risk of pneumothorax development, followed by intermediate and lower PEEP, and finally ZEEP (**Supplementary Figure 6B**).

DISCUSSION

We employed a Bayesian network meta-analysis to compare ZEEP levels in 28 RCTs (with 2,709 patients) that focused on ventilated patients without ARDS. Our results revealed that intermediate PEEP levels were associated with the highest decrease in the duration of mechanical ventilation, although there were no significant differences among PEEP levels based on direct and indirect comparisons. Meanwhile, higher PEEP levels were associated with significantly higher PFR and increased incidence of pneumothorax. Notably, we found no significant differences among the PEEP groups with regards to LOS of hospital and ICU, hospital, 28-day and ICU mortalities, occurrence of ARDS, atelectasis and hypoxemia. However, our results should be interpreted cautiously, owing to the TSA outcomes and presence of heterogeneity.

One meta-analysis published in 2016 (11) demonstrated that ventilation with higher PEEP levels in ICU patients without ARDS was not associated with neither reduced in-hospital mortality nor shorter ventilation duration, but with lower incidence of ARDS and hypoxemia, as well as higher PaO_2/FiO_2. Notably, the study had a moderate to high heterogeneity, while its quality of evidence was low to very low. Consequently, the authors could not address the effects of moderate levels of PEEP (11). When compared to the aforementioned meta-analysis, our study had several strengths. Firstly, we included seven recent studies, which included one large RCT describing use of high PEEP in patients without ARDS. The lower and higher PEEP groups in the former study corresponded to low and intermediate PEEP groups, respectively, in our study (10). This could also explain why our results were not completely consistent with previous meta-analyses. Secondly, we employed a novel

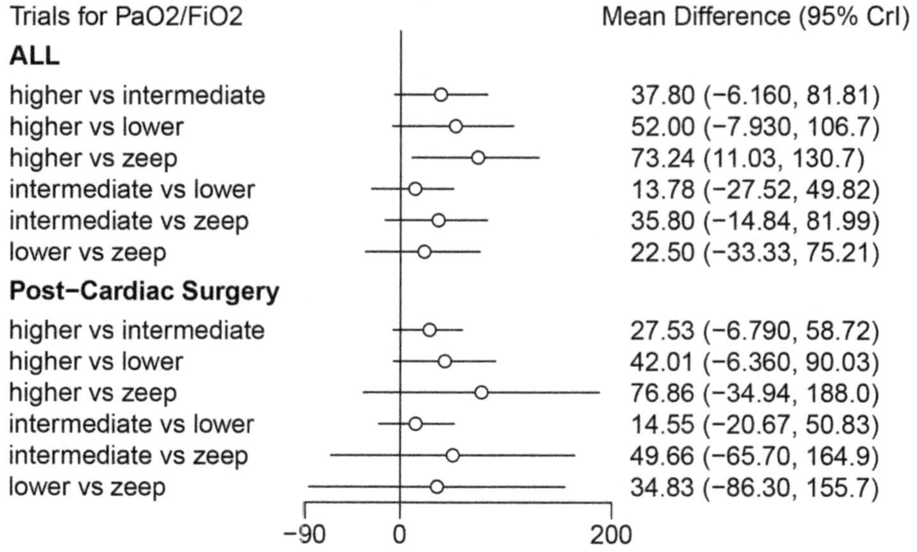

FIGURE 8 | Forest plot of Network Meta-Analysis for PaO_2/FiO_2.

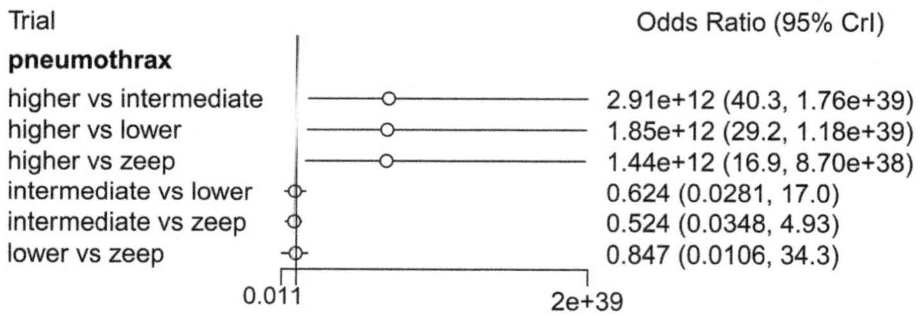

FIGURE 9 | Forest plot of Network Meta-Analysis for the incidence of pneumothorax.

classification, and divided the patients into four groups according to the specific PEEP levels. The ZEEP and very high PEEP (>10 cm H_2O) groups are not routine choices across clinical practice for non-ARDS patients, and these 2 extreme PEEP levels have always been applied in post cardiac surgery patients in our included studies. Moreover, since most of these studies were published 20 years ago, our novel classification allowed us to address the effects of moderate PEEP levels closer to clinical practice. Thirdly, a previous meta-analysis reported PEEP levels that ranged from 0 to10 cm H_2O for the low group, and 5 to 30 cm H_2O for the high group, while the heterogeneity was so large that the authors could not make a definite conclusion. Our novel classification solved this problem to a certain extent, and made the conclusion more credible.

Although previous studies have demonstrated the potential benefits and adverse effects of PEEP in ARDS, selecting appropriate PEEP levels seems to be a complex process in patients without ARDS owing to a huge heterogeneity in this population. Although an increase in PEEP levels has been reported in such population in the real-world, evidence of how to choose an optimal concentration was lacking (6, 41). In our study, Bayesian analysis revealed that intermediate PEEP (PEEP = 7–10 cm H_2O) was associated with shorter duration of mechanical ventilation, whereas network meta-analysis found no significant differences among the studied PEEP levels, which was partially in line with the RELAx trial (10). Interestingly, one study demonstrated that a higher PEEP could reduce the duration of mechanical ventilation (16), was although this corresponded to the intermediate PEEP group in our study. To our knowledge, there were many confounding factors that affected the duration of mechanical ventilation, affirming PEEP's lack of significant impact observed herein.

Our results further showed that PFR was positively correlated with PEEP levels, which was consistent with a previous meta-analysis (11). In ARDS patients, PEEP has been shown to recruit the collapse alveoli, maintain the end expiratory lung volume and improve gas exchange (3). Interestingly, the same principle seems to work in patients without ARDS. On the other hand, inadequate elevated PEEP has been found to cause alveoli overdistension in ARDS patients, thereby causing barotrauma (42, 43). In our opinion, this challenge might be even more pronounced in non-ARDS patients as the collapse alveoli in these patients might be less than those in ARDS patients. This explains why higher PEEP levels were associated with significantly increased incidence of pneumothorax relative to the other PEEP levels in our study. Although the meta-analysis published in 2016 demonstrated that high PEEP was associated with a lower incidence of ARDS and hypoxemia (11), we found no evidence to support this finding.

Although our findings provide evidence of the potential benefits or harmful effects of different PEEP levels, PEEP should not just be applied according to its height, as many physiologic effects of PEEP could be U-shaped (44, 45), Individualized PEEP regimes should be optimized based on a specific patient's physiology rather than focusing simply on the dosage. To date, however, no trial has attempted to evaluate the efficacy of PEEP in patients without ARDS prior to randomization (4), which necessitates future trials.

CONCLUSION

In summary, results of our Bayesian network meta-analysis and systematic review revealed that intermediate PEEP levels are associated with the highest decrease in duration of mechanical ventilation in patients without ARDS. However, there were no significant differences among studied PEEP level groups based on both direct and indirect comparisons. Meanwhile, it is evident that higher PEEP levels are associated with significantly higher PFR and increased incidence of pneumothorax. Furthermore, the four studied PEEP levels have no significant impact on LOS of hospital, LOS of ICU, hospital mortality, 28-day mortality, ICU mortality, occurrence of ARDS, as well as atelectasis and hypoxemia.

AUTHOR CONTRIBUTIONS

YH and LS: conceptualization, methodology, and supervision. JZ and ZL: data curation and writing-original draft preparation. XD and BL: software and visualization. YZhang, YZheng, HZ, YW, YLai, and WH: writing-review. XL, WH, YX, and YLi: supervision. All authors contributed to the article and approved the submitted version.

REFERENCES

1. Dreyfuss D, Soler P, Basset G, Saumon G. High inflation pressure pulmonary edema. Respective effects of high airway pressure, high tidal volume, and positive end-expiratory pressure. *Am Rev Res Dis.* (1988) 137:1159–64. doi: 10.1164/ajrccm/137.5.1159
2. Slutsky AS, Ranieri VM. Ventilator-induced lung injury. *N Engl J Med.* (2013) 369:2126–36. doi: 10.1056/NEJMra1208707
3. cAshbaugh DG, Bigelow DB, Petty TL, Levine BE. Acute respiratory distress in adults. *Lancet.* (1967) 2:319–23. doi: 10.1016/S0140-6736(67)90168-7
4. Sahetya SK, Goligher EC, Slutsky AS. Searching for the optimal PEEP in patients without ARDS: high, low, or in between? *JAMA.* (2020) 324:2490–2. doi: 10.1001/jama.2020.23067
5. Manzano F, Fernandez-Mondejar E, Colmenero M, Poyatos ME, Rivera R, Machado J, et al. Positive-end expiratory pressure reduces incidence of ventilator-associated pneumonia in nonhypoxemic patients. *Cri Care Med.* (2008) 36:2225–31. doi: 10.1097/CCM.0b013e31817b8a92
6. Penuelas O, Muriel A, Abraira V, Frutos-Vivar F, Mancebo J, Raymondos K, et al. Inter-country variability over time in the mortality of mechanically ventilated patients. *Int Care Med.* (2020) 46:444–53. doi: 10.1007/s00134-019-05867-9
7. Vreugdenhil HA, Heijnen CJ, Plotz FB, Zijlstra J, Jansen NJ, Haitsma JJ, et al. Mechanical ventilation of healthy rats suppresses peripheral immune function. *Eur Res J.* (2004) 23:122–8. doi: 10.1183/09031936.03.00035003
8. Carvalho AR, Jandre FC, Pino AV, Bozza FA, Salluh JI, Rodrigues R, et al. Effects of descending positive end-expiratory pressure on lung mechanics and aeration in healthy anaesthetized piglets. *Cri Care.* (2006) 10:R122. doi: 10.1186/cc5030
9. Villar J, Herrera-Abreu MT, Valladares F, Muros M, Perez-Mendez L, Flores C, et al. Experimental ventilator-induced lung injury: exacerbation by positive end-expiratory pressure. *Anesthesiology.* (2009) 110:1341–7. doi: 10.1097/ALN.0b013e31819fcba9
10. Writing C, Steering Committee for the RCG, Algera AG, Pisani L, Serpa Neto A, den Boer SS, et al. Effect of a lower vs. higher positive end-expiratory pressure strategy on ventilator-free days in icu patients without ARDS: a randomized clinical trial. *JAMA.* (2020) 324:2509–20. doi: 10.1001/jama.2020.23517
11. Serpa Neto A, Filho RR, Cherpanath T, Determann R, Dongelmans DA, Paulus F, et al. Associations between positive end-expiratory pressure and outcome of patients without ARDS at onset of ventilation: a systematic review and meta-analysis of randomized controlled trials. *Ann Int Care.* (2016) 6:109. doi: 10.1186/s13613-016-0208-7
12. Hutton B, Salanti G, Caldwell DM, Chaimani A, Schmid CH, Cameron C, et al. The PRISMA extension statement for reporting of systematic reviews incorporating network meta-analyses of health care interventions: checklist and explanations. *Ann Int Med.* (2015) 162:777–84. doi: 10.7326/M14-2385
13. Sterne JAC, Savovic J, Page MJ, Elbers RG, Blencowe NS, Boutron I, et al. RoB 2: a revised tool for assessing risk of bias in randomised trials. *BMJ.* (2019) 366:l4898. doi: 10.1136/bmj.l4898
14. Hozo SP, Djulbegovic B, Hozo I. Estimating the mean and variance from the median, range, and the size of a sample. *BMC Med Res Methodol.* (2005) 5:13. doi: 10.1186/1471-2288-5-13
15. Borges DL, Nina VJ, Costa Mde A, Baldez TE, Santos NP, Lima IM, et al. Effects of different PEEP levels on respiratory mechanics and oxygenation after coronary artery bypass grafting. *Rev Bras Cir Cardiovasc.* (2013) 28:380–5. doi: 10.5935/1678-9741.20130058
16. Lago Borges D, José da Silva Nina V, Pereira Baldez TE, de Albuquerque Gonçalves Costa M, Pereira dos Santos N, Mendes Lima I, et al. Effects of positive end-expiratory pressure on mechanical ventilation duration after coronary artery bypass grafting: a randomized clinical trial. *Ann Thor Cardiovasc Surg.* (2014) 20:773–7. doi: 10.5761/atcs.cr.13-00069
17. Carroll GC, Tuman KJ, Braverman B, Logas WG, Wool N, Goldin M, et al. Minimal positive end-expiratory pressure (PEEP) may be "best PEEP." *Chest.* (1988) 93:1020–5. doi: 10.1378/chest.93.5.1020
18. Celebi S, Koner O, Menda F, Korkut K, Suzer K, Cakar N. The pulmonary and hemodynamic effects of two different recruitment maneuvers after cardiac surgery. *Anesth Analg.* (2007) 104:384–90. doi: 10.1213/01.ane.0000252967.33414.44
19. Collier B, Kolff J, Devineni R, Gonzalez LS, 3rd. Prophylactic positive end-expiratory pressure and reduction of postoperative blood loss in open-heart surgery. *Ann Thor Surg.* (2002) 74:1191–4. doi: 10.1016/S0003-4975(02)03879-1
20. Cordeiro ALL, Gruska CA, Ysla P, Queiroz A, Nogueira SCO, Leite MC, et al. Effect of different levels of peep on oxygenation

during non-invasive ventilation in patients submitted to CABG surgery: randomized clinical trial. *Bra J Cardiovasc Surg.* (2017) 32:295–300. doi: 10.21470/1678-9741-2016-0038

21. Cordeiro ALL, Carvalho S, Leite MC, Vila-Flor A, Freitas B, Sousa L, et al. Impact of lung expansion therapy using positive end-expiratory pressure in mechanically ventilated patients submitted to coronary artery bypass grafting. *Bra J Cardiovasc Surg.* (2019) 34:699–703. doi: 10.21470/1678-9741-2019-0016
22. Dyhr T, Laursen N, Larsson A. Effects of lung recruitment maneuver and positive end-expiratory pressure on lung volume, respiratory mechanics and alveolar gas mixing in patients ventilated after cardiac surgery. *Acta Anaesthesiol Scand.* (2002) 46:717–25. doi: 10.1034/j.1399-6576.2002.460615.x
23. Good Jr JT, Wolz JF, Anderson JT, Dreisin RB, Petty TL. The routine use of positive end-expiratory pressure after open heart surgery. *Chest.* (1979) 76:397–400. doi: 10.1378/chest.76.4.397
24. Holland A, Thuemer O, Schelenz C, van Hout N, Sakka SG. Positive end-expiratory pressure does not affect indocyanine green plasma disappearance rate or gastric mucosal perfusion after cardiac surgery. *Eur J Anaesthesiol.* (2007) 24:141–7. doi: 10.1017/S026502150600130X
25. Lima RO, Borges DL, Costa Mde A, Baldez TE, Barbosa e Silva MG, Sousa FA, et al. Relationship between pre-extubation positive end-expiratory pressure and oxygenation after coronary artery bypass grafting. *Rev Bras Cir Cardiovasc.* (2015) 30:443–8. doi: 10.5935/1678-9741.20150044
26. Marvel SL, Elliott CG, Tocino I, Greenway LW, Metcalf SM, Chapman RH. Positive end-expiratory pressure following coronary artery bypass grafting. *Chest.* (1986) 90:537–41. doi: 10.1378/chest.90.4.537
27. Michalopoulos A, Anthi A, Rellos K, Geroulanos S. Effects of positive end-expiratory pressure (PEEP) in cardiac surgery patients. *Res Med.* (1998) 92:858–62. doi: 10.1016/S0954-6111(98)90388-2
28. Murphy DA, Finlayson DC, Craver JM, Jones EL, Kopel M, Tobia V, et al. Effect of positive end-expiratory pressure on excessive mediastinal bleeding after cardiac operations. A controlled study. *J Thor Cardiovasc Surg.* (1983) 85:864–9. doi: 10.1016/S0022-5223(19)37475-6
29. Setak-Berenjestanaki M, Bagheri-Nesami M, Gholipour Baradari A, Mousavinasab SN, Ghaffari R, Darbeheshti M. The prophylactic effect of different levels of positive endexpiratory pressure on the incidence rate of atelectasis after cardiac surgery: a randomized controlled trial. *Med J Islam Repub Iran.* (2018) 32:20. doi: 10.14196/mjiri.32.20
30. Zurick AM, Urzua J, Ghattas M, Cosgrove DM, Estafanous FG, Greenstreet R. Failure of positive end-expiratory pressure to decrease postoperative bleeding after cardiac surgery. *Ann Thor Surg.* (1982) 34:608–11. doi: 10.1016/S0003-4975(10)60898-3
31. Cujec B, Polasek P, Mayers I, Johnson D. Positive end-expiratory pressure increases the right-to-left shunt in mechanically ventilated patients with patent foramen ovale. *Ann Int Med.* (1993) 119:887–94. doi: 10.7326/0003-4819-119-9-199311010-00004
32. Koutsoukou A, Perraki H, Raftopoulou A, Koulouris N, Sotiropoulou C, Kotanidou A, et al. Respiratory mechanics in brain-damaged patients. *Int Care Med.* (2006) 32:1947–54. doi: 10.1007/s00134-006-0406-0
33. Lesur O, Remillard MA, St-Pierre C, Falardeau S. Prophylactic positive end-expiratory pressure and postintubation hemodynamics: an interventional, randomized study. *Can Res J.* (2010) 17:e45–50. doi: 10.1155/2010/269581
34. Ma C, Liang D, Zheng F. [Effect of high positive end-expiratory pressure for mechanical ventilation in the treatment of neurological pulmonary edema]. *Zhonghua Wei Zhong Bing Ji Jiu Yi Xue.* (2014) 26:339–42. doi: 10.3760/cma.j.issn.2095-4352.2014.05.011
35. Nelson LD, Civetta JM, Hudson-Civetta J. Titrating positive end-expiratory pressure therapy in patients with early, moderate arterial hypoxemia. *Cri Care Med.* (1987) 15:14–9. doi: 10.1097/00003246-198701000-00003
36. Pepe PE, Hudson LD, Carrico CJ. Early application of positive end-expiratory pressure in patients at risk for the adult respiratory-distress syndrome. *N Engl J Med.* (1984) 311:281–6. doi: 10.1056/NEJM198408023110502
37. Vigil AR, Clevenger FW. The effects of positive end-expiratory pressure of intrapulmonary shunt and ventilatory deadspace in nonhypoxic trauma patients. *J Trauma.* (1996) 40:618–22; discussion 22–3. doi: 10.1097/00005373-199604000-00017
38. Weigelt JA, Mitchell RA, Snyder WH, 3rd. Early positive end-expiratory pressure in the adult respiratory distress syndrome. *Arch Surg.* (1979) 114:497–501. doi: 10.1001/archsurg.1979.01370280151024
39. Cao F, Chen RL, Liu XF, He R. [Effect of positive end-expiratory pressure on the pressure gradient of venous return in hypovolemic patients under mechanical ventilation]. *Zhongguo Wei Zhong Bing Ji Jiu Yi Xue.* (2009) 21:583–6.
40. Feeley TW, Saumarez R, Klick JM, McNabb TG, Skillman JJ. Positive end-expiratory pressure in weaning patients from controlled ventilation. A prospective randomised trial. *Lancet.* (1975) 2:725–9. doi: 10.1016/S0140-6736(75)90719-9
41. Neto AS, Barbas CSV, Simonis FD, Artigas-Raventos A, Canet J, Determann RM, et al. Epidemiological characteristics, practice of ventilation, and clinical outcome in patients at risk of acute respiratory distress syndrome in intensive care units from 16 countries (PRoVENT): an international, multicentre, prospective study. *Lancet Res Med.* (2016) 4:882–93. doi: 10.1016/S2213-2600(16)30305-8
42. Iwashyna TJ, Burke JF, Sussman JB, Prescott HC, Hayward RA, Angus DC. Implications of heterogeneity of treatment effect for reporting and analysis of randomized trials in critical care. *Am J Res Cri Care Med.* (2015) 192:1045–51. doi: 10.1164/rccm.201411-2125CP
43. Goligher EC, Kavanagh BP, Rubenfeld GD, Ferguson ND. Physiologic responsiveness should guide entry into randomized controlled trials. *Am J Res Cri Care Med.* (2015) 192:1416–9. doi: 10.1164/rccm.201410-1832CP
44. Gurudatt C. Perioperative fluid therapy: how much is not too much? *Indian J Anaesth.* (2012) 56:323–5. doi: 10.4103/0019-5049.100810
45. Li Y, Bai Z, Li M, Wang X, Pan J, Li X, et al. U-shaped relationship between early blood glucose and mortality in critically ill children. *BMC pediatrics.* (2015) 15:88. doi: 10.1186/s12887-015-0403-y

14

Neuromuscular Electrical Stimulation in Patients with Severe COVID-19 Associated with Sepsis and Septic Shock

*Renato Fraga Righetti, Samantha Torres Grams, Wesla Neves da Silva Costa, Leandro Teixeira Saraiva, Isabel Chateaubriand Diniz de Salles and Wellington Pereira Yamaguti**

Hospital Sírio-Libanês, São Paulo, Brazil

***Correspondence:**
Wellington Pereira Yamaguti
wellington.psyamaguti@hsl.org.br

Background: Neuromuscular electrical stimulation (NMES) can be applied to critically ill patients. However, its results on muscle strength and functionality in patients with COVID-19 are unknown.

Objective: Evaluate the effects of intervention with NMES on muscle mass and functionality of patients with severe COVID-19 associated with sepsis and septic shock.

Methods: Seven patients with COVID-19 associated with sepsis or septic shock were selected, but only 5 patients completed all days of the intervention with NMES. The intervention was performed by a single physiotherapist on 7 consecutive days in a daily session of 40 min. The outcome measures were the femoris cross-sectional area; thickness of the anterior compartment of the quadriceps muscle; rectus femoris echogenicity; International Classification of Functioning, Disability, and Health (ICF)-muscle strength; PFIT-s, DEMMI, and the SOMS; feasibility, and safety. The patients were evaluated on days 1, 5, and 8.

Results: The rectus femoris cross-sectional area decreased significantly from days 1 to 8, but showed maintenance of the thickness of the anterior compartment of the quadriceps muscle from days 1 to 8. The MRC score increased significantly from days 1 to 5 and kept this improvement until day 8. All patients showed an increase in the MRC score and reduction of the ICF-muscle strength, meaning improved muscle strength from days 1 to 8. The PFIT-s increased significantly from days 1 to 5 and improved until day 8 compared to day 5. DEMMI and SOMS score increased significantly on day 8 compared to days 1 and 5.

Conclusion: Rehabilitation with NMES showed improvement in muscle strength and functionality of patients in this study with a potential protective effect on muscle mass loss in patients with critical COVID-19 associated with sepsis and septic shock. This study is the first report of the potential effects of neuromuscular electrical stimulation in patients with severe COVID-19 associated with sepsis and septic shock.

Keywords: COVID-19, sepsis, physiotherapy, neuromuscular electrical stimulation, muscle mass

INTRODUCTION

The Coronavirus disease 2019 (COVID-19) is caused by novel Severe Acute Respiratory Syndrome Coronavirus 2 (SARS-CoV-2) (1). The virus spread rapidly through the world population and several hospitals have produced guidelines for the respiratory management of these patients (2, 3). Most patients have a mild form of the disease, but 5% of patients present severe lung injury and required intensive care (4). These patients may develop ICU-acquired weakness (5).

Early mobilization in the intensive care unit (ICU) is proven to be effective in preventing muscle atrophy and functional disability. However, it is not necessarily applicable to all patients (6). Therefore, neuromuscular electrical stimulation (NMES) has been used as an additional rehabilitation strategy for critically ill patients (7). Studies using electrical muscle stimulation in septic patients have conflicting results depending on the titred stimulation frequency used. These studies showed that low stimulation frequency electrical stimulation was ineffective to preserve muscle mass (8) and high stimulation frequency electrical stimulation was able to increase strength (9). Carraro et al. (10) suggest that frail persons post-COVID-19 infection with muscle weakness or persons in prolonged inactivity for pandemic-related restriction may benefit from the full-body exercise program associated with NMES. However, these effects are unknown in patients in the acute phase of the disease with severe COVID-19.

The present study aims to describe our clinical protocol in the treatment with neuromuscular electrical stimulation of patients with COVID-19 associated with sepsis and septic shock during their acute intensive care unit stay and to discuss intervention responses in skeletal muscle mass and functional performance.

METHODS

All participants signed the Informed Consent Term, previously approved by the Ethics Committee of the Hospital Sírio-Libanês (number 3,999,139). This case series was conducted at the adult intensive care units of Hospital Sírio-Libanês, São Paulo, Brazil, and all approved ethical protocols were followed.

Patients

Seven patients with COVID-19 associated with sepsis or septic shock with age $\geq$ 18 years were selected. Sepsis diagnosis was defined by the Third International Consensus Definitions for Sepsis and Septic Shock (Sepsis-3) (11). Furthermore, patients should have the capacity to walk independently before hospitalization classified by mean of the Expanded Disability Status Score (EDSS) $\leq$ 6 (12) and immobilization period without walking $\leq$7 days.

Candidate Patients for Neuromuscular Electrical Stimulation

The inclusion criteria for starting NMES to critically ill patients include body mass index (BMI) $\leq$ 35 kg/m^2; without skin lesions, cardiac pacemaker, infection or trauma in lower limbs, neuromuscular diseases, use of neuromuscular blockers, polyneuropathy, and imminent risk of death in less than 48 hours (Simplified Acute Physiology Score III - SAPS III $\leq$ 80). The exclusion criteria for intervention were infarction and/or need for mechanical cardiopulmonary bypass devices or the need for intra-aortic balloon during ICU hospitalization.

Clinical Assessment

In the ICU admission, patients were evaluated and classified to clinical severity according to the Simplified Acute Physiology Score III (SAPS III) (13) and the Sequential Organ Failure Assessment (SOFA) (14). In addition, we collected clinical and neurological parameters. SAPS III and SOFA assessments were performed by the medical team of the intensive care unit.

Outcome Measures

Muscle mass was assessed using ultrasonography. Patients were evaluated concerning rectus femoris cross-sectional area (cm^2), the thickness of the anterior compartment of the quadriceps muscle (rectus femoris and vastus intermedius) (cm), and rectus femoris echogenicity (pixels) (5). The transducer was positioned perpendicular to the longitudinal axis of the thigh in 80% of the distal distance between the anterosuperior iliac spine and the upper midpoint of the patella to obtain measurements of the rectus femoris cross-sectional area, and thickness of the anterior compartment of the quadriceps muscle (rectus femoris and vastus intermedius). The measurements were performed using B-mode ultrasound (Logiq e ultrasound, GE Healthcare, USA) (**Figure 1**).

Functionality was assessed by the International Classification of Functioning, Disability, and Health (ICF) using the muscle strength domains (b730) based on the Medical Research Council (MRC) score for global strength (5). The ICF scores used were: 0–58 to 60 (without significant changes); 1–48 to 57 (slight loss); 2–31 to 47 (moderate loss); 3–4 to 30 (severe loss); and 4–0 to 3 (maximum loss). The MRC score is a voluntary method and depends on the understanding and collaboration of the patients. For this reason, in the case of patients on mechanical ventilation, it was evaluated only after interrupting sedation (15). In addition, we assessed functionality by the Physical Function ICU Test-scored (PFIT-s), Morton Mobility Index (DEMMI), and the Surgical Intensive Care Unit Optimal Mobilization Score (SOMS).

PFIT-s examine the capacity of the patient in the sit-to-stand level of assistance; maximal marching on the spot duration and number of steps; and shoulder flexion strength, and knee extension strength. The PFIT-s score ranges from 0 (unable to perform activities) to 10 (high physical functioning) (16). DEMMI is composed of 15 hierarchical mobility activities (bed-based, chair-based, static balance, walking-related, and dynamic balance). The total score is converted with Rasch Analysis with a score range from 0 (poor mobility) to 100 (high levels of independent mobility) (16). PFIT-s and DEMMI depend on the understanding and collaboration of the patients, and it was performed after interrupting the sedation. The SOMS score ranges from 0 (indicating that no mobilization should be considered since deemed to be futile, as for patients in a terminal unstable clinical condition such as those with intracranial

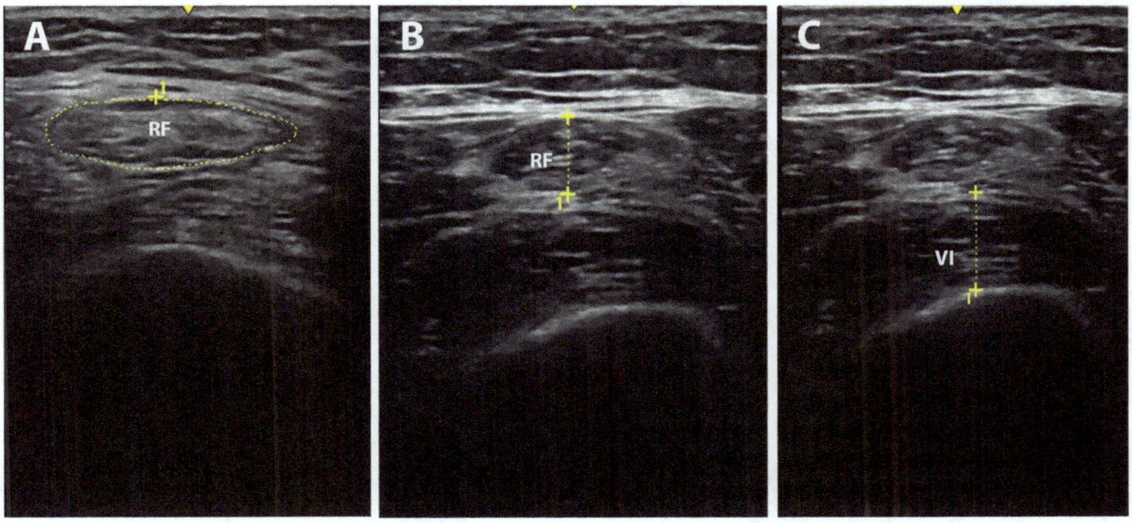

FIGURE 1 | Representative muscle ultrasound image methods: rectus femoris cross-section area **(A)**, the thickness of the anterior compartment of the quadriceps muscle [rectus femoris **(B)** and vastus intermedius **(C)**].

hypertension or severe systemic hemodynamic and respiratory insufficiency) to 4 (patients able to ambulate) (17).

The rectus femoris cross-sectional area (cm^2), the thickness of the anterior compartment of the quadriceps muscle, ICF-muscle strength, PFIT-s, DEMMI, and SOMS were evaluated on days 1, 5, and 8 of start intervention with neuromuscular electrical stimulation. All measurements were performed by the same physiotherapist on days 1, 5, and 8 and was blind to the interventions that were applied to the patients.

Neuromuscular Electrical Stimulation

The NMES was performed after interrupting the neuromuscular blocker with the patient in the supine position in the ICU bed with 30–60 degrees of the hips and knees joint flexion. The ICU bed itself was used to achieve the positioning of the patient necessary for intervention with NMES. Two pairs of self-adhesive electrodes (size 9 × 5 cm, SPES Medica Brazil Ltda, São Paulo, Brazil) were positioned distally over the motor area of vastus medialis and vastus lateralis muscles, and the other two were placed 5 cm below the inguinal region. The location of the electrodes was marked on the skin with a surgical marking pen to ensure application in the same location on subsequent days. This position of the NMES electrodes is capable of stimulating the motor points of the quadriceps muscles (18).

The parameters used were stimulation frequency of 100 Hz, a stimulation pulse width of 350 μs, a ramp-up time of 1 s, time on of 4 s, ramp-dow of the stimulation of the 1 s, and time off of 12 s. The stimulation pulse width was performed with charge-balanced biphasic pulses and trapezoidal waves. In awake patients, the intensity was established with the maximum muscle contraction tolerated by the patient. In sedated patients, it NMES was adjusted with 50% above the minimum necessary to generate a visible contraction (8). The stimulation frequency was based on Rodriguez et al. (9) that showed that the high stimulation frequency electrical stimulation presented a preventive effect in the progression of muscle weakness in patients having severe sepsis requiring mechanical ventilation. During the intervention with NMES, no voluntary muscle movement was requested.

The treatment with NMES was interrupted if the patient presented cardiorespiratory instability, high fever (above 39°C), development of muscle fatigue, pain above 7 on the Visual Analog Scale (VAS), or pain above 2 on the Pain Assessment in Advanced Dementia (PAINAD) scale (19).

The application of NMES was carried out by the same physiotherapist on 7 consecutive days in a daily session of 40 minutes. For the treatment, we used the NMES device (Neurodyn II; IBRAMED; Amparo; São Paulo; Brazil). The physiotherapist involved in the NMES intervention did not participate in the outcome assessment and was blind to the results.

Feasibility and Safety

Feasibility was determined based on adherence and safety was evaluated based on the incidence of adverse events. Adverse events were considered: hemodynamic instability, respiratory instability, skin injury, and bruises.

Statistical Analysis

Data were assessed for normality using the Shapiro-Wilk test. Parametric variables are presented as mean and standard error. Categorical data are presented as the absolute (*n*) and relative frequency (%). Change in the muscle mass and functional capacity was assessed by repeated measure analysis of variance. Statistical significance was indicated by a $P < 0.05$.

RESULTS

Seven patients attended the NMES sessions. One patient stopped the treatment of NMES and one patient died on day 8 (patients 4 and 6); therefore, data for these patients were not included in the outcomes of all patients; only their data are displayed in the

TABLE 1 | Characteristics of patients with COVID-19 associated with sepsis and septic shock during ICU and hospital stay.

Demographic characteristics and clinical characteristics													
Patient	**Age (y)**	**Gender**	**BMI**	**SOFA**	**SAPS III**	**COVID-19 severity**	**Sedation**	**Vasoactive drug**	**Neuromuscular blocker**	**Hydrocortisone**	**IMV days**	**ICU stay**	**Hospital stay**
1	67	Female	28.9	8	67	Critical illness	Yes	Yes	Yes	Yes	6	11	24
2	65	Female	30.2	0	38	Critical illness	Yes	Yes	Yes	Yes	4	15	22
3	72	Male	30.9	7	57	Critical illness	Yes	Yes	Yes	Yes	8	12	27
4	61	Male	31.7	0	46	Critical illness	Yes	Yes	Yes	Yes	6	28	28
5	67	Male	32.6	5	50	Critical illness	No	No	No	Yes	0	9	14
6	75	Male	31.2	7	90	Critical illness	Yes	Yes	Yes	Yes	9	9	21
7	70	Male	25.8	3	55	Critical illness	No	No	No	Yes	0	3	11
Mean ± SD	68.1 ± 4.6	–	30.2 ± 2.3	4.2 ± 3.3	57.5 ± 16.9	–	–	–	–	–	4.7 ± 3.5	12.4 ± 7.7	21.0 ± 6.3

Neurologic characteristics and comorbidities													
Patient	**EDSS ≤6**	**RASS (D1/D5/D8)**	**Glasgow (D1/D5/D8)**	**CAM (D1/D5/D8)**	**Oxygen therapy**	**NIV**	**Hypertension**	**Diabetes mellitus**	**Obesity**	**Dyslipidemia**	**Anxiety**	**Hypothyroidism**	**COPD**
1	Yes	−2/0/0	•/15/15	–/–/–	Yes	Yes	No	No	Yes	No	No	Yes	No
2	Yes	1/0/0	•/15/15	–/–/–	Yes	Yes	Yes	No	Yes	No	No	No	No
3	Yes	1/0/0	•/15/15	+/–/–	Yes	No	No	No	No	Yes	No	Yes	No
4	Yes	−4/0/•	•/15/•	–/–/•	Yes	No	No	No	No	No	No	No	No
5	Yes	0/0/0	15/15/15	–/–/–	Yes	No	Yes	Yes	Yes	Yes	No	No	No
6	Yes	−5/−5/•	•/•/•	–/–/•	Yes	Yes	Yes	No	Yes	Yes	No	No	No
7	Yes	0/0/0	15/15/15	–/–/–	Yes	Yes	Yes	No	No	No	No	No	Yes

BMI, body mass index; CAM, Confusion Assessment Method; COPD, chronic obstructive pulmonary disease; EDSS, Expanded Disability Status Score; ICU, intensive care unit; IMV, invasive mechanical ventilation; NIV, non-invasive ventilation; RASS, Richmond Agitation Sedation Scale; SAPS III, Simplified Acute Physiology Score III; SOFA, Sequential Organ Failure Assessment; •, not applicable.

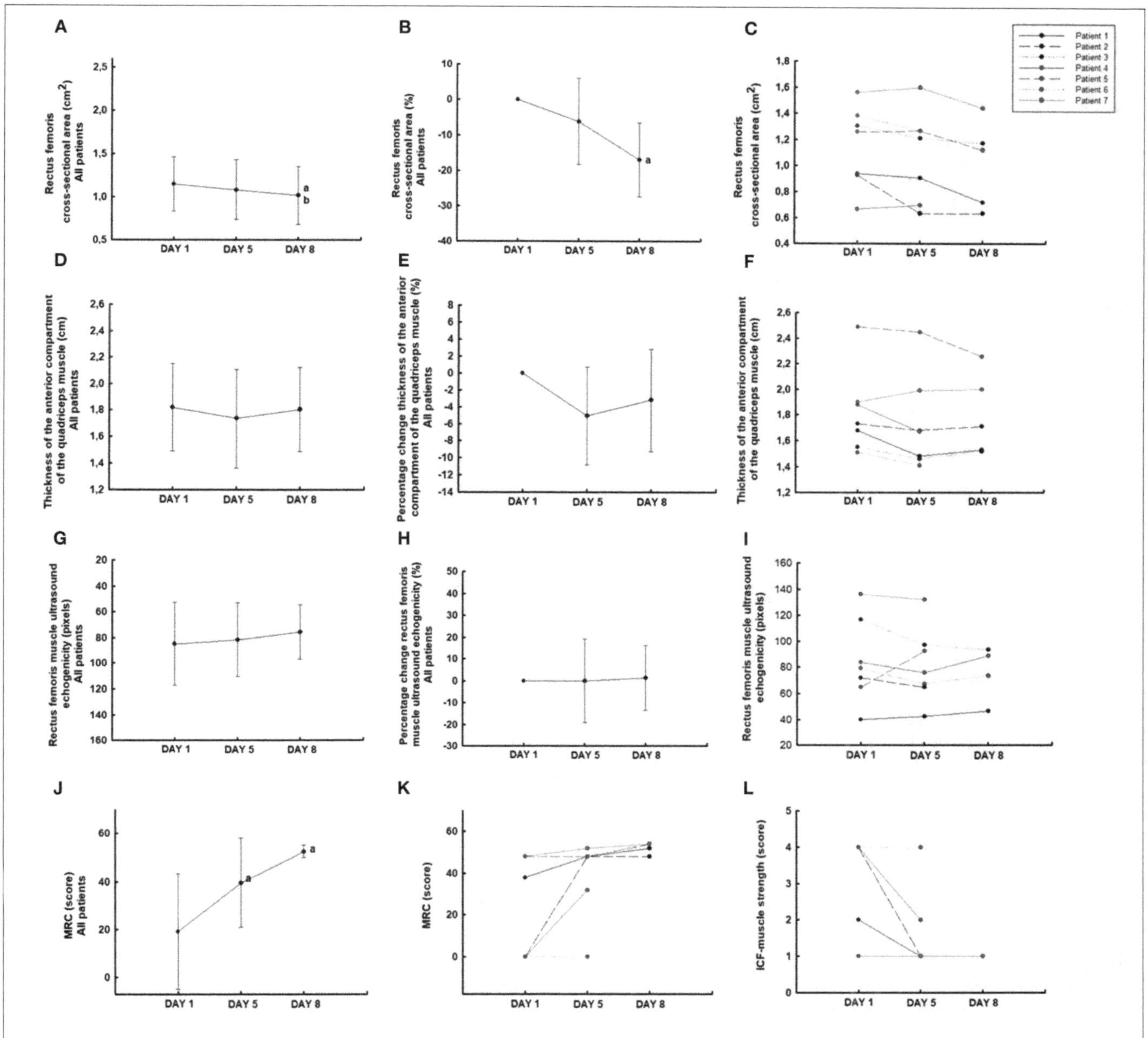

FIGURE 2 | Ultrasound muscle assessement of the rectus femoris cross-section área **(A–C)**; the thickness of the anterior compartment of the quadriceps muscle (rectus femoris and vastus intermedius) **(D–F)**; rectus femoris echogenicity **(G–I)**; MRC score **(J,K)**; and International Classification of Functioning, Disability, and Health (ICF)-muscle strength **(L)**. [a]$P < 0.05$ compared to day 1; [b]$P < 0.05$ compared to day 5.

individual patient values graph. The demographic characteristics of the patients are shown in **Table 1**.

Muscle Mass Outcomes

The rectus femoris cross-sectional area decreased significantly (−16.9% [95% CI, −29.8 to −3.9]; $P < 0.05$) from days 1 to 8 (**Figures 2A–C**), but showed maintenance of the thickness of the anterior compartment of the quadriceps muscle (−3.20% [95% CI, −10.6 to 4.2]; $P = 0.3$) from days 1 to 8 (**Figures 2D–F**). These patients showed a reduction of 2.1% [95% CI, −3.7 to −0.5] per day in the rectus femoris cross-sectional area and 0.3% [95% CI, −1.3 to 0.5] per day in the thickness of the anterior compartment of the quadriceps muscle during 8 days. Furthermore, patients showed maintenance of the echogenicity (1.3% [95% CI, −17.1 to 19.7%]; $P = 0.8$) from days 1 to 8 with an increase of 0.16% per day (**Figures 2G–I**).

Peripheral Muscle Strength and Functional Outcomes

The MRC score increased significantly from days 1 to 5 ($P < 0.05$) and kept this improvement until day 8 ($P = 0.5$) (**Figure 2J**). In the five patients evaluated, all (100%) showed an increase in the MRC score (**Figure 2K**) and reduction of the ICF-muscle strength, meaning improved muscle strength from days 1 to 8

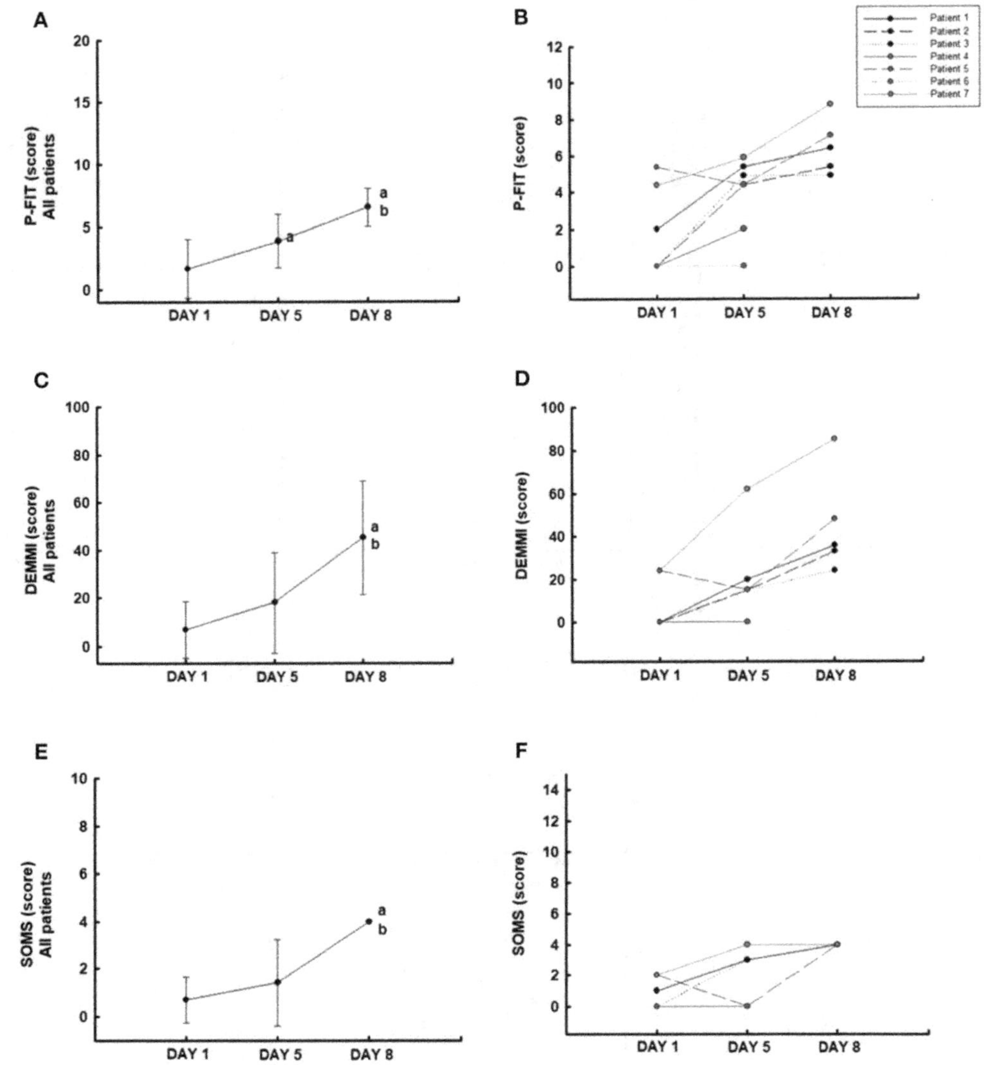

FIGURE 3 | Functionality: Physical Function ICU Test-scored (PFIT-s) **(A,B)**, Morton Mobility Index (DEMMI) **(C,D)**, and the Surgical Intensive Care Unit Optimal Mobilization Score (SOMS) **(E,F)**. [a]$P < 0.05$ compared to day 1; [b]$P < 0.05$ compared to day 5.

(**Figure 2L**). Four (80%) patients evaluated showed an increase in the MRC score and one (20%) maintained the MRC score values from days 5 to 8. Three patients (60%) showed a decrease in the ICF-muscle strength from days 1 to 5 and these values were maintained on day 8. Two patients (40%) maintained the ICF-muscle strength on days 5 and 8 compared with the baseline values (day 1).

The PFIT-s increased significantly from days 1 to 5 and improved until day 8 compared to day 5 ($P < 0.05$) (**Figure 3A**). All patients (100%) showed an increase in the PFIT-s on day 5 compared to day 1 and improvement on day 8 compared to day 5 (**Figure 3B**). DEMMI (**Figure 3C**) and SOMS (**Figure 3E**) scores increased significantly on day 8 compared to days 1 and 5 ($P < 0.05$). In the five patients evaluated, the individual data present that all (100%) patients showed an increase in the DEMMI (**Figure 3D**) and SOMS (**Figure 3F**) scores on days 5 and 8 compared with the baseline values (day 1).

Feasibility and Safety

No adverse events were reported during the case series. Five patients completed the assessments and intervention. One patient interrupted the NMES intervention but did not claim intolerance during the application, and one patient died due to worsening pulmonary and respiratory conditions. None of the NMES intervention sessions were interrupted by pain.

DISCUSSION

Patients with COVID-19 associated with sepsis and septic shock treated with NMES presented a reduction of 16.9% in the rectus femoris cross-sectional area, but with no significant reduction in the thickness of the anterior compartment of the quadriceps muscle (3.2%) and no significant increase of rectus femoris echogenicity on day 8 (1.3%). The magnitude of these alterations was 2.1, 0 3, and 0.16% per day, respectively. We emphasize that these reported values in the present case series are smaller than those found compared to another study conducted at the same hospital and research group that evaluated severe COVID-19 patients without NMES intervention. This study showed a reduction of 30.1% in the rectus femoris cross-sectional area, 18.6% in the thickness of the anterior compartment of the quadriceps muscle, and increase of 16.8% in the echogenicity on day 10 with themagnitude of these alterations being about 3.7, 2.1, and 1.68% per day, respectively (5).

The ability of electrical muscle stimulation to improve or maintain strength, muscle mass, and functionality in ICU patients with sepsis is controversial. However, the results seem to be related to the type of stimulation frequency involved in muscle stimulation. Rodriguez et al. (9) used high stimulation frequency in the neuromuscular electrical stimulation and showed a preventive effect in the progression of muscle weakness in patients having severe sepsis requiring mechanical ventilation. On the other hand, when Poulsen et al. (8) used low stimulation frequency in the patients with septic shock admitted to the ICU, and showed that loss of muscle mass was unaffected by electrical muscle stimulation. Our results corroborate with the Rodriguez et al. (9) study and enhance the possible benefit of using high stimulation frequency for muscle electrical stimulation.

The effect of electrical muscle stimulation on muscle mass and strength can be explained by several factors. Nuhr et al. (20) and Hambrecht et al. (21) showed that NMES induces an increase in oxidative capacity with the transition from fast to slow fiber types associated with a decrease in anaerobic enzymes levels. All physiological muscle changes found with the use of electrical muscle stimulation in critically ill patients suggest that the origin is a systemic effect on microcirculation (22). Vanderthommen et al. (23) showed that in the identical levels of workload (10% of the quadriceps maximum isometric voluntary torque), the muscle reaches higher values in blood flow and oxygen consumption during NMES compared with voluntary muscle contractions. Moreover, a single session of NMES is sufficient to stimulate the increased levels of mRNA for IGF binding protein-4 (84%), MyoD (83%), myogenin (~3-fold), cyclin D1 (50%), and p21-Waf1 (16-fold), which are indicative of the initiation of myogenic processes in skeletal muscle. In the same study, an additional NMES session (a total of 14 min spread over 2 days), was sufficient to induce an increase in the concentration of total skeletal muscle ribonucleic acid (RNA) (24), most likely representing an increase in muscle protein synthesis. These results indicate that molecular adaptations of skeletal muscle to loading respond in a very short time.

Neuromuscular blocking agents cause skeletal muscle relaxation by blocking the transmission of impulses at the neuromuscular junction (25). NMES evokes a muscle contraction by activating intramuscular branches of the nerve to the muscle and not the muscle fibers directly (26) and selected brain regions in a dose-response manner (27). The use of neuromuscular blocking agents during NMES intervention may interfere with the performance of muscle contraction. However, neuromuscular blockers present a recovery time of 8–40 min after their interruption (28). Therefore, we performed NMES intervention after interrupting the neuromuscular blocking agents.

Sedation is commonly used in patients admitted to the intensive care unit (29). Dirkes et al. (30) showed that NMES represents an effective and feasible interventional strategy to prevent skeletal muscle atrophy in a fully sedated patient with critically ill. In the same study, the non-stimulated leg showed substantial type 1 and type 2 muscle fiber atrophy (a 16 ± 9 and 24 ± 7% decline in muscle fiber; respectively). In contrast, no atrophy was observed in the muscle fibers collected from the stimulated leg. Although sedation does not interfere with NMES intervention, it can compromise functional assessments. Therefore, in the present study, the MRC score, P-FITs, and DEMMI evaluations were performed only after sedation withdrawal.

The limitation of this study is that it is a single-center study design and there is no control group to compare the efficacy. In addition, the number of cases is small and it is unclear whether the results can be generalized. Mateo et al. (31) used functional electrical stimulation associated with cycling in patients post-hospitalization in the ICU for a critical form of COVID-19. However, the present case series is the first report of the effects of neuromuscular electrical stimulation intervention in patients with severe COVID-19 in the acute phase of the disease associated with sepsis and septic shock. Randomized clinical trials with more patients reporting the efficacy of electrical stimulation using NMES in patients with COVID-19 associated with sepsis and septic shock are needed to confirm our findings.

CONCLUSION

Rehabilitation with NMES showed improvement in muscle strength and functionality of patients in this case series with a potential protective effect on muscle mass loss in patients with critical COVID-19 associated with sepsis and septic shock.

DATA AVAILABILITY STATEMENT

The raw data supporting the conclusions of this article will be made available by the authors, without undue reservation.

AUTHOR CONTRIBUTIONS

SG, WC, LS, IS, and WY: study design. SG, WC, and LS: data collection. RR and WY: data analysis and draft manuscript. RR, SG, WC, LS, IS, and WY: manuscript review. All authors contributed to the article and approved the submitted version.

ACKNOWLEDGMENTS

The authors thank the Fundação de Amparo à Pesquisa do Estado de São Paulo FAPESP, number 18/16832-9) and Hospital Sírio-Libanês.

REFERENCES

1. World Health Organization. *Clinical Management of COVID-19. May 14, 2020.* (2020). Available online at: https://www.who.int/publications/i/item/clinical-management-of-covid-19 (accessed October 1, 2020)
2. Lazzeri M, Lanza A, Bellini R, Bellofiore A, Cecchetto S, Colombo A, et al. Respiratory physiotherapy in patients with COVID-19 infection in acute setting: a Position Paper of the Italian Association of Respiratory Physiotherapists (ARIR). *Monaldi Arch Chest Dis.* (2020) 90:163–168. doi: 10.4081/monaldi.2020.1285
3. Righetti RF, Onoue MA, Politi FVA, Teixeira DT, Souza PN, Kondo CS, et al. Physiotherapy care of patients with coronavirus disease 2019. (COVID-19) - a Brazilian experience. *Clinics.* (2020) 75:e2017. doi: 10.6061/clinics/2020/e2017
4. Guan WJ, Ni ZY, Hu Y, Liang WH, Ou CQ, He JX, et al. Clinical characteristics of Coronavirus Disease 2019 in China. *New Engl J Med.* (2020) 382:1708–20. doi: 10.1056/NEJMoa2002032
5. de Andrade-Junior MC, de Salles ICD, de Brito CMM, Pastore-Junior L, Righetti RF, Yamaguti WP. Skeletal muscle wasting and function impairment in intensive care patients with severe COVID-19. *Front Physiol.* (2021) 12:640973. doi: 10.3389/fphys.2021.640973
6. Vanhorebeek I, Latronico N, Van den Berghe G. ICU-acquired weakness. *Intensive Care Med.* (2020) 46:637–53. doi: 10.1007/s00134-020-05944-4
7. Nakanishi N, Oto J, Tsutsumi R, Yamamoto T, Ueno Y, Nakataki E, et al. Effect of electrical muscle stimulation on upper and lower limb muscles in critically ill patients: a two-center randomized controlled trial. *Crit Care Med.* (2020) 48:e997–e1003. doi: 10.1097/CCM.0000000000004522
8. Poulsen JB, Møller K, Jensen CV, Weisdorf S, Kehlet H, Perner A. Effect of transcutaneous electrical muscle stimulation on muscle volume in patients with septic shock. *Crit Care Med.* (2011) 39:456–61. doi: 10.1097/CCM.0b013e318205c7bc
9. Rodriguez PO, Setten M, Maskin LP, Bonelli I, Vidomlansky SR, Attie S, et al. Muscle weakness in septic patients requiring mechanical ventilation: protective effect of transcutaneous neuromuscular electrical stimulation. *J Crit Care.* (2012) 27:319.e1-8. doi: 10.1016/j.jcrc.2011.04.010
10. Carraro U, Marcante A, Ravara B, Albertin G, Maccarone MC, Piccione F, et al. Skeletal muscle weakness in older adults home-restricted due to COVID-19 pandemic: a role for full-body in-bed gym and functional electrical stimulation. *Aging Clin Exp Res.* (2021) 33:2053–9. doi: 10.1007/s40520-021-01885-0
11. Singer M, Deutschman CS, Seymour CW, Shankar-Hari M, Annane D, Bauer M, et al. The third international consensus definitions for sepsis and septic shock (Sepsis-3). *JAMA.* (2016) 315:801–10. doi: 10.1001/jama.2016.0287
12. Kurtzke JF. Rating neurologic impairment in multiple sclerosis: an expanded disability status scale (EDSS). *Neurology.* (1983) 33:1444–52. doi: 10.1212/WNL.33.11.1444
13. Moreno RP, Metnitz PG, Almeida E, Jordan B, Bauer P, Campos RA, et al. SAPS 3–From evaluation of the patient to evaluation of the intensive care unit. Part 2: development of a prognostic model for hospital mortality at ICU admission. *Intensive Care Med.* (2005) 31:1345–55. doi: 10.1007/s00134-005-2763-5
14. Vincent JL, Moreno R, Takala J, Willatts S, De Mendonça A, Bruining H, et al. The SOFA (Sepsis-related Organ Failure Assessment) score to describe organ dysfunction/failure. on behalf of the working group on sepsis-related problems of the European society of intensive care medicine. *Intensive Care Med.* (1996) 22:707–10. doi: 10.1007/BF01709751
15. Hermans G, Clerckx B, Vanhullebusch T, Segers J, Vanpee G, Robbeets C, et al. Interobserver agreement of Medical Research Council sum-score and handgrip strength in the intensive care unit. *Muscle Nerve.* (2012) 45:18–25. doi: 10.1002/mus.22219
16. Silva VZMD, Lima AS, Nadiele H, Pires-Neto R, Denehy L, Parry SM. Brazilian versions of the physical function icu test-scored and de morton mobility index: translation, cross-cultural adaptation, and clinimetric properties. *J Bras Pneumol.* (2020) 46:e20180366. doi: 10.36416/1806-3756/e20180366
17. Kasotakis G, Schmidt U, Perry D, Grosse-Sundrup M, Benjamin J, Ryan C, et al. The surgical intensive care unit optimal mobility score predicts mortality and length of stay. *Crit Care Med.* (2012) 40:1122–8. doi: 10.1097/CCM.0b013e3182376e6d
18. Botter A, Oprandi G, Lanfranco F, Allasia S, Maffiuletti NA, Minetto MA. Atlas of the muscle motor points for the lower limb: implications for electrical stimulation procedures and electrode positioning. *Eur J Appl Physiol.* (2011) 111:2461–71. doi: 10.1007/s00421-011-2093-y
19. Valera GG, Carezzato NL, Vale FA, Hortense P. Adaptação cultural para o Brasil da escala Pain Assessment in Advanced Dementia - PAINAD* [Cultural adaptation of the scale Pain Assessment in Advanced Dementia - PAINAD to Brazil]. *Rev Esc Enferm USP.* (2014) 48:462–8. doi: 10.1590/S0080-623420140000300011
20. Nuhr M, Crevenna R, Gohlsch B, Bittner C, Pleiner J, Wiesinger G, et al. Functional and biochemical properties of chronically stimulated human skeletal muscle. *Eur J Appl Physiol.* (2003) 89:202–8. doi: 10.1007/s00421-003-0792-8
21. Hambrecht R, Fiehn E, Yu J, Niebauer J, Weigl C, Hilbrich L, et al. Effects of endurance training on mitochondrial ultrastructure and fiber type distribution in skeletal muscle of patients with stable chronic heart failure. *J Am Coll Cardiol.* (1997) 29:1067–73. doi: 10.1016/S0735-1097(97)00015-6
22. Gerovasili V, Tripodaki E, Karatzanos E, Pitsolis T, Markaki V, Zervakis D, et al. Short-term systemic effect of electrical muscle stimulation in critically ill patients. *Chest.* (2009) 136:1249–56. doi: 10.1378/chest.08-2888
23. Vanderthommen M, Duteil S, Wary C, Raynaud JS, Leroy-Willig A, Crielaard JM, et al. A comparison of voluntary and electrically induced contractions by interleaved 1H- and 31P-NMRS in humans. *J Appl Physiol.* (2003) 94:1012–24. doi: 10.1152/japplphysiol.00887.2001
24. Bickel CS, Slade J, Mahoney E, Haddad F, Dudley GA, Adams GR. Time course of molecular responses of human skeletal muscle to acute bouts of resistance exercise. *J Appl Physiol.* (2005) 98:482–8. doi: 10.1152/japplphysiol.00895.2004
25. Renew JR, Ratzlaff R, Hernandez-Torres V, Brull SJ, Prielipp RC. Neuromuscular blockade management in the critically Ill patient. *J Intensive Care.* (2020) 8:37. doi: 10.1186/s40560-020-00455-2
26. Collins DF. Central contributions to contractions evoked by tetanic neuromuscular electrical stimulation. *Exerc Sport Sci Rev.* (2007) 35:102–9. doi: 10.1097/jes.0b013e3180a0321b
27. Smith GV, Alon G, Roys SR, Gullapalli RP. Functional MRI determination of a dose-response relationship to lower extremity neuromuscular electrical stimulation in healthy subjects. *Exp Brain Res.* (2003) 150:33–9. doi: 10.1007/s00221-003-1405-9
28. Moore EW, Hunter JM. The new neuromuscular blocking agents: do they offer any advantages? *Br J Anaesth.* (2001) 87:912–25. doi: 10.1093/bja/87.6.912
29. Marra A, Ely EW, Pandharipande PP, Patel MB. The ABCDEF bundle in critical care. *Crit Care Clin.* (2017) 33:225–43. doi: 10.1016/j.ccc.2016.12.005

30. Dirks ML, Hansen D, Van Assche A, Dendale P, Van Loon LJ. Neuromuscular electrical stimulation prevents muscle wasting in critically ill comatose patients. *Clin Sci (Lond).* (2015) 128:357–65. doi: 10.1042/CS20140447
31. Mateo S, Bergeron V, Cheminon M, Guinet-Lacoste A, Pouget MC, Jacquin-Courtois S, et al. Functional electrical stimulation-cycling favours erectus position restoration and walking in patients with critical COVID-19. a proof-of-concept controlled study. *Ann Phys Rehabil Med.* (2021) 64:101516. doi: 10.1016/j.rehab.2021.101516

15

Low Vitamin D Levels at Birth and Early Respiratory Outcome in Infants with Gestational Age Less than 29 Weeks

Honoré Papalia[1†], Anais Samonini[1†], Christophe Buffat[2], E. Gras[1], Clotilde des Robert[1], Jean-Francois Landrier[3], Vanessa Pauly[4] and Farid Boubred[1,3]*

[1] Neonatal Unit, Hospital University La Conception, APHM, Marseille, France, [2] Laboratory of Biochemistry and Molecular Biology, Hospital University la Conception, APHM, Marseille, France, [3] Aix-Marseille University, INSERM, INRAE, C2VN, Marseille, France, [4] EA 3279, CEReSS—Health Service Research and Quality of Life Center, Public Health and Medical Information Department, APHM, Marseille, France

***Correspondence:**
Farid Boubred
farid.boubred@ap-hm.fr

† These authors have contributed equally to this work and share first authorship

Background: Vitamin D (VitD) is involved in lung development but its influence on respiratory distress syndrome of extremely preterm (EPT) infants have been little investigated. In this study, we examined the influence of low vitamin D status at birth on early respiratory outcomes of this vulnerable infant population.

Methods: Cord blood 25(OH)D levels ≤75 nmol/L were considered as Low vitamin D levels. Stepwise logistic regression and classification regression-tree analyses were used and the primary outcome was the combined outcome of death or mechanical ventilation need by the end of the first week (death or MV DoL7) as a marker od RDS severity.

Results: The mean (SD) GA and birth weight were 26 (1.4) weeks and 801 (212) gr, respectively; 81/109 (74%) infants had low 25(OH)D levels. Infants with low VitD levels had 25% higher initial FiO_2 levels (p < 0.05) and were more likely to be mechanically ventilated on DoL7 (36 vs. 7%, p <0.05). Adjusted for gestational age, they had 10-fold higher odds of death or MV DoL7 (p < 0.01). By regression tree analysis, the rate of death or MV DoL7 increased from 18 to 71% in infants with GA < 26 weeks and with cord blood 25(OH)D levels higher and lower than 74 nmol/L, respectively (p < 0.05).

Conclusion: Low vitamin D levels at birth are associated with early adverse respiratory outcomes in infants with GA less 29 weeks. Further largest studies are needed to confirm this association.

Keywords: extremely preterm infants, RDS—respiratory distress syndrome, surfactant, vitamin D, bronchopulmonary dysplasia, LISA (less invasive surfactant administration), nasal CPAP (continuous positive airway pressure), SGA (samll for gestational age)

INTRODUCTION

Respiratory distress syndrome (RDS) can be considered as a developmental disease which predominantly concerned extremely preterm (EPT) infants. These infants often have severe form of RDS with early high oxygen needs, multiple surfactant administration and prolonged mechanical ventilation. Early markers of RDS severity may help to better identify high risk infants and provide optimal care to prevent short and long term RDS complications such as bronchopulmonary dysplasia (BPD).

Vitamin D is well known for its major role in fetal bone metabolism, but recent evidence also shows a biological role in normal lung development and in surfactant synthesis (1–4). In animals, maternal gestational vitamin D depletion affects fetal lung development with reduced alveolar numbers and impaired bronchial structure (2, 4). Children born to vitamin D-deficient mothers are more likely to have respiratory symptoms such as wheezing events, asthma, respiratory tract infections or lung dysfunction (5–9). In premature infants, with immature lungs, the optimal dose of vitamin D supply is still under investigation. The few randomized clinical studies looking into the effects of vitamin D supply on respiratory outcomes have shown variable effects with either no effects or decreased RDS severity (10–12).

Preterm infants are at high risk of vitamin D deficiency at birth, with observational studies showing a prevalence as high as 90% (13–15). A part of that deficient state may result from limited vitamin D transfer from the mother. Indeed, the fetus entirely depends on the maternal vitamin D status, and placental transfer mainly occurs in the third trimester (16). Furthermore, the leading obstetrical causes of prematurity, including preeclampsia, gestational diabetes, small for gestational age (SGA) and threatened preterm delivery, are often associated with maternal vitamin D deficiency (17–19). However, the adverse effects of maternal/fetal vitamin D deficiency on neonatal outcomes remain conflicting in very preterm infants and still need to be further investigated in extremely preterm (EPT) infants, in particular.

The objective of the study was to examine the association between vitamin D status at birth and early respiratory outcomes of infants with GA <29 weeks.

METHODS

This observational and retrospective study included preterm infants born with GA between 24 weeks^{+0} and 28 weeks^{+6} between November 1, 2018 and April 31, 2020 that were admitted to the Neonatal Intensive Care Unit (NICU), Hospital University La Conception, Marseilles, France. This study was part of a quality improvement initiative aimed at optimizing vitamin D supplementation in preterm infants. All infants followed the same postnatal vitamin D supply protocol during the study period; no changes have been made between the two groups. Blood 25 hydroxyvitamin D [25(OH)D] concentration was measured at birth from umbilical cord blood. This study was approved by local ethical and privacy health data protection committees (N°. DSN_2019-06-20_7706). Clinical and biological data collection were anonymized. Parents were informed of the study and were not required to sign informed consent, but they could oppose data collection. For this study, preterm infants born at our institution and with specifically cord blood 25(OH)D measurements were eligible; infants with congenital or genetic abnormalities or whose parents refused to participate in the study were excluded. Cord blood 25(OH)D levels were determined by chemiluminescence (Roche Diagnostics, Mannheim, Germany). This method has been calibrated to liquid chromatography–mass spectrometry. In preterm infants, the optimal 25(OH)D levels for adequate respiratory outcome are unknown. We used the Endocrine Society recommendations for defining vitamin D status that are made for healthy bone growth (20). For this study, two groups of infants were compared: infants with cord blood 25(OH)D levels ≤75 nmol/L (LowVitD status group) and infants with cord blood 25(OH)D levels >75 nmol/L (SufficientVitD status).

Early Respiratory Outcome

The primary outcome was the combined outcome of death in the first week of life or the need for mechanical ventilation (MV) on day of life (DoL) 7 (death or MV DoL7). We also compared other respiratory outcomes, such as delivery room intubation within 15 mins of life (MV DR), need for MV on DoL3 (MV DoL3) and 7 (MV DoL7) and any need for MV in the first week of life (MV W1). Respiratory management was standardized; all spontaneously breathing infants were initially managed with nasal continuous positive airway pressure (NCPAP). Surfactant was indicated when the fractional inspired oxygen concentration (FiO_2) reached 30% or when the infant required mechanical ventilation (21, 22). Observational studies have confirmed that FiO_2 exceeding 0.30 in infants initially managed on NCPAP for RDS predicted NCPAP failure (22). Timing and FiO_2 levels immediately before surfactant administration were collected. The less invasive surfactant administration (LISA) technique or surfactant administration after a brief intubation procedure (intubation, surfactant and extubation, INSURE procedure) were compared between the two groups.

Data Collection and Statistical Analysis

Maternal and neonatal outcomes were collected from infant medical charts. Gestational age (GA) was calculated from first trimester obstetrical ultrasound, and small for gestational age (SGA) was determined using Fenton growth charts (23). At birth, umbilical cord milking or delayed cord clamping for at least 30 s defined placental transfusion. Severe cerebral injury included stage 3 and 4 intraventricular hemorrhage (Papile's classification), periventricular leukomalacia and isolated ventricular dilatation at term. The variable of severe digestive disease included necrotizing enterocolitis (NEC) stage 2 or more (Bell's classification) and isolated intestinal perforation. Late onset sepsis after DoL3 and severe retinopathy (stage 3 and more) were noted as well. Bronchopulmonary dysplasia (BPD) was defined as the need for oxygen supplementation or respiratory support at 36 weeks postmenstrual age. We used Jensen et al.'s definition to classify BPD severity: infants who required nasal cannula flow rate >2 L/min, non-invasive positive airway pressure, or invasive mechanical ventilation were classified as grade 2–3 BPD (24).

To compare both infant vitamin D status groups, we performed univariate statistical tests: Chi-squared (or Fischer's exact tests) and Student's *t* tests (or Mann-Whitney test) were used as appropriate to compare groups for categorical and

TABLE 1 | Obstetrical and neonatal characteristics according to vitamin D status at birth.

Characteristics, n (%)	All population (*N* = 109)	SufficientVitD status (*N* = 28)	LowVitD status (*N* = 81)	*P* value
Obstetrical data				
Multiple gestation	29 (27)	8 (28)	21 (26)	0.78
PPROM	21 (19)	5 (18)	16 (20)	0.82
Preeclampsia	22 (20)	5 (18)	17 (21)	0.79
MTR/PA	19 (17)	5 (18)	14 (17)	1.00
GD	4 (3.6)	0 (0)	4 (5)	0.57
Chorioamnionitis	25 (23)	5 (18)	20 (25)	0.60
Antenatal steroids	85 (78)	22 (78)	63 (78)	0.93
Mg^{2+} sulfate	81 (74)	23 (82)	58 (72)	0.27
Cesarean section	88 (81)	20 (71)	68 (84)	0.68
Neonatal data				
GA, mean (SD), weeks	26 (1.4)	26.5 (1.5)	26 (1.4)	0.11
BW, mean (SD), g	801 (212)	828 (198)	792 (217)	0.40
SGA	23 (21)	6 (21)	17 (21)	0.96
Female	60 (55)	19 (68)	41 (51)	0.11
5 min Apgar score < 7	24 (22)	4 (14)	20 (25)	0.27
Placental transfusion	66 (60)	19 (68)	47 (58)	0.17
Digestive disease	8 (7)	3 (11)	5 (6)	0.42
Severe cerebral injury	10 (9)	2 (7)	8 (10)	1.00
Early onset sepsis	9 (8)	2 (7)	7 (9)	1.00
Late onset sepsis	56 (51)	12 (43)	44 (54)	0.29
Treatment for PDA	38 (35)	8 (28)	30 (37)	0.41
Severe ROP	12/103 (12)	2/26 (8)	10/77 (13)	0.72
BPD any grade	59/97 (61)	12/25 (48)	47/72 (65)	0.12
BPD stage 2 – 3	31/97 (32)	5/25 (20)	26/72 (36)	0.21
Death before discharge	12 (11)	3 (11)	9 (11)	1.00

BPD, bronchopulmonary dysplasia; BW, birth weight (gr); GA, gestational age (weeks); GD, gestational diabetes mellitus; MTR/PA, metrorrhagia/placental abruption; PDA, patent ductus arteriosus; PPROM, preterm premature rupture of membranes; ROP, retinopathy of prematurity; SGA: small for gestational age; SufficientVitD status, infants with cord blood 25(OH)D levels > 75 nmol/L; LowVitD status, infants with cord blood 25(OH)D levels ≤ 75 nmol/L.

TABLE 2 | Early respiratory outcomes according to vitamin D status at birth.

Characteristics, *n* (%)	All population (*N* = 109)	SufficientVitD status (*N* = 28)	LowVitD status (*N* = 81)	*P* value
Surfactant	83 (76)	21 (75)	62 (76)	0.87
Timing (min)*	50 (25–90)	62 (30–90)	41 (25–60)	0.09
FiO_2 (%), mean (SD)	51 (22)	41 (18)	54 (22)	0.02
≥ 2 doses	19 (17)	3 (11)	16 (20)	0.39
LISA/INSURE procedure	46 (42)	14 (50)	32 (39)	0.33
MV W1	52 (48)	9 (32)	43 (53)	0.05
MV W1 duration (h)*	120 (24–168)	72 (15–144)	144 (14–168)	0.24
HFO	21 (40)	1 (11)	20 (46)	0.06
MV DR	24 (39)	4 (14)	20 (25)	0.30
MV DoL3	35 (32)	6 (21)	29/80 (36)	0.15
MV DoL7	28/106 (26)	2 (7)	26/78 (33)	0.007
Death or MV DoL7	31 (28)	2 (7)	29 (36)	0.003

**Median (IQR); HFO, high frequency oscillation; MV W1, mechanical ventilation in the first week of life; MV DR, mechanical ventilation in the first 15 min after birth (delivery room); MV DoL3, mechanical ventilation on day of life 3; MV DoL7, mechanical ventilation on day of life 7; SufficientVitD status, infants with cord blood 25(OH)D levels > 75 nmol/L; LowVitD status, infants with cord blood 25(OH)D levels ≤ 75 nmol/L.*

quantitative variables, respectively. All statistical tests were two-sided. To analyze factors associated with the combined variable of death or MV DOL7, we performed univariate and multivariate logistic regression analyses. We included variables with $p < 0.20$ in univariate analyses into a step-by-step backward multivariable analysis. We also used Firth's penalized estimation using logistic regression to account for the low number, which led to imprecisions in parameter estimation. The results are presented as odds ratios (ORs) and their 95% confidence intervals (CIs).

Then, as an explanatory analysis, we performed a classification regression tree analysis (CART) to identify an easy-to-understand algorithm for predicting the primary outcome of death or MV at DoL7. This analysis allows automatic selection of categorical variables and of optimal cutoff points of continued variables and generates a classification tree when the more important variable in relation to outcome is at the top of the decision tree (25). Variables initially entered for consideration into the CART analysis were the following: GA, sex, multiple pregnancies, preterm premature rupture of membranes, chorioamnionitis, antenatal corticosteroid therapy, cesarean section, placental transfusion and cord blood 25(OH)D levels. This CART analysis was mainly performed to reveal an optimal threshold for blood 25(OH)D levels. Due to the low number of subjects involved in the analysis, it was performed on the whole dataset; the accuracy was tested using three-fold cross validation repeated 200 times. The analyses were performed using IBM SPSS Statistics for Windows (IBM Company, Chicago, IL, USA), Version 20.0, and SAS®, Version 9.4 (SAS Institute Inc, Cary, NC, USA). In this study, $p < 0.05$ were considered statistically significant. The CART tree was generated using the RPART package in R® Software.

RESULTS

During the study period, 112 infants met the eligibility criteria, and 3 infants were excluded: 2 for congenital and genetic anomalies and 1 for parental refusal (**Supplementary Figure**). The mean (SD) GA and birth weight were 26 (1.4) weeks and 801 (212) gr, respectively. The mean (SD) cord blood 25(OH)D level was 53 (32) nmol/L. A total of 81 (74%) infants had low cord blood 25(OH)D levels (≤75 nmol/L) and 56 (51%) infants had cord blood 25(OH)D levels <50 nmol/L.

Obstetrical and neonatal characteristics, in particular GA, birth weight, SGA, sex ratio and exposure to antenatal corticosteroids, were comparable between infants with low and sufficient cord blood 25(OH)D levels (**Table 1**). However, early respiratory outcomes differed between the two groups of infants

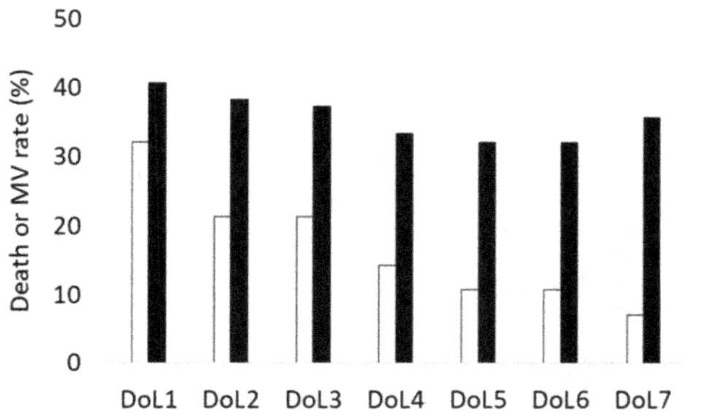

FIGURE 1 | Daily combined death or mechanical ventilation (death or MV) rate in the first week of life between LowVitD status and SufficientVitD status infants. During the first week of life, the rate of the combined outcome of death or MV need were high in infants with low vitamin D levels ≤ 75 nmol/L (black bars).

TABLE 3 | Regression analysis: factors associated with the combined outcome of death or mechanical ventilation on the 7th day after birth (death or MV DOL7).

	Adjusted OR (95%IC)	*P* value
GA	0.39 (0.25–0.60)	< 0.0001
LowVitD status	10.6 (1.13–65.1)	0.01

GA, gestational age (weeks); LowVitD status, infants with cord blood 25(OH)D levels ≤ 75 nmol/L.

(**Table 2**). The timing, dose number and technique procedure (LISA or INSURE) of surfactant administration were not different, but FiO_2 levels at the time of surfactant administration were 25% higher in LowVitD status infants ($p = 0.02$). At DoL7, the rate of the combined outcome of death or MV requirement was higher in LowVitD status infants (36 vs. 7%, $p < 0.01$). These infants were also more likely to receive MV during the first week (MV W1) (53 vs. 32%, $p = 0.05$) than the group of SufficientVitD status infants (**Figure 1**) and tended to be more frequently ventilated by high frequency oscillation (46 vs. 11%, $p = 0.06$). At DoL7, 93% of infants who died or needed MV were from the LowVitD status group.

In the multivariate analyses, and after backward elimination of variables, adjusted for GA, infants with LowVitD status had higher odds of death or being mechanically ventilated at DoL7 with an adjusted OR (95% CI) of 10.6 (1.13–65.1) ($p < 0.05$) (**Table 3**). The same association was found with the outcome of MV DoL7 with an adjusted (on GA) OR (95% CI) of 8.14 (1.37–48.5) ($p < 0.05$).

The CART analysis revealed GA, with the threshold value at 26 weeks, and cord blood 25(OH)D levels <74 nmol/L were important variables to predict the combined outcome of death or VM DoL7 (**Figure 2**). The rate was 10% in infants with GA above 26 weeks and reached 71% in infants with GA < 26 weeks who had cord blood 25(OH)D levels lower than 74 nmol/L. The mean accuracy of this algorithm was estimated to be equal to 0.77 CI 95% [0.64-0.89].

DISCUSSION

In this study, we found an association between vitamin D status at birth and early respiratory outcome in infants with GA <29 weeks. Infants who had low blood 25(OH)D levels ≤75 nmol/L at birth had early adverse outcomes with higher oxygen need for RDS and prolonged mechanical ventilation by the end of the first week of life compared to their counterparts that had adequate blood vitamin D levels.

Studies that evaluated the influence of vitamin D status on early respiratory outcome of very preterm infants have shown conflicted findings (15, 26–28). The makers used to define RDS severity and vitamin D deficiency varied between the studies. Some of them have found a high rate of RDS and markers of severe respiratory disease while others did not (15, 26–30). Onwuneme C et al. have found in a population of very preterm infants (GA <32 weeks) an association between vitamin D deficiency at birth [25(OH)D levels < 30 nmol/L] and clinical signs of acute respiratory morbidity with higher oxygen needs and a greater rate of MV in the delivery room and during the neonatal period (15). We also found higher FiO_2 levels at surfactant administration while the timing to administration tended to be shorter, and higher need of high frequency oscillation; these results can be considered marker of respiratory disease severity. In contrast to these previous studies, we included a population of more premature infants who are particularly vulnerable to a severe form of RDS with high needs of intubation and prolonged mechanical ventilation. We also included infants with higher prevalence (26%) of sufficient vitamin D concentrations (above 75 nmol/L); while this prevalence was usually reported <5–10%. Including infants with higher cord blood 25(OH)D levels may have revealed the adverse consequences of vitamin D deficiency in our study. Our study adds further evidence on the influence of vitamin D status at birth on early respiratory outcomes in preterm infants.

Although we used the international vitamin D definition to classify infants, the CART analysis identified optimal cutoff points for 25(OH)D of 74 nmol/L, which is the threshold level commonly used in pediatric and adult medicine to define vitamin D sufficiency (20). In this method, the more important variables are ranked early on the classification tree, showing the important influence of vitamin D on early respiratory outcome, especially in infants with GA < 26 weeks; the rate of death or MV DoL7 fourfold increased between SufficientVitD infants and their counterpart infants who had low 25(OH)D levels ($p < 0.05$). While the adequate vitamin D status is unknown in preterm infants; our study provides useful insights on the optimal 25(OH)D levels at birth.

Recent evidence suggests a biological role of vitamin D in normal lung development and maturation (2, 4, 30, 31). Vitamin D also contributes to surfactant synthesis and secretion by alveolar type II cells (31). The fetus is exclusively dependent on maternal vitamin D status, and transfer from the mother mainly occurs during the third trimester. The umbilical cord blood 25(OH)D level at birth is therefore representative of fetal vitamin D stores. Endothelial and alveolar type II cells

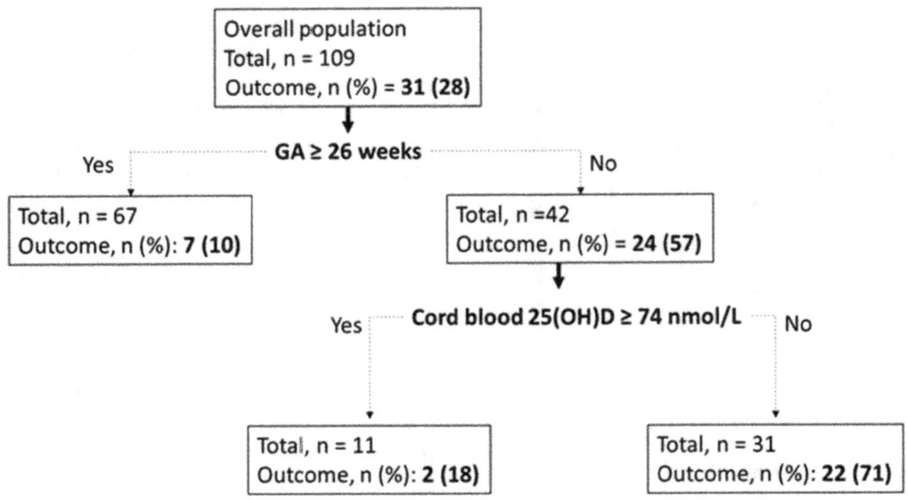

FIGURE 2 | CART model for death or MV DoL7 outcome. In each node (rectangle), the category "Outcome" refers to the presence of the combined outcome of death or MV DoL7, with *n* and percentage of related infants.

express a nuclear receptor specific for the bioactive form of vitamin D [1,25 $(OH)_2D_3$], named vitamin D receptor (VDR). VDR response elements are also present in a subset of more than 500 genes involved in lung development in humans and rodents (32, 33). In animals, maternal gestational vitamin D depletion impairs fetal lung development with reduced alveolar numbers, decreased vascular density, altered pneumocyte type II differentiation, decreased tracheal size, and increased airway smooth muscle mass (2, 31). In the neonatal lungs of vitamin D-depleted rats, genes involved in the inflammatory response and vascular development, such as VEGF, have been found to be up- and downregulated, respectively (34). These functional and structural alterations are responsible for increased neonatal mortality with lower oxygen saturation, reported in preterm pups (35). In the long term, the offspring displayed increased airway resistance and low tidal volume (2). Some of these functional alterations, including frequent wheezing events, asthma, lung dysfunctions and respiratory tract infections, were also observed in children of vitamin D-deficient mothers (7–9). Finally, in rodents, maternal gestational vitamin D administration prevents neonatal mortality and lung injury induced by intrauterine exposure to endotoxin, which is a model of bronchopulmonary dysplasia (36). Based on these preclinical data, we can hypothesize that high oxygen and sustained MV needs for RDS observed in LowVitD status preterm infants result from delayed lung maturation.

This study had some intrinsic limitations due to the study design. Some commonly used markers of RDS severity such as respiratory severity score and ventilator settings are lacking; but high initial FiO_2 levels, prolonged mechanical ventilation needs or frequently use of high frequency oscillation could be considered surrogate marker of RDS severity. Our sample size was too small to investigate the influence of vitamin D status at birth on other neonatal outcomes, especially BPD. Moreover, although our single-center experience may have limited bias linked to differences in health care practices, further multicenter studies with sufficient size are needed to confirm our findings.

In conclusion, in this study, we found that preterm infants with GA <29 weeks that had 25(OH)D levels at birth ≤75 nmol/L had early adverse outcomes. Our findings provide additional evidence for the important role of fetal vitamin D on lung development and provide new insights into optimal 25(OH)D levels. In very and extremely preterm infants early vitamin D status, and thus maternal vitamin D status, can be considered marker of respiratory disease including RDS and BPD. Early respiratory outcomes could be improved by preventing maternal gestational vitamin D deficiency. Larger studies should be performed to confirm these findings and to investigate the influence of vitamin D on other neonatal outcomes and especially on long-term respiratory functions.

AUTHOR CONTRIBUTIONS

HP and AS collected data, drafted the initial manuscript, and reviewed and revised the manuscript. EG collected data and reviewed and revised the manuscript. CB collected data, carried out vitamin D analyses, and reviewed and revised the manuscript. CR designed the data collection instruments and reviewed and revised the manuscript. J-FL participated to analysis and interpretation of data and critically reviewed the manuscript for important intellectual content. VP designed the data collection instruments and carried out the statistical analyses. FB conceptualized and designed the study and reviewed and revised the manuscript. All authors approved the final manuscript as submitted and agreed to be accountable for all aspects of the work.

REFERENCES

1. DeLuca HF. Overview of general physiologic features and functions of vitamin D. *Am J Clin Nutr.* (2004) 80:689S–1696S. doi: 10.1093/ajcn/80.6.1689S
2. Lykkedegn S, Sorensen GL, Beck-Nielsen SS, Christesen HT. The impact of vitamin D on fetal and neonatal lung maturation. A systematic review. *Am J Physiol Lung Cell Mol Physiol.* (2015) 308, L587–602. doi: 10.1152/ajplung.00117.2014
3. Chen L, Wilson R, Bennett E, Zosky GR. Identification of vitamin D sensitive pathways during lung development. *Respir Res.* (2016) 17:47. doi: 10.1186/s12931-016-0362-3
4. Wang P, Tan ZX, Fu L, Fan YJ, Luo B, Zhang ZH, et al. Gestational vitamin D deficiency impairs fetal lung development through suppressing type II pneumocyte differentiation. *Reprod Toxicol.* (2020) 94:40–7. doi: 10.1016/j.reprotox.2020.03.008
5. Thorsteinsdottir F, Cardoso I, Keller A, Stougaard M, Frederiksen P, Cohen AS, et al. Neonatal vitamin D status and risk of asthma in childhood: results from the D-Tect study. *Nutrients.* (2020) 12:842. doi: 10.3390/nu12030842
6. Pacheco-González RM, García-Marcos L, Morales E. Prenatal vitamin D status and respiratory and allergic outcomes in childhood: a meta-analysis of observational studies. *Pediatr Allergy Immunol.* (2018) 29:243–53. doi: 10.1111/pai.12876
7. Hart PH, Lucas RM, Walsh JP, Zosky GR, Whitehouse AJ, Zhu K, et al. Vitamin D in fetal development: findings from a birth cohort study. *Pediatrics.* (2015) 135:167–73. doi: 10.1542/peds.2014-1860
8. Lai SH, Liao SL, Tsai MH, Hua MC, Chiu CY, Yeh KW, et al. Low cord-serum 25-hydroxyvitamin D levels are associated with poor lung function performance and increased respiratory infection in infancy. *PLoS ONE.* (2017) 12:173268. doi: 10.1371/journal.pone.0173268
9. Zosky GR, Hart PH, Whitehouse AJ, Kusel MM, Ang W, Foong RE, et al. Vitamin D deficiency at 16 to 20 weeks' gestation is associated with impaired lung function and asthma at 6 years of age. *Ann Am Thorac Soc.* (2014) 11, 571–577. doi: 10.1513/AnnalsATS.201312-423OC
10. Fort P, Salas AA, Nicola T, Craig CM, Carlo WA, Ambalavanan N, et al. Comparison of 3 vitamin D dosing regimens in extremely preterm infants: a randomized controlled trial. *J Pediatr.* (2016) 174:132–8. doi: 10.1016/j.jpeds.2016.03.028
11. Al-Beltagi M, Rowiesha M, Elmashad A, Elrifaey SM, Elhorany H, Koura HG. Vitamin D status in preterm neonates and the effects of its supplementation on respiratory distress syndrome. *Pediatr Pulmonol.* (2020) 55:108–15. doi: 10.1002/ppul.24552
12. Salas AA, Woodfin T, Phillips V, Peralta-Carcelen M, Carlo WA, Ambalavanan N. Dose-response effects of early vitamin D supplementation on neurodevelopmental and respiratory outcomes of extremely preterm infants at 2 years of age: a randomized trial. *Neonatology.* (2018) 113:256–62. doi: 10.1159/000484399
13. Burris HH, Van Marter LJ, McElrath TF, Tabatabai P, Litonjua AA, Weiss ST, et al. Vitamin D status among preterm and full-term infants at birth. *Pediatr Res.* (2014) 75:75–80. doi: 10.1038/pr.2013.174
14. Matejek T, Navratilova M, Zaloudkova L, Malakova J, Maly J, Skalova S, et al. Vitamin D status of very low birth weight infants at birth and the effects of generally recommended supplementation on their vitamin D levels at discharge. *J Matern Fetal Neonatal Med.* (2020) 33:3784–90. doi: 10.1080/14767058.2019.1586873
15. Onwuneme C, Martin F, McCarthy R, Carroll A, Segurado R, Murphy J, et al. The association of vitamin D status with acute respiratory morbidity in preterm infants. *J Pediatr.* (2015) 166:1175–80. doi: 10.1016/j.jpeds.2015.01.055
16. Karras SN, Wagner CL, Castracane VD. Understanding vitamin D metabolism in pregnancy: from physiology to pathophysiology and clinical outcomes. *Metabolism.* (2018) 86:112–23. doi: 10.1016/j.metabol.2017.10.001
17. Miliku K, Vinkhuyzen A, Blanken LM, McGrath JJ, Eyles DW, Burne TH, et al. Maternal vitamin D concentrations during pregnancy, fetal growth patterns, and risks of adverse birth outcomes. *Am J Clin Nutr.* (2016) 103:1514–22. doi: 10.3945/ajcn.115.123752
18. Sadeghian M, Asadi M, Rahmani S, Akhavan Zanjani M, Sadeghi O, Hosseini SA, et al. Circulating vitamin D and the risk of gestational diabetes: a systematic review and dose-response meta-analysis. *Endocrine.* (2020) 70:36–47. doi: 10.1007/s12020-020-02360-y
19. Qin LL, Lu FG, Yang SH, Xu HL, Luo BA. Does maternal vitamin D deficiency increase the risk of preterm birth: a meta-analysis of observational studies. *Nutrients.* (2016) 8:301. doi: 10.3390/nu8050301
20. Holick MF, Binkley NC, Bischoff-Ferrari HA, Gordon CM, Hanley DA, Heaney RP, et al. Evaluation, treatment, and prevention of vitamin D deficiency: an endocrine Society clinical practice guideline. *J Clin Endocrinol Metab.* (2011) 96, 1911–1930. doi: 10.1210/jc.2011-0385
21. Templin L, Grosse C, Andres V, Robert CD, Fayol L, Simeoni U, et al. A quality improvement initiative to reduce the need for mechanical ventilation in extremely low gestational age neonates. *Am J Perinatol.* (2017) 34, 759–764. doi: 10.1055/s-0037-1598106
22. Dargaville PA, Aiyappan A, De Paoli AG, Dalton RG, Kuschel CA, Kamlin CO, et al. Continuous positive airway pressure failure in preterm infants: incidence, predictors and consequences. *Neonatology.* (2013) 104:8–14. doi: 10.1159/000346460
23. Fenton TR, Kim JH, A. systematic review and meta-analysis to revise the Fenton growth chart for preterm infants. *BMC Pediatr.* (2013) 13:59. doi: 10.1186/1471-2431-13-59
24. Jensen EA, Dysart K, Gantz MG, McDonald S, Bamat NA, Keszler M, et al. The diagnosis of bronchopulmonary dysplasia in very preterm infants. An evidence-based approach. *Am J Respir Crit Care Med.* (2019) 200:751–9. doi: 10.1164/rccm.201812-2348OC
25. Ambalavanan N, Baibergenova A, Carlo WA, Saigal S, Schmidt B, Thorpe KE, et al. Early prediction of poor outcome in extremely low birth weight infants by classification tree analysis. *J Pediatr.* (2006) 148:438–444. doi: 10.1016/j.jpeds.2005.11.042
26. Kazzi SNJ, Karnati S, Puthuraya S, Thomas R. Vitamin D deficiency and respiratory morbidity among African American very low birth weight infants. *Early Hum Dev.* (2018) 119:19–24. doi: 10.1016/j.earlhumdev.2018.02.013
27. Kim I, Kim SS, Song JI, Yoon SH, Park GY, Lee YW. Association between vitamin D level at birth and respiratory morbidities in very-low-birth-weight infants. *Korean J Pediatr.* (2019) 62:166–72. doi: 10.3345/kjp.2018.06632
28. Matejek T, Zemankova J, Malakova J, Cermakova E, Skalova S, Palicka V. Severe vitamin D deficiency in preterm infants: possibly no association with clinical outcomes? *J Matern Fetal Neonatal Med.* (2020) 2021:1–9. doi: 10.1080/14767058
29. Fettah ND, Zenciroglu A, Dilli D, Beken S, Okumuş N. Is higher 25-hydroxyvitamin D level preventive for respiratory distress syndrome in preterm infants? *Am J Perinatol.* (2015) 32:247–50. doi: 10.1055/s-0034-1383849
30. Shah BA, Padbury JF, Anderson MP, Holick MF, Szyld E, Gordon CM. Vitamin D and associated perinatal-neonatal outcomes among extremely low-birth-weight infants. *J Perinatol.* (2018) 38:1318–23. doi: 10.1038/s41372-018-0203-y
31. Foong RE, Bosco A, Jones AC, Gout A, Gorman S, Hart PH, et al. The effects of in utero vitamin D deficiency on airway smooth muscle mass and lung function. *Am J Respir Cell Mol Biol.* (2015) 53, 664–675. doi: 10.1165/rcmb.2014-0356OC
32. Phokela SS, Peleg S, Moya FR, Alcorn JL. Regulation of human pulmonary surfactant protein gene expression by 1alpha,25-dihydroxyvitamin D3. *Am J Physiol Lung Cell Mol Physiol.* (2005) 289:L617–626. doi: 10.1152/ajplung.00129.2004
33. Kho AT, Bhattacharya S, Tantisira KG, Carey VJ, Gaedigk R, Leeder JS, et al. Transcriptomic analysis of human lung development. *Am J Respir Crit Care Med.* (2010) 181, 54–63. doi: 10.1164/rccm.200907-1063OC
34. Mandell E, Ryan S, Seedorf GJ, Gonzalez T, Abman SH, Fleet JC. Maternal vitamin D deficiency induces transcriptomic changes in newborn rat lungs. *J Steroid Biochem Mol Biol.* (2020) 199:105613. doi: 10.1016/j.jsbmb.2020.105613
35. Lykkedegn S, Sorensen GL, Beck-Nielsen SS, Pilecki B, Duelund L, Marcussen N, et al. Vitamin D depletion in pregnancy decreases survival time, oxygen saturation, lung weight and body weight in preterm rat offspring. *PLoS ONE.* (2016) 11:e0155203. doi: 10.1371/journal.pone.0155203

36. Mandell E, Seedorf G, Gien J, Abman SH. Vitamin D treatment improves survival and infant lung structure after intra-amniotic endotoxin exposure in rats: potential role for the prevention of bronchopulmonary dysplasia. *Am J Physiol Lung Cell Mol Physiol.* (2014) 306:L420–8. doi: 10.1152/ajplung.00344.2013

16

Comparative Efficacy and Safety of Four Different Spontaneous Breathing Trials for Weaning from Mechanical Ventilation

Li-Juan Yi [1†], Xu Tian [2†], Min Chen [1†], Jin-Mei Lei [1], Na Xiao [1] and Maria F. Jiménez-Herrera [2]*

[1] Nursing Department, Hunan Traditional Chinese Medical College, Zhuzhou, China, [2] Nursing Department, Universitat Rovira i Virgili, Tarragona, Spain

Correspondence:
Maria F. Jiménez-Herrera
maria.jimenez@urv.cat

† These authors have contributed equally to this work and share first authorship

Background: Spontaneous breathing trial (SBT) has been used to predict the optimal time of weaning from ventilator. However, it remains controversial which trial should be preferentially selected. We aimed to compare and rank four common SBT modes including automatic tube compensation (ATC), pressure support ventilation (PSV), continuous positive airway pressure (CPAP), and T-piece among critically ill patients receiving mechanical ventilation (MV).

Methods: We searched PubMed, EMBASE, and the Cochrane Central Register of Controlled Trials (CENTRAL) to identify studies that investigated the comparative efficacy and safety of at least two SBT strategies among critically ill patients up to May 17, 2020. We estimated the surface under the cumulative ranking curve (SUCRA) to rank SBT techniques, and determined the certainty of evidence using the Grading of Recommendations Assessment, Development and Evaluation method. Primary outcome was weaning success. Secondary outcomes were reintubation, SBT success, duration of acute care, and intensive care unit (ICU) mortality. Statistical analysis was conducted by using RevMan 5.4, Stata, and R software.

Results: We enrolled 24 trials finally. Extubation success rate was significantly higher in ATC than that in T-piece (OR, 0.28; 95% CI, 0.13–0.64) or PSV (OR, 0.53; 95% CI, 0.32–0.88). For SBT success, ATC was better than other SBT techniques, with a pooled OR ranging from 0.17 to 0.42. For reintubation rate, CPAP was worse than T-piece (OR, 2.76; 95% CI, 1.08 to 7.06). No significant difference was detected between SBT modes for the length of stay in ICU or long-term weaning unit (LWU). Similar result was also found for ICU mortality between PSV and T-piece. Majority direct results were confirmed by network meta-analysis. Besides, ATC ranks at the first, first, and fourth place with a SUCRA of 91.7, 99.7, and 39.9%, respectively in increasing weaning success and SBT success and in prolonging ICU or LWU length of stay among four SBT strategies. The confidences in evidences were rated as low for most comparisons.

Conclusion: ATC seems to be the optimal choice of predicting successful weaning from ventilator among critically ill patients. However, randomized controlled trials (RCTs) with high quality are needed to further establish these findings.

Keywords: spontaneous breathing trials, weaning, mechanical ventilation, meta-analysis, systematic review

INTRODUCTION

Successful weaning from mechanical ventilation (MV) refers to the gradual transition from total artificial ventilation support to spontaneous breathing. Delayed disconnection from ventilator can be associated with numerous complications, such as ventilator-associated pneumonia, airway trauma, and multiple-organ failure (MOF) (1–3). The risk of complications and mortality may accrue with increasing duration of MV (4). Therefore, it is essential to timely and safely liberate patients from mechanical ventilator when they have restored the ability of spontaneous breathing (5–8).

Spontaneous breathing trial (SBT) is one of the most common approaches to facilitate the disconnection from MV (9). Evidence-based guidelines have also recommended to conduct SBT immediately before extubation for the purpose of assessing whether a patient is able to restore the ability of spontaneous breath, and thus determine the optimal time for disconnecting from ventilator (10–14). At present, T-piece, continuous positive airway pressure (CPAP), pressure support ventilation (PSV), and automatic tube compensation (ATC) are the most common ventilation techniques (11, 12, 15–20). SBT strategies focused in this study can be categorized into three categories as follows: (a) providing constant or dynamic ventilatory support to counteract the resistance of the endotracheal tube such as PSV and ATC (21–23), (b) providing continuous positive pressure in both inspiration and expiration to enhance breathing mechanics and reduce the effort needed by mechanically ventilated patients with airflow obstruction such as CPAP (24–27), and (c) accelerating spontaneous breath of patients without positive pressure support such as T-piece, which is related to more frequent respiratory activity and consumption of more oxygen (28, 29).

Disconnection from mechanical ventilator should be conducted when patients do not experience any intolerable events after accomplishing SBT (5). However, it is still conflicting as to which SBT should be preferentially selected in route daily practice. Although many studies comparing the efficacy and safety of more than two SBT strategies have been published (21, 22, 30–40, 94), only one (32) investigated the comparative efficacy and safety of all available SBT modes simultaneously at one analysis and suggested that ATC might be superior to T-tube or CPAP for extubation success and tolerance. It must be noted that the reliability of these findings should be interpreted cautiously because these findings were generated from a single-center trial with a limited sample size. Moreover, standard ventilators were utilized in this study, which deeply compromised the accurate compensation of ATC, provided an for the workload imposed by the tube (32). Furthermore, a direct meta-analysis (41) evaluated the efficacy of common types of SBTs, and revealed that patients receiving PSV (vs. T-tube) were more likely to obtain successful extubation. However, this meta-analysis ignored the variations in populations (children and adult) and study design (randomized and quasi-randomized trials) and only provided fragmentary pairwise results, all of which limited the value of pooled results.

As an expansion of direct meta-analysis, network meta-analysis (NMA) can simultaneously combine multiple treatments (more than two) in an individual analysis at one time. Consequently, it can make comprehensive assessments of the differences between all available treatments and clearly display the hierarchies of available treatments (42, 43). We therefore conducted the present NMA of randomized controlled trials (RCTs) to comprehensively compare and rank four common SBT strategies among critically ill patients who required invasive MV for at least 24 h through evaluating weaning success, reintubation, SBT success, duration of acute care, and ICU mortality.

METHODS

We conducted the present study and reported all pooled results according to the preferred reporting items for systematic review and meta-analysis for NMA (PRISMA-NMA) (44). The completed PRISMA-NMA checklist is available in **Supplementary Table 1**. No informed consent and institutional ethical approval if the patients were required because all analyses were completed based on published data.

Information Sources

We conducted a systematic literature search in PubMed, EMBASE, and CENTRAL from their inception until to May 17, 2020, and the latest search was updated on May 28, 2021. No restriction on language was imposed. The following terms were used to construct search strategy based on principle of combination of medical subject heading (MeSH) and text words: "ventilator weaning," "spontaneous breathing trial," "artificial respiration," "random," and various SBT techniques. Details of electronic search strategies and results identified are summarized in **Supplementary Table 2**. Any disagreements about study retrieval were solved based on consensus between two authors.

Study Selection

All identified potentially eligible records were firstly imported into EndNote to develop a literature database, and then duplicate records were automatically eliminated by software.

In the next step, two authors (LJY and XT) independently evaluated eligibility of unique records through screening titles and abstracts. Finally, they retrieved full-texts of all potentially relevant studies for further checking eligibility. To avoid literature omissions, clinical trial registry (such as www.clinicaltrials.gov) was also searched for unpublished and undergoing trials. Moreover, reference lists of included studies and relevant reviews were also manually screened to identify additional studies. Any controversies were solved based on consensus or adjudication with a third author (MC).

Selection Criteria

For inclusion, a study should meet the following criteria: (a) enrolled adult patients suffering from respiratory failure who received invasive MV for at least 24 h regardless of gender; (b) compared at least two SBT techniques (T-piece, CPAP, ATC, or PSV); (c) reported at least one of the following outcomes including weaning success, reintubation, SBT success, duration of acute care, and ICU mortality; (d) used a RCT design with full-text. Moreover, abstract with sufficient information was also considered. A study was excluded if it covered at least one of the following criteria: (a) evaluated SBT methods in tracheostomized patients or in patients receiving noninvasive ventilation; (b) SBTs was only used as a part of the comprehensive weaning strategy; (c) with insufficient information and additional data cannot be added from authors; (d) used ineligible study design such as crossover design, quasi-randomized trials, observational studies, and commentary; and (e) duplicate study with poor methodology and insufficient data.

Definition of Outcome

Our primary outcome was weaning success, which was defined as the absence of reintubation and/or resumption of ventilatory support for 48 h after extubation (45, 94). Secondary outcomes included reintubation rate (which was defined as the rate of reintubation within 48 h following extubation) (45, 94), successful SBT (if the patient showed no signs of intolerance when the SBT was performed, the SBT was considered successful) (45, 94), duration of ICU or long-term weaning unit (defined as the time from randomization to ICU or LWU) (46), and ICU mortality (defined as rate of the number of deaths during staying in ICU was divided by the number of all patients) (46).

Data Extraction

Two authors independently extracted the following relevant information from eligible studies with a predesigned standard information extraction sheet:(a) details of the studies including the first author's name, publication year, country, publication type, study design, types of intervention and control;(b) population characteristics including ventilation time before SBT, age, and severity of the disease; (c) reported outcomes including primary and secondary outcomes. What's more, we also extracted the information about quality of included studies. Discrepancies were resolved through consulting a third author. Leading author was contacted *via* email if the information of interest is absent.

Risk of Bias Assessment

Two independent authors assessed the methodological quality by using the Cochrane risk of bias assessment tool from the following seven items (47, 48): random sequence generation, allocation concealment, blinding of participants and personnel, blinding of outcome assessors, incomplete outcome data, selective reporting, and other bias. Each item was labeled as low, unclear, or high risk of bias according to the evaluation criteria (47). Among these target outcomes, all except for two (ICU mortality and ICU duration) depended on subjective judgement, which means the existence of different detection bias; therefore we performed risk of bias assessment respectively. We usually assume that blinding of outcome assessment was generally low risk of bias for objective outcomes.

Geometry of the Network

Network plots were produced to visualize the body of available evidence. In network geometry, each node represents a treatment and each line between the nodes represents a direct comparison. The size of the nodes and the thickness of the lines are proportional to total sample size and precision, respectively.

Statistical Analysis

All analyses were done using RevMan 5.3 (used for pairwise meta-analysis) and R version 3.6.1 (used for conducting NMA with gemtc package, assessing global heterogeneity, and calculating the surface under the cumulative ranking curve [SUCRA]) and STATA version 15.0 (used for estimation of inconsistency and local heterogeneity, funnel plot, and contribution plot).

Methods for Direct Treatment Comparisons

We conducted a pairwise meta-analysis for all comparisons by using the DerSimonian–Laird (DL) random-effects model. Odds ratio (OR) with 95% confidence interval (CI) was calculated for dichotomous outcome, whereas standardized mean difference with 95% CI was calculated for continuous outcome. We used Chi square and I^2 statistic simultaneously to evaluate the heterogeneity across studies. I^2 statistic measures the proportion of the overall variation that is attributable to between-study heterogeneity and $I^2 \geq 50\%$ was deemed as substantial heterogeneity (49, 50). For studies with multiple arms, outcome data were extracted from each group that meets the inclusion criteria, and then were created independent pairwise comparisons (43).

Methods for Indirect and Mixed Comparisons

For each endpoint, a Bayesian random-effects NMA (51, 52) was conducted to combine direct and indirect results. We calculated the relative ranking probabilities of being the best, second best for each weaning method, and so on. What's more, we also employed the SUCRA to estimate the ranking probabilities for available weaning methods on various outcomes (53). When one weaning technique is regarded as the best one without uncertainty, SUCRA value equals 1. If not, we draw an opposite conclusion (53, 54).

Assessment of Consistency and Heterogeneity

To explore the inconsistency of the entire network, the design-by treatment interaction model was used (55, 56). By using the "ifplot" command, inconsistency factor (IF) was calculated in each closed loop (a loop is made up of three technologies) to estimate the local inconsistencies, with values near 1 denoting statistical consistency (57, 58). Besides, a node-splitting method was undertaken to assess the potential inconsistency between the direct and indirect evidence for each comparison, which is a node in a direct acyclic graph (59). A *P* of more than 0.05 was deemed as consistent, which implied that the information from both sources of evidence contains enough similarities to be combined (60). A global heterogeneity was quantified using the I^2-statistic. The prediction intervals for the pooled ORs provided a limited range in which the relative effect of a future similar study is expected to be involved (61, 62). The predictive interval plot, considering the extent of heterogeneity, was used to assess the magnitude of uncertainty in the estimated effect size for the NMA (63). If uncertainty is affected by heterogeneity, discordances exist between the confidence intervals of relative treatment effects and their predictive intervals.

Contribution Plot and Publication Bias

A contribution plot revealed the influence of each direct comparison to the estimation of the network summary effects, which helped to make an objective appraisal of the overall quality of evidence from NMA (58, 64). A comparison-adjusted funnel plot was constructed to inspect the small-study effects when sufficient number of eligible studies were analyzed in a single pair of comparison (<10) (65).

GRADE Evaluation on Quality of Evidence

We evaluated the certainty of evidence contributing to all network estimates of the primary outcomes by using the Grading of Recommendations Assessment, Development, and Evaluation (GRADE) framework (66). Disagreements,, if any, were resolved by consulting a third researcher.

RESULTS

Study Selection and Characteristics

After assessment of 105 full-text articles, 24 publications involving 4,241 subjects were included to investigate the efficacy of T-piece, PSV, CPAP, and ATC in critically ill patients weaning from MV (21, 22, 30–40, 45, 67–75, 94). We designed **Figure 1** to outline the details of capturing and selecting studies.

The baseline characteristics of included articles are summarized in **Supplementary Table 3**. The majority of the studies were designed double-arm trials (21/24, 87.5%) (21, 30, 31, 33–37, 39, 40, 45, 67–75, 94). Publication year was between 1991 and 2020, and the number of participants of individual study ranged from 14 to 578. To illustrate the head-to-head comparisons involved in the NMA, network plots for four outcomes were delineated in **Figure 2**. T-piece (20 studies) (21, 22, 31–33, 35, 37–40, 45, 67–73, 75, 94) and PSV (20 studies) (22, 31–33, 35–39, 45, 67, 69–75, 94) were the most frequently investigated SBT methods, whereas CPAP (six studies) (21, 22, 30, 32, 34, 38, 40, 68) and ATC(six studies) (32, 34, 36, 74) acquired fewer samples, thus suggesting a higher potential deviation in traditional meta-analysis.

Methodological Quality of Studies

Out of 24 RCTs, seven (29.1%) (32, 33, 35, 36, 45, 74, 75) did not describe the method of generating random sequence. Eight RCTs (33.3%) (33, 35, 36, 38, 39, 71, 74, 75) did not report the details of allocation concealment, which could cause potential selection bias. Besides, one study (34) stated that personnel supervising of the SBTs failed to conceal allocation, and was therefore considered to present a high risk of bias. For subjective outcomes (weaning success, reintubation, and SBT success), eight studies (21, 22, 30, 31, 34, 38, 68, 94) provided details on blinding of outcome assessors, and three articles (37, 67, 71) did not evaluate outcomes in a blinded manner. Since all studies stated a clear patient flow or used intention-to-treat analysis, there was no hint of attrition bias. What's more, no study selectively reported results. Risk of bias summary was documented in **Supplementary Table 4.**

Weaning Success

The effects of four extubation strategies on weaning success from pairwise metaanalyses can be found in **Figure 2A**. Among six direct comparisons in direct random-effects meta-analysis, ATC was associated with increased weaning success rate compared with T-piece (OR, 0.28; 95% CI, 0.13 to 0.64) and PSV (OR, 0.53; 95% CI, 0.32 to 0.88), respectively. Remaining comparisons were not statistically significant (see **Supplementary Figure 1**).

In NMA, ATC was superior to the T-piece (OR, 0.34; 95% CI, 0.17 to 0.65) and PSV (OR, 0.5; 95% CI, 0.27 to 0.92) in terms of weaning success, respectively. Besides, an improvement effect of weaning success was detected for the comparison between PSV and T-piece (OR, 0.68; 95% CI, 0.45 to 0.98). **Figure 3A** reported all pooled results of the NMA.

Reintubation

Of all 24 eligible RCTs, 17 (21, 22, 30–32, 37–40, 45, 67–69, 71–73, 94) reported the reintubation within 48 h following extubation, which included six direct comparisons (**Figure 2B**). CPAP could slightly decrease reintubation compared with T-piece (OR, 2.76; 95% CI, 1.08 to 7.06). All pooled results from traditional meta-analysis can be found in **Supplementary Figure 2.**

In NMA, all comparisons did not show significant effects on reintubation. All pooled results can be found in **Figure 3B.**

SBT Success

Of all eligible RCTs, 13 (21, 22, 32, 34, 39, 45, 67, 68, 70–73, 94) reported SBT success, which included six direct comparisons (**Figure 2C**). In all direct comparisons, the comparative efficacy of T-piece vs. PSV (OR, 0.61; 95% CI, 0.46 to 0.80), T-piece vs. ATC (OR, 0.17; 95% CI, 0.06 to 0.50), PSV vs. ATC (OR, 0.42; 95% CI, 0.20 to 0.90), and CPAP vs. ATC (OR, 0.21; 95% CI, 0.08 to 0.58) reached statistical significance. All pooled results from direct comparisons can be obtained in **Supplementary Figure 3.**

The results of comparisons of SBT success in our NMA are presented in **Figure 3C**. ATC exerted a trend of high SBT success

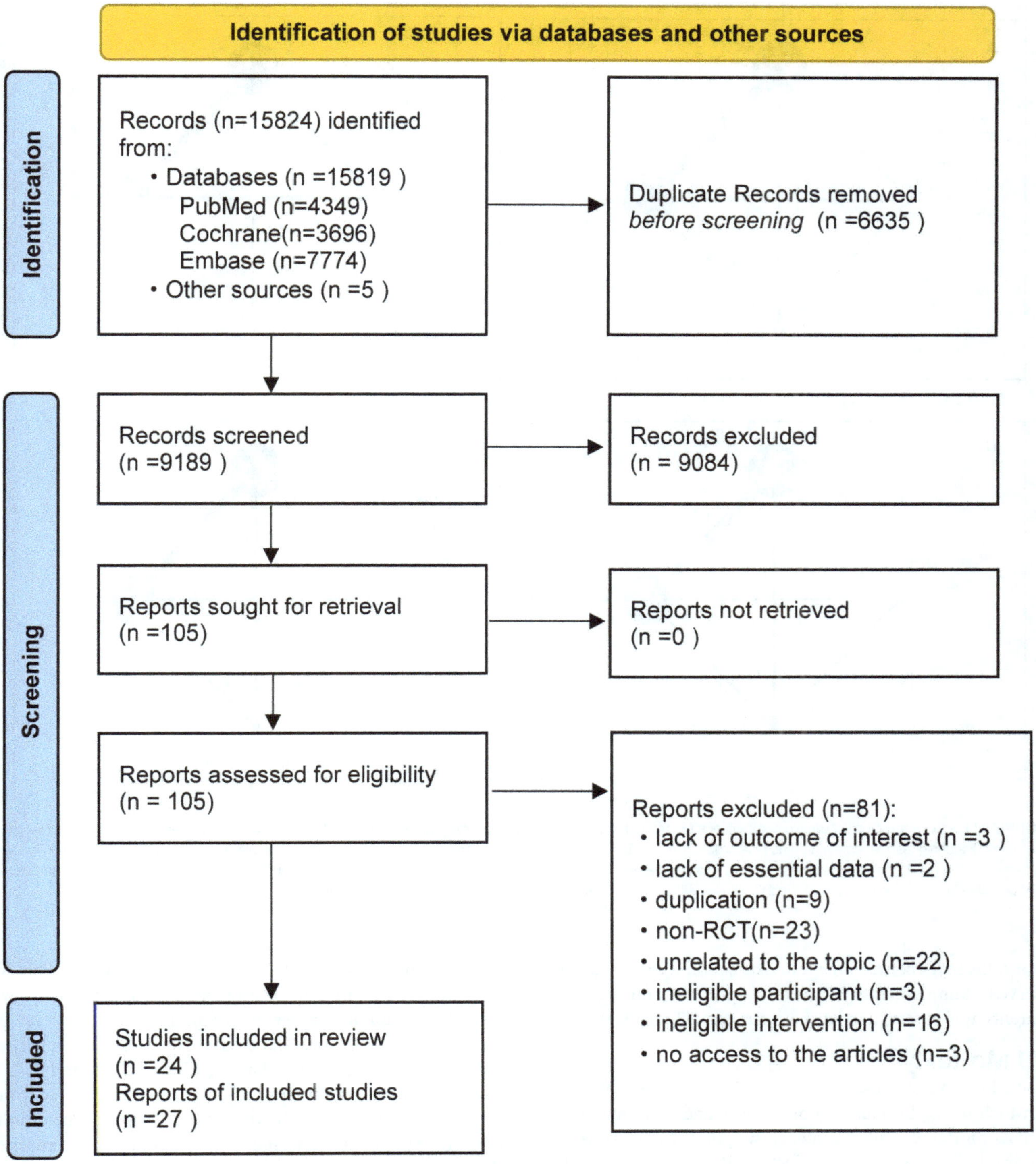

FIGURE 1 | PRISMA flow diagram of retrieval and selection of studies.

when compared with T-piece (OR, 0.21; 95% CI, 0.1–0.45), PSV (OR, 0.35; 95% CI, 0.16–0.73), and CPAP (OR, 0.22; 95% CI, 0.08–0.52), respectively. PSV had significant superiority over T-piece in SBT success (OR, 0.59; 95% CI, 0.43–0.84).

ICU or LWU Length of Stay

Of all included RCTs, seven (31, 32, 36, 39, 69–71) reported ICU or LWU length of stay, which included six direct-comparisons (**Figure 2D**). In all six direct-comparisons, no

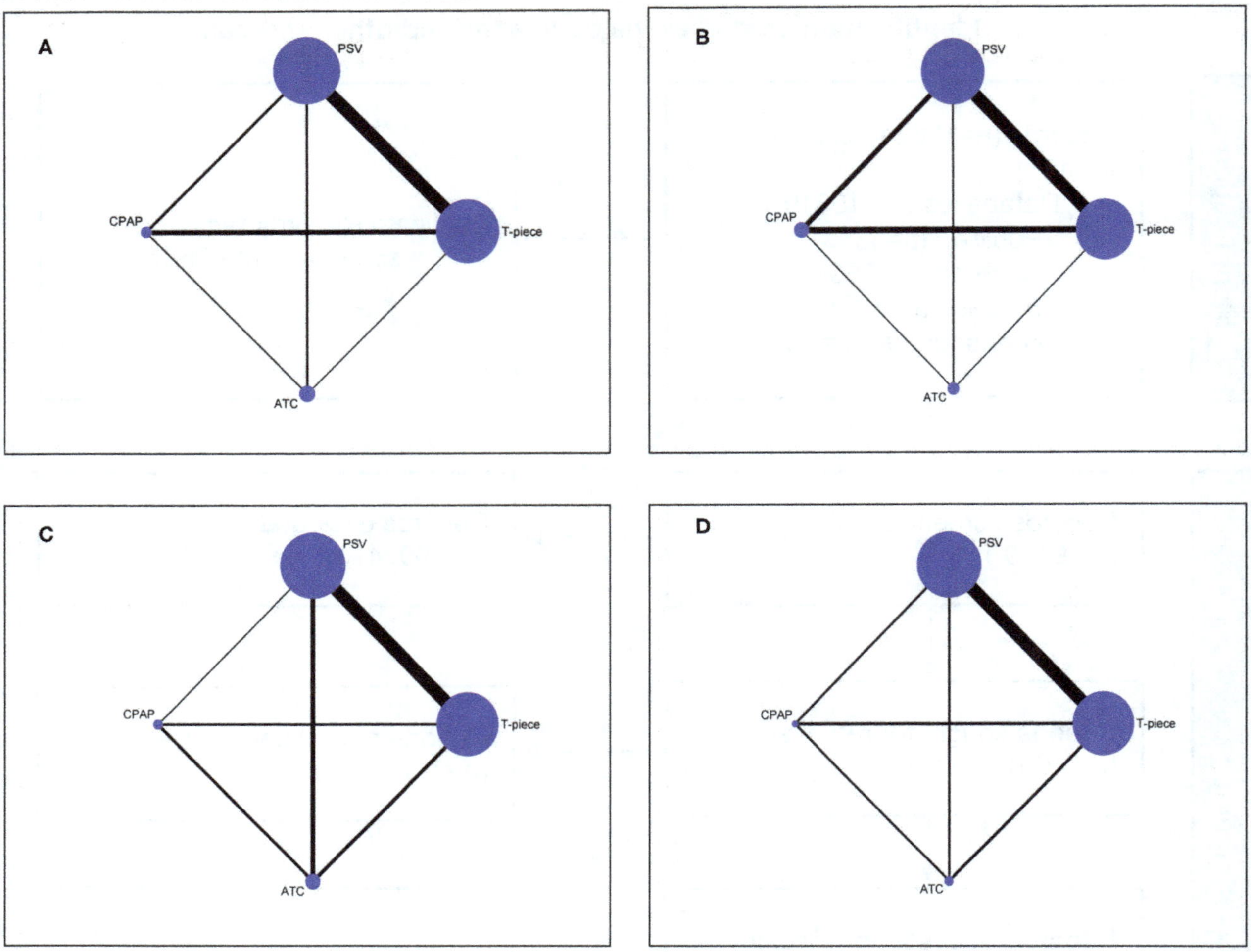

FIGURE 2 | Evidence structure of eligible comparisons for network meta-analysis. **(A)** weaning success. **(B)**. reintubation. **(C)** SBT success. **(D)** ICU or LWU length of stay. All SBT techniques are represented as blue solid circles, and existing head-to-head (direct) comparisons are drawn as black solid lines. The size of every node is proportion to the number of randomly assigned participants (sample size) and the width of the lines is proportion to the number of RCTs for each pairwise comparison. PSV, pressure support ventilation; CPAP, continuous positive airway pressure; ATC, automatic tube compensation.

major differences between the four extubation technologies were observed (**Supplementary Figure 4**). In NMA, no significant difference was observed in any comparisons (**Figure 3D**).

ICU Mortality

Of all 24 eligible studies, 10 RCTs (31, 35, 39, 45, 67, 69–71, 73, 94) which focused exclusively on T-piece and PSV investigated the ICU mortality. Direct evidence supports that there was no significant difference in the effect of PSV and T-piece (OR, 1.19; 95% CI, 0.89 to 1.59) without heterogeneity ($I^2 = 0\%$) (**Supplementary Figure 5**).

Assessment of Consistency and Heterogeneity

The test of global inconsistency detected no significant difference between the consistency and inconsistency models for four outcomes ($P = 0.690$ for weaning success, $P = 0.523$ for reintubation, $P = 0.951$ for STB success, and $P = 0.308$ for ICU or LWU length of stay, respectively). For four outcomes, test for local inconsistency showed that all loops were consistent (**Supplementary Figure 6**). Predictive interval plot indicated 33.3%, 0.00%, 33.3%, and 0.00% of the comparisons for weaning success, reintubation, SBT success, and ICU or LWU length of stay respectively, and therefore no outcomes was substantially affected by the estimated heterogeneity in the network (**Supplementary Figure 7**). The common heterogeneity through the Bayesian meta-analysis was 0.224 for weaning success, 0.020 for reintubation, 0.036 for SBT success, and 0.000 for ICU or LWU length of stay.

SUCRA and Ranking of all Treatments

We showed the mean values of SUCRA for providing the hierarchy ranking of different weaning technologies on weaning success, reintubation, SBT success, and ICU or LWU length of stay. According to SUCRA, T-piece ranked fourth, second, third, and second on increase of weaning success, reintubation, SBT

A

T-piece	1.46 (1.02, 2.24)	1.53 (0.72, 3.42)	2.93 (1.53, 5.98)
0.68 (0.45, 0.98)	PSV	1.05 (0.46, 2.35)	2 (1.08, 3.76)
0.65 (0.29, 1.38)	0.95 (0.42, 2.17)	CPAP	1.92 (0.79, 4.74)
0.34 (0.17, 0.65)	0.5 (0.27, 0.92)	0.52 (0.21, 1.27)	ATC

B

T-piece	1.05 (0.81, 1.36)	**2.76 (1.08, 7.06)**	1.00 (0.23, 4.43)
1.17 (0.83, 1.85)	PSV	0.81 (0.23, 2.77)	0.67 (0.32, 1.38)
2.04 (0.82, 5.78)	1.73 (0.69, 4.79)	CPAP	0.72 (0.15, 3.54)
0.85 (0.36, 2.37)	0.72 (0.31, 1.79)	0.42 (0.12, 1.42)	ATC

C

T-piece	**0.61 (0.46, 0.80)**	0.85 (0.38, 1.88)	**0.17 (0.06, 0.50)**
0.59 (0.43, 0.84)	PSV	2.51 (0.83, 7.64)	**0.42 (0.20, 0.90)**
0.99 (0.45, 2.16)	1.66 (0.74, 3.71)	CPAP	**0.21 (0.08, 0.58)**
0.21 (0.1, 0.45)	**0.35 (0.16, 0.73)**	**0.22 (0.08, 0.52)**	ATC

D

T-piece	0.10 (0.01, 0.19)	-0.24 (-0.75, 0.27)	0.00 (-0.51, 0.51)
1.52 (0.74, 6.87)	PSV	0.08 (-0.43, 0.58)	-0.02 (-0.58, 0.54)
0.81 (0.08, 12.3)	0.51 (0.04, 5.39)	CPAP	0.13 (-0.37, 0.64)
1.39 (0.12, 21.42)	0.87 (0.07, 9.89)	1.7 (0.08, 38.98)	ATC

FIGURE 3 | Summary for four outcomes of different SBT techniques. **(A)** weaning success. **(B)** reintubation. **(C)** SBT success. **(D)**. ICU or LWU length of stay. If available, the upper right half presented results from pairwise meta-analysis and the left lower half showed the results from network meta-analysis. For direct comparison, odds ratios (ORs) below 1 favor the row-defining treatment. For indirect comparison, ORs below 1 favor the column-defining treatment. For numerical data, the number in each cell represented the effect size of the treatment in upper left area minus the treatment in bottom right area. Significant results are in bold print. PSV: pressure support ventilation, CPAP: continuous positive airway pressure, ATC: automatic tube compensation.

success and ICU or LWU length of stay, among all strategies, with a probability of 85.2%, 51.7%, 49.8%, and 44.3%, respectively. Whereas ATC had a probability of 91.7%, 62.1%, 99.7% and 39.9% to rank first, first, first, and fourth for each corresponding outcome above (**Supplementary Table 5**). However, considering that the sample sizes of different interventions varied greatly, the results might be highly biased and should be interpreted with caution. The ranking of all SBT technologies is depicted in **Supplementary Figure 8**.

Contribution Plot and Publication Bias

According to the contribution plots of the network (see **Supplementary Figure 9**), the comparison of T-piece (mode A) vs. PSV (mode B) or PSV (mode B) vs. ATC (mode D) in the four entire networks showed 26.4% and 24.3% for weaning success, 32.7% and 23.9% for reintubation, 31.0% and 18.5% for SBT success, 29.5% and 19.2% for ICU or LWU length of stay, respectively.

We performed comparison-adjusted funnel-plot analysis for four outcomes (**Supplementary Figure 10**). The funnel plots were relatively asymmetric, highlighting that there is a significant risk of publication bias in our study.

GRADE Evaluation on Quality of Evidence

According to GRADE, the quality of evidence ranged from very low to high, but was rated as low and as very low for most comparisons. In terms of T-piece vs. PSV, the quality was low for ICU or LWU length of stay and weaning success, and was very low for SBT success and reintubation, whereas moderate for ICU mortality. Quality of evidence was low for the overall ranking of treatment for weaning success, reintubation, ICU or LWU length of stay, and SBT success (**Supplementary Table 6**).

DISCUSSION

Summary of Main Findings

This is the first NMA on this topic. After completing all analyses, we obtained several important findings: (a) Evidence from direct and NMA showed that ATC obtained superior weaning success compared to T-piece and PSV. Besides, the direct evidence demonstrated patients receiving PSV (vs. T-piece) appeared to be more likely to be extubated successfully; (b) Direct evidence suggested that T-piece had higher reintubation rate vs. CPAP, but these findings were not be supported by network evidence; (c) Direct evidence indicated that ATC was superior to others in SBT success, PSV was also better than T-piece in terms of this given outcome, and all statistically significant findings were detected in network meta-analyses; (d) In terms of prolonging ICU or LWU length of stay, no weaning technologies have been shown superior to another which were determined both directly and thorough NMA; (e) Compared with T-piece, PSV did not show different effects on the ICU mortality, whereas this conclusion was supported by direct evidence only; (f) The ranking of all weaning modes was ATC, CPAP, PSV, and T-piece in enhancing weaning success; (g) For increasing SBT success, the ranking of all weaning modes was ATC, PSV, T-piece, and CPAP; (h) The ranking of all weaning modes was ATC, T-piece, PSV, and CPAP in terms of reintubation rate; and (i) For prolonging ICU or LWU length of stay, the ranking of all weaning modes was CPAP, T-piece, PSV, and ATC.

Automatic tube compensation is a new mode of ventilatory assistance. It potentially simulates spontaneous breathing without the endotracheal tube, and so it has been called as "electronic extubation" (76, 77). There are several possible explanations for this clinical observation that ATC might be more efficacious than other investigated SBT techniques performed before extubation in critical patients. First and foremost, according to the actual flow that assists the spontaneously breathing intubated patient (78), ATC gives dynamic pressure support during the breathing cycle, which can automatically compensate for the non-linear resistance added by the artificial airway (21, 76, 79). This characteristic of ATC causes a reduction in the work of breathing (17, 80), and thus increases the probability of successful extubation (81). Secondly, ATC is able to maintain the natural and variable breathing pattern to the greatest extent (82, 83), which can more closely represent the postextubation scenario. This potential advantage of ATC can improve synchronization between patient and ventilator, and then promote respiratory comfort (82, 84, 85). Meanwhile, it can result in more significant predictive values for successful weaning and extubation (23). Last but not least, as a result of auto-positive end expiratory pressure (PEEP), ineffective ventilator-triggering is more likely to be less common with ATC than with PSV (77). Hence, ATC is ideally suitable for the weaning process (24).

Though direct evidence suggested that T-piece had higher reintubation rate when compared with CPAP, this finding was not supported by network evidence. Since network evidence combined the direct and indirect evidence in the same analytical model and more eligible RCTs were included, these results were more reliable and accurate.

Pressure support ventilation is widely used to overcome the additional work of breathing and pressure–time product exerted by the endotracheal tubes (18, 22, 86). Consequently, it can significantly decrease the endocrine stress response and relieve the clinical picture of intolerance (37, 38, 87). Furthermore, PSV allows patients to control the respiratory rate and the inspiratory flow during the spontaneous inspiration, thereby diminishing the oxygen consumption of respiratory muscles and preventing fatigue (88–90). These may be the primary reasons why PSV SBTs result in both higher SBT and extubation success rates compared with a T-piece SBT. This finding is broadly in line with previous work. A moderate-quality evidence (91) demonstrated that some intubated subjects who previously failed a weaning trial through the T-tube but continued a weaning trial with PSV were extubated successfully. A latest large-scale multicenter trial also compared PSV and T-piece ventilation in adults and noted that PSV SBT produced significantly higher rates of successful extubation, not adversely influencing reintubation rates (70).

Agreements and Disagreements in the Current Literature

It was worth mentioning that several studies have exclusively investigated the efficacy and safety of at least two modalities of ventilator weaning, but primary studies comparing all the approaches have but one and cannot identify subtle clinical differences due to small sample size. To date, three traditional pairwise metaanalyses with full-text have been performed to evaluate the comparative efficacy of PSV vs. T-piece (46, 92)and PSV vs. other alternative SBT techniques (41) in patients ready to be liberated from MV. However, no head-to-head meta-analysis comparing all SBTs with each other has been reported. Consequently, that in which SBT technique is superior remains to be elucidated.

The results of Ladeira et al. (46) indicated an improvement in PSV group for successful SBTs among patients with simple weaning, but no difference between these two strategies for weaning success, ICU mortality, reintubation, ICU and LWU length of stay was found. Li et al. (92) found no difference between PSV SBT mode and T-piece SBT mode in all outcomes reported in the above-mentioned trial. Burns et al. (41)verified that extubation only tended to be more successful during PSV as compared with T-piece, but there was no difference between PSV vs. CPAP and PSV vs. ATC. After excluding an outlier trial, authors observed that patients undergoing PSV are more likely to pass an SBT. In contrast to previous metaanalyses, we comprehensively evaluated four common SBT technologies and obtained more informative findings. Firstly, we found that PSVs were associated with higher weaning success and SBT success, which is in agreement with previous results, but only these findings were confirmed by network metaanalyses. In addition, our analysis supported that ATC is an important weaning alternative for critically ill patients. Without increasing the reintubation rate and ICU or LWU length of stay, ATC provides clinical benefits in improving weaning success and SBT success. We also firstly make hierarchies of four different SBT technologies including T-piece, PSV, CPAP, and TAC, all of which were not reported in previous studies.

Strengths and Limitations

Our NMA has certain important strengths including (a) We designed comprehensive search algorithms to obtain and identified eligible studies in critically ill patients, thereby minimizing information bias and enhancing generalizability; (b) NMA method allowed us to assess the results from both direct comparison and mixed-treatment comparisons, and thus optimally addressing the relative effectiveness of those SBT techniques; (c) We just included RCTs, which were the highest level of evidence; so we deemed that our pooled results can reflect closely the true effectiveness of the four most commonly performed SBT modes; and (d) We rated the certainty of evidence by the GRADE approach when explaining each unique comparison and across the network.

Nevertheless, some limitations in this study merited further discussion, including (a) Due to paucity of available data, we introduced criteria for pooling ventilation techniques. Many of the trials included varied in the level of pressure or did not specify whether PEEP was added; however, when implementing similar weaning strategies, we considered them to be in a clinically similar condition and combined them into a single group. This action may induce potential heterogeneity. (b) Since few publications existed, it is impossible to assess the impact of the mode of ventilation on other important indicators, such as hospital length of stay, hospital mortality, total duration of MV, and adverse events. Currently, most of the researchers monitored patients only during ICU stay, and very little data was available when they moved into the general ward. Further studies with a larger number of patients are warranted to consider these problems to gain full insight into the real effect of various extubation strategies. (c) No trials were designed to evaluate the impact of ATC and CPAP on ICU mortality in present. Also, we only captured 10 RCTs by directly comparing PSV and T-piece focusing on this parameter; thus larger studies with excellent designs are warranted to make up the gap. (d) It is important that neither patients nor personnel could be blinded after randomization as different SBT technologies had different requirements at the different preparation stages. We believe that this factor has potential influence on the results. However, the majority of weaning and extubation studies were not free from this limitation. (e) We did not specifically stratify all interventions in the current study, which may introduce a potential bias. However, the major aim of this NMA is to generally determine the comparative efficacy and safety of available macroscopic SBT techniques. Certainly, we suggest conducting future studies to further specifically differentiate the efficacy and safety of different regimes (e.g., low, middle, or high PSV) of each SBT technique.

Implications for Further Research

Spontaneous breathing trials are an integrated component of the weaning assessment, so the "weaning condition" of a patient entering to SBT will influence the accuracy of different SBT methods. On the basis of the difficulty and duration of the weaning process, patients are divided into three categories: simple weaning, difficult weaning, and prolonged weaning (12, 93). In this review, the target patients in most of the studies included belonged to simple weaning, and our analysis supported the selection of ATC as an important alternative for this group. Hence, if one method to perform SBT has any superiority over the other, improvement in weaning outcome is more likely to be expected in selected populations at higher risk for prolonged weaning and difficult weaning. Further studies should be conducted to establish this classification and to confirm how related clinical outcomes are affected in each category of weaning, finalizing the optimal weaning strategy in specific weaning situations. Meanwhile, researchers should pay more attention to ATC weaning mode to clarify its role in weaning patients off mechanical ventilation.

It must be noted that, as an objective marker of identifying the severity, the MV duration before conducting SBT can reflect the demands for ventilation, the risk of suffering from infection, and refractory bronchospasm, all of which were positively associated with worse prognosis. A previous study (69) has revealed that the MV duration before conducting SBT may greatly increase the risk of weaning failure within 48 h. However, the role of this factor under the different SBT modes (PSV, T-piece, CPAP, and ATC) and among specific populations is unclear, which should be further clarified in future studies.

CONCLUSIONS

In summary, the present NMA demonstrated that ATC is an alternative mode of ventilation for critically ill patients. Our finding should be interpreted with caution as it generates from RCT with small sample sizes. Further large scale and well-designed studies are needed to confirm this point.

AUTHOR CONTRIBUTIONS

L-JY, XT, MC, and MJ-H: conception and design. XT and MJ-H: administrative support. L-JY, XT, and MC: provision of study materials or patients. L-JY, XT: collection and assembly of data. L-JY and XT: data analysis and interpretation. L-JY, XT, MC, J-ML, NX, and MJ-H: manuscript writing and final approval of manuscript. All authors contributed to the article and approve the submitted version.

ACKNOWLEDGMENTS

I would like to acknowledge my teammates for their wonderful collaboration. In addition, we would particularly like to express our appreciation to all authors listed in all the primary studies that were included in the current review.

REFERENCES

1. Esteban A, Anzueto A, Alía I, Gordo F, Apezteguía C, Pálizas F, et al. How is mechanical ventilation employed in the intensive care unit? An international utilization review. *Am J Respir Crit Care Med.* (2000) 161:1450–8. doi: 10.1164/ajrccm.161.5.9902018
2. Esteban A, Anzueto A, Frutos F, Alía I, Brochard L, Stewart TE, et al. Characteristics and outcomes in adult patients receiving mechanical ventilation: a 28-day international study. *JAMA.* (2002) 287:345–55. doi: 10.1001/jama.287.3.345
3. Tomicic V, Espinoza M, Andresen M, Molina J, Calvo M, Ugarte H, et al. [Characteristics and factors associated with mortality in patients receiving mechanical ventilation: first Chilean multicenter study]. *Rev Med Chil.* (2008) 136:959–67. doi: 10.4067/S0034-98872008000800001
4. Dasta JF, McLaughlin TP, Mody SH, Piech CT. Daily cost of an intensive care unit day: the contribution of mechanical ventilation. *Crit Care Med.* (2005) 33:1266–71. doi: 10.1097/01.CCM.0000164543.14619.00
5. Epstein SK. Weaning from ventilatory support. *Curr Opin Crit Care.* (2009) 15:36–43. doi: 10.1097/MCC.0b013e3283220e07
6. Frutos-Vivar F, Ferguson ND, Esteban A, Epstein SK, Arabi Y, Apezteguía C, et al. Risk factors for extubation failure in patients following a successful spontaneous breathing trial. *Chest.* (2006) 130:1664–71. doi: 10.1378/chest.130.6.1664
7. Jindal SK, Aggarwal AN, Gupta D. Adult respiratory distress syndrome in the tropics. *Clin Chest Med.* (2002) 23:445–55. doi: 10.1016/S0272-5231(01)00009-0
8. Meade M, Guyatt G, Sinuff T, Griffith L, Hand L, Toprani G, et al. Trials comparing alternative weaning modes and discontinuation assessments. *Chest.* (2001) 120(Suppl. 6):425s_37s. doi: 10.1378/chest.120.6_suppl.425S
9. Pellegrini J, Moraes RB, Mac Ca Ri JG, Oliveira R, Teixeira C. Spontaneous breathing trials with t-piece or pressure support ventilation. *Respir Care.* (2016) 61:1693–703. doi: 10.4187/respcare.04816
10. Thille AW, Harrois A, Schortgen F, Brun-Buisson C, Brochard L. Outcomes of extubation failure in medical intensive care unit patients. *Crit Care Med.* (2011) 39:2612–8. doi: 10.1097/CCM.0b013e3182282a5a
11. MacIntyre NR, Cook DJ, Ely EW, Jr., Epstein SK, Fink JB, Heffner JE, et al. Evidence-based guidelines for weaning and discontinuing ventilatory support: a collective task force facilitated by the American College of Chest Physicians; the American Association for Respiratory Care; and the American College of Critical Care Medicine. *Chest.* (2001) 120(Suppl. 6):375s_95s. doi: 10.1378/chest.120.6_suppl.375S
12. Boles JM, Bion J, Connors A, Herridge M, Marsh B, Melot C, et al. Weaning from mechanical ventilation. *Eur Respir J.* (2007) 29:1033–56. doi: 10.1183/09031936.00010206
13. Tobin MJ, Jubran A. Variable performance of weaning-predictor tests: role of Bayes' theorem and spectrum and test-referral bias. *Intensive Care Med.* (2006) 32:2002–12. doi: 10.1007/s00134-006-0439-4
14. Alía I, Esteban A. Weaning from mechanical ventilation. *Crit Care.* (2000) 4:72–80. doi: 10.1186/cc660
15. Bien MY, Hseu SS, Yien HW, Kuo BI, Lin YT, Wang JH, et al. Breathing pattern variability: a weaning predictor in postoperative patients recovering from systemic inflammatory response syndrome. *Intensive Care Med.* (2004) 30:241–7. doi: 10.1007/s00134-003-2073-8
16. El-Khatib M, Jamaleddine G, Soubra R, Muallem M. Pattern of spontaneous breathing: potential marker for weaning outcome. Spontaneous breathing pattern and weaning from mechanical ventilation *Intensive Care Med.* (2001) 27:52–8. doi: 10.1007/s001340000758
17. Fabry B, Haberthür C, Zappe D, Guttmann J, Kuhlen R, Stocker R. Breathing pattern and additional work of breathing in spontaneously breathing patients with different ventilatory demands during inspiratory pressure support and automatic tube compensation. *Intensive Care Med.* (1997) 23:545–52. doi: 10.1007/s001340050371
18. Kuhlen R, Max M, Dembinski R, Terbeck S, Jürgens E, Rossaint R. Breathing pattern and workload during automatic tube compensation, pressure support and T-piece trials in weaning patients. *Eur J Anaesthesiol.* (2003) 20:10–6. doi: 10.1097/00003643-200311000-00014
19. MacIntyre N. Discontinuing mechanical ventilatory support. *Chest.* (2007) 132:1049–56. doi: 10.1378/chest.06-2862
20. Wysocki M, Cracco C, Teixeira A, Mercat A, Diehl JL, Lefort Y, et al. Reduced breathing variability as a predictor of unsuccessful patient separation from mechanical ventilation. *Crit Care Med.* (2006) 34:2076–83. doi: 10.1097/01.CCM.0000227175.83575.E9
21. Cohen J, Shapiro M, Grozovski E, Fox B, Lev S, Singer P. Prediction of extubation outcome: a randomised, controlled trial with automatic tube compensation vs. pressure support ventilation. *Crit Care (London, England).* (2009) 13:R21. doi: 10.1186/cc7724
22. Haberthür C, Mols G, Elsasser S, Bingisser R, Stocker R, Guttmann J. Extubation after breathing trials with automatic tube compensation, T-tube, or pressure support ventilation. *Acta Anaesthesiol Scand.* (2002) 46:973–9. doi: 10.1034/j.1399-6576.2002.460808.x
23. G.Ferreyra S, Weber-Cartens V, Aquadrone. Comparison of automatic tube compensation (ATC) with pressure support ventilation (PSV) during spontaneous breathing trials. *Int Care Med.* (2007) 33:s57.
24. Cohen JD, Shapiro M, Grozovski E, Lev S, Fisher H, Singer P. Extubation outcome following a spontaneous breathing trial with automatic tube compensation versus continuous positive airway pressure. *Crit Care Med.* (2006) 34:682–6. doi: 10.1097/01.CCM.0000201888.32663.6A
25. Petrof BJ, Legaré M, Goldberg P, Milic-Emili J, Gottfried SB. Continuous positive airway pressure reduces work of breathing and dyspnea during weaning from mechanical ventilation in severe chronic obstructive pulmonary disease. *Am Rev Respir Dis.* (1990) 141:281–9. doi: 10.1164/ajrccm/141.2.281
26. Smith TC, Marini JJ. Impact of PEEP on lung mechanics and work of breathing in severe airflow obstruction. *J Appl Physiol.* (1988) 65:1488–99. doi: 10.1152/jappl.1988.65.4.1488
27. Lago AF, Goncalves EC, Silva EC, Menegueti MG, Nicolini EA, Auxiliadora-Martins M, et al. Comparison of energy expenditure and oxygen consumption of spontaneous breathing trial conducted with and without automatic tube compensation. *J Clin Med Res.* (2015) 7:700–5. doi: 10.14740/jocm r2250w
28. Pinsky MR. Breathing as exercise: the cardiovascular response to weaning from mechanical ventilation. *Intensive Care Med.* (2000) 26:1164–6. doi: 10.1007/s001340000619
29. Walsh TS. Recent advances in gas exchange measurement in intensive care patients. *Br J Anaesth.* (2003) 91:120–31. doi: 10.1093/bja/aeg128
30. Cekmen N, Erdemli O. The comparison of the effects of T-piece and CPAP on hemodynamic parameters, arterial blood gases and success of weaning. *Bratisl Lek Listy.* (2011) 112:512–6.
31. Chittawatanarat K, Orrapin S, Jitkaroon K, Mueakwan S, Sroison U. An open label randomized controlled trial to compare low level pressure support and T-piece as strategies for discontinuation of mechanical ventilation

in a general surgical intensive care unit. *Med Arch.* (2018) 72:51–7. doi: 10.5455/medarh.2018.72.51-57

32. E.Zanfaly H. Automatic Tube Compensation versus Pressure Support Ventilation, Continuous Positive Airway Pressure and T-Tube during Spontaneous Breathing Trial. *Res Opin Anesth Intensive Care.* (2014) 2:35–42.
33. Faleh K, Fredj H, Maayouf H, Mokline A, Jami I, Saad MB, et al. Weaning from mechanical ventilation in burns: which weaning test in clinical practice? *Ann Intensive Care.* (2020) 10:105.
34. Figueroa-Casas JB, Ricardo M, Alejandro A, Connery SM. Comparison between automatic tube compensation and continuous positive airway pressure during spontaneous breathing trials. *Respir Care.* (2010) 55:549–54.
35. Jamoussi A, Jarraya F, Ayed S, Merhabene T, Khelil JB, Besbes M. T-piece versus sub-therapeutic pressure support for weaning from invasive mechanical ventilation in patients with chronic obstructive pulmonary disease: a comparative prospective study. *Ann Intensive Care.* (2020) 10:58
36. Kashefi P, Abbasi S, Katiraei F, Alikiaii B. Comparison of the weaning rate in three mechanical ventilation methods, automatic tube compensation and pressure support ventilation with airway pressure of five and eight centimeters of water. *J Isfahan Med Sch.* (2017) 34:1297–303.
37. Koh Y, Hong SB, Lim CM, Lee SD, Kim WS, Kim DS, et al. Effect of an additional 1-hour T-piece trial on weaning outcome at minimal pressure support. *J Crit Care.* (2000) 15:41–5. doi: 10.1053/jcrc.2000.7898
38. Koksal GM, Sayilgan C, Sen O, Oz H. The effects of different weaning modes on the endocrine stress response. *Crit Care.* (2004) 8:R31–4. doi: 10.1186/cc2671
39. Lourenço IS, Franco AM, Bassetto S, Rodrigues AJ. Pressure support-ventilation versus spontaneous breathing with "T-tube" for interrupting the ventilation after cardiac operations. *Braz J Cardiovasc Surg.* (2013) 28:455–61. doi: 10.5935/1678-9741.20130075
40. Jones DP, Byrne P, Morgan C, Fraser I, Hyland R. Positive end-expiratory pressure vs T-piece: extubation after mechanical ventilation. *Chest.* (1991) 100:1655–9. doi: 10.1378/chest.100.6.1655
41. Burns KEA, Soliman I, Adhikari NKJ, Zwein A, Wong JTY, Gomez-Builes C, et al. Trials directly comparing alternative spontaneous breathing trial techniques: a systematic review and meta-analysis. *Crit Care.* (2017) 21:127. doi: 10.1186/s13054-017-1698-x
42. Mavridis D, Giannatsi M, Cipriani A, Salanti G. A primer on network meta-analysis with emphasis on mental health. *Evid Based Ment Health.* (2015) 18:40–6. doi: 10.1136/eb-2015-102088
43. Higgins JP, Green S. *Cochrane Handbook for Systematic Review of Interventions Version 5.1.0. The Cochrane Collaboration.* (2011). Available online at: http://handbook.cochrane.org
44. Hutton B, Salanti G, Caldwell DM, Chaimani A, Schmid CH, Cameron C, et al. The PRISMA extension statement for reporting of systematic reviews incorporating network meta-analyses of health care interventions: checklist and explanations. *Ann Intern Med.* (2015) 162:777–84. doi: 10.7326/M14-2385
45. Matić I, Majerić-Kogler V. Comparison of pressure support and T-tube weaning from mechanical ventilation: randomized prospective study. *Croat Med J.* (2004) 45:162–6.
46. Ladeira M, Vital F, Andriolo R, Andriolo B, Atallah A, Peccin M. Pressure support versus T-tube for weaning from mechanical ventilation in adults. *Cochrane Database Syst Rev.* (2014) 2014:CD006056. doi: 10.1002/14651858.CD006056.pub2
47. Higgins JP, Altman DG, Gøtzsche PC, Jüni P, Moher D, Oxman AD, et al. The Cochrane Collaboration's tool for assessing risk of bias in randomised trials. *BMJ.* (2011) 343:d5928. doi: 10.1136/bmj.d5928
48. Zeng X, Zhang Y, Kwong JS, Zhang C, Li S, Sun F, et al. The methodological quality assessment tools for preclinical and clinical studies, systematic review and meta-analysis, and clinical practice guideline: a systematic review. *J Evid Based Med.* (2015) 8:2–10. doi: 10.1111/jebm.12141
49. Bowden J, Tierney JF, Copas AJ, Burdett S. Quantifying, displaying and accounting for heterogeneity in the meta-analysis of RCTs using standard and generalised Q statistics. *BMC Med Res Methodol.* (2011) 11:41. doi: 10.1186/1471-2288-11-41
50. Higgins JP, Thompson SG. Quantifying heterogeneity in a meta-analysis. *Stat Med.* (2002) 21:1539–58. doi: 10.1002/sim.1186
51. Ades AE, Sculpher M, Sutton A, Abrams K, Cooper N, Welton N, et al. Bayesian methods for evidence synthesis in cost-effectiveness analysis. *Pharmacoeconomics.* (2006) 24:1–19. doi: 10.2165/00019053-200624010-00001
52. Lumley T. Network meta-analysis for indirect treatment comparisons. *Stat Med.* (2002) 21:2313–24. doi: 10.1002/sim.1201
53. Salanti G, Ades AE, Ioannidis JP. Graphical methods and numerical summaries for presenting results from multiple-treatment meta-analysis: an overview and tutorial. *J Clin Epidemiol.* (2011) 64:163–71. doi: 10.1016/j.jclinepi.2010.03.016
54. Lu G, Ades AE. Assessing evidence inconsistency in mixed treatment comparisons. *J. Am. Stat. Assoc.* (2006) 101:447–59. doi: 10.1198/016214505000001302
55. Higgins JP, Jackson D, Barrett JK, Lu G, Ades AE, White IR. Consistency and inconsistency in network meta-analysis: concepts and models for multi-arm studies. *Res Synth Methods.* (2012) 3:98–110. doi: 10.1002/jrsm.1044
56. Ansai JH, Aurichio TR, Gonçalves R, Rebelatto JR. Effects of two physical exercise protocols on physical performance related to falls in the oldest old: a randomized controlled trial. *Geriatr Gerontol Int.* (2016) 16:492–9. doi: 10.1111/ggi.12497
57. White IR, Barrett JK, Jackson D, Higgins JP. Consistency and inconsistency in network meta-analysis: model estimation using multivariate meta-regression. *Res Synth Methods.* (2012) 3:111–25. doi: 10.1002/jrsm.1045
58. Chaimani A, Higgins JP, Mavridis D, Spyridonos P, Salanti G. Graphical tools for network meta-analysis in STATA. *PLoS ONE.* (2013) 8:e76654. doi: 10.1371/journal.pone.0076654
59. Dias S, Welton NJ, Caldwell DM, Ades AE. Checking consistency in mixed treatment comparison meta-analysis. *Stat Med.* (2010) 29:932–44. doi: 10.1002/sim.3767
60. van Valkenhoef G, Dias S, Ades AE, Welton NJ. Automated generation of node-splitting models for assessment of inconsistency in network meta-analysis. *Res Synth Methods.* (2016) 7:80–93. doi: 10.1002/jrsm.1167
61. Dias S, Sutton AJ, Welton NJ, Ades AE. Evidence synthesis for decision making 3: heterogeneity–subgroups, meta-regression, bias, and bias-adjustment. *Med Decis Making.* (2013) 33:618–40. doi: 10.1177/0272989X13485157
62. Guddat C, Grouven U, Bender R, Skipka G, A. note on the graphical presentation of prediction intervals in random-effects meta-analyses. *Syst Rev.* (2012) 1:34. doi: 10.1186/2046-4053-1-34
63. Riley RD, Higgins JP, Deeks JJ. Interpretation of random effects meta-analyses. *BMJ.* (2011) 342:d549. doi: 10.1136/bmj.d549
64. Chaimani ASG. Visualizing assumptions and results in network meta-analysis: the network graphs package. *Stata J.* (2015) 15:905–50. doi: 10.1177/1536867X1501500402
65. Chen LX, Zhou ZR Li YL, Ning GZ, Zhang TS, Zhang D, et al. Comparison of bone mineral density in lumbar spine and fracture rate among eight drugs in treatments of osteoporosis in men: a network meta-analysis. *PLoS ONE.* (2015) 10:e0128032. doi: 10.1371/journal.pone.0128032
66. Salanti G, Del Giovane C, Chaimani A, Caldwell DM, Higgins JP. Evaluating the quality of evidence from a network meta-analysis. *PLoS ONE.* (2014) 9:e99682. doi: 10.1371/journal.pone.0099682
67. Matić I, Danić D, Majerić-Kogler V, Jurjević M, Mirković I, Vučinić NM. Chronic obstructive pulmonary disease and weaning of difficult-to-wean patients from mechanical ventilation: randomized prospective study. *Croat Med J.* (2007) 48:51–8.
68. Molina-Saldarriaga FJ, Fonseca-Ruiz NJ, Cuesta-Castro DP, Esteban A. Frutos-Vivar F. Spontaneous breathing trial in chronic obstructive pulmonary disease: continuous positive airway pressure (CPAP) versus T-piece. *Med Intensiva.* (2010) 34:453–8. doi: 10.1016/j.medin.2010.03.007
69. Pellegrini JAS, Boniatti MM, Boniatti VC, Zigiotto C, Viana MV, Nedel WL, et al. Pressure-support ventilation or T-piece spontaneous breathing trials for patients with chronic obstructive pulmonary disease - a randomized controlled trial. *PLoS ONE.* (2018) 13:e0202404. doi: 10.1371/journal.pone.0202404
70. Subirà C, Hernández G, Vázquez A, Rodríguez-Garciá R, González-Castro A, Garciá C, et al. Effect of pressure support vs T-piece ventilation strategies during spontaneous breathing trials on successful extubation among patients receiving mechanical ventilation: a randomized clinical trial. *JAMA.* (2019) 321:2175–82. doi: 10.1001/jama.2019.7234

71. Teixeira SN, Osaku EF, de Macedo Costa CRL, Toccolini BF, Costa NL, Cândia MF, et al. Comparison of proportional assist ventilation plus, T-tube ventilation, and pressure support ventilation as spontaneous breathing trials for extubation: a randomized study. *Respir Care.* (2015) 60:1527–35. doi: 10.4187/respcare.03915
72. Vats N. Khanna GL, Goyal, R. Improved extubation outcome with breathing exercises during spontaneous breathing trials with t-tube/pressure support ventilation, decreased pulmonary complications in thoracic cancers: a clinical trial. *Indian J Physiother Occup Ther.* (2016) 10:46–51. doi: 10.5958/0973-5674.2016.00081.2
73. Vats N, Singh J, Kaira S. Extubation outcome after spontaneous breathing trials with T-tube or pressure support ventilation. *Indian J Physiother Occup Ther.* (2012) 6:86–9.
74. Wafy S, El-Shahat H, Salama S, Bayoumi H. Automatic tube compensation versus pressure support ventilation as a weaning mode, does it make a difference? *Chest.* (2015) 148:312A. doi: 10.1378/chest.2250779
75. Zhang B, Qin YZ. Comparison of pressure support ventilation and T-piece in determining rapid shallow breathing index in spontaneous breathing trials. *Am J Med Sci.* (2014) 348:300–5. doi: 10.1097/MAJ.0000000000000286
76. Fabry B, Guttmann J, Eberhard L, Wolff G. Automatic compensation of endotracheal tube resistance in spontaneously breathing patients. *Technol Health Care.* (1994) 1:281–91. doi: 10.3233/THC-1994-1405
77. Stocker R, Fabry B, Haberthür C. *New Modes of Ventilatory Support in Spontaneously Breathing Intubated Patients.* Berlin, Heidelberg: Springer (1997). doi: 10.1007/978-3-662-13450-4_43
78. Kuhlen R, Rossaint R. Electronic extubation–is it worth trying? *Intensive Care Med.* (1997) 23:1105–7. doi: 10.1007/s001340050464
79. Kuhlen R, Guttmann J, Nibbe L, Max M, Reyle-Hahn S, Rossaint R, et al. Proportional pressure support and automatic tube compensation: new options for assisted spontaneous breathing. *Acta Anaesthesiol Scand Suppl.* (1997) 111:155–9.
80. Haberthür C, Elsasser S, Eberhard L, Stocker R, Guttmann J. Total versus tube-related additional work of breathing in ventilator-dependent patients. *Acta Anaesthesiol Scand.* (2000) 44:749–57. doi: 10.1034/j.1399-6576.2000.440615.x
81. Aggarwal AN, Agarwal R, Gupta D. Automatic tube compensation as an adjunct for weaning in patients with severe neuroparalytic snake envenomation requiring mechanical ventilation: a pilot randomized study. *Respir Care.* (2009) 54:1697–702.
82. Haberthür C, Fabry B, Zappe D, Guttmann J. Effects of mechanical unloading/loading on respiratory loop gain and periodic breathing in man. *Respir Physiol.* (1998) 112:23–36. doi: 10.1016/S0034-5687(98)00015-2
83. Haberthür C, Fabry B, Zappe D, Eberhard L, Trüeb K. Stulz P. Automatic tube compensation (ATC) und proportional assist V entilation (PA V) klinische erfahrungen mit einem neuen modus zur unterstützung von intubierten, spontanatmenden patienten. *Intensivmed.* (1996) 33:282–92.
84. Guttmann J, Bernhard H, Mols G, Benzing A, Hofmann P, Haberthür C, et al. Respiratory comfort of automatic tube compensation and inspiratory pressure support in conscious humans. *Intensive Care Med.* (1997) 23:1119–24. doi: 10.1007/s001340050467
85. Mols G, Rohr E, Benzing A, Haberthür C, Geiger K, Guttmann J. Breathing pattern associated with respiratory comfort during automatic tube compensation and pressure support ventilation in normal subjects. *Acta Anaesthesiol Scand.* (2000) 44:223–30. doi: 10.1034/j.1399-6576.2000.440302.x
86. Cabello B, Thille AW, Roche-Campo F, Brochard L, Gómez FJ, Mancebo J. Physiological comparison of three spontaneous breathing trials in difficult-to-wean patients. *Intensive Care Med.* (2010) 36:1171–9. doi: 10.1007/s00134-010-1870-0
87. Farias JA, Retta A, Alía I, Olazarri F, Esteban A, Golubicki A, et al. A comparison of two methods to perform a breathing trial before extubation in pediatric intensive care patients. *Intensive Care Med.* (2001) 27:1649–54. doi: 10.1007/s001340101035
88. Mancebo J, Amaro P, Mollo JL, Lorino H, Lemaire F, Brochard L. Comparison of the effects of pressure support ventilation delivered by three different ventilators during weaning from mechanical ventilation. *Intensive Care Med.* (1995) 21:913–9. doi: 10.1007/BF01712332
89. Brimacombe J, Keller C, Hörmann C. Pressure support ventilation versus continuous positive airway pressure with the laryngeal mask airway: a randomized crossover study of anesthetized adult patients. *Anesthesiology.* (2000) 92:1621–3. doi: 10.1097/00000542-200006000-00019
90. Brochard L, Harf A, Lorino H, Lemaire F. Inspiratory pressure support prevents diaphragmatic fatigue during weaning from mechanical ventilation. *Am Rev Respir Dis.* (1989) 139:513–21. doi: 10.1164/ajrccm/139.2.513
91. Ezingeard E, Diconne E. Guyomarc'h S, Venet C, Page D, Gery P, et al. Weaning from mechanical ventilation with pressure support in patients failing a T-tube trial of spontaneous breathing. *Intensive Care Med.* (2006) 32:165–9. doi: 10.1007/s00134-005-2852-5
92. Li Y, Li H, Zhang D. Comparison of T-piece and pressure support ventilation as spontaneous breathing trials in critically ill patients: a systematic review and meta-analysis. *Crit Care.* (2020) 24:67. doi: 10.1186/s13054-020-2764-3
93. Tonnelier A, Tonnelier JM, Nowak E, Gut-Gobert C, Prat G, Renault A, et al. Clinical relevance of classification according to weaning difficulty. *Respir Care.* (2011) 56:583–90. doi: 10.4187/respcare.00842
94. Esteban A, Alía I, Gordo F, Fernández R, Solsona JF, Vallverdú I, et al. Extubation outcome after spontaneous breathing trials with T-tube or pressure support ventilation. The Spanish Lung Failure Collaborative Group. *Am J Respir Crit Care Med.* (1997) 156:459–65. doi: 10.1164/ajrccm.156.2.9610109
95. Thille AW, Cortés-Puch I, Esteban A. Weaning from the ventilator and extubation in ICU. *Curr Opin Crit Care.* (2013) 19:57–64. doi: 10.1097/MCC.0b013e32835c5095

17

Impact of Plasma 5 Hydroxyindoleacetic Acid, a Serotonin Metabolite, on Clinical Severity in Acute Respiratory Distress Syndrome

Takeshi Tanaka[1*], *Masahiko Mori*[2], *Masato Tashiro*[1,3] *and Koichi Izumikawa*[1,3]

[1] *Infection Control and Education Center, Nagasaki University Hospital, Nagasaki, Japan,* [2] *Department of Paediatrics, University of Oxford, Oxford, United Kingdom,* [3] *Department of Infectious Diseases, Nagasaki University Graduate School of Biomedical Sciences, Nagasaki, Japan*

***Correspondence:**
Takeshi Tanaka
ttakeshi@nagasaki-u.ac.jp

Acute respiratory distress syndrome (ARDS) is characterized by dysregulated vascular permeability. The clinical outcomes remain poor, and the disease burden is widespread. We demonstrated that plasma 5-hydroxyindoleacetic acid (5-HIAA), a serotonin metabolite, is a pivotal severity indicator of ARDS. Serotonin is an effector of cellular contraction and a modulator of vascular permeability. Plasma 5-HIAA levels were significantly elevated in severe ARDS cases with shock status ($p = 0.047$) and positively correlated with SOFA ($p < 0.0001$) and APACHE-II score ($p < 0.0001$). In the longitudinal analysis, plasma 5-HIAA levels were also a strong independent predictor of mortality rate ($p = 0.005$). This study indicates that plasma 5-HIAA is a biomarker of ARDS severity and highlights the importance of evaluating vascular leakage levels for ARDS treatment.

Keywords: ARDS, serotonin, 5-HIAA (5-hydroxyindoleacetic acid), vascular permeability, shock

INTRODUCTION

The concept of acute respiratory distress syndrome (ARDS) was first introduced over 50 years ago (1); however, its mechanism of pathogenesis remains poorly understood, while its disease burden is substantial. In addition, a large number of cases are complicated by septic shock, which further increases morbidity and mortality. ARDS and septic shock are characterized by dysregulated vascular permeability (2). One of the major mechanisms that regulate vascular permeability is cellular contraction (3), which can be induced via the serotonin and RhoA/Rho-associated protein kinase (ROCK) signaling pathway in certain cell types (4). Serotonin (5-hydroxytryptamine [5-HT]) is a classical neurotransmitter in the central nervous system; however, 95% of 5-HT production in the body is generated in peripheral tissues, where a variety of pleiotropic effects are elicited, including vasoconstriction, proliferation, and inflammation (5).

We recently reported the effect of plasma 5-hydroxyindoleacetic acid (5-HIAA), a serotonin metabolite, on the clinical outcomes of sepsis (6), with an increase in plasma 5-HIAA levels in patients with severe septic shock. In addition, we demonstrated the potential role of serotonin in vascular permeability through *in vitro* ROCK activation experiments (6). Burdens of vascular leak remain a large issue in several diseases, such as ARDS (any etiology including COVID-19), viral hemorrhagic fever, and dengue fever. Our conceptual hypothesis of the serotonin-ROCK pathway approach to regulating vascular permeability could be a common approach for all types of these diseases. In this study, plasma 5-HIAA measurements were performed using high-performance liquid chromatography on plasma samples from 157 ARDS patients. In addition, we statistically analyzed its association with disease severity and mortality.

METHODS

Plasma samples were collected on day 0 from 157 randomly selected ARDS patients, and the SAILS Research Materials dataset was obtained from the National Heart, Lung, and Blood Institute (NHLBI) Biologic Specimen and Data Repository Information Coordinating Center, USA. Data sets that were analyzed in this report were from patients who were diagnosed with ARDS on day 0, had a ratio of the partial pressure of arterial oxygen (PaO_2) to the fraction of inspired oxygen (FiO_2) of 300 or less, and had bilateral infiltrates on chest radiography that were consistent with pulmonary edema without evidence of left atrial hypertension (7). Plasma 5-HIAA levels were measured by high-performance liquid chromatography at the SRL laboratory (Tokyo, Japan). Baseline information and disease severity indices of the Sequential Organ Failure Assessment (SOFA) score from 137 subjects, and Acute Physiology and Chronic Health Evaluation (APACHE) II score from 157 subjects were obtained from the NHLBI dataset. Statistical analysis was performed using GraphPad Prism, version 6.07 (San Diego, CA, USA). Between alive and death groups during 90 days of follow-up, Fisher's exact tests were used for sex and shock distribution difference analyses, and Mann–Whitney *U*-tests were used for age, SOFA score, APACHE II score, and plasma 5-HIAA level difference analyses. Analysis of plasma 5-HIAA level differences between ARDS patients with and without shock was performed using the Mann–Whitney *U*-test. Spearman's correlation test was used to analyze the correlations between disease severity indices (SOFA score and APACHE II score) and plasma 5-HIAA levels. Further, for the survival rate analyses, we constructed a binary logistic regression model for cross-sectional analysis and a Cox hazard model for longitudinal analysis.

RESULTS

Baseline clinical characteristics are shown in **Table 1**. Between alive and death groups, significant differences were identified in age (median 55 years old in alive group vs. median 63 years old in death group, $p = 0.004$), shock status (61 vs. 87%, $p < 0.001$), APACHE-II score (24 vs. 26, $p = 0.004$), and plasma 5-HIAA level (8.6 ng/ml vs. 14.6 ng/ml, $p < 0.001$). The plasma 5-HIAA levels were higher in the ARDS/shock+ group compared to the ARDS/shock- group (11.5 ng/mL vs. 7.1 ng/mL, $p = 0.047$) (**Figure 1**). Plasma 5-HIAA levels were positively correlated with SOFA scores ($r = 0.40$, $p < 0.0001$) (**Figure 2A**) and APACHE II scores ($r = 0.40$, $p < 0.0001$; **Figure 2B**). In the cross-sectional survival rate analysis, age (odds ratio [OR] 1.03, $p = 0.005$), shock status (OR 4.1, $p = 0.002$), APACHE-II score (OR 1.1, $p = 0.005$), and plasma 5-HIAA level (OR 1.03, $p < 0.001$) were significantly associated with mortality (**Table 2**), while shock (OR 3.7, $p = 0.008$) and plasma 5-HIAA levels (OR 1.02, $p = 0.005$) remained significant in the multivariate analysis (**Table 2**). In the longitudinal analysis, age (hazard ratio [HR] 1.03, $p = 0.004$), shock status (HR 3.3, $p = 0.003$), APACHE-II score (HR 1.06, $p = 0.004$), and plasma 5-HIAA level (HR 1.01, $p < 0.001$) were significantly associated with mortality in the univariate analyses (**Table 3**). In multivariate analysis, plasma 5-HIAA level (adjusted hazard ratio [aHR] 1.01, $p = 0.005$) as well as shock status (aHR 2.7, $p = 0.02$) remained significantly associated with mortality (**Table 3**). These results strongly suggest that plasma 5-HIAA levels could be an indicator of disease severity in patients with ARDS.

TABLE 1 | Characteristics of 157 ARDS patients.

Characteristics	All ($n = 157$)	Alive ($n = 105$)	Death ($n = 52$)	p
Sex (female)	82 (52%)	56 (53%)	26 (50%)	0.7
Age	[a]59 (46–68)	[a]55 (43–65)	[a]63 (55–71)	0.004
Shock	109 (69%)	64 (61%)	45 (87%)	<0.001
SOFA score ($n = 137$)	[a]11 (8–13)	[a]11 (8–13) ($n = 89$)	[a]11 (9–13) ($n = 48$)	0.2
APACHE II score	[a]25 (20–30)	[a]24 (18–29)	[a]26 (24–32)	0.004
Plasma 5-HIAA (ng/ml)	[a]9.4 (5.5–24.3)	[a]8.6 (5–16.5)	[a]14.6 (6.9–49.7)	<0.001

Characteristics of all ($n = 157$), alive ($n = 105$), and death ($n = 52$) during 90 days of follow-up are shown. Between alive and death groups, Fisher's exact tests were used for sex and shock distribution difference analyses, and Mann–Whitney U-tests were used for age, SOFA score, APACHE II score, and plasma 5-HIAA level difference analyses.
[a]Median (interquartile range) are shown.

DISCUSSION

The pathogenesis of ARDS consists of endothelial-epithelial injury, a dysregulated inflammatory response, and fibrosis. To address its inherent heterogeneity, several studies have focused on categorizing the disease by phenotyping based on clinical characteristics and associated blood biomarkers (2, 8). Although the etiologies of ARDS are diverse and complex, supportive treatments are provided, and the clinical effects of these interventions are often limited. In this study, we revealed that plasma 5-HIAA levels were significantly higher in ARDS cases with shock compared to ARDS cases without shock and its was positively correlated with SOFA score and APACHE-II. Such a strong association between plasma 5-HIAA levels and ARDS disease severity was also identified in the longitudinal mortality rate analysis.

An ideal disease biomarker should have a clear correlation with the disease's pathophysiological factors, and must provide specific contexts such as early diagnosis and guide the successful

Abbreviations: ARDS, acute respiratory distress syndrome; 5-HIAA, 5-hydroxyindoleacetic acid; ROCK, RhoA/Rho-associated protein kinase; 5-HT, 5-hydroxytryptamine; SOFA, Sequential Organ Failure Assessment; APACHE, Acute Physiology and Chronic Health Evaluation; SSRIs, selective serotonin reuptake inhibitors; POC, point-of-care; Ang-2, angiopoietin 2; eNAMPT, extracellular nicotinamide phosphoribosyltransferase; sRAGE, soluble receptor for advanced glycation endproducts; miRNAs, microRNAs.

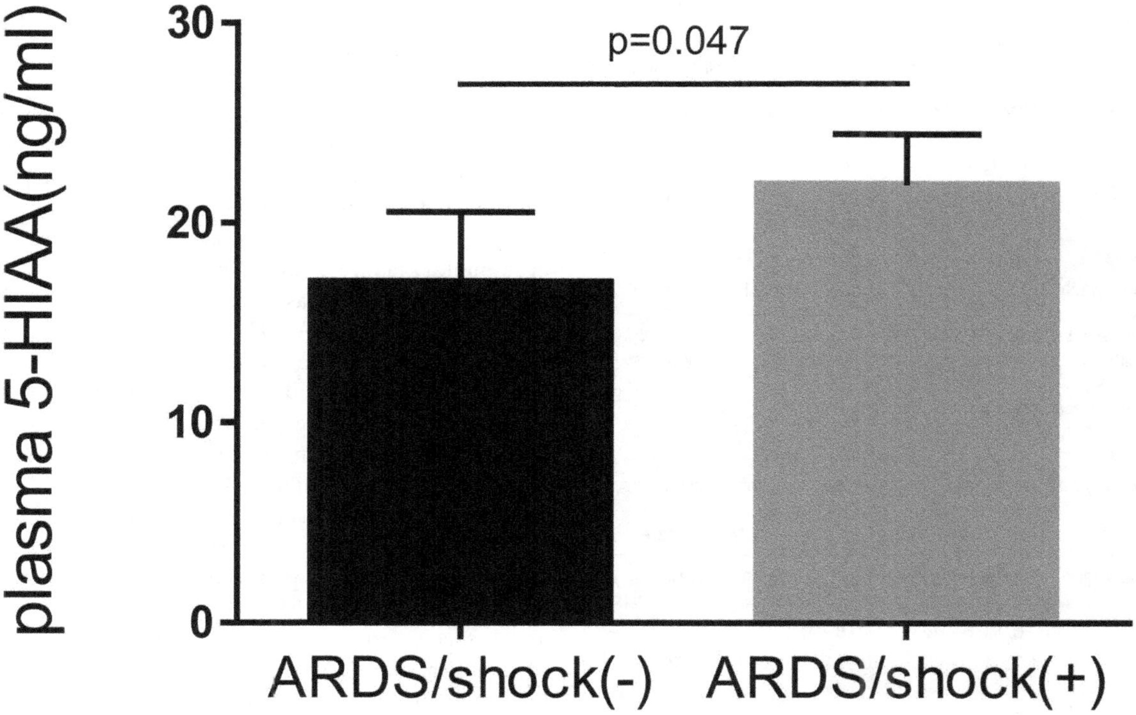

FIGURE 1 | Plasma 5-HIAA levels in patients with ARDS. Comparison of plasma 5-HIAA levels between ARDS/shock+ and ARDS/shock- patients was performed using the Mann–Whitney *U*-test the 5-HIAA levels were higher in the ARDS/shock+ group compared to the ARDS/shock- group (median 7.1 ng/mL vs. 11.5 ng/mL, $p = 0.047$).

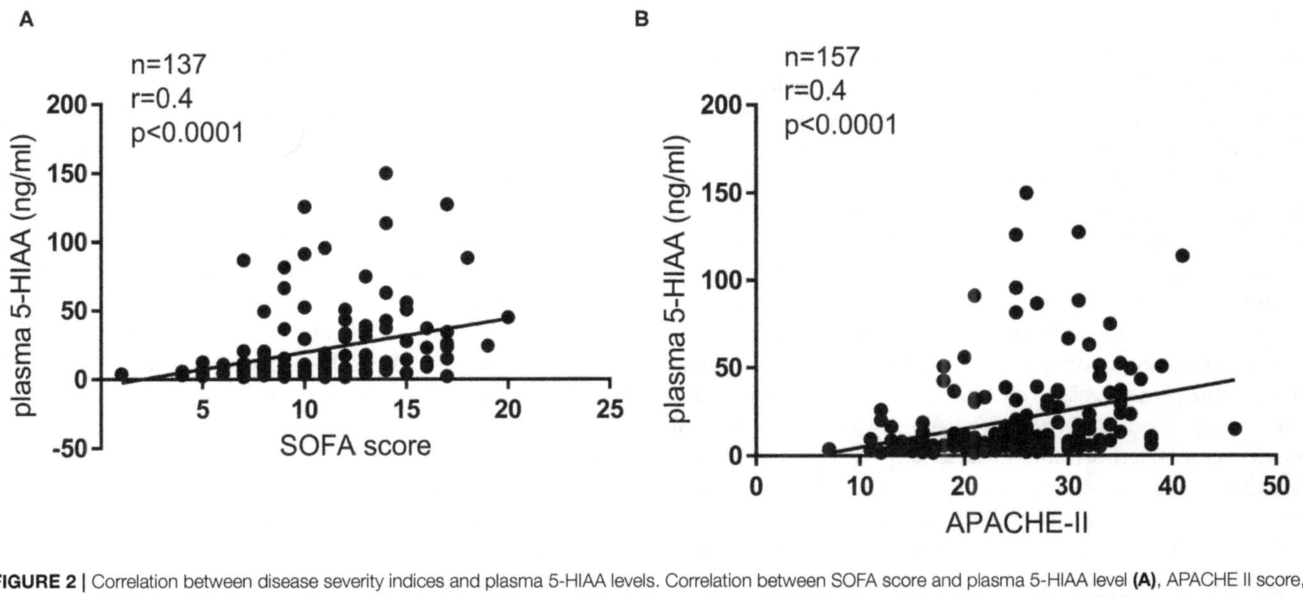

FIGURE 2 | Correlation between disease severity indices and plasma 5-HIAA levels. Correlation between SOFA score and plasma 5-HIAA level **(A)**, APACHE II score, and plasma 5-HIAA level **(B)**; Spearman's correlation test. A positive correlation between plasma 5-HIAA levels and clinical disease severity indices was observed ($r = 0.40$, $p < 0.0001$, $r = 0.40$, $p < 0.0001$).

development of novel therapeutic strategies. However, although numerous studies have been conducted, there are no targeted therapies to treat ARDS. There exists a critical gap between biomarker discovery and translation to clinical use. The clinical and biological heterogeneity of ARDS is a pivotal barrier in identifying effective treatments. However, the development of rapid point-of-care (POC) tests remains a priority. Introducing novel POC tests for biomarkers in blood or other body

TABLE 2 | Differences in mortality rate based on clinical variables evaluated by cross-sectional analysis.

	Univariate analysis		Multivariate analysis	
Variables (*n* = 157)	**[a]OR (95% [b]CI)**	***p***	**[a]OR (95% [b]CI)**	***p***
Sex (female)	0.9 (0.4–1.7)	0.7	–	–
Age	1.03 (1.01–1.06)	0.005	1.02 (0.9–1.04)	0.1
Shock	4.1 (1.7–10)	0.002	3.7 (1.4–9.5)	0.008
APACHE-II score	1.1 (1.02–1.1)	0.005	1.03 (0.9–1.1)	0.3
Plasma 5-HIAA (ng/ml)	1.03 (1.01–1.04)	<0.001	1.02 (1.007–1.04)	0.005

Binary logistic regression model analyses of the mortality rate during 90 days of follow-up are shown. Variables with significance ($p < 0.05$) in the univariate analysis were used for multivariate analysis.

[a]OR, odds ratio; [b]CI, confidential interval range.

TABLE 3 | Mortality rate difference in clinical variables, by longitudinal analysis.

	Univariate		Multivariate	
Variables (*n* = 157)	**[a]HR (95% [b]CI)**	**p**	**[c]aHR (95% CI)**	***p***
Sex (female)	0.9 (0.5–1.6)	0.8	–	–
Age	1.03 (1.01–1.05)	0.004	1.01 (0.9–1.03)	0.2
Shock	3.3 (1.5–7.3)	0.003	2.7 (1.2–6.0)	0.02
APACHE-II score	1.06 (1.02–1.09)	0.004	1.02 (0.9–1.1)	0.3
Plasma 5-HIAA (ng/ml)	1.01 (1.007–1.02)	<0.001	1.01 (1.003–1.02)	0.005

Cox hazard model analyses of the mortality rate during 90 days of follow-up are shown. Variables with significance ($p < 0.05$) in the univariate analysis were used for multivariate analysis.

[a]HR, hazard ratio; [b]CI, confidential interval range; [c]aHR, adjusted hazard ratio.

fluids could lead to potentially significant clinical trials for biomarker-guided, cell-specific therapies (e.g., epithelial targeted therapies or endothelial barrier permeability modifiers) (9).

Recently, ARDS biomarkers have been categorized based on their possible pathogenesis and pathways, and have mostly been assessed as diagnostic and prognostic biomarkers. Candidate diagnostic biomarkers that have been well studied include the following: angiopoietin 2 (Ang-2), high mobility group box nuclear protein 1, interleukin 1 beta, interleukin 1 receptor antagonist, interleukin 6, interleukin 8, macrophage inflammatory protein-1a, extracellular nicotinamide phosphoribosyltransferase (eNAMPT), soluble receptor for advanced glycation end products (sRAGE), vascular endothelial growth factor, selectins, and surfactants (8, 10). Furthermore, researchers have thoroughly investigated candidate prognostic biomarkers, including Ang-2, eNAMPT, sRAGE, protein C, and soluble intercellular adhesion molecule-1 (8, 10). To pursue breakthrough therapeutic strategies, the role of microRNAs (miRNAs) as biomarkers or pharmacologic targets has been increasingly investigated (11). In addition, contrary to conventional chemical detection methods for biomarker candidates, recently, a new method, metabolomics, has been applied, allowing for the simultaneous detection of a large set of metabolites from a single sample (12). However, these markers are still far from successfully transitioning to clinical therapeutic development.

In this study, we adopted the coupled hypothesis from our previous study (6), focusing on the serotonin-ROCK pathway approach for the regulation of vascular permeability in ARDS. Several studies have revealed that ROCK inhibition leads to the attenuation of endothelial vascular hyperpermeability in lung injury (13, 14). Several studies have focused on the analysis of the involvement of serotonin in the pathology of ARDS and targeted serotonin as a therapeutic intervention and have shown that serotonin antagonism improves the clinical efficacy of respiratory failure in animal models and human cases. Serum serotonin levels may be associated with pulmonary hypertension in patients with septic ARDS (15). Serotonin receptor blockage contributes to favorable outcomes in a porcine ARDS model (16). One study indicated that platelet entrapment in the lungs and 5-HT release are in part responsible for early respiratory failure. 5-HT inhibition contributes to a favorable outcome of acute respiratory failure (17). These studies indicate the feasibility of the involvement of serotonin in the pathology of ARDS and targeted serotonin as a therapeutic intervention. In addition, from various perspectives, ARDS research has been drawn into focus by the SARS-CoV-2/COVID-19 pandemic and has come to be conducted based on the recent analysis of severe cases of COVID-19; thus, several papers focusing on the action of selective serotonin reuptake inhibitors (SSRIs) have been published. Fluvoxamine [SSRI and a sigma-1 receptor (S1R) agonist] prevented clinical deterioration of symptomatic COVID-19 in a small placebo-controlled randomized trial in the United States. The authors mentioned that the rationale for administering fluvoxamine is its agonistic effect in attenuating the damaging effects of the inflammatory response (18). A larger randomized placebo-controlled study conducted in Brazil found that patients administered fluvoxamine had a lower risk of hospitalization in a COVID-19 emergency setting or transfer to a tertiary hospital due to COVID-19 deterioration (19). Further, a large observational study conducted in France showed that the use of antidepressants (SSRIs) was significantly and substantially associated with a reduced risk of intubation or death (20). The mechanism underlying the role of SSRIs in these results remains uncertain. However, several hypotheses were discussed in these reports, such as its anti-inflammatory action, antiplatelet activity, and antiviral effects on SARS-CoV-2. Serum serotonin levels were increased in COVID-19 cases, including COVID-19-related ARDS. They focused on platelet hyperreactivity in the pathogenesis of COVID-19. However, COVID-19 non-related ARDS is inconclusive because of the small number and heterogeneity of patients for assessment (21). In addition, one review mentioned a potential benefit of SSRIs in the treatment and prevention of inflammatory lung diseases (e.g., COVID-19, ARDS, COPD, and pneumonia) (22), since SSRIs have anti-inflammatory properties. Serotonin transporter inhibitors and ROCK inhibitors have already been approved and applied for treatment, including certain diseases, depression worldwide, and vasospasm of subarachnoid hemorrhage complications in Japan and China, respectively. As mentioned above, ROCK inhibitors have been applied to animal models of lung injury. However, from the viewpoint of clinical application to humans, approved drugs are limited to Japan and China. As for serotonin antagonism, SSRIs are strongly recognized as drugs in the central nervous system, and the function of peripheral serotonin has been attracting attention, but there are few demonstrative cases in animal experiments targeting lung disorders. For these reasons, the application has not yet progressed to clinical applications. However, as mentioned above, there is a growing body of evidence in COVID-19 clinical studies to promote the application of SSRIs to human patients.

Serotonin storage is abundant in platelets, and activation of platelets is induced by inflammation, and the release of serotonin from platelets increases (23). In addition, since it is stored mostly in the enterochromaffin cells of the intestinal tract (24), the release of serotonin is a possible event due to intestinal barrier dysfunction during septic shock (25, 26). If these two factors are proposed as clinical evaluation indicators in the future, they may become more sensitive to the indicators of the combination of plasma 5-HIAA, platelet activation, and intestinal barrier dysfunction. Clinical indicators that may reflect vascular permeability may be the doses of vasopressors and fluid balance, so attempts to quantify these two indicators and combine the evaluation with plasma 5-HIAA might be more accurate in the evaluation in the future.

In this study, plasma 5-HIAA levels were measured using HP liquid chromatography. However, it is technically possible to perform mass analysis (TOF-MAS) as well. Recently, since more hospital laboratories are introducing TOF-MAS for bacterial identification, measurement of plasma 5-HIAA levels by TOF-MAS, with more rapid time would be available.

Our study has several limitations: First, the involvement of 5-HT-ROCK signaling is highly assumed in the clinical observations of these results in our study; however, the complete mechanism of 5-HT or ROCK-associated vascular permeability regulation could not be evaluated using a molecular basis approach. In our previous study, we demonstrated that plasma 5-HIAA levels can be a predominant biomarker of septic shock severity and a novel role of 5-HT in vascular permeability via the ROCK activation pathway. Given that we showed partial elucidation of the involvement of serotonin/ROCK in the regulation of *in vitro* experiments in our previous study (6), additional work should consider the feasibility of clinical trials using these inhibitors to examine the effect on the regulation of vascular permeability in the lung of ARDS. Second, since this data set provided only ARDS patients, comparative analyses including healthy controls or non-ARDS ICU patients were not available. Third, serotonin levels were not directly measured in the present study. Another study in which plasma serotonin and 5HIAA were measured simultaneously in septic shock subjects revealed that more severe cases showed low-serotonin and high-5-HIAA results over time (27). This trend may be because activated serotonin is immediately metabolized to 5-HIAA, which matches with our hypotheses and results. Fourth, the changes in plasma 5-HIAA levels over time were not monitored because of limited data sources. The trend in the time course of plasma 5-HIAA levels would have revealed a more precise understanding of the association between serotonin and vascular leakage in the treatment clinical course.

As a general perception of the pathophysiology of ARDS, there is considerable crosstalk in its pathogenesis (2, 8), and a variety of causes of ARDS also make it difficult to discuss its pathogenesis in a simple manner. We think that the results of our study do not necessarily reflect the whole and accurate phenomenon of ARDS, possibly reflecting one aspect among many. We believe that the same composition of difficulties in showing a positive result study of ARDS in several clinical trials. We would like to emphasize that the biomarkers (plasma 5-HIAA) demonstrated in this study could be used as prognostic factors, in addition to the existing therapeutic drug candidates (SSRIs or ROCK inhibitors) that can directly regulate vascular hyperpermeability.

In this study, we demonstrated the possibility of using plasma 5-HIAA as a prognostic biomarker of ARDS severity. Plasma 5-HIAA (a serotonin metabolite) could be an ideal and unique target to allow the successful transition of a novel clinical treatment targeting the serotonin-ROCK pathway through biomarker development. Furthermore, comprehensive *in vitro* experiments and clinical data assessment are required to reveal the detailed involvement of the serotonin and ROCK pathways in ARDS pathogenesis.

ETHICS STATEMENT

The studies involving human participants were reviewed and approved by the Institutional Review Board of Nagasaki University Hospital (approval number 16072514). The NHLBI Research Materials Distribution Agreement (RMDA) was concluded between Nagasaki University Hospital and NHLBI. Written informed consent for participation was not required for this study in accordance with the national legislation and the institutional requirements.

AUTHOR CONTRIBUTIONS

TT designed the study and wrote and edited the original draft of the manuscript. MM performed statistical analyses. TT and MM acquired the data set. MT reviewed the study design and edited the manuscript. KI supervised the study and edited the manuscript. All authors approved the study design and manuscript.

ACKNOWLEDGMENTS

This manuscript was prepared using SAILS Research Materials obtained from the NHLBI Biologic Specimen and Data Repository Information Coordinating Center and does not necessarily reflect the opinions or views of the SAILS or the NHLBI. We would like to thank Editage (www.editage.com) for English language editing.

REFERENCES

1. Ashbaugh DG, Bigelow DB, Petty TL, Levine BE. Acute respiratory distress in adults. *Lancet.* (1967) 2:319–23. doi: 10.1016/s0140-6736(67)90168-7
2. Han S, Mallampalli RK. The acute respiratory distress syndrome: from mechanism to translation. *J Immunol.* (2015) 194:855–60. doi: 10.4049/jimmunol.1402513
3. Hardin C, Rajendran K, Manomohan G, Tambe DT, Butler JP, Fredberg JJ, et al. Glassy dynamics, cell mechanics, and endothelial permeability. *J Phys Chem B.* (2013) 117:12850–6. doi: 10.1021/jp4020965
4. Guilluy C, Eddahibi S, Agard C, Guignabert C, Izikki M, Tu L, et al. RhoA and Rho kinase activation in human pulmonary hypertension: Role of 5-HT signaling. *Am J Respir Crit Care Med.* (2009) 179:1151–8. doi: 10.1164/rccm.200805-691OC
5. Wu H, Denna TH, Storkersen JN, Gerriets VA. Beyond a neurotransmitter: The role of serotonin in inflammation and immunity. *Pharmacol Res.* (2019) 140:100–14. doi: 10.1016/j.phrs.2018.06.015
6. Tanaka T, Mori M, Sekino M, Higashijima U, Takaki M, Yamashita Y, et al. Impact of plasma 5-hydroxyindoleacetic acid, a serotonin metabolite, on clinical outcome in septic shock, and its effect on vascular permeability. *Sci Rep.* (2021) 11:14146. doi: 10.1038/s41598-021-93649-z
7. National Heart, Lung, and Blood Institute ARDS Clinical Trials Network, Truwit JD, Bernard GR, Steingrub J, Matthay MA, Liu KD, et al. Rosuvastatin for sepsis-associated acute respiratory distress syndrome. *N Engl J Med.* (2014) 370:2191–200. doi: 10.1056/NEJMoa1401520
8. Bime C, Camp SM, Casanova N, Oita RC, Ndukum J, Lynn H, et al. The acute respiratory distress syndrome biomarker pipeline: crippling gaps between discovery and clinical utility. *Transl Res.* (2020) 226:105–5. doi: 10.1016/j.trsl.2020.06.010
9. Mekontso Dessap A, Ware LB, Bagshaw SM. How could biomarkers of ARDS and AKI drive clinical strategies? *Intensive Care Med.* (2016) 42:800–2. doi: 10.1007/s00134-016-4231-9
10. Mokra D, Kosutova P. Biomarkers in acute lung injury. *Respir Physiol Neurobiol.* (2015) 209:52–8. doi: 10.1016/j.resp.2014.10.006
11. Lee LK, Medzikovic L, Eghbali M, Eltzschig HK, Yuan X. The role of MicroRNAs in acute respiratory distress syndrome and sepsis, from targets to therapies: a narrative review. *Anesth Analg.* (2020) 131:1471–84. doi: 10.1213/ANE.0000000000005146
12. Metwaly S, Cote A, Donnelly SJ, Banoei MM, Mourad AI, Winston BW. Evolution of ARDS biomarkers: Will metabolomics be the answer? *Am J Physiol Lung Cell Mol Physiol.* (2018) 315:L526–L34. doi: 10.1152/ajplung.00074.2018
13. Siddiqui MR, Akhtar S, Shahid M, Tauseef M, McDonough K, Shanley TP. miR-144-mediated inhibition of ROCK1 protects against LPS-induced lung endothelial hyperpermeability. *Am J Respir Cell Mol Biol.* (2019) 61:257–65. doi: 10.1165/rcmb.2018-0235OC
14. Tasaka S, Koh H, Yamada W, Shimizu M, Ogawa Y, Hasegawa N, et al. Attenuation of endotoxin-induced acute lung injury by the Rho-associated kinase inhibitor, Y-27632. *Am J Respir Cell Mol Biol.* (2005) 32:504–10. doi: 10.1165/rcmb.2004-0009OC
15. Sibbald W, Peters S, Lindsay RM. Serotonin and pulmonary hypertension in human septic ARDS. *Crit Care Med.* (1980) 8:490–4. doi: 10.1097/00003246-198009000-00003
16. Sielaff TD, Kellum JM, Sugerman HJ, Kuemmerle JF, Tatum JL. Serotonin receptor blockade improves cardiac output and hypoxia in porcine ARDS. *J Surg Res.* (1987) 43:118–27. doi: 10.1016/0022-4804(87)90153-3
17. Huval WV, Lelcuk S, Shepro D, Hechtman HB. Role of serotonin in patients with acute respiratory failure. *Ann Surg.* (1984) 200:166–72. doi: 10.1097/00000658-198408000-00008
18. Lenze EJ, Mattar C, Zorumski CF, Stevens A, Schweiger J, Nicol GE, et al. Fluvoxamine vs. placebo and clinical deterioration in outpatients with symptomatic COVID-19: A randomized clinical trial. *JAMA.* (2020) 324:2292–300. doi: 10.1001/jama.2020.22760
19. Reis G, Dos Santos Moreira-Silva EA, Silva DCM, Thabane L, Milagres AC, Ferreira TS, et al. Effect of early treatment with fluvoxamine on risk of emergency care and hospitalisation among patients with COVID-19: the TOGETHER randomised, platform clinical trial. *Lancet Glob Health.* (2021) S2214–109X:00448–4. doi: 10.1016/S2214-109X(21)00448-4
20. Hoertel N, Sánchez-Rico M, Vernet R, Beeker N, Jannot AS, Neuraz A, et al. Association between antidepressant use and reduced risk of intubation or death in hospitalized patients with COVID-19: results from an observational study. *Mol Psychiatry.* (2021) 26:5199–212. doi: 10.1038/s41380-021-01021-4
21. Zaid Y, Guessous F, Puhm F, Elhamdani W, Chentoufi L, Morris AC, et al. Platelet reactivity to thrombin differs between patients with COVID-19 and those with ARDS unrelated to COVID-19. *Blood Adv.* (2021) 5:635–9. doi: 10.1182/bloodadvances.2020003513
22. Meikle CKS, Creeden JF, McCullumsmith C, Worth RG. SSRIs: Applications in inflammatory lung disease and implications for COVID-19. *Neuropsychopharmacol Rep.* (2021) 41:325–35. doi: 10.1002/npr2.12194
23. Caranobe C, Sie P, Boneu B. Serotonin uptake and storage in human platelet density subpopulations. *Br J Haematol.* (1982) 52:253–8. doi: 10.1111/j.1365-2141.1982.tb03887.x
24. Gershon MD, Tack J. The serotonin signaling system: from basic understanding to drug development for functional GI disorders. *Gastroenterology.* (2007) 132:397–414. doi: 10.1053/j.gastro.2006.11.002
25. Zhang K, Li X, Wang X, Zheng H, Tang S, Lu L, et al. Gut barrier proteins mediate liver regulation by the effects of serotonin on the non-alcoholic fatty liver disease. *Curr Protein Pept Sci.* (2020) 21:978–84. doi: 10.2174/138920372166620061517192817
26. Ha S, Jin B, Clemmensen B, Park P, Mahboob S, Gladwill V, et al. Serotonin is elevated in COVID-19-associated diarrhoea. *Gut.* (2021) 70:2015–17. doi: 10.1136/gutjnl-2020-323542
27. Troché G, Henry-Lagarrigue M, Soppelsa F, Legriel S, Yehia A, Bruneel F, et al. Tryptophan pathway catabolites (serotonin, 5-hydroxyindolacetic acid, kynurenine) and enzymes (monoamine oxidase and indole amine 2,3 dioxygenase) in patients with septic shock: A prospective observational study versus healthy controls. *Medicine.* (2020) 99:e19906. doi: 10.1097/MD.0000000000019906

18

Risk Factors and Clinical Characteristics of Neonatal Acute Respiratory Distress Syndrome Caused by Early Onset Sepsis

Ting You[1†], Yan-Rong Zhou[2†], Xiao-Chen Liu[1] and Lu-Quan Li[1]*

[1] Department of Neonatology, National Clinical Pesearch Center for Child Health and Disorders, Ministry of Education Key Laboratory of Child Development and Disorders, Chongqing Key Laboratory of Pediatrics, Children's Hospital of Chongqing Medical University, Chongqing, China, [2] Jiulongpo People's Hospital of Chongqing, Chongqing, China

***Correspondence:**
Lu-Quan Li
liluquan123@163.com

† These authors have contributed equally to this work

Purpose: To identify risk factors associated with the development of acute respiratory distress syndrome (ARDS) in infants with early onset sepsis (EOS) and to describe the clinical features.

Methods: A retrospective study was conducted at the Children's Hospital of Chongqing Medical University between January 2000 and October 2020. The infants were divided into ARDS and non-ARDS groups. Clinical characteristics and risk factors were compared between the two groups.

Results: Two hundred fifty infants (58 with ARDS) were included. Smaller gestational age, lower birth weight (LBW), lower serum albumin level, a higher rate of preterm birth, premature rupture of membranes, antenatal steroid exposure, and lower Apgar score were associated with an increased development of ARDS by univariate analysis ($P < 0.05$). LBW ($\beta = -0.001$, $P = 0.000$, *OR*: 0.999, 95% *CI*: 0.998–0.999) and low serum albumin levels ($\beta = -0.063$, $P = 0.022$, *OR*: 0.939, 95% *CI*: 0.889–0.991) were identified as independent risk factors for the development of ARDS by logistic regression analysis. A higher frequency of complications, including persistent pulmonary hypertension, intraventricular hemorrhage, pulmonary hemorrhage, septic shock, and bronchopulmonary dysplasia, was found in the ARDS group ($P < 0.05$). The rate of mortality was higher for those in the ARDS group than for those in the non-ARDS group (46.6% vs. 15.6%, $\chi^2 = 24.205$, $P = 0.000$).

Conclusion: Acute respiratory distress syndrome (ARDS) in EOS could lead to a higher frequency of complications and mortality. The risk factors for the development of ARDS were LBW and low serum albumin levels.

Keywords: early onset sepsis, acute respiratory distress syndrome, clinical characteristics, risk factors, neonate

INTRODUCTION

Although advances in medical technology have improved over the past several decades, early onset sepsis (EOS), defined as sepsis occurring within 72 h after birth, still remains one of the most common causes of neonatal morbidity and mortality (1). The survivors of EOS have a high incidence of various complications and poor outcomes in very low birth weight infants

(2). EOS may present just as a gradual onset of signs (such as lethargy, apnea, cyanosis, hypo- or hyperthermia, and poor feeding) or as rapid progression featuring acute respiratory distress syndrome (ARDS) soon after birth (3, 4). The characteristics of sepsis complicated with ARDS in adults and children have been well studied (5–7) and yield greater complications, such as neurological dysfunction, septic shock, renal injury, and cardiac damage. In addition, ARDS is correlated with high mortality in infants with sepsis (7–9). In neonates, previous studies have shown that early onset *group B Streptococcus* (GBS) infection can manifest as ARDS (3, 10) and may be associated with the highest case-fatality rate (11, 12).

In addition to GBS, organisms such as *Klebsiella pneumoniae*, *Escherichia coli*, *Staphylococcus aureus*, and *Listeria monocytogenes* are involved in EOS (13). Thus, a more comprehensive understanding of the risk factors and clinical features of EOS complicated with ARDS is still needed to develop better treatment strategies. The aim of this study was to identify the risk factors associated with the development of ARDS in EOS infants and to describe their clinical features.

MATERIALS AND METHODS

Study Population

This retrospective study was conducted at the Children's Hospital of Chongqing Medical University (CHCMU) between January 2000 and October 2020. The infants who were diagnosed with EOS were included in this study. EOS was defined as a sepsis occurring within 72 h of birth (14). The definition of sepsis was proven by positive blood or cerebrospinal fluid culture with clinical manifestations such as lethargy, hypothermia (<36.5°C), poor feeding, apnea [a pause of breathing for more than 15–20 s or accompanied by oxygen desaturation (peripheral capillary oxygen saturation ≤80%) and bradycardia], tachypnea (an increase in the sinus rate of above 160–180 beats/min), grunting, nasal flaring, cyanosis, desaturation (peripheral capillary oxygen saturation <85%), bradycardia (heart rate <100 bpm for more than 5 s), and poor perfusion, which were in accordance with the diagnostic criteria of EOS (15). Two successive positive blood cultures with the same antibiotic susceptibility pattern were required for the diagnosis of *coagulase-negative Staphylococcus* infection. Neonatal ARDS was defined using the Montreux definition published in 2017 (16). The diagnostic criteria of intraventricular hemorrhage (IVH) were graded according to the Papile criteria (17). This study received an ethics approval from the Institutional Review Board of CHCMU (No: 2016-16), and the use of the database housing the evaluated data was permitted by the ethics committees of CHCMU.

Inclusion and Exclusion Criteria

The inclusion criteria included the infants who had positive blood or cerebrospinal fluid cultures with clinical manifestations of sepsis, in accordance with the diagnostic criteria of neonatal sepsis (15), and infants who were admitted within 24 h after birth. The exclusion criteria included the infants with incomplete records or a lack of infectious clinical manifestations, although they were combined with a positive blood culture.

Data Collection

Medical record data were extracted from the medical record management system and included the gender, birth weight, gestational age (GA), Apgar score, mode of delivery and pregnancy-induced hypertension, diabetes, prenatal corticosteroids, intrahepatic cholestasis of pregnancy, a premature rupture of membranes (PROM) ≥18 h, and chorioamnionitis. The information on laboratory tests (within 24 h after birth), clinical complications, therapeutic strategies, and outcomes were also reviewed.

Statistical Analysis

All analyses were performed by the SPSS statistical software (version 17; SPSS, Chicago, IL, United States). Continuous data were reported as means and standard deviations and were analyzed by means of *Student's t-test*. Non-normally distributed measurement data were presented as the median (M) and interquartile range (IQR) and were analyzed by means of the *Wilcoxon rank-sum test*. Categorical data were reported as counts and percentages, and chi-square tests were used to compare characteristics. Logistic regression analyses were performed to determine the risk factors for the development of ARDS. $P < 0.05$ was considered statistically significant.

RESULTS

Baseline Information

During the study period, 273 infants had positive cultures in the Neonatal Diagnosis and Treatment Center of CHCMU. Among them, twenty-three were excluded from further study due to incomplete records ($n = 3$) and the contamination of blood samples ($n = 20$). Therefore, 250 cases were included in the final analysis. A total of 58 (23.20%) infants had cases complicated with ARDS, 96 (38.4%) infants were preterm, and 80 (32.0%) infants had low birth weight (LBW). PROM and chorioamnionitis were found in 59 (23.6%) and 46 (18.4%) infants, respectively, and antenatal steroid exposure was found in 33 (13.2%) infants. *K. pneumoniae* (27.6%), *E. coli* (26.0%), and *S. epidermidis* (15.6%) remain the principal organisms responsible for EOS. Among the Gram-negative bacteria (GNB), *K. pneumoniae* (43.7%) and *E. coli* (41.1%) were the main pathogens. Meanwhile, among Gram-positive bacteria (GPB), *S. epidermidis* (54.2%), *Enterococcus faecium* (20.7%), and *S. haemolyticus* (15.2%) were major pathogens (**Figure 1**).

Identification of Risk Factors for the Development of Acute Respiratory Distress Syndrome in Early Onset Sepsis Infants by Univariate Analysis

In order to determine which factors are related to the occurrence of ARDS, we compared the baseline data and laboratory results of the two groups. Compared with infants without ARDS, infants

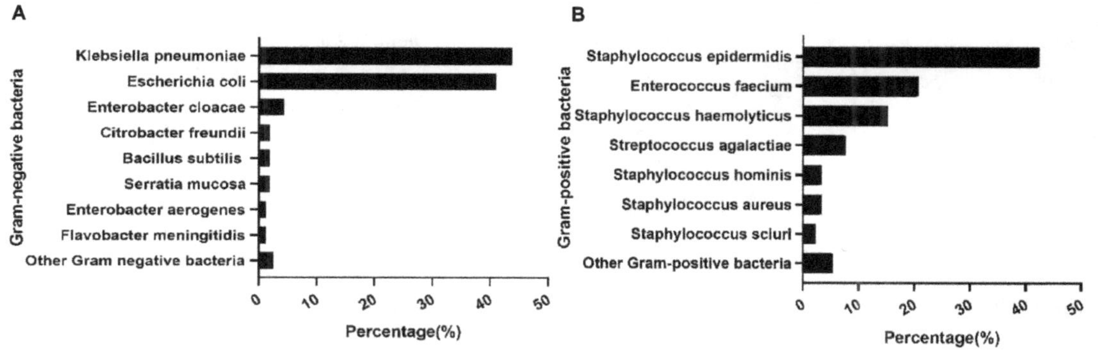

FIGURE 1 | Distribution of pathogens. Composition of major Gram-positive bacteria **(A)**. Composition of major Gram-negative bacteria **(B)**.

with ARDS had LBW, a higher rate of preterm birth, PROM, and antenatal steroid exposure and a lower Apgar score ($P < 0.05$). Other parameters, such as gender and the mode of delivery, were not significantly different between the two groups (**Table 1**). Meanwhile, low serum albumin levels were found in infants with ARDS ($P < 0.05$), and other hematologic parameters, such as white blood cell counts, immature/total neutrophil ratio, C-reactive protein, platelet counts, and hemoglobin concentrations showed no significant difference between the ARDS and non-ARDS groups (**Table 2**).

Identification of Independent Risk Factors of Acute Respiratory Distress Syndrome in Early Onset Sepsis Infants by Multivariate Analysis

Low birth weight ($\beta = -0.001$, $P = 0.000$, *OR*: 0.999, 95% CI: 0.998–0.999) and low serum albumin levels ($\beta = -0.063$, $P = 0.022$, *OR*: 0.939, 95% CI: 0.889–0.991) were independently associated with an increased morbidity of ARDS in EOS infants by logistic regression analysis. The development of ARDS at different birth weights and serum albumin levels is shown in **Figure 2**.

Clinical Complications in Infants With Acute Respiratory Distress Syndrome

Overall, significantly higher rates of complications, including persistent pulmonary hypertension (PPHN), IVH, pulmonary hemorrhage, hypoglycemia, septic shock, renal insufficiency, bronchopulmonary dysplasia (BPD), and coagulation disorders, were found in the ARDS group ($P < 0.05$) (**Table 3**).

Antimicrobial Susceptibility to Different Types of Pathogens of Early Onset Sepsis-Related Acute Respiratory Distress Syndrome

No statistically significant difference was found in most antibiotic resistance rates between the two groups. GNB showed a low degree of sensitivity to common antibiotics, such as penicillin (21.8%), beta-lactams (45.2%–73.5%) and cephalosporins (31.1–59.7%), while a relatively high sensitivity to quinolones (86.1–87.8%) and aminoglycosides (76.8–96.5%) was observed among GNB. Furthermore, in this study, in a cohort of newborns with GNB, the incidence of ESBL was 53.3% (**Table 4**).

The total antibiotic resistance rates to the following drugs were high among GPB strains: ampicillin (63.8%), erythromycin (70.1%), azithromycin (68.4%), and amoxicillin-clavulanic acid (74.4%). However, all GPBs were sensitive to vancomycin, teicoplanin, linezolid, and tigecycline (**Table 5**).

All infants were treated with antibiotics according to drug sensitivity. The rate of mortality was higher for those in the ARDS group than for those in the non-ARDS group (46.6 vs. 15.6%, $\chi^2 = 24.205$, $P = 0.000$). In infants with ARDS, no significant difference in the use of a pulmonary surfactant (PS) between the survivor group and the non-survivor group was found (53.6 vs. 46.4%, $\chi^2 = 0.000$, $P = 0.986$).

DISCUSSION

In recent years, with the rapid development of maternal fetal medicine and neonatal intensive care medicine, the ARDS of neonates has received increasing attention (18). ARDS has long been recognized as a devastating complication of sepsis (19). We found that ARDS developed rapidly in EOS infants and was associated with more complications and higher mortality. Therefore, identifying early independent risk factors for the development of ARDS in EOS infants might be helpful for optical therapeutic strategies.

Risk Factors for the Development of Acute Respiratory Distress Syndrome in Early Onset Sepsis Infants

Our findings suggested that LBW and low serum albumin levels are independent risk factors for the development of ARDS in EOS infants. The incidence of ARDS increased gradually with decreasing birth weight in the present study. ARDS has long been recognized as a devastating complication of sepsis (19); it develops because sepsis can initiate a systemic inflammatory response that releases proinflammatory cytokines

TABLE 1 | Demographic characteristics of infants enrolled in the present study.

Variable	ARDS (*n* = 55)	Non-ARDS (*n* = 195)	Statistic	*P*
Gestational age, M (IQR), w	33.86 (31.29–38.00)	38.57 (36.43–39.86)	5.390	0.000
Birth weight, M (IQR), g	2,000 (1,510–2,800)	2,995 (2,519–3,400)	5.268	0.000
Apgar 1 min, M (IQR)	8 (7–9)	9 (8–10)	2.744	0.006
Apgar 5 min, M (IQR)	9 (8–10)	10 (9–10)	4.014	0.000
Male,% (*n*)	49.1 (27)	60.5 (118)	2.298	0.130
Age of admission, M (IQR), h	0.85 (0.08–4.67)	4.97 (2.11–8.53)	3.975	0.000
Low birth weight,% (*n*)	61.8 (34)	24.1 (47)	27.862	0.000
Prematurity,% (*n*)	70.9 (39)	29.2 (57)	31.504	0.000
Meconium-stained amniotic fluid,% (*n*)	16.4 (9)	19.0 (37)	0.195	0.659
PROM,% (*n*)	43.6 (24)	17.9 (35)	15.700	0.000
Maternal hypertension,% (*n*)	5.5 (3)	4.1 (8)	0.004	0.953
GDM,% (*n*)	9.1 (5)	8.2 (16)	0.000	1.000
Antenatal steroid use,% (*n*)	30.9 (17)	8.2 (16)	19.300	0.000
Cesarean section, *n* (%)	50.9 (28)	46.7 (91)	0.310	0.578
Twins, *n* (%)	34.5 (19)	17.9 (35)	0.978	0.008
ICP, *n* (%)	3.6 (2)	1.5 (3)	0.190	0.663
Total volume within 24 h after birth, (± SD), ml/kg	84.41 ± 15.18	81.39 ± 17.23	0.914	0.473

PROM: premature rupture of membranes >18 h; GDM: gestational diabetes mellitus; ICP: intrahepatic cholestasis of pregnancy; M: median; IQR: interquartile range.

such as interleukin 6 (IL-6), IL-1β, IL-8, and tumor necrosis factor, and high levels of these cytokines can damage the alveolar-capillary barrier and alveolar type II cells (20, 21). Then, plasma, large proteins, and cellular blood components leak from the pulmonary capillary into the lung tissues and cause acute pulmonary edema, which accelerates the inactivation of PS (22–24). Meanwhile, oxidation and hydrolysis activated by inflammatory reactions can increase the degradation of PS, eventually leading to hyaline membrane formation and alveolar collapse (25). The lower the birth weight, the less mature the lung type II epithelial cells, and the less PS secreted, which will seriously hinder the expansion of the lung, leading to severe respiratory distress.

Low serum albumin levels were also independently associated with the development of ARDS in EOS infants in the current study. The association between low serum albumin levels and the development of ARDS in EOS infants may be due to the following reasons. First, low serum albumin levels are a marker of malnutrition (18). Malnutrition leads to respiratory muscle dysfunction, which decreases oxygenation (26, 27). Second, serum albumin plays an essential role in maintaining the regulation of intravascular volume and fluid balance (28, 29). Low serum albumin levels cause a lower lung oncotic pressure, which contributes to the leakage of fluid into the pulmonary interstitial tissues and leads to a decrease in lung compliance, inefficient gas exchange, and the inactivation of PS (30, 31). Furthermore, it has been postulated that albumin has the antioxidant capability of scavenging free radicals and preventing apoptosis in the respiratory tract (31). Hence, low serum albumin levels reduce the ability to combat oxidative stress and further increase the risk of lung oxidative injury, which increases the degradation of PS and eventually leads to the development of ARDS (18, 30, 32, 33).

TABLE 2 | Comparison of laboratory results between the two groups of infants.

Variable	ARDS (*n* = 55)	Non-ARDS (*n* = 195)	Statistic	*P*
Albumin, M (IQR), g/L	27.35 (24.70–32.63)	32.60 (28.30–36.60)	3.998	0.000
WBC < 5 or > 30 (× 10^9/L),% (n)	30.8 (16)	21.2 (41)	2.082	0.149
Hemoglobin (± SD), g/L	144.1 ± 30.51	153.23 ± 36.08	1.653	0.100
I/T > 0.16,% (*n*)	13.7 (7)	11.9 (20)	0.011	0.918
Platelet count < 100 × 10^9/L,% (*n*)	21.2 (11)	20.7 (40)	0.005	0.946
CRP > 10 mg/L,% (*n*)	42.3 (22)	43.6 (79)	0.029	0.864
Gram-negative bacteria,% (*n*)	69.1 (38)	62.1 (121)	0.918	0.388

WBC: white blood cell count; I/T: immature/total neutrophil; CRP: C-reactive protein; M: median; IQR: interquartile range.

Other potential possible risk factors for ARDS in EOS infants include preterm birth, PROM, and a low Apgar score. PROM increases the risk of intrauterine infection, which may lead to systemic fetal inflammatory response syndrome (FIRS) (34). FIRS has been implicated as a cause of long-term fetal lung and eventually drives the development of ARDS (35). A low Apgar score might also be responsible for the development of ARDS in EOS infants. Animal experiments have shown that hypoxia can reduce the content of phospholipids and PS protein and decrease the blood vessel density of alveolar interstitial tissues in fetal rats (36, 37), which can cause vasospasm and lead to an increase in pulmonary capillary permeability and the formation of hyaline membranes. Asphyxia at birth can directly damage alveolar type II epithelial cells, reduce PS production, and inhibit the activity of PS (38).

High Complications and Mortality of Acute Respiratory Distress Syndrome in Early Onset Sepsis Infants

Early onset sepsis could increase the risk of respiratory failure, IVH, pulmonary hemorrhage, and severe retinopathy of prematurity (1, 14, 39). In this study, we further found that infants with ARDS had more multiple organ complications

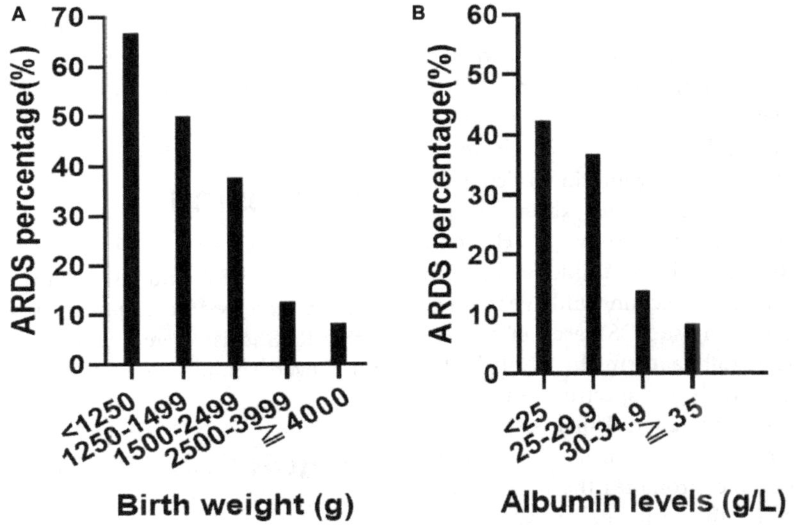

FIGURE 2 | Relationship between birth weight, serum albumin level, and the incidence of acute respiratory distress syndrome (ARDS). With the decrease of birth weight, the incidence of ARDS increased gradually **(A)**. With the decrease of plasma albumin level, the incidence of ARDS increased gradually **(B)**.

and more than threefold higher mortality than infants who did not develop ARDS. Similar high mortality was observed in a previous study in adults or children with sepsis-related ARDS (7, 8). Higher occurrence rates of IVH, PPHN, BPD, coagulation disorders, hypoglycemia, renal insufficiency, septic shock and pulmonary hemorrhage were found in infants with ARDS. The possible explanation is that ARDS leads to more severe lung compliance reduction, low gas exchange efficiency, and increased physiological dead space, which lead to multiple organ hypoxia and dysfunction.

Low Sensitivity to the Most Commonly Used Antibiotics in Early Onset Sepsis Infants With Acute Respiratory Distress Syndrome

In the current study, *K. pneumoniae*, *E. coli*, and *S. epidermidis* remained the principal organisms responsible for EOS. This result is similar to the previously reported pathogen composition of EOS in China (40), while it seemed to differ from those in developed countries whose main pathogens of EOS were *E. coli* and GBS (1, 41, 42). This difference might be partly attributed

TABLE 3 | Comparison of neonatal complications between the two groups of infants.

Variable	ARDS (*n* = 55)	Non-ARDS (*n* = 195)	Statistic	*P*
IVH,% (*n*)	40.0 (22)	15.4 (30)	15.779	0.000
PPNH,% (*n*)	30.9 (17)	5.6 (11)	27.540	0.000
BPD,% (*n*)	7.3 (4)	0.5 (1)	6.850	0.009
Septic shock,% (*n*)	16.4 (9)	3.[illegible] (61)	11.176	0.001
Pulmonary hemorrhage,% (*n*)	21.8 (12)	1.5 (3)	27.790	0.000
NEC,% (*n*)	7.3 (4)	11.8 (23)	0.921	0.340
Hypoglycemia,% (*n*)	21.8 (12)	7.7 (15)	8.886	0.003
Renal insufficiency,% (*n*)	40.0 (22)	12.3 (24)	21.911	0.000
Coagulation dysfunction,% (*n*)	58.1 (32)	29.7 (58)	15.058	0.000
Heart failure,% (*n*)	3.6 (2)	0.0 (0)	–	0.048

IVH: intraventricular hemorrhage; PPHN: persistent pulmonary hypertension; BPD: bronchopulmonary dysplasia; NEC: necrotizing enterocolitis.

TABLE 4 | Rates of Gram-negative bacteria susceptibility to different antibiotics [% (*n*)].

Variable	Total (*N* = 159)	ARDS (*N* = 38)	Non-ARDS (*N* = 121)	Statistics	*P*
Penicillin					
Piperacillin	21.8 (26)	15.4 (4)	23.7 (22)	0.814	0.367
Beta-lactam					
Ampicillin + Sulbactam	45.2 (66)	48.6 (17)	44.1 (49)	0.211	0.646
Piperacillin + Tazobactam	73.5 (108)	72.2 (26)	73.9 (82)	0.038	0.845
Cephalosporin					
Cefazolin	31.1 (47)	33.3 (12)	30.4 (35)	0.107	0.743
Ceftazidime	59.7 (92)	55.6 (20)	61.0 (72)	0.342	0.559
Cefotaxime	39.9 (61)	30.6 (11)	42.7 (50)	1.703	0.192
Carbapenem					
Imipenem	91.9 (143)	91.7 (33)	90.9 (110)	0.00	1.000
Quinolone					
Levofloxacin	87.8 (130)	75.0 (27)	92.0 (103)	5.837	0.016
Ciprofloxacin	86.1 (130)	77.8 (28)	88.7 (102)	2.730	0.099
Aminoglycoside					
Amikacin	96.5 (138)	94.3 (33)	97.2 (105)	0.676	0.770
Gentamicin	76.8 (116)	63.9 (23)	80.9 (93)	4.440	0.035
Others					
ESBL (+),% (*n*)	53.3 (72)	66.7 (22)	49.0 (50)	3.120	0.077

Partial strains were not tested for sensitivity to this drug; the denominator inside parentheses comprises the actual bacterial strains tested for sensitivity to this drug. ESBL: extended-spectrum β -lactamases.

to different population characteristics and intrapartum/postnatal healthcare strategies (43).

Our study showed that the majority of GNBs had high resistance to commonly used antibiotics, such as semisynthetic penicillin and cephalosporins, and exhibited the highest sensitivity rates to imipenem and amikacin. GPB showed a high resistance to penicillin and erythromycin. Teicoplanin and vancomycin were the most efficacious drugs in our study, which was similar to a previous study (7). However, a study from the Eunice Kennedy Shriver National Institute of Child Health showed that ampicillin and gentamicin remained effective antibiotics in most EOS cases in western countries (42). This significant difference might be attributed to (1) the overuse and misuse of broad-spectrum antibiotics, particularly cephalosporins, in neonates in China (44) and (2) the routine feeding of antibiotics to healthy farm animals, which occurs without a prescription and promotes the development of antibiotic-resistant bacteria that can be transferred to humans (45).

There are some limitations in this study, including the errors and bias inherent to the nature of a retrospective study. Additionally, the number of subjects was relatively small in this single-center study, and multicenter studies are therefore recommended. In this study, the GA of some infants was less than 34 weeks, which was also a risk factor for neonatal respiratory distress syndrome (NRDS). Therefore, it is difficult to completely rule out the possibility of NRDS + EOS in some infants. However, the application of PS did not improve the prognosis of these infants with respiratory distress, which was obviously inconsistent with the consensus that PS has a significant effect on NRDS (46).

TABLE 5 | Rates of gram-positive bacteria susceptibility to different antibiotics [% (*n*)].

Variable	Total (*N* = 91)	ARDS (*N* = 14)	Non-ARDS (*N* = 79)	Statistics	*P*
Penicillin					
Ampicillin	36.2 (17)	62.5 (5)	30.8 (39)	1.684	0.194
Glycopeptide					
Teicoplanin	100.0 (74)	100.0 (12)	100.0 (62)	–	–
Vancomycin	100.0 (88)	100.0 (14)	100.0 (71)	–	–
Macrolides					
Azithromycin	31.6 (12)	33.3 (2)	31.3 (10)	0.000	1.000
Erythromycin	29.9 (26)	33.3 (5)	29.2 (21)	0.000	0.991
Quinolone					
Levofloxacin	61.8 (40)	64.3 (9)	68.9 (31)	0.000	1.000
Ciprofloxacin	61.8 (47)	61.5 (8)	61.9 (39)	0.000	1.000
Aminoglycoside					
Amikacin	58.8 (20)	62.5 (5)	57.7 (15)	0.000	1.000
Gentamicin	70.5 (55)	62.2 (9)	70.8 (46)	0.000	1.000
Oxazolidinones					
Linezolid	100.0 (84)	100.0 (14)	100.0 (76)	–	–
Others					
Tigecycline	100.0 (47)	100.0 (9)	100.0 (38)	–	–
Amoxicillin-clavulanic acid	25.6 (20)	28.6 (4)	25.0 (16)	0.000	1.000
Rifampicin	86.6 (58)	88.9 (8)	86.2 (50)	0.000	1.000

Partial strains were not tested for sensitivity to this drug; the denominator inside parentheses comprises the actual bacterial strains tested for sensitivity to this drug.

CONCLUSION

In summary, LBW and low serum albumin levels are associated with an increased development of ARDS in EOS infants. EOS with ARDS is associated with a higher overall disease severity, more severe complications, and higher case-fatality rate.

AUTHOR CONTRIBUTIONS

TY contributed to the acquisition, analysis and interpretation of the data and the drafting, and final approval of the manuscript. Y-RZ contributed to the acquisition, analysis and interpretation of the data. X-CL contributed to the acquisition of the data. L-QL supervised the project and contributed to the conception and design of the study, analysis and interpretation of the data, and critical revision and final approval of the manuscript. All authors made substantial contributions to the study and manuscript and met the criteria for authorship defined in the author instructions and reviewed the manuscript, provided feedback and approved the manuscript in its final form.

ACKNOWLEDGMENTS

We are grateful to the patients for their consent to publish this case series. We thank all the nurses and clinical staff who provided care for these patients and who are providing continuous care to other patients in China.

REFERENCES

1. Schrag SJ, Farley MM, Petit S, Reingold A, Weston EJ, Pondo T, et al. Epidemiology of invasive early-onset neonatal sepsis, 2005 to 2014. *Pediatrics.* (2016) 138:e20162013. doi: 10.1542/peds.2016-2013
2. Rodríguez-Trujillo A, Ríos J, Ángeles MA, Posadas DE, Murillo C, Rueda C, et al. Influence of perinatal inflammation on the neurodevelopmental outcome of premature infants. *J Matern Fetal Neonatal Med Off J Eur Assoc Perinatal Med Federat Asia Oceania Perinatal Soc Int Soc Perinatal Obstetricians.* (2019) 32:1069–77. doi: 10.1080/14767058.2017.1399118
3. Dong Y, Jiang S-Y, Zhou Q, Cao Y. Group B Streptococcus causes severe sepsis in term neonates: 8 years experience of a major Chinese neonatal unit. *World J Pediatr WJP.* (2017) 13:314–20. doi: 10.1007/s12519-017-0034-5
4. Pokhrel B, Koirala T, Shah G, Joshi S, Baral P. Bacteriological profile and antibiotic susceptibility of neonatal sepsis in neonatal intensive care unit of a tertiary hospital in Nepal. *BMC Pediatr.* (2018) 18:208. doi: 10.1186/s12887-018-1176-x
5. Yehya N, Thomas NJ. Sepsis and pediatric acute respiratory distress syndrome. *J Pediatr Intens Care.* (2019) 8:32–41. doi: 10.1055/s-0038-1676133

6. Ishaque S. Sepsis induced pediatric acute respiratory distress syndrome (PARDS) - Are biomarkers the answer in a resource limited setting? *Ind Pediatr.* (2020) 57:1090.
7. Li S, Zhao D, Cui J, Wang L, Ma X, Li Y. Prevalence, potential risk factors and mortality rates of acute respiratory distress syndrome in Chinese patients with sepsis. *J Int Med Res.* (2020) 48:300060519895659. doi: 10.1177/0300060519895659
8. Mikkelsen ME, Shah CV, Meyer NJ, Gaieski DF, Lyon S, Miltiades AN, et al. The epidemiology of acute respiratory distress syndrome in patients presenting to the emergency department with severe sepsis. *Shock (Augusta, GA).* (2013) 40:375–81. doi: 10.1097/SHK.0b013e3182a64682
9. Nam H, Jang SH, Hwang YI, Kim J-H, Park JY, Park S. Nonpulmonary risk factors of acute respiratory distress syndrome in patients with septic bacteraemia. *Korean J Int Med.* (2019) 34:116–24. doi: 10.3904/kjim.2017.204
10. Oh W. Early onset neonatal group B streptococcal sepsis. *Am J Perinatol.* (2013) 30:143–7. doi: 10.1055/s-0032-1332804
11. Centers for Disease Control and Prevention [CDC]. Early-onset and late-onset neonatal group B streptococcal disease–United States, 1996-2004. *MMWR Morb Mortal Wkly Rep.* (2005) 54:1205–8.
12. Asghar S, Khan JA, Mahmood MS, Arshad MI. A cross-sectional study of group B streptococcus-associated sepsis, coinfections, and antibiotic susceptibility profile in neonates in Pakistan. *Adv Neonatal Care Off J Natl Assoc Neonatal Nurses.* (2020) 20:E59–69. doi: 10.1097/ANC.0000000000000701
13. Simonsen KA, Anderson-Berry AL, Delair SF, Davies HD. Early-onset neonatal sepsis. *Clin Microbiol Rev.* (2014) 27:21–47. doi: 10.1128/CMR.00031-13
14. Lee SM, Chang M, Kim K-S. Blood culture proven early onset sepsis and late onset sepsis in very-low-birth-weight infants in Korea. *J Korean Med Sci.* (2015) 30(Suppl. 1):S67–74. doi: 10.3346/jkms.2015.30.S1.S67
15. Khaertynov KS, Boichuk SV, Khaiboullina SF, Anokhin VA, Andreeva AA, Lombardi VC, et al. Comparative assessment of cytokine pattern in early and late onset of neonatal sepsis. *J Immunol Res.* (2017) 2017:8601063. doi: 10.1155/2017/8601063
16. De Luca D, van Kaam AH, Tingay DG, Courtney SE, Danhaive O, Carnielli VP, et al. The Montreux definition of neonatal ARDS: biological and clinical background behind the description of a new entity. *Lancet Respirat Med.* (2017) 5:657–66. doi: 10.1016/S2213-2600(17)30214-X
17. Papile LA, Burstein J, Burstein R, Koffler H. Incidence and evolution of subependymal and intraventricular hemorrhage: a study of infants with birth weights less than 1,500 gm. *J Pediatr.* (1978) 92:529–34.
18. Thongprayoon C, Cheungpasitporn W, Chewcharat A, Mao MA, Thirunavukkarasu S, Kashani KB. Impacts of admission serum albumin levels on short-term and long-term mortality in hospitalized patients. *QJM Monthly J Assoc Phys.* (2020) 113:393–8. doi: 10.1093/qjmed/hcz305
19. Kim W-Y, Hong S-B. Sepsis and acute respiratory distress syndrome: recent update. *Tuberculosis Respirat Dis.* (2016) 79:53–7. doi: 10.4046/trd.2016.79.2.53
20. Hammoud MS, Raghupathy R, Barakat N, Eltomi H, Elsori D. Cytokine profiles at birth and the risk of developing severe respiratory distress and chronic lung disease. *J Res Med Sci Off J Isfahan Univ Med Sci.* (2017) 22:62. doi: 10.4103/jrms.JRMS_1088_15
21. Huppert LA, Matthay MA. Alveolar fluid clearance in pathologically relevant conditions: and models of acute respiratory distress syndrome. *Front Immunol.* (2017) 8:371. doi: 10.3389/fimmu.2017.00371
22. Timmons O. Infection in pediatric acute respiratory distress syndrome. *Semin Pediatr Infect Dis.* (2006) 17:65–71.
23. Wohlrab P, Kraft F, Tretter V, Ullrich R, Markstaller K, Klein KU. Recent advances in understanding acute respiratory distress syndrome. *F1000Research.* (2018) 7:F1000FacultyRev–263. doi: 10.12688/f1000research.11148.1
24. Englert JA, Bobba C, Baron RM. Integrating molecular pathogenesis and clinical translation in sepsis-induced acute respiratory distress syndrome. *JCI Insight.* (2019) 4:e124061. doi: 10.1172/jci.insight.124061
25. Dushianthan A, Cusack R, Goss V, Postle AD, Grocott MPW. Clinical review: exogenous surfactant therapy for acute lung injury/acute respiratory distress syndrome–where do we go from here? *Crit Care (London, England).* (2012) 16:238. doi: 10.1186/cc11512
26. Lippi G, Plebani M. Laboratory abnormalities in patients with COVID-2019 infection. *Clin Chem Lab Med.* (2020) 58:1131–4. doi: 10.1515/cclm-2020-0198
27. Thongprayoon C, Cheungpasitporn W, Chewcharat A, Mao MA, Thirunavukkarasu S, Kashani KB. Risk of acute respiratory failure among hospitalized patients with various admission serum albumin levels: a cohort study. *Medicine.* (2020) 99:e19352. doi: 10.1097/MD.0000000000019352
28. Farrugia A. Albumin usage in clinical medicine: tradition or therapeutic? *Trans Med Rev.* (2010) 24:53–63. doi: 10.1016/j.tmrv.2009.09.005
29. Garcia-Martinez R, Caraceni P, Bernardi M, Gines P, Arroyo V, Jalan R. Albumin: pathophysiologic basis of its role in the treatment of cirrhosis and its complications. *Hepatology (Baltimore, Md.).* (2013) 58:1836–46. doi: 10.1002/hep.26338
30. Ñamendys-Silva SA, González-Herrera MO, Texcocano-Becerra J, Herrera-Gómez A. Hypoalbuminemia in critically ill patients with cancer: incidence and mortality. *Am J Hospice Palliative Care.* (2011) 28:253–7. doi: 10.1177/1049909110384841
31. Taverna M, Marie A-L, Mira J-P, Guidet B. Specific antioxidant properties of human serum albumin. *Ann Intens Care.* (2013) 3:4. doi: 10.1186/2110-5820-3-4
32. Yu M-Y, Lee SW, Baek SH, Na KY, Chae D-W, Chin HJ, et al. Hypoalbuminemia at admission predicts the development of acute kidney injury in hospitalized patients: a retrospective cohort study. *PLoS One.* (2017) 12:e0180750. doi: 10.1371/journal.pone.0180750
33. Thongprayoon C, Cheungpasitporn W, Mao MA, Sakhuja A, Kashani K. U-shape association of serum albumin level and acute kidney injury risk in hospitalized patients. *PLoS One.* (2018) 13:e0199153. doi: 10.1371/journal.pone.0199153
34. Clark EAS, Varner M. Impact of preterm PROM and its complications on long-term infant outcomes. *Clin Obstetr Gynecol.* (2011) 54:358–69. doi: 10.1097/GRF.0b013e318217ee18
35. Villamor-Martinez E, Álvarez-Fuente M, Ghazi AMT, Degraeuwe P, Zimmermann LJI, Kramer BW, et al. Association of chorioamnionitis with bronchopulmonary dysplasia among preterm infants: a systematic review, meta-analysis, and metaregression. *JAMA Netw Open.* (2019) 2:e1914611. doi: 10.1001/jamanetworkopen.2019.14611
36. Tang JR, Le Cras TD, Morris KG, Abman SH. Brief perinatal hypoxia increases severity of pulmonary hypertension after reexposure to hypoxia in infant rats. *Am J Physiol. Lung Cell Mol Physiol.* (2000) 278:L356–64.
37. Schmiedl A, Roolfs T, Tutdibi E, Gortner L, Monz D. Influence of prenatal hypoxia and postnatal hyperoxia on morphologic lung maturation in mice. *PLoS One.* (2017) 12:e0175804. doi: 10.1371/journal.pone.0175804
38. Kim SS, Park IS, Hong HS. Neonatal arterial thromboembolism and limb loss following respiratory distress syndrome: case report. *Arch Argentinos Pediatr.* (2015) 113:e157–60. doi: 10.1590/S0325-00752015000300018
39. Klinger G, Levy I, Sirota L, Boyko V, Lerner-Geva L, Reichman B. Outcome of early-onset sepsis in a national cohort of very low birth weight infants. *Pediatrics.* (2010) 125:e736–40. doi: 10.1542/peds.2009-2017
40. Jiang S, Hong L, Gai J, Shi J, Yang Y, Lee SK, et al. Early-onset sepsis among preterm neonates in China, 2015 to 2018. *Pediatr Infect Dis J.* (2019) 38:1236–41. doi: 10.1097/INF.0000000000002492
41. Stoll BJ, Hansen NI, Sánchez PJ, Faix RG, Poindexter BB, Van Meurs KP, et al. Early onset neonatal sepsis: the burden of group B Streptococcal and E. coli disease continues. *Pediatrics.* (2011) 127:817–26. doi: 10.1542/peds.2010-2217
42. Stoll BJ, Puopolo KM, Hansen NI, Sánchez PJ, Bell EF, Carlo WA, et al. Early-Onset neonatal sepsis 2015 to 2017, the Rise of *Escherichia coli*, and the need for novel prevention strategies. *JAMA Pediatr.* (2020) 174:e200593. doi: 10.1001/jamapediatrics.2020.0593
43. Dong Y, Basmaci R, Titomanlio L, Sun B, Mercier J-C. Neonatal sepsis: within and beyond China. *Chin Med J.* (2020) 133:2219–28. doi: 10.1097/CM9.0000000000000935
44. Li J-Y, Chen S-Q, Yan Y-Y, Hu Y-Y, Wei J, Wu Q-P, et al. Identification and antimicrobial resistance of pathogens in neonatal septicemia in China-A meta-analysis. *Int J Infect Dis Ijid Off Publ Int Soc Infect Dis.* (2018) 71:89–93. doi: 10.1016/j.ijid.2018.04.794

45. Qiao M, Ying G-G, Singer AC, Zhu Y-G. Review of antibiotic resistance in China and its environment. *Environ Int.* (2018) 110:160–72. doi: 10.1016/j.envint.2017.10.016

46. Sweet DG, Carnielli V, Greisen G, Hallman M, Ozek E, Te Pas A, et al. European consensus guidelines on the management of respiratory distress syndrome - 2019 update. *Neonatology.* (2019) 115:432–50. doi: 10.1159/000499361

19

Impact of Succinylcholine vs. Rocuronium on Apnea Duration for Rapid Sequence Induction

Lijun Tang[1†], Xiao Zhao[2†], Shitong Li[2], Lina Huang[2], Jinbao Li[2], Lianhua Chen[1] and Shiwei Huang[2*]*

[1] Department of Anesthesiology, Shanghai General Hospital of Nanjing Medical University, Shanghai, China, [2] Department of Anesthesiology, Shanghai General Hospital, Shanghai Jiao Tong University, Shanghai, China

***Correspondence:**
Lianhua Chen
chenlianhua@aliyun.com
Shiwei Huang
huangshiwei@sina.com

[†] These authors have contributed equally to this work

Objective: The present study aimed to evaluate the impact of 1.5 mg/kg succinylcholine or 1.2 mg/kg rocuronium, vs. 1.0 mg/kg succinylcholine on apnea duration in patients underwent rapid sequence induction (RSI).

Methods: This prospective cohort study was conducted in the Department of Anesthesiology in Shanghai General Hospital from July 2020 to November 2020. Apnea duration was defined as the time from apnea prompted by the $P_{ET}CO_2$ waveform to the time the point of oxygen saturation declined to 90% (T90) and 95% (T95) after succinylcholine or rocuronium administration. The primary outcome included T90 and T95 changes in 1.5 mg/kg vs. 1.0 mg/kg succinylcholine groups and 1.5 mg/kg succinylcholine vs. 1.2 mg/kg rocuronium groups.

Results: A total of 265 participants were subjected for analysis. The succinylcholine (1.0 mg/kg) group had a significantly longer T90 (50.72, 95% confidence interval [CI, 7.60, 94.38], $P = 0.015$) and T95 (48.09, 95% CI [7.11, 89.07], $P = 0.012$) than the succinylcholine (1.5 mg/kg) group. In addition, significantly longer T90 (56.84, 95% CI [16.24, 97.44], $P = 0.003$) and T95 (50.57, 95% CI [12.58, 88.57], $P = 0.003$) were observed in the rocuronium (1.2 mg/kg) group than those in the succinylcholine (1.5 mg/kg) group. No severe side events were observed during the operation.

Conclusion: Rocuronium and the lower dose of succinylcholine may be recommended to patients underwent RSI.

Keywords: rapid sequence induction intubation, succinylcholine, rocuronium, apnea duration, oxygen saturation

INTRODUCTION

Rapid sequence induction (RSI) is a special technique of anesthetic induction designed to reduce the risk of aspiration of secretions of any kind, e.g., regurgitated or vomited gastric contents. This is done by shortening the normal sequence of intubation procedures and omitting certain steps to minimize the time between loss of consciousness and swallowing reflexes until the airway is secured by tracheal intubation (1). In particular, RSI involves not using mask ventilation, at least for adults.

Neuromuscular blockade agents (NMBAs) are used to facilitate endotracheal intubation (2). Succinylcholine is a short-acting depolarizing NMBA that is the most commonly conventionally used NMBA in RSI because of its fast onset and short duration (3). Unfortunately, it can have serious side effects (4, 5). Rocuronium, a steroidal non-depolarizing NMBA, is an alternative to succinylcholine due to its fast onset (6, 7). However, the 1.0–1.2 mg/kg dose recommended for RSI has too long a duration of action that fatal hypoxia is imminent if the airway is difficult, especially if intubation and mask ventilation fail simultaneously. This disadvantage of rocuronium is not eliminated by the very rapid reversal with sugammadex (8), because this drug is often not available fast enough in emergency situations (9). Therefore, the selection of succinylcholine or rocuronium in RSI should be carefully considered and tailored to the specifics of each patient and their clinical indications and medical conditions.

Apnea caused from not using mask ventilation, however, includes the risk of hypoxemia. Therefore, "non-hypoxic apnea," defined as duration of apnea with SpO2 > 90%, is relevant to patient safety (10). Previous studies focused mainly on increasing oxygen storage to prolong non-hypoxic apnea duration (10, 11), whereas few studies have been performed on approaches to decrease oxygen consumption. Two aspects should be considered in the assessment of the optimal dose of succinylcholine and rocuronium in RSI: prolonging the non-hypoxic apnea duration (without additional oxygen consumption) and shortening the apnea interval (fast onset and good intubation conditions). Succinylcholine may lead to increased dose-dependent oxygen consumption (12). Our previous study showed that in obese patients the non-hypoxic apnea duration in the treatment with 1.5 mg/kg succinylcholine was shorter than that in the treatment with 0.9 mg/kg rocuronium (13), we assumed that fasciculation may be a potential cause of the shorter non-hypoxic apnea. However, poor intubation conditions and repeated intubation may also increase oxygen consumption. Succinylcholine is superior to rocuronium in terms of muscle relaxation effects in both good intubation conditions and clinically acceptable intubation conditions at quantities of 2–3 times the ED95 dose (6). Similar onset times and intubation conditions were achieved at doses higher than 3 times the ED95 dose (1.0 mg/kg−1.5 mg/kg succinylcholine and 1.0 mg/kg−1.2 mg/kg rocuronium) (7, 14–16). Therefore, the optimal doses of succinylcholine and rocuronium for application in RSI are still inconclusive.

Therefore, the aim of the present study was to compare the non-hypoxic apnea duration of the administration of 1.5 mg/kg succinylcholine, 1.0 mg/kg succinylcholine, and 1.2 mg/kg rocuronium during RSI.

MATERIALS AND METHODS

Study Design

This prospective cohort study was conducted in the Department of Anesthesiology in Shanghai General Hospital from July 2020 to November 2020. This study was approved by the Ethics Committee of Shanghai General Hospital ([2020]54) and was registered in the Chinese Clinical Trial Registration Center (http://www.chictr.org.cn/index.aspx) with the registration number ChiCTR2000034769. Written informed consent was obtained from all individual participant.

Participants

Patients who underwent elective surgery requiring RSI were enrolled. The following inclusion criteria were used: (1) American Society of Anesthesiologists (ASA) physical status I or II and (2) Age between 18 and 65 years. The exclusion criteria were as follows: (1) Unwilling to provide written informed consent; (2) Pregnancy; (3) Patients with a history of difficulty in intubation or failed intubation; (4) Obstructive sleep apnea syndrome; (5) A history of respiratory tract infection within a month; (6) Smoking cessation <2 months before surgery; (7) History of alcohol or drug abuse; (8) Cerebrovascular disease and increased intracranial pressure; (9) Drugs antagonists of rocuronium (such as phenytoin, carbamazepine, or protease inhibitors). In case one of the following conditions was present, the observation was to be suspended and the participant withdrawn from the study: (1) After preoxygenation, the end-tidal oxygen concentration was <90%; (2) Coughing during tracheal intubation; (3) Failed tracheal intubation twice times or more; (4) Recovery from spontaneous breathing before mechanical ventilation; (5) Severe allergic reactions; (6) Patients with circulatory fluctuations that were difficult to correct after 5 min of using vasoactive drugs. The participants were not compensated for their study participation.

Grouping and Masking

General anesthesia drugs and treatment strategies were selected based on clinical needs. The choice of a muscle relaxant was jointly decided by the anesthetist and the participants. As an observational exploratory study, no blindness was applied.

Typical Procedures

All subjects fasted for more than 8 h before surgery. After entering the operation room, a 20G indwelling vein cannula was placed in the median vein of the left antecubital fossa, and 10 mL/kg of sodium lactate Ringer's solution was infused to substitute for the fasting-induced fluid deficit. Then, 2% local lidocaine anesthesia was administered for the puncture and the placement of the left radial artery. Next, a pressure sensor was connected to the patient to measure the direct arterial pressure and perform blood gas analysis. If the left radial artery puncture and placement failed, the right forearm was used to measure the non-invasive blood pressure with a measurement interval of 1 min. Further, the subjects were connected to a GE CARESCAPE Monitor B650 (GE Healthcare Finland OY, Helsinki, Finland) to monitor the heart rate (HR), mean arterial pressure (MAP), finger pulse oxygen saturation (SpO_2), bispectral index (BIS) and nasopharyngeal temperature (Temp). The subject lied in the supine position and was kept warm using a medical insulation blanket. The oxygen flow rate used was 10 L/min; the oxygen concentration reached was 100%. The airway pressure-limiting valve of the anesthesia machine was fully opened, the breathing circuit was pre-filled, and the subject was instructed to breathe calmly under a closed mask for 3 min.

Then, an intravenous injection of fentanyl 3 μg/kg and propofol 2 mg/kg was administered. After the eyelash reflex disappeared and the subject ceased respond to the patting call, the muscle relaxant was administered (following the decision previously made by the anesthetist and the participants). Before the spontaneous breathing disappeared, the subject was to fasten the mask to avoid inhaling air; the mandible had to be unsupported before intubation, and any manual or mechanical ventilation was not to be applied. Fifty seconds after the administration of the muscle relaxant, the mask was removed, and a video laryngoscope (UETDC-K3) was utilized to perform a laryngoscopy to expose the glottis. Next, 60 s after the administration of the muscle relaxant, endotracheal intubation was conducted (7.5-mm cuffed tracheal tube for men and 7-mm cuffed tracheal tube for women). The insertion depth of the tracheal tube was 1 cm after the cuff was fully inserted into the glottis. After the tracheal intubation, a fiberoptic bronchoscope (UESCOPETIC-I1) was used to check whether the tracheal tube position is correct. The tracheal tube was opened in the air, without mechanical ventilation, and the end-expiratory carbon dioxide output was observed to monitor the recovery of spontaneous breathing. After tracheal intubation, to prevent the recovery of spontaneous breathing, intravenous bolus of rocuronium (0.6 mg/kg) was given to maintain muscle relaxation in the succinylcholine (1.5

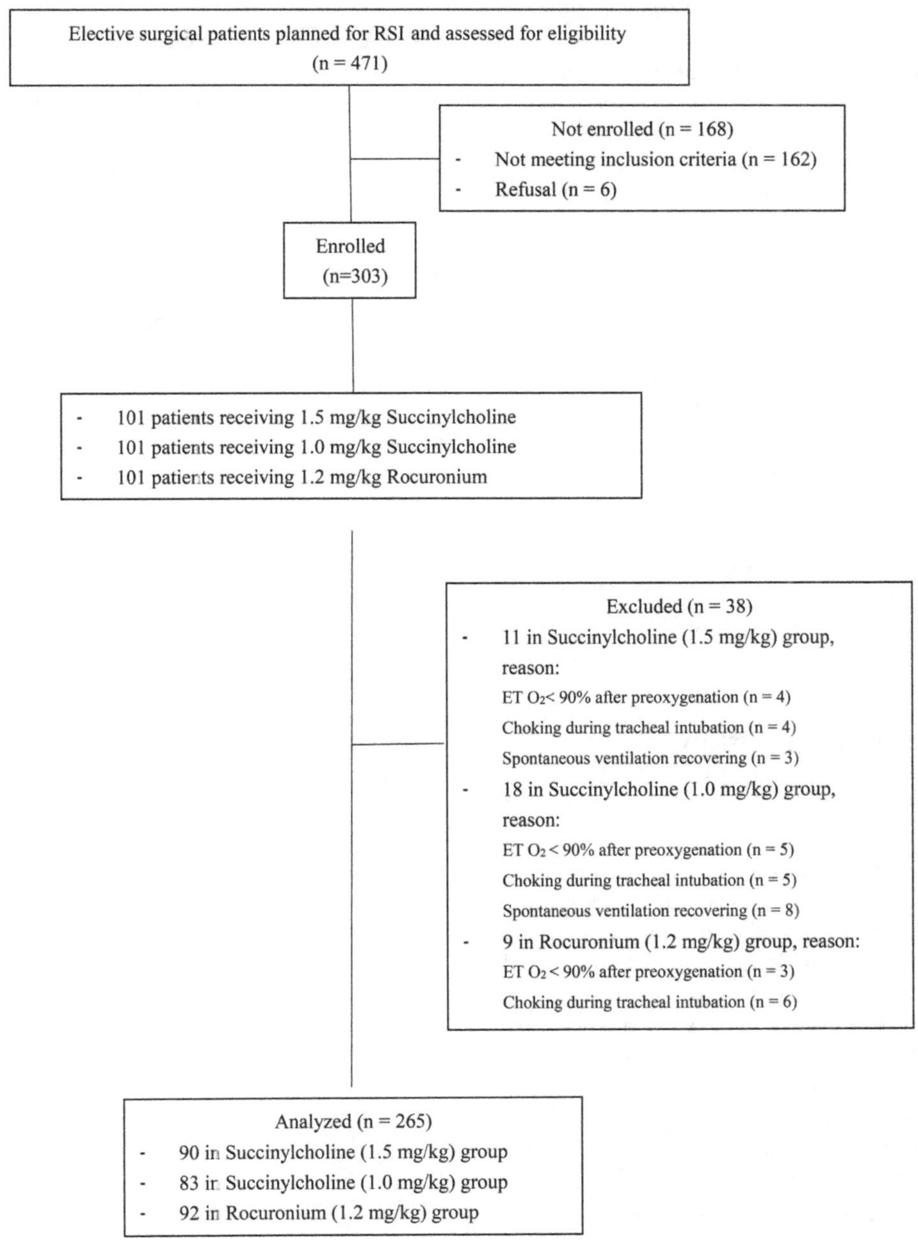

FIGURE 1 | Flow chart.

mg/kg) and succinylcholine bromide (1.0 mg/kg) groups. To prevent consciousness restoration during anesthesia, propofol was intravenously injected at a rate of 5 mg /kg/h (Willi's Ark CONCERT-III infusion pump). In case BIS was >60, intravenous injection of 20 mg of propofol was applied. When SpO_2 dropped to 90%, the tracheal tube was immediately connected to the anesthesia machine (GE Carestation 620) for mechanically controlled mechanical ventilation (parameter settings: oxygen concentration 100%, oxygen flow 1 L/min, tidal volume 8 mL/kg, frequency 16 beats/min, inhale-to-exhale ratio 1:2).

During the anesthesia, the hemodynamic parameters were monitored in real time. If HR > 110 beats/min, intravenous bolus of 1 mg of esmolol was administrated; if HR < 50 beats/min, an intravenous bolus injection of atropine 0.5 mg was given. If SBP > 170 mmHg, intravenous bolus injection of 1 mg perdipine was administered, and if SBP < 80 mmHg or MAP dropped more than 25% of the baseline value, 50 μg oxypinephrine was applied as an intravenous bolus injection.

Outcomes

The primary outcome was the non-hypoxic apnea duration. That is, the time interval between $P_{ET}CO_2$ waveform area prompts apnea to oxygen saturation declined to 95% (T95) and 90% (T90) of 1.5 mg/kg succinylcholine vs. 1.0 mg/kg succinylcholine groups, and 1.5 mg/kg succinylcholine vs. 1.2 mg/kg rocuronium groups.

Prespecified secondary outcomes included the T95 and T90 of the 1.0 mg/kg succinylcholine and 1.2 mg/kg rocuronium groups and adverse events. The exploratory outcomes included the exploration of factors that correlated with T90, and the variation of blood gas analysis, BIS, temperature, HR, MAP, SpO_2, ETO_2, and $P_{ET}CO_2$.

Any adverse reactions, such as laryngospasm, bronchospasm, and masseter spasm, or muscle rigidity during intubation, were recorded during the surgery operation. Any adverse events found were followed up before improvement or discharge.

Data Collection and Definition

The data collected included gender, age, ASA classification, preoperative hemoglobin (Hb), hematocrit (Hct), weight, height, body-mass index (BMI, kg/m^2), smoking history, Mallampati score, T95, T90, duration of muscle fibrillation (TF, the time from the onset of muscle fibrillation to the disappearance of muscle fibrillation after intravenous injection of muscle relaxants), classification of the degree of muscle fibrillation, and the conditions of tracheal intubation. In addition, the laryngoscope exposure classification, number of intubation attempts, HR, MAP, SpO_2, Temp, BIS, ETO_2, as well as for at room entry, 3 min after oxygen inhalation, 30 s after muscle relaxant administration, 50 s after muscle relaxant administration, 2 min after intubation, SpO_2 reduction to 95%, SpO_2 decrease to 90%, SpO_2 increase to 96%. Moreover, blood gas analysis was performed of pH, pO_2, pCO_2, cLac at room entry, 3 min after oxygen inhalation, and SpO2 decrease to 90%.

Muscle fibrillation was classified using the scale scores described in a previous report (17): 0 = No muscle tremor; 1 = Mild: slight muscle tremor in eyes, neck, face, or fingers, no limb movement; 2 = Moderate: moderate muscle tremor or obvious limb movement on both sides; 3 = Severe: severe or continuous and extensive muscle fibrillation. Endotracheal intubation condition was evaluated by Copenhagen score (18): 1 = excellent; 2 = good, and 3 = poor. Laryngoscope exposure classification (Cormack-Lehane classification) was defined as follows: 1 = the glottis was mostly visible; 2 = only the posterior union of the glottis could be seen, but not the glottis; 3 = only the epiglottis was visible; 4 = no glottal epiglottis could be seen. We used the World Health Organization classification for BMI: <18.5 (underweight), 18.5–24.9 (normal range), 25–29.9 (overweight), and >30 (obesity).

Sample Size Calculation

Preliminary analysis revealed that T90 in the succinylcholine (1.5 mg/kg), succinylcholine (1.0 mg/kg), and rocuronium (1.2 mg/kg) groups was 475.9 ± 64.7, 534.7 ± 64.7, and 528.7 ± 52.5, respectively. Therefore, an estimated sample size of 91

TABLE 1 | Clinical characteristics.

	Succinylcholine (1.5 mg/kg) (*n* = 90)	Rocuronium (1.2 mg/kg) (*n* = 92)	Succinylcholine (1.0 mg/kg) (*n* = 83)
Age, median (IQR)	39 (32, 52)	41 (32, 51)	43 (33, 52)
Gender			
Male	31 (34.4%)	43 (46.7%)	24 (28.9%)
Female	59 (65.6%)	49 (53.3%)	59 (71.1%)
Hemoglobin (g/L)	135 ± 13	137 ± 13	134 ± 11
Hematocrit	0.41 ± 0.04	0.41 ± 0.04	0.41 ± 0.03
Body weight (kg), median (IQR)	60 (54, 69)	65 (55, 72)	61 (54, 67)
Height (m)	1.63 ± 0.08	1.66 ± 0.09	1.63 ± 0.08
BMI (kg/m^2)	23.3 ± 3.0	23.4 ± 3.0	23.0 ± 2.8
<18.5	3 (3.3%)	3 (3.2%)	3 (3.61%)
18.5–24.9	65 (72.2%)	61 (66.3%)	62 (74.7%)
25–29.9	21 (23.3%)	27 (29.4%)	16 (19.3%)
≥30.0	1 (1.1%)	1 (1.1%)	2 (2.4%)
ASA			
1	70 (77.8%)	69 (75.0%)	63 (75.9%)
2	20 (22.2%)	23 (25.0%)	20 (24.1%)
Mallampati			
1	25 (27.8%)	27 (28.3%)	24 (28.9%)
2	47 (52.2%)	52 (56.5%)	46 (55.4%)
3	18 (20.0%)	13 (14.1%)	13 (15.7%)
Smoking No	87 (96.7%)	82 (89.1%)	70 (84.3%)
Yes	3 (3.3%)	10 (10.9%)	13 (15.7%)
Medical history None	70 (77.8%)	69 (75%)	63 (75.9%)
High blood pressure	11 (12.2%)	8 (8.7%)	6 (7.2%)
Diabetic mellitus	4 (4.4%)	5 (5.4%)	8 (9.6%)
Hypothyroidism	3 (23.1%)	6 (6.5%)	4 (4.8%)
Hepatitis B	2 (2.2%)	4 (4.3%)	2 (3.0%)

BMI, body-mass index; IQR, interquartile range.

TABLE 2 | Non-hypoxic apnea duration.

	Succinylcholine (1.5 mg/kg) (*n* = 90)	Rocuronium (1.2 mg/kg) (*n* = 92)	Succinylcholine (1.0 mg/kg) (*n* = 83)	
T90 (s)	404 (310, 511)	487 (385, 578)	446 (385, 551)	
T95 (s)	354 (267, 450)	420 (333, 513)	392 (337, 493)	
Primary outcome				
	Rocuronium vs. Succinylcholine (1.5 mg/kg)	**P**	**Succinylcholine (1.0 mg/kg) vs. Succinylcholine (1.5 mg/kg)**	**P**
T90 Change (95% CI)	56.84 s (16.24, 97.44)	0.003	50.72 s (7.06, 94.38)	0.015
T95 Change (95% CI)	50.57 s (12.58, 88.57)	0.003	48.09 s (7.11, 89.07)	0.012
Secondery outcome				
	Rocuronium vs. Succinylcholine (1.0 mg/kg)	**P**		
T90 Change (95% CI)	6.12 s (−34.58, 46.82)	0.48		
T95 Change (95% CI)	2.48 s (−35.74, 40.70)	0.54		

T90, oxygen saturation declined to 90%; T95, oxygen saturation declined to 95%. CI, confidence interval.

patients per group could provide 80% power to detect a between-group difference, assuming a two-sided significance level of 2.5%. Considering a loss of follow-up of 10%, a number of 101 subjects per group are required.

Statistical Analysis

Continuous variables that follow normal distribution was expressed with mean ± Standard deviation (SD), otherwise presented as median and interquartile range (IQR). Categorical variables were displayed using number and percentages. For multiple demographic characteristics comparison, nonparametric test was applied for continuous variables that not conformed to normal distribution. The comparison between the 1.5 mg/kg succinylcholine vs. 1.0 mg/kg succinylcholine and 1.5 mg/kg succinylcholine vs. 1.2 mg/kg rocuronium groups were analyzed using student *t* test. Two-way repeated measurement ANOVA was used to detect the effects of treatment and time interaction on HR and MAP. In addition, categorical variable comparison was conducted using Chi-square or Fisher exact tests. Pearson correlation analysis was employed to assess the correlation between T90 and the interested variables. All data were analyzed using SPSS 22.0 (IBM Corp., Armonk, NY, USA). $P < 0.05$ was considered statistically significant.

Patient and Public Involvement

Not applicable.

RESULTS

A total of 471 patients were assessed for eligibility, of which 162 failed to meet the inclusion criteria, and 6 refused to participate. Of the enrolled 303 patients, 38 were excluded because of incomplete data for T90 and T95. Therefore, a total number of 265 subjects were analyzed: 90 cases in the 1.5 mg/kg succinylcholine, 83 in the 1.0 mg/kg succinylcholine, and 92 in the 1.2 mg/kg rocuronium groups (**Figure 1**). The demographic data are presented in **Table 1**.

TABLE 3 | Adverse events.

	Succinylcholine (1.5 mg/kg) (*n* = 90)	Rocuronium (1.2 mg/kg) (*n* = 92)	Succinylcholine (1.0 mg/kg) (*n* = 83)
Overall	23	13	19
Type of adverse events			
Sore throat	17	13	14
Myalgia	10	0	6
Degree of adverse events			
Mild	23	13	19
Severe	0	0	0

T90 in the 1.2 mg/kg rocuronium group was significantly longer (56.84 [95% CI 16.24–97.44], $P = 0.003$) than that in the 1.5 mg/kg succinylcholine group. Additionally, T90 in the 1.0 mg/kg succinylcholine group was statistically significantly longer (50.72 [95% CI 7.06–94.38], $P = 0.015$) than that in the 1.5 mg/kg succinylcholine group. Compared with the 1.5 mg/kg succinylcholine group, the 1.2 mg/kg rocuronium group had a significant longer T95 (50.57 [95% CI 12.58–88.57], $P = 0.003$). When compared with the succinylcholine (1.5 mg/kg) group, the succinylcholine (1.0 mg/kg) exhibited a significant longer T90 (48.09 [95% CI 7.11–89.07], $P = 0.012$).

For secondary outcome comparison, the T90 (6.12 [95% CI −34.58–46.82], $P = 0.48$) and T95 (2.48 [95% CI 35.74–40.70], $P = 0.54$) values were comparable between the 1.0 mg/kg succinylcholine and 1.2 mg/kg rocuronium groups (**Table 2**). No severe adverse events were observed during the surgery and during follow-up in all groups. A total number of 23, 13, and 19 mild adverse reactions occurred in the 1.5 mg/kg succinylcholine, 1.2 mg/kg rocuronium, and 1.0 mg/kg succinylcholine groups, respectively. Among them, sore throat and myalgia were the most common side effects (**Table 3**).

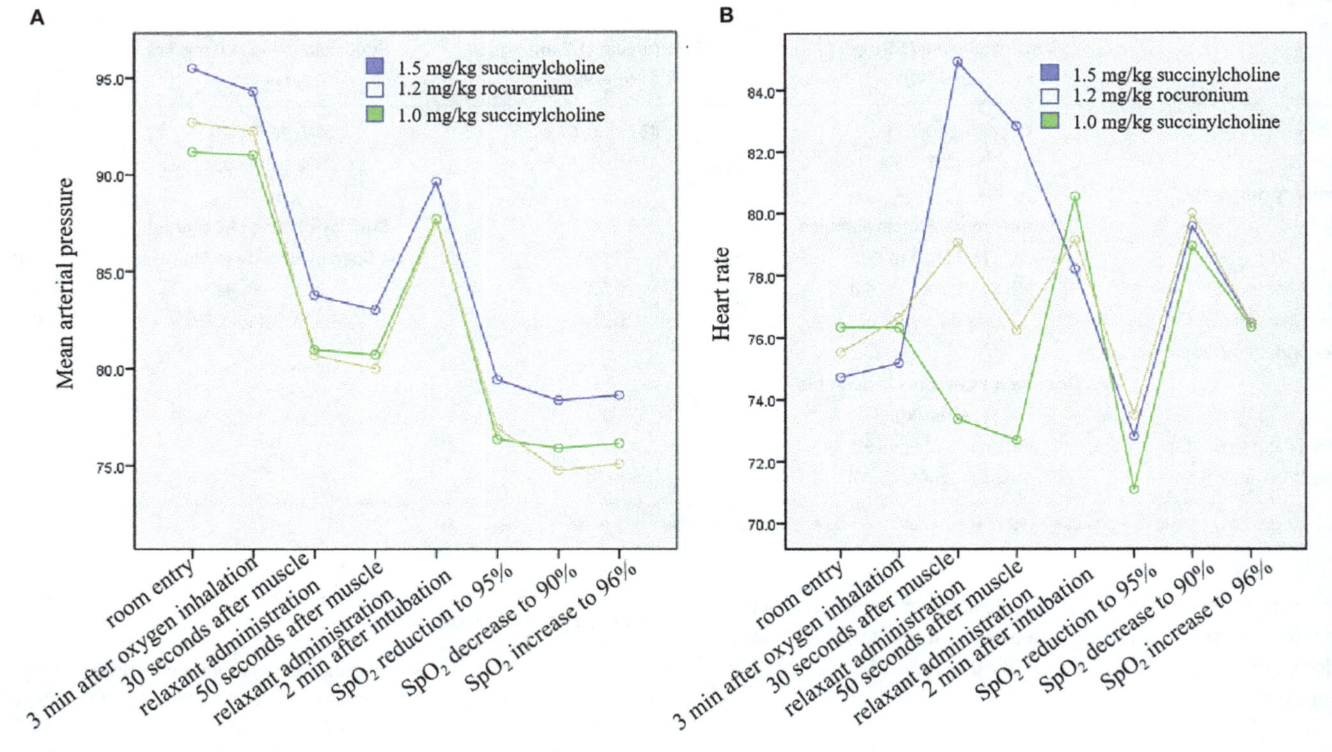

FIGURE 2 | Mean arterial pressure and heart rate variation. **(A)** Mean arterial pressure. Two-way repeated measurement ANOVA suggested that time and treatment interaction was comparable ($P = 0.279$). **(B)** Heart rate. Two-way repeated measurement ANOVA suggested that time and treatment interaction showed statistical significance among the groups ($P < 0.001$), though no clinical significance was observed.

One incubation attempt was successfully performed in all patients. Tracheal intubation evaluation revealed that the incubation conditions, C-L classification, and incubation number were comparable among the groups. The time for muscle fibrillation was comparable between the 1.5 mg/kg and 1.0 mg/kg succinylcholine groups ($P = 0.73$) (**Supplementary Table 1**). The degrees of muscle fibrillation in these two groups were also similar ($P = 0.11$) (**Supplementary Table 2**).

Moreover, the variation ratio of MAP and HR were within 30% at each time point (**Figures 2A,B**). In addition, the BIS variation among the three groups showed no clinical significance (**Supplementary Table 3**). The temperature during RSI was relatively stable, ranging from 36.0 °C to 37.1 °C.

Blood gas analysis showed a significantly different pH between room entry and 3 min after oxygen inhalation ($P < 0.01$) among the groups, despite no clinical significance. pO_2 at 3 min after oxygen inhalation time point was highest in the 1.0 mg/kg succinylcholine group ($P = 0.005$). The pCO_2 and cLac values significantly differed among the groups at room entry, 3 min after oxygen inhalation, and SpO_2 decrease to 90% time points (all $P < 0.01$) (**Table 4**). The SpO_2 in room entry and the minimum SpO_2 time points were comparable among the groups (all $P > 0.05$). In addition, ETO_2 was comparable among the groups, and $P_{ET}CO_2$ at 3 min after oxygen inhalation ($P = 0.013$) and SpO_2 increase to 96% time points ($P = 0.002$) were significantly differed (**Supplementary Table 4**).

Correlation analysis was used to explore the potential factors that might affect T90. As depicted in **Supplementary Table 5**, BMI, age, and hemoglobin were significantly correlated with T90 (all $P < 0.001$). Gender, smoking, muscle fibrillation time period, and muscle fibrillation degree were not correlated with T90.

DISCUSSION

In the present study, compared with 1.5 mg/kg succinylcholine group, both 1.0 mg/kg succinylcholine and 1.2 mg/kg rocuronium groups had significantly longer T90 and T95. These findings may provide evidence that lower dose succinylcholine and 1.2 mg/kg rocuronium may be feasible in clinical practice.

RSI is a critical medical measure that facilitates intubation. The selection of neuromuscular relaxants has been extensively studied, but there is no consensus. One of the highest risks of RSI comes from hypoxemia and reducing hypoxemia risk should be considered in the choice of muscle relaxants. Nevertheless, the available evidence on non-hypoxic apnea duration is limited. A meta-analysis showed that succinylcholine was superior to rocuronium in achieving excellent clinically acceptable intubation conditions (6). However, no statistical difference in the intubation conditions achieved was found between rocuronium and succinylcholine (19). In terms of non-hypoxic apnea duration, it was suggested that 1.0 mg/kg succinylcholine and 1.2 mg/kg rocuronium were superior to 1.5 mg/ kg succinylcholine in T90 and T95. These findings suggested

TABLE 4 | Blood gas analysis.

	Succinylcholine (1.5 mg/kg) (*n* = 90)	Rocuronium (1.2 mg/kg) (*n* = 92)	Succinylcholine (1.0 mg/kg) (*n* = 83)	P
pH				
Room entry	7.40 (7.39, 7.42)	7.42 (7.40, 7.43)	7.41 (7.40, 7.43)	0.002
3 min after oxygen inhalation	7.40 (7.38, 7.42)	7.42 (7.40, 7.43)	7.41 (7.39, 7.42)	0.005
SpO_2 decrease to 90%	7.30 (7.28, 7.33)	7.30 (7.28, 7.31)	7.31 (7.29, 7.32)	0.24
pO_2 (mmHg)				
Room entry	86 (85, 88)	85 (82, 87)	86 (84, 87)	0.051
3 min after oxygen inhalation	457 (413, 493)	445 (401, 482)	479 (432, 517)	0.005
SpO_2 decrease to 90%	63 (62, 65)	63 (62, 65)	63 (62, 65)	0.83
pCO_2 (mmHg)				
Room entry	36.1 (34.7, 38.2)	37.4 (36.6, 38.5)	36.8 (35.4, 38.8)	0.003
3 min after oxygen inhalation	35.6 (32.7, 37.7)	39.15 (36.7, 41.6)	38.1 (35.7, 40.9)	<0.001
SpO_2 decrease to 90%	52.8 (47.4, 57.7)	55.9 (51.4, 59.5)	57.2 (53.5, 62.4)	<0.001
cLac (mmol/L)				
Room entry	0.9 (0.8, 1.0)	1.0 (0.9, 1.2)	0.9 (0.7, 1.1)	<0.001
3 min after oxygen inhalation	0.9 (0.8, 1.1)	1.1 (1, 1.2)	0.9 (0.8, 1.1)	<0.001
SpO_2 decrease to 90%	1.0 (0.9, 1.1)	1.1 (1, 1.2)	1.0 (0.8, 1.1)	<0.001

that the administration of 1.0 mg/kg succinylcholine may be safer than higher doses. We noted that apneic oxygenation during the apnea period in RSI did not prevent desaturation as compared with conventional care measures in cardiac or traumatic arrest patients (20).

In the present study, the T95 and T90 in the 1.0 mg/kg succinylcholine and 1.2 mg/kg rocuronium groups were significantly longer than that in the 1.5 mg/kg succinylcholine group. In a previous study, Taha et al. reported that the T95 value in 1.5 mg/kg rocuronium-treated patients was 378 (370–393), which was lower than that in the present study. This discrepancy may be attributed to the differences in the fentanyl dose, start time points, and sample sizes (21). Our previous study compared the time of oxygen saturation decline to 92% (T92) in 0.9 mg/kg rocuronium- and 1.5 mg/kg succinylcholine-treated obese patients, in which rocuronium showed a significantly longer T92 (13), which in agreement with the present study.

Succinylcholine can trigger muscle fibrillation and increase muscle fibrillation-related metabolism. In this study, the degree and duration in the 1.5 mg/kg succinylcholine and 1.0 mg/kg succinylcholine groups were comparable, which may be explained with the supply of oxygen by myoglobin, which minimized its effect on systemic oxygen reservation (22). Moreover, the heart rate was significantly accelerated in the 1.5 mg/kg succinylcholine group, whereas mild effect was observed in the 1.0 mg/kg succinylcholine and 1.2 mg/kg rocuronium groups. Previous study suggested that succinylcholine increased anaerobic metabolism and disturbed the tissue oxygen supply and demand balance, and that high-dose succinylcholine elevated the risk of hemoglobin desaturation (12). In animal experiments, continuous infusion of succinylcholine augmented oxygen consumption (23). These previous results together with our findings suggest that a high dose of succinylcholine during RSI may need to be avoided.

This study is not without limitations. Although there were no significant differences in the intubation conditions, due to the observational nature of the study, we could not conclude whether they showed comparable effects. Additionally, elder adults and obese patients, as well as such with lung-related diseases were not included, which limited the representativeness of the conclusion. We noted that gender and height significantly differed among the three groups, and whether these two parameters affect oxygenation desaturation needs further investigation. Moreover, patients failed to complete RSI, coughing during intubation, or spontaneous breathing before mechanical ventilation were excluded for analysis, which may introduce selection bias, so the interpretation of results should be cautious.

CONCLUSION

In conclusion, this study revealed that a relatively low dose of succinylcholine and rocuronium led to a longer non-hypoxic apnea duration. Therefore, 1.0 mg/kg succinylcholine or 1.2 mg/kg rocuronium may be recommended for RSI to satisfy the required intubation conditions. Further large-scale randomized control studies are needed to validate these findings.

AUTHOR CONTRIBUTIONS

LT and XZ conceived and coordinated the study, designed, performed and analyzed the experiments, and wrote the paper. SL, LH, JL, LC, and SH carried out the data collection, data analysis, and revised the paper. All authors reviewed the results and approved the final version of the manuscript.

REFERENCES

1. H.J. Morton, and W.D. Wylie. Anaesthetic deaths due to regurgitation or vomiting. Anaesthesia. (1951) 6:190–201. doi: 10.1111/j.1365-2044.1951.tb01388.x
2. Gray TC, Halton JA. Milestone in Anaesthesia?: (d-Tubocurarine Chloride). *Proc R Soc Med.* (1946) 39:400–10. doi: 10.1177/003591574603900716
3. Foldes FF, McNall PG, Borrego-Hinojosa JM. Succinylcholine: a new approach to muscular relaxation in anesthesiology. *N Engl J Med.* (1952) 247:596–600. doi: 10.1056/NEJM195210162471603
4. G.A. Gronert. A possible mechanism of succinylcholine-induced hyperkalemia. *Anesthesiology.* (1980) 53:356. doi: 10.1097/00000542-198010000-00027
5. J.M. Hunter. Adverse effects of neuromuscular blocking drugs. *Br J Anaesth.* (1987) 59:46–60. doi: 10.1093/bja/59.1.46
6. Tran DTT, Newton EK, Mount VAH, Lee JS, Mansour C, Wells GA. et al. Rocuronium vs succinylcholine for rapid sequence intubation: a Cochrane systematic review. *Anaesthesia.* (2017) 72:765–77. doi: 10.1111/anae.13903
7. Guihard B, Chollet-Xémard C, Lakhnati P, Vivien B, Broche C, Savary D. et al. Effect of Rocuronium vs Succinylcholine on Endotracheal Intubation Success Rate Among Patients Undergoing Out-of-Hospital Rapid Sequence Intubation: A Randomized Clinical Trial. *JAMA.* (2019) 322:2303–12. doi: 10.1001/jama.2019.18254
8. Lee C, Jahr JS, Candiotti KA, Warriner B, Zornow MH, Naguib M. Reversal of profound neuromuscular block by sugammadex administered three minutes after rocuronium: a comparison with spontaneous recovery from succinylcholine. *Anesthesiology.* (2009) 110:1020–5. doi: 10.1097/ALN.0b013e31819dabb0
9. Bisschops MM, Holleman C, Huitink JM. Can sugammadex save a patient in a simulated 'cannot intubate, cannot ventilate' situation? *Anaesthesia.* (2010) 65:936–41. doi: 10.1111/j.1365-2044.2010.06455.x
10. Herriger A, Frascarolo P, Spahn DR, Magnusson L. The effect of positive airway pressure during pre-oxygenation and induction of anaesthesia upon duration of non-hypoxic apnoea. *Anaesthesia.* (2004) 59:243–7. doi: 10.1111/j.1365-2044.2004.03615.x
11. Dixon BJ, Dixon JB, Carden JR, Burn AJ, Schachter LM, Playfair JM, et al. Preoxygenation is more effective in the 25 degrees head-up position than in the supine position in severely obese patients: a randomized controlled study. *Anesthesiology.* (2005) 102:1110–5. doi: 10.1097/00000542-200506000-00009
12. Naguib M, Samarkandi AH, Abdullah K, Riad W, Alharby SW. Succinylcholine dosage and apnea-induced hemoglobin desaturation in patients. *Anesthesiology.* (2005) 102:35–40. doi: 10.1097/00000542-200501000-00009
13. Tang L, Li S, Huang S, Ma H, Wang Z. Desaturation following rapid sequence induction using succinylcholine vs. rocuronium in overweight patients. *Acta anaesthesiologica Scandinavica.* (2011) 55:203–8. doi: 10.1111/j.1399-6576.2010.02365.x
14. Stourac P, Adamus M, Seidlova D, Pavlik T, Janku P, Krikava I, et al. Low-dose or high-dose rocuronium reversed with neostigmine or sugammadex for cesarean delivery anesthesia: a randomized controlled noninferiority trial of time to tracheal intubation and extubation. *Anesth Analg.* (2016) 122:1536–45. doi: 10.1213/ANE.0000000000001197
15. Andrews JI, Kumar N, van den Brom RH, Olkkola KT, Roest GJ, Wright PM. A large simple randomized trial of rocuronium vs. succinylcholine in rapid-sequence induction of anaesthesia along with propofol. *Acta anaesthesiologica Scandinavica.* (1999) 43:4–8. doi: 10.1034/j.1399-6576.1999.430102.x
16. Sluga M, Ummenhofer W, Studer W, Siegemund M, Marsch SC. Rocuronium vs. succinylcholine for rapid sequence induction of anesthesia and endotracheal intubation: a prospective, randomized trial in emergent cases. *Anesth Analg.* (2005) 101:1356–61. doi: 10.1213/01.ANE.0000180196.58567.FE
17. Kararmaz A, Kaya S, Turhanoglu S, Ozyilmaz MA. Effects of high-dose propofol on succinylcholine-induced fasciculations and myalgia. *Acta anaesthesiologica Scandinavica.* (2003) 47:180–4. doi: 10.1034/j.1399-6576.2003.00052.x
18. Fuchs-Buder T, Claudius C, Skovgaard LT, Eriksson LI, Mirakhur RK, Viby-Mogensen J. Good clinical research practice in pharmacodynamic studies of neuromuscular blocking agents II: the Stockholm revision. *Acta anaesthesiologica Scandinavica.* (2007) 51:789–808. doi: 10.1111/j.1399-6576.2007.01352.x
19. Tran DT, Newton EK, Mount VA, Lee JS, Wells GA, Perry JJ. Rocuronium vs. succinylcholine for rapid sequence induction intubation. *Cochrane Database Syst Rev.* (2015) 2015:Cd002788. doi: 10.1002/14651858.CD002788.pub3
20. Caputo N, Azan B, Domingues R, Donner L, Fenig M, Fields D. et al. Emergency department use of apneic oxygenation vs. usual care during rapid sequence intubation: a randomized controlled trial (The ENDAO Trial) academic emergency medicine: official journal of the society for academic emergency. *Medicine.* (2017) 24:1387–94. doi: 10.1111/acem.13274
21. Taha SK, El-Khatib MF, Baraka AS, Haidar YA, Abdallah FW, Zbeidy RA, et al. Effect of suxamethonium vs rocuronium on onset of oxygen desaturation during apnoea following rapid sequence induction. *Anaesthesia.* (2010) 65:358–61. doi: 10.1111/j.1365-2044.2010.06243.x
22. Erbguth PH, Bergman NA. The effect of a single dose of succinylcholine on oxygen consumption and carbon dioxide production in man. *Anesthesiology.* (1973) 39:447–9. doi: 10.1097/00000542-197310000-00023
23. Prakash S, Barde S, Thakur P, Gogia AR, Singh R. Intubating conditions following rapid sequence induction with three doses of succinylcholine. *Indian J Anaesth.* (2012) 56:139–44. doi: 10.4103/0019-5049.96309

20

Relevant Outcomes in Pediatric Acute Respiratory Distress Syndrome Studies

Nadir Yehya[1] and Neal J. Thomas[2]*

[1] Department of Anesthesiology and Critical Care Medicine, Children's Hospital of Philadelphia, University of Pennsylvania, Philadelphia, PA, USA, [2] Department of Pediatrics and Public Health Science, Division of Pediatric Critical Care Medicine, Penn State Hershey Children's Hospital, Hershey, PA, USA

***Correspondence:**
Nadir Yehya
yehyan@email.chop.edu

Despite distinct epidemiology and outcomes, pediatric acute respiratory distress syndrome (PARDS) is often managed based on evidence extrapolated from treatment of adults. The impact of non-pulmonary processes on mortality as well as the lower mortality rate compared to adults with acute respiratory distress syndrome (ARDS) renders the utilization of short-term mortality as a primary outcome measure for interventional studies problematic. However, data regarding alternatives to mortality are profoundly understudied, and proposed alternatives, such as ventilator-free days, may be themselves subject to hidden biases. Given the neuropsychiatric and functional impairment in adult survivors of ARDS, characterization of these morbidities in children with PARDS is of paramount importance. The purpose of this review is to frame these challenges in the context of the existing pediatric literature, and using adult ARDS as a guide, suggest potential clinically relevant outcomes that deserve further investigation. The goal is to identify important areas of study in order to better define clinical practice and facilitate future interventional trials in PARDS.

Keywords: pediatrics, ARDS, outcomes, acute respiratory distress syndrome, children, acute lung injury

INTRODUCTION

Pediatric intensivists were not present for either the 1994 American-European Consensus Conference (AECC) (1) or the 2012 Berlin re-definition (2) of acute respiratory distress syndrome (ARDS), and so pediatric considerations were not addressed. Despite this limitation, AECC and Berlin definitions were historically applied to children without modification, despite the different epidemiology and outcomes of pediatric ARDS. To address this deficiency, the Pediatric Acute Lung Injury Consensus Conference (PALICC) was convened to propose specific definitions for pediatric acute respiratory distress syndrome (PARDS) (3). Notable differences in the PALICC definition are use of oxygenation index (OI) instead of PaO_2/FiO_2, the ability to diagnose PARDS in the absence of arterial blood gas analysis by using non-invasive measures of hypoxemia based on SpO_2 [oxygen saturation index (OSI)], and less restrictive radiographic criteria.

Irrespective of definitions utilized, cohort studies and clinical trials have generally demonstrated lower mortality for PARDS (relative to adult ARDS), as well as an appreciable decrease in mortality over time (4, 5). Adult studies have demonstrated decreased pulmonary capacity, decreased quality of life, and worsened neurocognition among survivors of ARDS (6–8); however, comparable studies are lacking in PARDS. An appreciation of long-term sequelae is important for characterizing the epidemiology of this syndrome. Additionally, the already low and further decreasing mortality rate makes short-term survival an impractical endpoint for most clinical trials in PARDS, necessitating the identification of clinically relevant patient-centered outcomes to test future interventions. The purpose of this review is to identify the challenges in identifying appropriate outcomes for current and future studies in PARDS, framed in the context of the existing literature. Additionally, using adult ARDS studies as a guide, potential alternative outcomes that deserve further investigation in PARDS are suggested.

MORTALITY

Pediatric acute respiratory distress syndrome has lower mortality than adult ARDS (4, 5), with mortality decreasing over time. Unfortunately, short-term mortality – such as 28- to 60-day mortality, pediatric intensive care unit (PICU) mortality, and hospital mortality – remains an objective, easily obtained, clinically relevant, and patient-centered outcome. As such, it is the most consistently reported endpoint in cohort studies (**Table 1**) (5, 9–23) and in clinical trials (**Table 2**) (24–32). However, predictors of mortality in PARDS are often not specific to PARDS but are characteristic of risk factors in several conditions that result in critical illness. Notably, immunocompromised status (5, 21, 26) and multisystem organ failure (MSOF) (5, 12, 17) are associated with increased mortality risk in several PARDS studies, including clinical trials (26). However, immunocompromised status and MSOF have little pulmonary specificity, are associated with mortality in sepsis, and are component variables of severity of illness scoring systems. Thus, a generalization of this observation states that children die *with* PARDS, rather than *because of* PARDS. In such cases, the associated PARDS has resolved at the time of death, despite the persistence of mechanical ventilation. Further complicating the use of mortality as an endpoint is elective withdrawal of potentially futile care, either for persistent MSOF, underlying refractory malignancy, or for presumed poor neurologic prognosis, none of which are specific for PARDS.

One example is worth examining in further detail. A multicenter randomized controlled trial (RCT) of exogenous surfactant (calfactant) in moderate and severe PARDS (OI > 7) demonstrated improved mortality associated with calfactant treatment (26). However, imbalance in the proportion of immunocompromised patients, with over-representation in the placebo arm, likely contributed to this effect, and after adjustment for immunocompromised status, the association between calfactant treatment and improved mortality was no longer evident ($p = 0.07$). Furthermore, patients received treatment within 48 h of intubation, but the proportion of patients successfully extubated did not differ between the groups and curves for cumulative successful extubation did not begin to diverge until 12 days after intubation, suggesting that factors unrelated to the initial PARDS insult, such as immunocompromised status, may have been responsible for mortality and prolonged ventilation. A follow-up trial of calfactant was restricted to immunocompromised children [Calfactant for Acute Lung Injury in Pediatric Stem Cell Transplant and Oncology Patients (CALIPSO)] using mortality as the primary outcome.

While mortality may be problematic as a primary endpoint for a general PARDS population, there remain subgroups of children with PARDS who still have a substantial mortality risk, yet with a reasonable chance of survival. CALIPSO is an example of limiting an intervention to a subgroup of PARDS with substantial mortality (>50%), albeit at the risk of difficult recruitment and reduced generalizability. Indeed, recently, successful trials in adult ARDS of neuromuscular blockade (33) and prone positioning (34) employed this strategy, as ARDS et Curarisation Systematique (ACURASYS) limited enrollment to patients with $PaO_2/FiO_2 \leq 150$, rather than the typical ≤ 300. Prone position in severe ARDS (PROSEVA) required even more stringent enrollment criteria, as it requires $PaO_2/FiO_2 \leq 150$ *after* 12–24 h of initial stabilization, thereby excluding patients who rapidly improved with standard ventilator management. In both cases, the goal was enrichment of a higher risk population in which the tested intervention could plausibly impact mortality with a reasonable sample size. This, simultaneously, avoids unnecessarily exposing patients to treatment when they have low risk of mortality and high probability of survival irrespective of randomization arm, thereby diluting any potential treatment effect. For PARDS to reproduce this, predictors of mortality risk need to be identified and validated. These predictors need to be available early in the PARDS course to allow enrollment within a timeframe amenable for interventions to work, ideally within 48 h of PARDS onset. This strategy has particular appeal for testing interventions for "refractory" PARDS, such as high-frequency oscillatory ventilation (HFOV), prone positioning, methylprednisolone, inhaled nitric oxide (iNO), and extracorporeal membrane oxygenation (ECMO).

DURATION OF MECHANICAL VENTILATION

Duration of ventilation is a common outcome described in PARDS studies, especially when this outcome is limited to survivors. This outcome has face validity, as more severe PARDS can reasonably be expected to require a longer duration of mechanical ventilation. The 2012 Berlin definition (2) demonstrated an increase in duration of mechanical ventilation in survivors across increasing severity classes of ARDS, which was confirmed in LUNG SAFE (Large Observational Study to Understand the Global Impact of Severe Acute Respiratory Failure) (35). This observation has been corroborated in PARDS when using oxygenation at 24 h, rather than at PARDS onset (5).

To be used as a valid endpoint, the definition of "duration of mechanical ventilation" needs to be limited to survivors, given the risk of contamination of this endpoint with non-survivors with a short-duration of ventilation. Alternatively, liberation from ventilation can be analyzed as the primary outcome of interest, with death treated as a competing outcome. Appropriate statistical techniques must be employed for quantifying the effect of an intervention while accounting for competing events (36). Furthermore, given the increased utilization of non-invasive ventilation both prior to (37–39) and after endotracheal intubation, duration of mechanical ventilation requires clear definition

TABLE 1 | Reported outcomes in cohorts using PARDS-type inclusion criteria and ≥100 patients.

Years	Centers	Countries	Cases	Outcomes	Comments	Reference
1986–1990	1	USA	100	Mortality (72%)	PaO_2 ≤75 with FiO_2 ≥0.5; bilateral infiltrates; 74% immunocompromised	(9)
1990–1991	14	France	123	Mortality (60%)	Intubated; FiO_2 ≥0.5 on PEEP; bilateral infiltrates	(10)
1993–1995	1	Canada	131	Mortality (27%) Ventilator days survivors (8, range 1–27)	Intubated; PEEP ≥6 and FiO_2 ≥0.5 for 12 h	(11)
1997–1998	10	USA, Canada	232	Mortality (40%)	Intubated; HFOV	(22)
1996–2000	2	USA	328	Mortality (22%) VFD (15 ± 11)	Non-invasive and intubated; AECC ALI with PF ≤300	(12)
2004–2005	12	Australia, New Zealand	117	Mortality (35%)	Non-invasive and intubated; AECC ALI with PF ≤300	(13)
2005–2006	26	China	358	Mortality (44%)	Any respiratory support; AECC ALI with PF ≤300	(14)
2000–2007	1	USA	398	Mortality (20%) VFD (17, IQR 0–24)	Intubated; PF ≤300; 192 with bilateral infiltrates	(15)
2007–2010	5	USA	168	Mortality (11%) VFD (20, IQR 10–23)	Intubated; AECC ALI with PF ≤300; excluded SCT	(16)
2009–2010	7	USA, Canada, Belgium, Switzerland, Netherlands	328	Mortality (38%)	Intubated; HFOV	(23)
2010–2011	21	Spain	146	Mortality (26%)	Intubated; AECC ARDS with PF ≤200	(17)
2009–2011	7	Italy, Spain, France, Austria, Netherlands	221	Mortality (17%) ECMO/death (19%)	Intubated; Berlin ARDS with PF ≤300; age 1–18 months	(18)
2009–2013	1	USA	312	Mortality (22%)	Intubated; Berlin ARDS with SpO_2 cutoffs	(19)
2008–2014	5	USA	299	Mortality (13%)	Non-invasive and intubated; AECC ARDS with PF ≤200	(20)
2009–2014	12	USA	222	Mortality (60%) Ventilator days survivors (9, IQR 4–16)	Intubated; SCT	(21)
2011–2014	1	USA	283	Mortality (13%) VFD (17, IQR 3–21) Ventilator days survivors (10, IQR 7–17)	Intubated; AECC ALI and Berlin ARDS with PF ≤300	(5)

AECC, American-European Consensus Conference; ALI, acute lung injury; ARDS, acute respiratory distress syndrome; HFOV, high-frequency oscillatory ventilation; PEEP, positive end-expiratory pressure; PF, PaO_2/FiO_2; SCT, stem cell transplant; VFD, ventilator-free days.

regarding whether non-invasive support is included. Both Berlin (mild) ARDS (2) and PALICC PARDS (3) definitions make allowances for non-invasive support, suggesting that screening for studies based on these criteria would allow for inclusion of a substantial number of non-intubated patients. This potential for increased enrollment needs consistent and well-delineated reporting of what is meant by "duration of mechanical ventilation."

Therefore, while the endpoint "duration of ventilation in survivors" retains face validity and likely reflects the severity of PARDS, it is unclear exactly how "patient-centric" this outcome is. Specifically, it is unclear whether a given child would be better served with 10 days of invasive mechanical ventilation and extubated to high-flow cannula or whether 8 days of invasive ventilation followed by 4 days of non-invasive bi-level positive airway pressure (BiPAP) with full-facemask interface. Indeed, the answer likely varies between patients for a multitude of variables, including sedation requirements, strength, airway status, and indication for intubation.

Finally, duration of ventilation in survivors is complicated by the prevalence of subglottic stenosis, poor secretion tolerance, or severe upper airway obstruction from poor airway tone as an indication for prolonged intubation. Such patients may wean appropriately to minimal invasive support given their underlying PARDS severity, but the actual act of removing the endotracheal tube may be delayed, or ultimately attempted and unsuccessful, for reasons related primarily to their airway. Given the substantial number of comorbidities described in PARDS, reasons for prolonged intubation unrelated to the actual PARDS risk factor have the potential to confound the utility of duration of ventilation as an endpoint. An alternative has been proposed to only count the duration of time until successful completion of an extubation readiness test, irrespective of whether or not the patient is actually extubated (40). However, this has not been validated nor described in an actual practice or trial and does not address the prior criticism of not being patient-centered, as the child remains intubated.

VENTILATOR-FREE DAYS

Perhaps, the most commonly adopted surrogate endpoint in PARDS trials, recently (**Table 2**), is ventilator-free days (VFD) at some arbitrary endpoint (e.g., at 28 days). VFD at 28 days are typically derived by subtracting duration of ventilation in survivors from 28 and scoring non-survivors and those requiring

TABLE 2 | Reported outcomes in select placebo-controlled randomized clinical trials in acute respiratory failure and PARDS.

Trial	Years	Intervention	Total subjects	Primary outcome	Other reported outcomes	Reference
HFOV	1990–1994	HFOV versus conventional	58	Mortality (34% HFOV; 41% conventional)	Ventilator days in survivors; supplemental O_2 requirement; chronic lung disease	(24)
Weaning protocol	1999–2001	Protocolized PSV or VSV versus no protocol	179	Days to extubation (median 2 for no protocol; 1.6 PSV; 1.8 VSV)	Successful extubation	(25)
Calfactant	2000–2003	Intratracheal calfactant versus air placebo	152	VFD (13 ± 8 for calfactant; 12 ± 11 for air)	Mortality; failure of conventional ventilation; oxygenation; supplemental O_2 requirement; PICU and hospital LOS	(26)
Prone position	2001–2004	Prone versus supine position	101	VFD (16 ± 8 for supine; 16 ± 8 for prone)	Mortality; organ failure-free days; supplemental O_2 requirement; PCPC; POPC	(27)
Inhaled nitric oxide	2003–2005	iNO versus nitrogen placebo	53	VFD (15 ± 8 for iNO; 9 ± 9 for placebo)	Mortality; ECMO/death	(28)
Lucinactant	2007–2010	Intratracheal lucinactant versus air placebo	165	Adjusted LSM of ventilator days (4 for lucinactant; 4.5 for air)	Mortality; VFD; PICU and hospital LOS	(29)
PED-CARDS	2008–2010	Intratracheal calfactant versus air placebo	109	Mortality (12% for calfactant; 9% for air)	VFD; oxygenation; PICU and hospital LOS	(30)
RESTORE	2009–2013	Protocolized sedation versus usual care	2449	Ventilator days (median 6.5 for protocol; 6.5 for usual care)	Mortality; duration of weaning; duration of non-invasive ventilation; PICU and hospital LOS	(31)
Steroids	2010–2014	Methylprednisolone versus placebo	35	Ventilator days (10 ± 7 for steroids; 10 ± 5 for placebo)	Mortality; VFD; oxygenation; PICU and hospital LOS	(32)

ECMO, extracorporeal membrane oxygenation; HFOV, high-frequency oscillatory ventilation; LSM, least squares means; LOS, length of stay; PCPC, pediatric cerebral performance category; PED-CARDS, pediatric calfactant in acute respiratory distress syndrome; POPC, pediatric overall performance category; PICU, pediatric intensive care unit; PSV, pressure-support ventilation; RESTORE, randomized evaluation of sedation titration for respiratory failure; VFD, ventilator-free days; VSV, volume support ventilation.

≥28 ventilator days as 0 (41). It has also been defined as "days alive and free of mechanical ventilation" (42), which creates confusion for cases where the patient is extubated on day 10, but dies on day 20 (10 days alive and free of mechanical ventilation is VFD = 10; non-survival at day 28 suggests VFD = 0). This composite endpoint combines mortality and duration of ventilation by penalizing non-survivors, unlike duration of ventilation. Similar to duration of ventilation in survivors, VFD at 28 days has demonstrated correlation across severity of Berlin ARDS (2) and PALICC PARDS (3) categories, with worse oxygenation categories associated with fewer VFD. This composite endpoint potentially represents efficiency, as an outcome of an intervention, which both reduces mortality and duration of ventilation, can be detected with a smaller sample size (42).

The same caveats regarding clarity of non-invasive support are required for VFD as mentioned for duration of ventilation (41). However, VFD has a major limitation as a composite endpoint, as the merged individual endpoints (mortality and ventilator duration) are *not* equivalent and interchangeable. A child requiring 30 days of mechanical ventilation, but surviving, cannot be considered identical to a child who dies after 7 days of ventilation, although both would be recorded as VFD = 0. Composite endpoints are best utilized when the separate endpoints are of equivalent importance for the patient, such as stroke or myocardial infarction in hypertensive adults. When initially described for adult ARDS, VFD was demonstrated to be useful only when the more pejorative outcome of mortality was improved alongside duration of ventilation (42). Given the >30% mortality in adult ARDS (35), this is a reasonable expectation: interventions which shorten ventilation *should* improve mortality, assuming mechanical ventilation and ARDS are in the causal pathway for non-survival. However, even in adults, this assumption can be problematic. The ARDSNet corticosteroid trial (43) failed to demonstrate superiority of methylprednisolone for persistent ARDS for the primary outcome of mortality at 60 days (29.2% mortality in methylprednisolone, 28.6% in placebo, $p = 1$). However, methylprednisolone treatment was associated with 4.4 additional VFD and 2.7 additional ICU-free days at 28 days. Significantly, more patients in the methylprednisolone arm required re-initiation of ventilation (28 versus 9%, $p = 0.006$). These discrepant results make interpretation of the trial difficult: mortality is reported at 60 days, but VFD at 28 days. Mortality is nominally higher in the methylprednisolone group, but VFD are also more favorable for methylprednisolone. Thus, in this case, the reporting of VFD offers no advantages or power relative to reporting on mortality alone: when an intervention has opposite effects on duration of ventilation and mortality, VFD merely confuses the interpretation.

In pediatrics, the utilization of VFD at 28 days is potential suspect for these same reasons, as PARDS mortality is much lower, and persistent hypoxemia is unlikely to be the cause of mortality. Thus, the effect on mortality is less certain to be in the same direction as duration of ventilation. For instance, a trial of ECMO for severe refractory PARDS may result in improved nominal mortality rates but would likely result in prolonged duration of ventilation, thereby complicating the interpretation and utility of VFD. Finally, several interventions sorely in need of testing in PARDS, including fluid management, sedation protocols, weaning, and extubation readiness all clearly impact length of ventilation much more so than they will impact mortality, hampering the utility of

VFD as an outcome unless these parameters are protocolized in the context of the trial.

NEED FOR EXTRACORPOREAL SUPPORT AS AN OUTCOME

A more recently reported composite outcome for PARDS investigations has been the composite of need for ECMO or death (18, 28). This attempts to address the limitations of VFD and the low mortality (and thus difficult to adequately power) of PARDS. The underlying assumption is that lung injury severe enough to require ECMO is essentially refractory to conventional mechanical ventilation, and thus need for ECMO would be a death in any center unable to provide ECMO. Therefore, "ECMO" is close enough to "death" to justify combination as a composite endpoint.

The European Society for Pediatric and Neonatal Intensive Care (ESPNIC) used this definition to test the utility of the Berlin criteria in children (18) and demonstrated that the inclusion of a "severe" ARDS category improved validity with an increased risk of ECMO/death in children with Berlin-defined severe ARDS, whereas risks were similar when defined using AECC definitions. It should be noted, however, that the incidence of ECMO/death (18.6%) was only marginally increased over the incidence of mortality (17.2%), and that comparable analyses for the outcome mortality yielded identical conclusions.

A recently published RCT (28) for iNO (total $n = 53$) reported both mortality (28% placebo, 8% iNO, χ^2 $p = 0.07$) and ECMO/death (48% placebo, 8% iNO, $p < 0.01$). The trial was powered for a difference in VFD at 28 days, for which it required a sample size of 169 children, and was stopped early for slow enrollment. Of note, the difference in the reported VFD in this trial was also significant. While the primary outcome of more VFD was achieved despite the small sample size, the reporting of ECMO/death in this study points to a potential mechanism, whereby iNO improved VFD. Specifically, exposure to iNO appeared to decrease the rate of ECMO utilization, suggesting an improvement in hypoxemia, thereby reducing total ventilator days and potentially impacting mortality. This is significant, as it implies a connection between improvement in hypoxemia and better outcomes in PARDS, a connection which is not consistently corroborated in adult ARDS trials (44). For certain trials of salvage therapy, such as methylprednisolone, iNO, prone positioning, and HFOV, the use of ECMO/death as a primary outcome may be rational. However, as in the example above, there is little information added by this specific reporting that was not also captured by the more conventional short-term outcome of VFD at 28 days. Additionally, as ECMO is not an outcome *per se* but simply an additional mode of supportive care, with subjective thresholds for its utilization among different centers and practitioners, the composite outcome of ECMO/death is difficult to standardize. Finally, the component variables of ECMO/death are not of equal importance to the patient, thus calling into question its validity as a patient-centered, clinically meaningful composite outcome.

POST-DISCHARGE OUTCOMES

There have been no studies examining long-term mortality in PARDS, but outcomes, such as 90-day, 6-month, or 12-month mortality, are unlikely to represent significant differences compared to short-term mortality. Additionally, long-term mortality is more likely to result from either the underlying condition or an unrelated cause and is unlikely to be a sequelae of PARDS. Therefore, alternative post-discharge outcomes are needed (**Table 3**). Recent attention has focused on the development of new morbidities in the PICU as a relevant outcome (45, 46), with up to twice the prevalence of mortality.

Few studies have investigated the physical or neurocognitive quality of life in survivors of PARDS (47–51). The existing studies are of extremely limited sample size (all $n \leq 11$) and outdated, with ventilator management not reflective of current PICU practices (52, 53). In 1985, Fanconi et al. (47) published on pulmonary function testing (PFT) of nine survivors of PARDS ventilated between 1978 and 1982 (five of whom experienced peak pressures >40 cmH_2O) at a mean 2.3-year follow-up. Seven of the nine were considered "hypoxemic," with PaO_2 <80 mmHg on room air, and eight of nine had ventilation inequalities on multibreath nitrogen washout. Increased peak pressures and increased exposure to FiO_2 >0.5 during PARDS correlated with increased ventilation inequalities, suggesting a potential association between ventilator management and long-term pulmonary outcome. In a separate study published in 1996, 11 PARDS survivors ventilated between 1986 and 1993 (mean PaO_2/FiO_2 160; 9 of 11 with peak pressures >40 cmH_2O) with PFT performed at a mean 23-month follow-up demonstrated obstructive physiology in three children and mixed obstruction and restrictive physiology in an additional four children (49). The most recent investigation of PARDS survivors (51) occurred in children ventilated between 1986 and 1998 (all experienced pressure-controlled ventilation, with all peak pressures <35 cmH_2O). These investigators were able to assess PFT in seven patients, finding one with an abnormal diffusion capacity, and a second with exercise-induced hypoxemia.

Based on these small case series, the PALICC group recommended that survivors of PARDS undergo screening for PFT abnormalities within 1 year of discharge (54). The small sample size of these existing studies, antiquated ventilator management, and variable follow-up time precludes any real assessment of the prevalence of pulmonary dysfunction in PARDS survivors. Larger scale, multicenter follow-up is sorely needed, potentially exploiting the infrastructure of existing pediatric critical care research networks and in collaboration with pediatric pulmonologists and rehabilitation providers.

Studies within this framework are becoming more common in pediatric critical care. The out-of-hospital arm of Therapeutic Hypothermia after Pediatric Cardia Arrest (THAPCA) trial (55) was powered for a primary outcome of a dichotomized (good versus bad) version of the Vineland Adaptive Behavior Scale, second edition (VABS-II). Ebrahim et al. (56) reported on the 1-month post-PICU admission outcome of 65 urgently admitted survivors using VABS-II, pediatric cerebral performance category

TABLE 3 | Potential outcomes for PARDS studies.

Outcome	Timeframe	Advantages	Disadvantages
Mortality	Short term 28 or 60 days PICU Hospital Medium and long term 90 days 1 year	Easy to obtain Fixed time-point Related to acute process Patient-centered Potentially captures longer period of risk for unfavorable outcomes	Impractical given low baseline mortality Similarly low rate Harder to obtain follow-up More related to underlying comorbidities
VFD	28 days	Easy to obtain Increases power to detect clinically meaningful improvements related to shortened ventilation	Imbalance in components of the composite outcome Only increases power if intervention benefits both mortality and ventilator days
Ventilator days	28 days PICU LOS	Easy to obtain Related to pulmonary nature of PARDS	Needs non-invasive support explicitly defined Unclear if patient-centered
ECMO/death	Short term	Increases power to detect efficacy of pre-ECMO "salvage therapies'	Subjective use of ECMO Imbalance in components of the composite outcome Unclear if patient-centered
Neurocognitive and functional (POPC/PCPC)	Medium and long term 90 days 1 year Pre-return to school	Rapid (POCP/PCPC) Patient-centered Potentially completed over telephone Potentially more practical, as it is a prevalent outcome	More thorough cognitive function requires longer testing Changes with developmental age and with comorbidities
Pulmonary outcomes	Medium and long term 90 days 1 year Pre-return to school	Patient-centered Related to pulmonary nature of PARDS	Requires infrastructure (expertise and equipment) for in-person follow-up
Biometric outcomes	Medium and long term 90 days 1 year Pre-return to school	Patient-centered Does not require return to clinic Potentially improved response rate	Requires development, testing and validation Requires expertise HIPAA concerns Ownership concerns (who owns the data and how will it be used?)
Psychiatric	Long term	Patient-centered Potentially completed over telephone	Requires infrastructure (expertise) for in-person follow-up
Health care utilization	Medium and long term 90 days and 1 year re-hospitalization	Patient-centered Does not require inpatient follow-up Related to pulmonary nature of PARDS Addresses cost to patient/family	Difficult to obtain Sensitive to local practices Potentially more related to underlying comorbidities than to PARDS

ECMO, extracorporeal membrane oxygenation; LOS, length of stay; PARDS, pediatric acute respiratory distress syndrome; PCPC, pediatric cerebral performance category; POPC, pediatric overall performance category; PICU, pediatric intensive care unit; VFD, ventilator-free days.

(PCPC), pediatric overall performance category (POPC), and overall pediatric quality of life inventory, fourth edition. They demonstrated an overall poor quality of life for these patients at 1-month post-PICU admission. A recent review article identified potentially useful health-related quality of life (HRQL) metrics for pediatric critical care (57). This review identified substantial morbidity for PICU survivors, some of which were associated with treatments received during their PICU stay, suggesting possible modifiable risk factors. Additionally, a recent review has also suggested significant psychiatric morbidity in PICU survivors (58), including post-traumatic stress disorder (PTSD), depression, and behavioral disorders, with prevalence of post-traumatic stress symptoms potentially as high as 62% (59). Finally, the ongoing multicenter Life after Pediatric Sepsis Evaluation (LAPSE) study is a prospective observational study collecting information on quality of life, family dynamics and stress, and health care utilization in survivors of pediatric severe sepsis.

ADULT ARDS INVESTIGATIONS OF ALTERNATIVE OUTCOMES

Seminal work in adult ARDS long-term outcome (6, 7) has paved the way for potentially comparable studies in PARDS. In 2002, adult survivors of moderate and severe ARDS were followed at 3, 6, and 12 months, with a primary outcome of 6-min walk distance (6). The authors found that survivors of ARDS (median age 45 years) had persistent physical limitations at all time-points tested, primarily due to muscle wasting and weakness. At 12 months, only 49% of patients had returned to work. In multivariable regression, use of corticosteroids and duration of mechanical ventilation both negatively affected 6-min walk distance, suggesting a possible relationship between modifiable risk factors and medium-term functional outcome. In the subsequent 5-year follow-up study, the median 6-min walk distance remained below predicted values (7). However, pulmonary function had returned to near normal, and persistent exercise limitations were attributed to continuing weakness and neuropsychological impairments. Health-care costs continued to be substantial for survivors up to 5 years after discharge, especially in those with pre-existing comorbidities.

For PARDS investigators, this experience is instructive. The major strengths of these studies are the well-characterized, multicenter cohort, the longitudinal study design, the high rates of follow-up, and the in-person data collection. The granularity of the data allowed significant associations to be made regarding ICU exposures (e.g., corticosteroids) and subsequent medium- and long-term outcomes. While these observations remain hypothesis-generating, these are still essential initial steps toward determining how to design future prospective trials with clinically meaningful, patient-centered outcomes.

An earlier study employing an alternative design is also worth considering (60). A prospective case control interview/questionnaire study was performed of adult ARDS survivors matched with non-ARDS survivors with similar severity of illness at a median of 23 months after discharge. ARDS survivors demonstrated worse HRQL in nearly all domains tested, including respiratory-specific domains. The most profound reductions in ARDS survivors were in the domains assessing either physical limitations or on the impact of pulmonary symptoms on activities of daily living. This was the first study to assess the HRQL in ARDS survivors matched to similarly ill non-ARDS patients, thus minimizing the possibility that observations were simply reflections of severity of illness; rather, this study design increased the plausibly that these associations were either actually caused by having ARDS specifically, or conversely, by the treatments used for it.

The significance of long-term, patient-centered outcomes is elegantly made when considering the neuropsychological function in adult ARDS survivors of the fluid and catheter treatment trial (FACTT). The initial trial used a 2 × 2 factorial design to test (separately) the utility of pulmonary-artery catheters versus central-venous catheters, and the effects of a conservative versus a liberal fluid management strategy on hemodynamically stable ARDS patients (61, 62). The trial failed to demonstrate superiority of either fluid strategy in its primary outcome of 60-day mortality (25.5% mortality in fluid conservative, 28.4% in fluid liberal, $p = 0.30$). However, the conservative arm resulted in 2.5 more VFD ($p < 0.001$) and 2.2 additional ICU-free days ($p < 0.001$) (61) without additional increase in non-pulmonary organ failures. Based on these findings, the FACTT investigators recommended a conservative fluid strategy in hemodynamically stable ARDS patients.

The follow-up ARDS cognitive outcome study (ACOS) conducted telephone interviews of FACTT survivors at 2 and 12 months post-discharge (8). Similar to prior investigations (6, 60), the investigators found that most survivors (55–60%, depending on metric used) experienced long-term cognitive impairment. Interestingly, lower PaO_2 ($p = 0.015$) and allocation to the conservative fluid arm ($p = 0.005$) were independently associated with long-term cognitive impairment. The PaO_2 during ARDS reported in ACOS survivors with cognitive impairment was median 71 (interquartile range 67–80), well within the ARDSNet recommended PaO_2 ranges of 55–80, suggesting that existing, arbitrary guidelines may be too permissive, and that this level of mild hypoxemia may be associated with long-term neurologic sequelae. Additionally, the conclusions of the FACTT trial that conservative fluid management resulted in 2.5 additional VFD without additional organ failures are now called into question, as 12-month neurologic function clearly suggests potential sub-clinical neurologic dysfunction, leading to long-term functional impairment. To date, no study in children with PARDS has investigated any sort of long-term outcome, and the efficacy of our interventions on long-term function in growing and developing children remains a mystery.

BIOMETRIC OUTCOMES

One of the disadvantages of the existing framework for evaluating long-term outcomes is the expense and expertise necessary to bring back patients to a follow-up clinic and conduct PFT and neuromuscular testing. An alternative strategy has been demonstrated by cardiologists with the embrace of remote telemonitoring (RTM) technology. These have taken the form of devices, which record heart rate, cardiac rhythm, pulse oximetry, and blood pressure, with wireless transmission to a data collection center (63). Devices can be modified to also include brief questionnaires, adding additional data regarding subjective experiencing of symptoms by the patient. Home spirometry adapted with an automated modem for data transmission has been used in a trial for management of children with asthma (64). Device modifications exist, which can additionally measure grip strength, as well as assess flexibility and reaction time using game-playing scenarios (65), which may be able to address certain neurocognitive and neuromuscular outcomes in PARDS survivors. RTM devices have already been incorporated as interventions in clinical trials in adult heart failure (66, 67). The use of RTM for patients with pacemakers and implantable cardioverter defibrillators by pediatric cardiologists was associated with fewer clinic visits (68), providing proof of concept for RTM to allow follow-up for patients at lower cost.

Remote telemonitoring remains unexplored in pediatric critical illness research, although it possesses significant potential. Some of the limitations regarding patient loss to follow-up are nicely addressed by RTM. Platforms which may only require smartphones and appropriate adaptors, or which utilize gaming, are intuitively appealing to a pediatric population, and may improve compliance. However, expertise in development and interpretation are still necessary, and validation will be required prior to implementation.

CONCLUSION

Mortality in PARDS is decreasing, and while it remains clinically relevant and patient-centered, it is impractical for most purposes, and its use should likely be limited to trials aimed at enrolling pre-determined higher risk groups. VFD is likely to remain the most common primary endpoint for clinical trials in the foreseeable future, but advocates should be aware of its limitations, and should ensure that the power of this composite outcome rests on whether the tested intervention improve *both* mortality and duration of ventilation in survivors. Finally, given the prevalence of long-term neuropsychiatric morbidity and functional impairment in adult ARDS survivors, it is imperative that these parameters are defined for children. After a better understanding of the burden of surviving PARDS on patients and families is obtained, studies can be designed to demonstrate a return to pre-morbid functioning, which is fundamentally most important to the child and family.

AUTHOR CONTRIBUTIONS

NY and NT researched the topic, reviewed the relevant source articles, and wrote the manuscript together.

REFERENCES

1. Bernard GR, Artigas A, Brigham KL, Carlet J, Falke K, Hudson L, et al. The American-European Consensus Conference on ARDS. Definitions, mechanisms, relevant outcomes, and clinical trial coordination. *Am J Respir Crit Care Med* (1994) **149**(3 Pt 1):818–24.
2. ARDS Definition Task Force, Ranieri VM, Rubenfeld GD, Thompson BT, Ferguson ND, Caldwell E, et al. Acute respiratory distress syndrome: the Berlin definition. *JAMA* (2012) **307**(23):2526–33. doi:10.1001/jama.2012.5669
3. Pediatric Acute Lung Injury Consensus Conference Group. Pediatric acute respiratory distress syndrome: consensus recommendations from the Pediatric Acute Lung Injury Consensus Conference. *Pediatr Crit Care Med* (2015) **16**(5):428–39. doi:10.1097/PCC.0000000000000350
4. Zimmerman JJ, Akhtar SR, Caldwell E, Rubenfeld GD. Incidence and outcomes of pediatric acute lung injury. *Pediatrics* (2009) **124**(1):87–95. doi:10.1542/peds.2007-2462
5. Yehya N, Servaes S, Thomas NJ. Characterizing degree of lung injury in pediatric acute respiratory distress syndrome. *Crit Care Med* (2015) **43**(5):937–46. doi:10.1097/CCM.0000000000000867
6. Herridge MS, Cheung AM, Tansey CM, Matte-Martyn A, Diaz-Granados N, Al-Saidi F, et al. One-year outcomes in survivors of the acute respiratory distress syndrome. *N Engl J Med* (2003) **348**(8):683–93. doi:10.1056/NEJMoa022450
7. Herridge MS, Tansey CM, Matté A, Tomlinson G, Diaz-Granados N, Cooper A, et al. Functional disability 5 years after acute respiratory distress syndrome. *N Engl J Med* (2011) **364**(14):1293–304. doi:10.1056/NEJMoa1011802
8. Mikkelsen ME, Christie JD, Lanken PN, Biester RC, Thompson BT, Bellamy SL, et al. The adult respiratory distress syndrome cognitive outcomes study: long-term neuropsychological function in survivors of acute lung injury. *Am J Respir Crit Care Med* (2012) **185**(12):1307–15. doi:10.1164/rccm.201111-2025OC
9. DeBruin W, Notterman DA, Magid M, Godwin T, Johnston S. Acute hypoxemic respiratory failure in infants and children: clinical and pathologic characteristics. *Crit Care Med* (1992) **20**(9):1223–34. doi:10.1097/00003246-199209000-00008
10. Costil J, Cloup M, Leclerc F, Devictor D, Beaufils F, Siméoni U, et al. Acute respiratory distress syndrome (ARDS) in children: multicenter collaborative study of the French Group of Pediatric Intensive Care. *Pediatr Pulmonol Suppl* (1995) **11**:106–7. doi:10.1002/ppul.1950191152
11. Trachsel D, McCrindle BW, Nakagawa S, Bohn D. Oxygenation index predicts outcome in children with acute hypoxemic respiratory failure. *Am J Respir Crit Care Med* (2005) **172**(2):206–11. doi:10.1164/rccm.200405-625OC
12. Flori HR, Glidden DV, Rutherford GW, Matthay MA. Pediatric acute lung injury: prospective evaluation of risk factors associated with mortality. *Am J Respir Crit Care Med* (2005) **171**(9):995–1001. doi:10.1164/rccm.200404-544OC
13. Erickson S, Schibler A, Numa A, Nuthall G, Yung M, Pascoe E, et al. Acute lung injury in pediatric intensive care in Australia and New Zealand: a prospective, multicenter, observational study. *Pediatr Crit Care Med* (2007) **8**(4):317–23. doi:10.1097/01.PCC.0000269408.64179.FF
14. Hu X, Qian S, Xu F, Huang B, Zhou D, Wang Y, et al. Incidence, management and mortality of acute hypoxemic respiratory failure and acute respiratory distress syndrome from a prospective study of Chinese paediatric intensive care network. *Acta Paediatr* (2010) **99**(5):715–21. doi:10.1111/j.1651-2227.2010.01685.x
15. Khemani RG, Conti D, Alonzo TA, Bart RD III, Newth CJ. Effect of tidal volume in children with acute hypoxemic respiratory failure. *Intensive Care Med* (2009) **35**(8):1428–37. doi:10.1007/s00134-009-1527-z
16. Valentine SL, Sapru A, Higgerson RA, Spinella PC, Flori HR, Graham DA, et al. Fluid balance in critically ill children with acute lung injury. *Crit Care Med* (2012) **40**(10):2883–9. doi:10.1097/CCM.0b013e31825bc54d
17. López-Fernández Y, Azagra AM, de la Oliva P, Modesto V, Sánchez JI, Parrilla J, et al. Pediatric Acute Lung Injury Epidemiology and Natural History study: incidence and outcome of the acute respiratory distress syndrome in children. *Crit Care Med* (2012) **40**(12):3238–45. doi:10.1097/CCM.0b013e318260caa3
18. De Luca D, Piastra M, Chidini G, Tissieres P, Calderini E, Essouri S, et al. The use of the Berlin definition for acute respiratory distress syndrome during infancy and early childhood: multicenter evaluation and expert consensus. *Intensive Care Med* (2013) **39**(12):2083–91. doi:10.1007/s00134-013-3110-x
19. Khemani RG, Rubin S, Belani S, Leung D, Erickson S, Smith LS, et al. Pulse oximetry vs. PaO_2 metrics in mechanically ventilated children: Berlin definition of ARDS and mortality risk. *Intensive Care Med* (2015) **41**(1):94–102. doi:10.1007/s00134-014-3486-2
20. Zinter MS, Spicer A, Orwoll BO, Alkhouli M, Dvorak CC, Calfee CS, et al. Plasma angiopoietin-2 outperforms other markers of endothelial injury in prognosticating pediatric ARDS mortality. *Am J Physiol Lung Cell Mol Physiol* (2016) **310**(3):L224–31. doi:10.1152/ajplung.00336.2015
21. Rowan CM, Gertz SJ, McArthur J, Fitzgerald JC, Nitu ME, Loomis A, et al. Invasive mechanical ventilation and mortality in pediatric hematopoietic stem cell transplantation: a multicenter study. *Pediatr Crit Care Med* (2016) **17**(4):294–302. doi:10.1097/PCC.0000000000000673
22. Arnold JH, Anas NG, Luckett P, Cheifetz IM, Reyes G, Newth CJ, et al. High-frequency oscillatory ventilation in pediatric respiratory failure: a multicenter experience. *Crit Care Med* (2000) **28**(12):3913–9. doi:10.1097/00003246-200012000-00031
23. Rettig JS, Smallwood CD, Walsh BK, Rimensberger PC, Bachman TE, Bollen CW, et al. High-frequency oscillatory ventilation in pediatric acute lung injury: a multicenter international experience. *Crit Care Med* (2015) **43**(12):2660–7. doi:10.1097/CCM.0000000000001278
24. Arnold JH, Hanson JH, Toro-Figuero LO, Gutiérrez J, Berens RJ, Anglin DL. Prospective, randomized comparison of high-frequency oscillatory ventilation and conventional mechanical ventilation in pediatric respiratory failure. *Crit Care Med* (1994) **22**(10):1530–9. doi:10.1097/00003246-199422100-00006
25. Randolph AG, Wypij D, Venkataraman ST, Hanson JH, Gedeit RG, Meert KL, et al. Effect of mechanical ventilator weaning protocols on respiratory outcomes in infants and children: a randomized controlled trial. *JAMA* (2002) **288**(20):2561–8. doi:10.1001/jama.288.20.2561
26. Willson DF, Thomas NJ, Markovitz BP, Bauman LA, DiCarlo JV, Pon S, et al. Effect of exogenous surfactant (calfactant) in pediatric acute lung injury: a randomized controlled trial. *JAMA* (2005) **293**(4):470–6. doi:10.1001/jama.293.4.470
27. Curley MA, Hibberd PL, Fineman LD, Wypij D, Shih MC, Thompson JE, et al. Effect of prone positioning on clinical outcomes in children with acute lung injury: a randomized controlled trial. *JAMA* (2005) **294**(2):229–37. doi:10.1001/jama.294.2.229
28. Bronicki RA, Fortenberry J, Schreiber M, Checchia PA, Anas NG. Multicenter randomized controlled trial of inhaled nitric oxide for pediatric acute respiratory distress syndrome. *J Pediatr* (2015) **166**(2):365–9. doi:10.1016/j.jpeds.2014.10.011
29. Thomas NJ, Guardia CG, Moya FR, Cheifetz IM, Markovitz B, Cruces P, et al. A pilot, randomized, controlled clinical trial of lucinactant, a

peptide-containing synthetic surfactant, in infants with acute hypoxemic respiratory failure. *Pediatr Crit Care Med* (2012) **13**(6):646–53. doi:10.1097/PCC.0b013e3182517bec
30. Willson DF, Thomas NJ, Tamburro R, Truemper E, Truwit J, Conaway M, et al. Pediatric calfactant in acute respiratory distress syndrome trial. *Pediatr Crit Care Med* (2013) **14**(7):657–65. doi:10.1097/PCC.0b013e3182917b68
31. Curley MA, Wypij D, Watson RS, Grant MJ, Asaro LA, Cheifetz IM, et al. Protocolized sedation vs usual care in pediatric patients mechanically ventilated for acute respiratory failure: a randomized clinical trial. *JAMA* (2015) **313**(4):379–89. doi:10.1001/jama.2014.18399
32. Drago BB, Kimura D, Rovnaghi CR, Schwingshackl A, Rayburn M, Meduri GU, et al. Double-blind, placebo-controlled pilot randomized trial of methylprednisolone infusion in pediatric acute respiratory distress syndrome. *Pediatr Crit Care Med* (2015) **16**(3):e74–81. doi:10.1097/PCC.0000000000000349
33. Papazian L, Forel JM, Gacouin A, Penot-Ragon C, Perrin G, Loundou A, et al. Neuromuscular blockers in early acute respiratory distress syndrome. *N Engl J Med* (2010) **363**(12):1107–16. doi:10.1056/NEJMoa1005372
34. Guérin C, Reignier J, Richard JC, Beuret P, Gacouin A, Boulain T, et al. Prone positioning in severe acute respiratory distress syndrome. *N Engl J Med* (2013) **368**(23):2159–68. doi:10.1056/NEJMoa1214103
35. Bellani G, Laffey JG, Pham T, Fan E, Brochard L, Esteban A, et al. Epidemiology, patterns of care, and mortality for patients with acute respiratory distress syndrome in intensive care units in 50 countries. *JAMA* (2016) **315**(8):788–800. doi:10.1001/jama.2016.0291
36. Varadhan R, Weiss CO, Segal JB, Wu AW, Scharfstein D, Boyd C. Evaluating health outcomes in the presence of competing risks: a review of statistical methods and clinical applications. *Med Care* (2010) **48**(6 Suppl):S96–105. doi:10.1097/MLR.0b013e3181d99107
37. Azevedo LC, Park M, Salluh JI, Rea-Neto A, Souza-Dantas VC, Varaschin P, et al. Clinical outcomes of patients requiring ventilatory support in Brazilian intensive care units: a multicenter, prospective, cohort study. *Crit Care* (2013) **17**(2):R63. doi:10.1186/cc12594
38. Azoulay E, Lemiale V, Mokart D, Pène F, Kouatchet A, Perez P, et al. Acute respiratory distress syndrome in patients with malignancies. *Intensive Care Med* (2014) **40**(8):1106–14. doi:10.1007/s00134-014-3354-0
39. Piastra M, De Luca D, Pietrini D, Pulitanò S, D'Arrigo S, Mancino A, et al. Noninvasive pressure-support ventilation in immunocompromised children with ARDS: a feasibility study. *Intensive Care Med* (2009) **35**(8):1420–7. doi:10.1007/s00134-009-1558-5
40. Khemani RG, Newth CJ. The design of future pediatric mechanical ventilation trials for acute lung injury. *Am J Respir Crit Care Med* (2010) **182**(12):1465–74. doi:10.1164/rccm.201004-0606CI
41. Contentin L, Ehrmann S, Giraudeau B. Heterogeneity in the definition of mechanical ventilation duration and ventilator-free days. *Am J Respir Crit Care Med* (2014) **189**(8):998–1002. doi:10.1164/rccm.201308-1499LE
42. Schoenfeld DA, Bernard GR; ARDS Network. Statistical evaluation of ventilator-free days as an efficacy measure in clinical trials of treatments for acute respiratory distress syndrome. *Crit Care Med* (2002) **30**(8):1772–7. doi:10.1097/00003246-200208000-00016
43. Steinberg KP, Hudson LD, Goodman RB, Hough CL, Lanken PN, Hyzy R, et al. Efficacy and safety of corticosteroids for persistent acute respiratory distress syndrome. *N Engl J Med* (2006) **354**(16):1671–84. doi:10.1056/NEJMoa051693
44. The Acute Respiratory Distress Syndrome Network. Ventilation with lower tidal volumes as compared with traditional tidal volumes for acute lung injury and the acute respiratory distress syndrome. *N Engl J Med* (2000) **342**(18):1301–8.
45. Pollack MM, Holubkov R, Funai T, Berger JT, Clark AE, Meert K, et al. Simultaneous prediction of new morbidity, mortality, and survival without new morbidity from pediatric intensive care: a new paradigm for outcomes assessment. *Crit Care Med* (2015) **43**(8):1699–709. doi:10.1097/CCM.0000000000001081
46. Holubkov R, Clark AE, Moler FW, Slomine BS, Christensen JR, Silverstein FS, et al. Efficacy outcome selection in the therapeutic hypothermia after pediatric cardiac arrest trials. *Pediatr Crit Care Med* (2015) **16**(1):1–10. doi:10.1097/PCC.0000000000000272
47. Fanconi S, Kraemer R, Weber J, Tschaeppeler H, Pfenninger J. Long-term sequelae in children surviving adult respiratory distress syndrome. *J Pediatr* (1985) **106**(2):218–22. doi:10.1016/S0022-3476(85)80290-0
48. Effmann EL, Merten DF, Kirks DR, Pratt PC, Spock A. Adult respiratory distress syndrome in children. *Radiology* (1985) **157**(1):69–74. doi:10.1148/radiology.157.1.4034980
49. Weiss I, Ushay HM, DeBruin W, O'Loughlin J, Rosner I, Notterman D. Respiratory and cardiac function in children after acute hypoxemic respiratory failure. *Crit Care Med* (1996) **24**(1):148–54. doi:10.1097/00003246-199601000-00024
50. Golder ND, Lane R, Tasker RC. Timing of recovery of lung function after severe hypoxemic respiratory failure in children. *Intensive Care Med* (1998) **24**(5):530–3. doi:10.1007/s001340050607
51. Ben-Abraham R, Weinbroum AA, Roizin H, Efrati O, Augarten A, Harel R, et al. Long-term assessment of pulmonary function tests in pediatric survivors of acute respiratory distress syndrome. *Med Sci Monit* (2002) **8**(3):CR153–7.
52. Santschi M, Jouvet P, Leclerc F, Gauvin F, Newth CJ, Carroll CL, et al. Acute lung injury in children: therapeutic practice and feasibility of international clinical trials. *Pediatr Crit Care Med* (2010) **11**(6):681–9. doi:10.1097/PCC.0b013e3181d904c0
53. Santschi M, Randolph AG, Rimensberger PC, Jouvet P; Acute Lung Injury Mechanical Ventilation Investigators, Pediatric Acute Lung Injury and Sepsis Investigators Network, et al. Mechanical ventilation strategies in children with acute lung injury: a survey on stated practice pattern*. *Pediatr Crit Care Med* (2013) **14**(7):e332–7. doi:10.1097/PCC.0b013e31828a89a2
54. Quasney MW, López-Fernández YM, Santschi M, Watson RS; Pediatric Acute Lung Injury Consensus Conference Group. The outcomes of children with pediatric acute respiratory distress syndrome: proceedings from the Pediatric Acute Lung Injury Consensus Conference. *Pediatr Crit Care Med* (2015) **16**(5 Suppl 1):S118–31. doi:10.1097/PCC.0000000000000438
55. Moler FW, Silverstein FS, Holubkov R, Slomine BS, Christensen JR, Nadkarni VM, et al. Therapeutic hypothermia after out-of-hospital cardiac arrest in children. *N Engl J Med* (2015) **372**(20):1898–908. doi:10.1056/NEJMoa1411480
56. Ebrahim S, Singh S, Hutchison JS, Kulkarni AV, Sananes R, Bowman KW, et al. Adaptive behavior, functional outcomes, and quality of life outcomes of children requiring urgent ICU admission. *Pediatr Crit Care Med* (2013) **14**(1):10–8. doi:10.1097/PCC.0b013e31825b64b3
57. Aspesberro F, Mangione-Smith R, Zimmerman JJ. Health-related quality of life following pediatric critical illness. *Intensive Care Med* (2015) **41**(7):1235–46. doi:10.1007/s00134-015-3780-7
58. Davydow DS, Richardson LP, Zatzick DF, Katon WJ. Psychiatric morbidity in pediatric critical illness survivors: a comprehensive review of the literature. *Arch Pediatr Adolesc Med* (2010) **164**(4):377–85. doi:10.1001/archpediatrics.2010.10
59. Judge D, Nadel S, Vergnaud S, Garralda ME. Psychiatric adjustment following meningococcal disease treated on a PICU. *Intensive Care Med* (2002) **28**(5):648–50. doi:10.1007/s00134-002-1237-2
60. Davidson TA, Caldwell ES, Curtis JR, Hudson LD, Steinberg KP. Reduced quality of life in survivors of acute respiratory distress syndrome compared with critically ill control patients. *JAMA* (1999) **281**(4):354–60. doi:10.1001/jama.281.4.354
61. National Heart, Lung, and Blood Institute Acute Respiratory Distress Syndrome (ARDS) Clinical Trials Network, Wiedemann HP, Wheeler AP, Bernard GR, Thompson BT, Hayden D, et al. Comparison of two fluid-management strategies in acute lung injury. *N Engl J Med* (2006) **354**(24):2564–75. doi:10.1056/NEJMoa062200
62. National Heart, Lung, and Blood Institute Acute Respiratory Distress Syndrome (ARDS) Clinical Trials Network, Wheeler AP, Bernard GR, Thompson BT, Schoenfeld D, Wiedemann HP, et al. Pulmonary-artery versus central venous catheter to guide treatment of acute lung injury. *N Engl J Med* (2006) **354**(21):2213–24. doi:10.1056/NEJMoa061895
63. Triantafyllidis A, Velardo C, Chantler T, Shah SA, Paton C, Khorshidi R, et al. A personalised mobile-based home monitoring system for heart failure: the SUPPORT-HF Study. *Int J Med Inform* (2015) **84**(10):743–53. doi:10.1016/j.ijmedinf.2015.05.003
64. Deschildre A, Béghin L, Salleron J, Iliescu C, Thumerelle C, Santos C, et al. Home telemonitoring (forced expiratory volume in 1 s) in children with severe asthma does not reduce exacerbations. *Eur Respir J* (2012) **39**(2):290–6. doi:10.1183/09031936.00185310
65. Tseng KC, Wong AM, Hsu CL, Tsai TH, Han CM, Lee MR. The iFit: an integrated physical fitness testing system to evaluate the degree of physical fitness of the elderly. *IEEE Trans Biomed Eng* (2013) **60**(1):184–8. doi:10.1109/TBME.2012.2211357

66. Bekelman DB, Plomondon ME, Carey EP, Sullivan MD, Nelson KM, Hattler B, et al. Primary results of the Patient-Centered Disease Management (PCDM) for heart failure study: a randomized clinical trial. *JAMA Intern Med* (2015) **175**(5):725–32. doi:10.1001/jamainternmed.2015.0315
67. Ong MK, Romano PS, Edgington S, Aronow HU, Auerbach AD, Black JT, et al. Effectiveness of remote patient monitoring after discharge of hospitalized patients with heart failure: the Better Effectiveness After Transition-Heart Failure (BEAT-HF) randomized clinical Trial. *JAMA Intern Med* (2016) **176**(3):310–8. doi:10.1001/jamainternmed.2015.7712
68. Boyer SL, Silka MJ, Bar-Cohen Y. Current practices in the monitoring of cardiac rhythm devices in pediatrics and congenital heart disease. *Pediatr Cardiol* (2015) **36**(4):821–6. doi:10.1007/s00246-014-1090-4

21

Nutrition: A Primary Therapy in Pediatric Acute Respiratory Distress Syndrome

Bryan Wilson[1] and Katri Typpo[2]*

[1] Department of Emergency Medicine, University of Arizona College of Medicine, Tucson, AZ, USA, [2] Department of Pediatrics, Steele Children's Research Center, University of Arizona College of Medicine, Tucson, AZ, USA

***Correspondence:**
Katri Typpo
ktyppo@email.arizona.edu

Appropriate nutrition is an essential component of intensive care management of children with acute respiratory distress syndrome (ARDS) and is linked to patient outcomes. One out of every two children in the pediatric intensive care unit (PICU) will develop malnutrition or have worsening of baseline malnutrition and present with specific micronutrient deficiencies. Early and adequate enteral nutrition (EN) is associated with improved 60-day survival after pediatric critical illness, and, yet, despite early EN guidelines, critically ill children receive on average only 55% of goal calories by PICU day 10. Inadequate delivery of EN is due to perceived feeding intolerance, reluctance to enterally feed children with hemodynamic instability, and fluid restriction. Underlying each of these factors is large practice variation between providers and across institutions for initiation, advancement, and maintenance of EN. Strategies to improve early initiation and advancement and to maintain delivery of EN are needed to improve morbidity and mortality from pediatric ARDS. Both, over and underfeeding, prolong duration of mechanical ventilation in children and worsen other organ function such that precise calorie goals are needed. The gut is thought to act as a "motor" of organ dysfunction, and emerging data regarding the role of intestinal barrier functions and the intestinal microbiome on organ dysfunction and outcomes of critical illness present exciting opportunities to improve patient outcomes. Nutrition should be considered a primary rather than supportive therapy for pediatric ARDS. Precise nutritional therapies, which are titrated and targeted to preservation of intestinal barrier function, prevention of intestinal dysbiosis, preservation of lean body mass, and blunting of the systemic inflammatory response, offer great potential for improving outcomes of pediatric ARDS. In this review, we examine the current evidence regarding dose, route, and timing of nutrition, current recommendations for provision of nutrition to children with ARDS, and the current literature for immune-modulating diets for pediatric ARDS. We will examine emerging data regarding the role of the intestinal microbiome in modulating the response to critical illness.

Keywords: pediatric, ARDS, nutrition, intensive care

INTRODUCTION

There are direct nutritive and non-nutritive benefits of feeding patients with pediatric acute respiratory distress syndrome (pARDS). Adequate nutrition therapy in support of protein, energy, and micronutrient needs prevents loss of lean body mass, improves protein turnover for production of acute phase and immune proteins, prevents depletion of tissue antioxidant systems which occur with starvation, and is associated with improved 60-day mortality in mechanically ventilated, critically ill children (1–3). Adequate protein delivery prevents loss of respiratory and cardiac muscle function and is associated with increased ventilator-free days and improved mortality in pARDS (4). And, yet, median delivery of enteral nutrition (EN) remains 40–75% of goal over the first week of pediatric intensive care unit (PICU) hospitalization (3, 5–10). In addition, as protein synthesis rates are reliant upon adequate protein delivery, patients may not realize benefits of adjuvant therapies that rely on protein signaling if they fail to meet goal EN.

The gastrointestinal tract is a primary lymphoid organ, housing 70% of all immune cells with the ability to alter systemic inflammatory responses (11–14). Non-nutritive benefits of feeding, therefore, include downstream reduction in pro-inflammatory signaling to the lung (11, 15, 16). The gastrointestinal tract is an important target to improve lung inflammation, during pARDS, and subsequent patient outcomes. The intestinal epithelial barrier is a single-cell monolayer, which must absorb fluids and nutrients, interact with commensal organisms, and prevent entrance of pathogens and their toxic products (17). Intestinal barrier dysfunction has many downstream negative consequences. It is associated with bacterial translocation, endotoxemia, organ failure, immune dysfunction, and lung inflammation (13, 18, 19). The intestinal epithelial barrier, the host microbiome, and intestinal immune system interaction contribute to the pathophysiology of pARDS and present novel therapeutic targets.

Specific nutrients provided at pharmacological doses or nutrition supplemented with immune-modulating factors may directly impact lung pro-inflammatory cytokines and neutrophil accumulation in the setting of pARDS (20–22). Non-nutritive goals of feeding with either a standard enteral formula or an immune-modulating formula include maintenance of intestinal barrier functions, to alter or attenuate the immune or inflammatory responses in pARDS, and to modulate microbiome and/or host–microbe interactions. The host microbiome is emerging as an important mediator in chronic as well as acute inflammatory states. An understanding of the necessary and sufficient nutrition for each of these nutritive and non-nutritive benefits is important to determine the minimum necessary macronutrient and micronutrient delivery during each phase of pARDS to optimize patient outcomes. Optimizing nutritional therapy to delivery the right nutrition to the right patient at the right time is an excellent opportunity to improve outcomes in pARDS.

METABOLISM DURING PEDIATRIC CRITICAL ILLNESS

Currently, knowledge of the normal nutritional needs of children and of the metabolic response to critical illness guides recommendations and goals for nutritional support in pediatric patients (**Figure 1**). Critical illness and the associated inflammation and tissue injury alter metabolism by inducing a catabolic state, which may exacerbate pre-existing malnutrition (1, 23). Metabolism

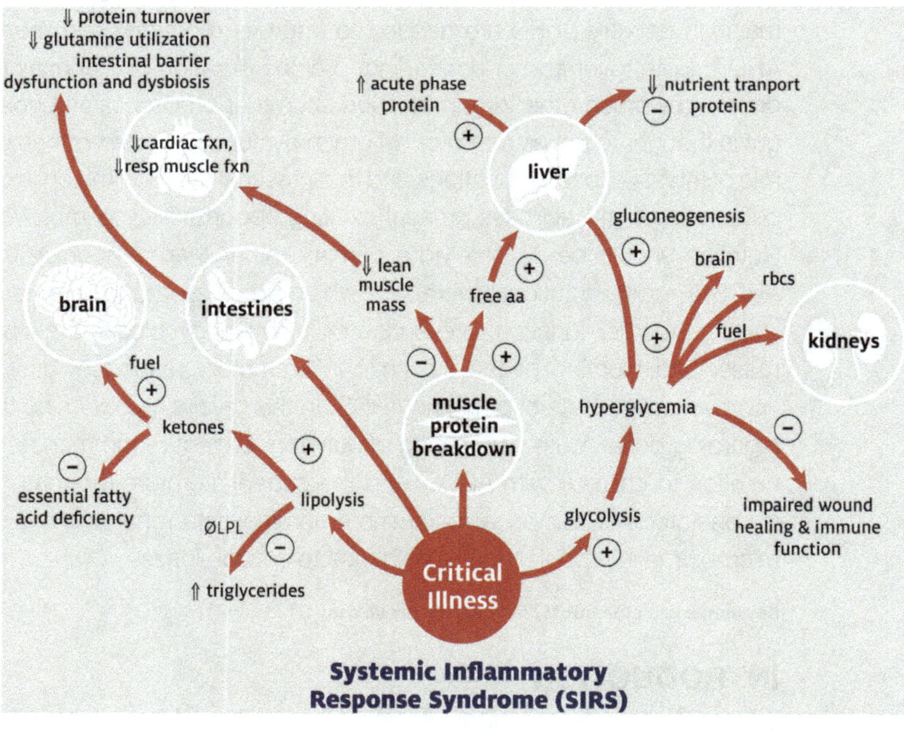

FIGURE 1 | Metabolic response to pediatric critical illness. + Acute adaptive response; – maladaptive consequence; ↑ increased; ↓ decreased. Abbreviations: LPL, lipoprotein lipase; aa, amino acids; resp, respiratory; rbc's, red blood cells. Adapted with permission from Graciano and Turner (25). Copyright from the Society of Critical Care Medicine.

shifts away from growth to support the production of acute phase proteins, enzymes, and glucose to facilitate recovery (23, 24). This is accomplished through glycolysis, lipolysis, and protein turnover with resulting hyperglycemia, ketone production, and breakdown of skeletal muscle protein (23, 24). This diversion of resources results in cessation of normal growth and development in pediatric patients (23, 24). Prolonged persistence of this catabolic state progressively depletes the body's nutritional resources, ultimately leading to muscle wasting, impaired cardiopulmonary function, decreased immune response, and poor wound healing (**Figure 1**). Pediatric patients (especially those with pre-existing nutritional, cardiopulmonary, or muscular disease) are particularly susceptible to these adverse sequelae due to their limited macronutrient and micronutrient reserves. In the setting of pARDS, this loss of lean body mass and diaphragmatic function is likely to amplify the severity of the patient's respiratory failure and prolong ventilator dependence.

PRE-EXISTING NUTRITIONAL STATUS MEDIATES PATIENT OUTCOMES

Patients who are undernourished prior to their critical illness experience worse outcomes (**Table 1**) (26). High quality research to understand how adequacy of nutrition delivery and premorbid nutritional status influences outcomes of pARDS is limited; however, pre-illness nutritional status and adequacy of macronutrient delivery early in critical illness are well established as risk factors for morbidity and mortality of critically ill patients in neonatal and pediatric populations (2, 3, 7, 10, 26–31). Malnutrition is both prevalent and incident in children hospitalized in the PICU; 30% of children admitted to the PICU have pre-existing acute or chronic malnutrition, and up to 58% of patients are discharged from the PICU malnourished (3, 6, 28). Even children who are well nourished prior to their critical illness may develop acute protein–energy malnutrition within 48 h of PICU admission due to limited protein and energy reserves in the setting of severe acute illness (6, 32–35). In a study of 1622 mechanically ventilated children, underweight nutritional status based on admission BMI *z*-score was associated with an increase in hospital-acquired infections, fewer ventilator-free days, and lower likelihood of hospital discharge (Hazard ratio 0.71, $p < 0.001$) (**Table 1**) (26). These high-risk patients may benefit from personalized nutritional strategies.

A growing percentage of children worldwide are now obese (39). While literature on the obese and critically ill pediatric patient is sparse, adult studies demonstrate a complex

TABLE 1 | Key observational studies of the impact of nutrition and nutritional status on patient outcomes in pediatric critical illness.

Study	Patient population	Exposure of interest	Outcomes
Timing, dose, route nutrition			
Wong et al. (4)	Multicenter study of 107 children with ARDS	Enteral calorie and protein adequacy	Reduction in ICU mortality in patients who received adequate calories (34.6 versus 60.5%, $p = 0.025$) and adequate protein (14.3 versus 60.2%, $P = 0.002$) compared with those who did not. Patients with adequate protein intake also had more VFDs [median (interquartile range), 12 (3.0–19.0) versus 0 (0.0–14.8) days; $p = 0.005$]
Mikhailov et al. (36)	Multicenter study of 5105 children 1 month to 18 years with PICU length of stay ≥96 h	Early enteral nutrition	Early EN was associated with lower odds of mortality (OR 0.52; 95% CI 0.34–0.76, $p = 0.001$). No significant differences in length of stay or duration of mechanical ventilation in patients exposed to early EN
Mehta et al. (2)	Multicenter study of 1245 children 1 month to 18 years requiring mechanical ventilation ≥48 h	Enteral protein adequacy	Adequacy of enteral protein intake was associated with lower 60-day mortality ($p < 0.001$)
Mehta et al. (3)	Multicenter study of 500 children 1 month to 18 years requiring mechanical ventilation >48 h	Enteral calorie adequacy	A higher percentage of goal energy intake *via* enteral nutrition route was significantly associated with lower 60-day mortality ($p = 0.002$). Mortality was higher in patients who received PN ($p = 0.008$). Patients admitted to units that utilized a feeding protocol had a lower prevalence of acquired infections and this association was independent of the amount of energy or protein intake
Nutritional status			
Bechard et al. (26)	Multicenter study of 1622 mechanically ventilated children from 2 study cohorts	Baseline nutritional status	BMI *z*-score classification as underweight or obese was associated with higher risk of hospital-acquired infections and lower likelihood of hospital discharge. Underweight children had a higher risk of mortality and fewer ventilator-free days
de Souza Menezes et al. (27)	Single-center prospective study of 385 critically ill children	Baseline nutritional status	Malnutrition (BMI *z*-score <−2 for weight for age, height for age, and BMI) was associated with greater length of mechanical ventilation and length of stay. Malnutrition was not a predictor of mortality
EN safety and complications			
Lopez-Herce et al. (37)	Single-center prospective, observational study of 526 critically ill children who received post-pyloric enteral nutrition (PEN)	Enteral nutrition	The stepwise multivariate logistic regression analysis showed that the most important factors associated with gastrointestinal complications were shock, epinephrine at a rate higher than 0.3 μg/kg/min and hypophosphatemia
Panchal et al. (38)	Multicenter study of 339 children admitted to PICU for ≥96 h and on vasoactive infusions	Enteral nutrition	Unadjusted mortality was lower in the patients exposed to EN (6.9 versus 15.9%, $p < 0.01$). Vasoactive-inotropic score did not differ between the two groups except on day 1. No difference in gastrointestinal outcomes between patients who did and did not receive enteral nutrition

VFD, ventilator-free days; BMI, body mass index.

relationship between obesity and clinical outcomes in critical illness and acute respiratory distress syndrome (ARDS) (40, 41). While overall morbidity, including ventilator days and length of hospitalization, is higher, mortality was lower (40, 41). A mortality benefit may be due to a higher nutritional reserve in the setting of prolonged catabolism (40, 41). Similar to risks in underweight children, obesity based on admission BMI *z*-score is associated with higher risk of hospital-acquired infections and lower likelihood of hospital discharge (hazard ratio 0.82, $p = 0.04$) (26). It is important to note, however, that obesity is not exclusive of malnutrition and that the obese child should receive the same consideration for nutritional supplementation (40). Both obese and underweight children are at increased risk compared with normal weight children for adverse outcomes while undergoing mechanical ventilation (26). For this reason, a nutritional support strategy should include early screening and diagnosis of malnutrition (42).

MACRONUTRIENT REQUIREMENTS DURING PEDIATRIC CRITICAL ILLNESS

Protein

Protein requirements during acute illness are increased secondary to the catabolic state generated to support the production of acute phase proteins, repair of tissue, and the production of immune proteins (1). Protein demands can be increased by as much as 100% in severe sepsis, and even mild stressors, such as routine surgery, may increase protein needs by 25% (1). Infants who require extracorporeal membrane oxygenation have the highest reported rates of protein turnover in the literature (43, 44). As discussed previously, prolongation of this catabolic state can result in decreased cardiopulmonary function secondary to breakdown of cardiac and respiratory muscle mass. While evidence currently suggests this catabolic process is not averted through protein intake but prevents recruitment of lean muscle mass as the major source of amino acids and increases protein production (44), and muscle mass can be preserved (45). Many adjuvant therapies, such as insulin for treatment of stress hyperglycemia, may be dependent upon adequate protein delivery to demonstrate efficacy. In 12 neonates on extracorporeal membrane oxygenation, Agus et al. found that improved protein balance as a result of insulin therapy was only seen in patients with adequate protein delivery (44). Liebau et al. was able to improve protein balance, but not protein breakdown, in 10 critically ill adults with sufficient enteral protein delivery (46). Concurrent supplementation with adequate carbohydrate and lipid energy sources improves protein turnover and synthesis, thereby potentiating this counterbalancing (47). The decrease in protein breakdown seen with glucose supplementation in simple starvation does not decrease muscle catabolism for gluconeogenesis in the response to critical illness (47). Excessive protein administration should also be avoided as it can result in morbidity, such as azotemia, metabolic acidosis, and neurologic dysfunction, particularly as the patient improves and catabolic turnover subsides (48, 49). Recommended protein requirements in critically ill children vary by age and range from 3 g/kg/day in infants to 1.5 g/kg/day in adolescents (50).

Energy

Energy sources in the form of lipids and carbohydrates are needed to facilitate protein synthesis and meet the patient's total energy expenditure, which includes the energy needed for basal metabolism, growth, physical activity, and thermogenesis. Critical illness induces an unpredictable metabolic state in children, which makes calculation of energy requirements challenging (51–53). Decisions regarding energy prescription are further complicated by the inherent variability both between patients and within the same patient over the course of their ICU stay, depending on ICU course and severity of illness (54–57). Age, anthropometric criteria, biochemical criteria, clinical exam, disease category, and stage of illness have all been demonstrated to be poor predictors of energy expenditure (51, 54). Other common factors that affect total energy expenditure and further complicate estimation are fever, sedation, temperature support, paralytics, and ventilator support. The variation in these factors requires frequent reassessment and adjustment of nutritional support to accurately meet but not exceed the patient's nutritional requirements.

Given the inaccuracy of estimating energy requirements and negative consequences of both over and underfeeding patients, PICU nutritional guidelines currently endorse precise and personalized determination of energy needs by indirect calorimetry (50). The ongoing physical growth and cognitive development of children suggest a need for early and adequate nutrition, supported by evidence that even short episodes of starvation during infancy result in permanent neurocognitive losses (29, 58, 59). One size does not fit most when it comes to delivery of calories and protein, and, in the absence of measured energy expenditure, patients may be easily misclassified as adequately fed when they are in fact over or underfed. This misclassification makes the relationship between energy adequacy and patient outcomes difficult to study. Indirect calorimetry is specifically recommended in the setting of outlier BMI (<5th percentile or >85th percentile), a >10% change in weight, prolonged ventilation, prolonged muscle relaxation, thermal injuries, oncologic diagnosis, or neurologic injury with dysautonomia (50). Indirect calorimetry is labor intensive, cannot be completed in all patients, and is poorly reimbursed but can be targeted to these high-risk populations, where precise nutritional support is likely to alter patient outcome (50). In the absence of measured resting energy expenditure, clinicians rely on predictive equations to assess calorie requirements and biomarkers to monitor for return of growth. Persistently elevated CRP and decreased prealbumin may indicate ongoing catabolism, while normalization may reflect transition to an anabolic state with a concurrent increase in energy requirements (60, 61).

Current recommendations are that energy should be prescribed as a balanced mixture of carbohydrates and lipids after appropriate provision of protein to preserve lean muscle mass (1). As previously discussed, the delivery of additional carbohydrates does not inhibit stress response gluconeogenesis and may result in hyperglycemia and its morbidities (poor wound healing, immune dysfunction, prolonged mechanical ventilation, and damage to the endothelial glycocalyx) (62–66). Lipid metabolism and turnover are increased in critical illness as fatty acids are used as a primary fuel source (64). Excessive carbohydrates are converted to lipids but generate carbon dioxide in the process, which may prolong mechanical ventilation (60). Infants and children generally have limited fat stores and are susceptible to the development of essential fatty acid deficiencies as early as 1 week into critical illness, if not receiving sufficient lipids. Lipids are generally limited to 30–40% of total calories. Balanced nutritional strategies provide sufficient macronutrients, while avoiding acute complications of excess protein, carbohydrate, and lipids.

ADEQUATE ENTERAL NUTRITION IS ASSOCIATED WITH REDUCED MORTALITY IN pARDS

Evidence for Early Nutritional Support

Prioritization of early EN is associated with improved tolerance of future EN and a reduction in morbidity from sepsis (3, 36). Murine studies demonstrated improved preservation of intestinal histoarchitecture and barrier function and improved local and remote organ immune function, with concurrent reduction in bacterial translocation and endotoxemia with the use of early EN (19, 67–70). Clinical research has demonstrated decreased mortality when EN is started within 48 h (30, 36). Specifically, one large study of >5000 patients with a PICU stay >96 h demonstrated a decrease in mortality associated with provision of at least 25% of goal calories within 48 h (**Table 1**) (36). Adult studies have examined starting EN within 6 h of ICU admission without complication (71). These lines of evidence support the preferential use of EN in pARDS when it is safe to do so, a recommendation supported by the 2015 Pediatric Acute Lung Injury Consensus Conference (72).

Evidence for Dose of Enteral Nutrition

Multiple retrospective studies demonstrate mortality benefit with improved adequacy of energy and protein provided during pediatric critical illness (**Table 1**) (2, 3, 36). In a prospective, international study of nutritional practices in 500 children ventilated for >48 h, Mehta et al. found that patients who received less than ⅓ of prescribed energy on average during the first 10 days after admission to the PICU had higher odds of mortality (3). An increase in prescribed energy by one tertile significantly decreased the odds of mortality. This relationship was only observed in patients with increased energy fed by the enteral route. ICUs, where a feeding guideline was in place, had overall lower hospital-acquired infection rates (3). Wong et al. examined 107 children with pARDS and identified that adequate energy and protein intake were associated with reduced mortality, while protein adequacy was also associated with increase ventilator-free days (4). These lines of evidence suggest that optimizing safe EN, rather than delivery of energy or protein *via* other routes of nutrition, is important for improving outcomes of pARDS.

Despite data regarding early nutritional adequacy and improved mortality, patients frequently fail to meet their calorie goals during the first week of illness with median intake generally falling at 40–75% due to multiple barriers to provision of EN (3, 5–10). Mechanisms for poor patient outcome in the setting of under nutrition relate to both nutritive and non-nutritive sequelae of inadequate EN. Direct nutritive consequences to under nutrition are largely due to inadequate protein substrate for production of acute phase and immune proteins, with subsequent loss of lean body mass. This may lead to loss of both respiratory and cardiac muscle and difficulty with ventilator weaning (**Figure 1**). Non-nutritive benefits of EN include improved intestinal barrier function, improved immune function, and maintenance of intestinal microbiome diversity. Appropriate targets to monitor these non-nutritive benefits are under development. Therefore, "optimal" nutrition can be defined in many ways depending on the target to define efficacy: sufficient energy and protein to meet metabolic demand, sufficient energy and protein to maintain lean body mass and functional recovery, sufficient energy and protein to maintain neurocognitive development, sufficient EN to maintain intestinal barrier functions, and adequate enteral composition to maintain microbiome diversity. The appropriate nutritional target in children with ARDS is not defined.

OVERFEEDING AND UNDERFEEDING ARE ASSOCIATED WITH WORSE OUTCOME IN PEDIATRIC CRITICAL ILLNESS

Studies in adults and animals suggest negative impact of excessive nutrition with difficulty with ventilator weaning and either a mortality benefit or non-inferiority with restricted caloric intake (**Table 2**) (73–79). Several retrospective studies in critically ill children identify overfeeding occurring in PICU patients with negative clinical consequences (53, 80). Overfeeding is associated with delayed ventilator weaning, lipogenesis, hepatic dysfunction, hyperglycemia, increased mortality, and prolonged hospitalization. Complications associated with underfeeding included delayed ventilator weaning, impaired protein synthesis, organ failure, and an increased risk of sepsis (7, 10, 24, 32). Several potential mechanisms exist for the negative impact of overfeeding on patient outcome, such as increase in carbon dioxide production, increased intolerance of EN and parenteral nutrition (PN), refeeding syndrome, azotemia and metabolic acidosis from excess protein administration, hepatic steatosis from excess glucose delivery, hyperglycemia, hypertriglyceridemia, and on the cellular level the suppression of autophagy (53, 62, 81, 82). Administration of PN early in the course of critical illness may suppress autophagy, a necessary form of programmed cell death, which aids in removal of damaged proteins and mitochondria and is thought to play a role in recovery after organ failure (83).

ADULT ICU GUIDELINES

American Society of Parenteral and Enteral Nutrition (ASPEN) Guidelines of the Provision and Assessment of Nutrition Support Therapy in the Adult Critically Ill Patient recommend that patients with ALI/ARDS receive either trophic or full EN over the first week of hospitalization. Even in adults, there is uncertainty regarding timing and dose of nutrition therapy. Evidence exists that hypocaloric nutritional strategies, experienced by the majority of patients, may not benefit specific subsets of the critically ill, such as in the setting of mechanical ventilation, severe burns, and surgery (111–113). Patients at high nutritional risk,

TABLE 2 | Key randomized, controlled trials in critical care nutrition 2006–2016.

Study	Patient population	Intervention/comparison	Outcomes
Dose, route, and timing			
Parenteral nutrition			
Fivez et al. (84)	Multicenter RCT involving 1440 critically ill children	PN at 24 h versus 1 week (EN initiated in both groups)	No difference in mortality. Fewer infections in late PN (10.7 versus 18.5%) group, shorter duration of mechanical ventilation ($p = 0.001$), fewer patients required renal replacement therapy ($p = 0.04$), shorter ICU stays ($p = 0.001$)
Harvey et al. (85)	Multicenter RCT of 2400 critically ill adults	Early PN versus Early EN up to 5 days after ICU admission in adults who could be enterally fed	No difference in 30- (33.1 versus 34.2%, $p = 0.57$) or 90-day mortality ($p = 0.4$). Reduced hypoglycemia, vomiting in the early PN group. No difference in treated infectious complications
Doig et al. (86)	Multicenter RCT of 1372 critically ill adults	Early PN versus standard care for patients with relative contraindications to early EN	No difference in 60-day mortality (21.5 versus 22.8%, $p = 0.6$). Early PN patients required fewer days of mechanical ventilation and experienced less muscle wasting
Heidegger et al. (87)	Multicenter RCT of 153 critically ill adults meeting <60% of caloric needs by EN on ICU day 3	Supplemental PN versus EN alone on days 4–8	Supplemental PN associated with higher percentage of energy target and fewer nosocomial infections
Casaer et al. (88)	Multicenter RCT of 2328 critically ill adults	PN at 48 h versus 1 week (EN initiated in both groups)	No difference in mortality. Fewer ICU infections (22.8 versus 26.2%, $p = 0.008$) in late PN group, smaller proportion of patients with >2 days of mechanical ventilation, median reduction of 3 days for renal replacement therapy ($p = 0.008$)
Dose of macronutrients			
Arabi et al. (89)	Multicenter RCT of 894 critically ill adults	Permissive underfeeding of non-protein calories (40 to 60% of goal) versus standard enteral feeding (75–100% of goal)	No difference in 90-day mortality (27.2 versus 28.9%, RR 0.94). No significant between-group differences for feeding intolerance, diarrhea, ICU-acquired infections, or length of stay
Braunschweig et al. (90)	Single-center RCT of 78 adults with acute lung injury	Intensive medical nutrition (>75% goal) versus standard nutritional support (~55% goal)	Significantly greater hospital mortality in intensive group (40 versus 16%, $p = 0.02$)
Rice et al. (91)	Multicenter RCT of 1000 adults with acute lung injury	Early trophic versus full enteral feeding	No difference in 28-day ventilator-free days (14.9 versus 15.0, $p = 0.89$) or 60-day mortality (23.2 versus 22.2%, $p = 0.77$). No differences in infectious complications between the groups. Initial trophic feeds were associated with less feeding intolerance
Gastric versus post-pyloric feeds			
Davies et al. (92)	Multicenter RCT of 181 critically ill and intubated adults with elevated gastric residuals	Continuation of gastric feeds versus transition to post-pyloric feeds	No clinically significant difference
Acosta-Escribano et al. (93)	Single-center RCT of 104 adults with severe traumatic brain injury	Gastric versus post-pyloric feeds	Lower incidence of pneumonia in post-pyloric groups OR 0.3 (95% CI 0.1–0.7, $p = 0.01$) and higher percentage of nutrional needs met (92 versus 84%, $p < 0.01$)
Hsu et al. (94)	Single-center RCT of 121 critically ill adults	Gastric versus post-pyloric feeds	Post-pyloric feeds associated with earlier achievement of nutritional goals, less vomiting, and less pneumonia
Early enteral nutrition			
Khorasani and Mansouri (95)	Single-center RCT of 688 burned children	EN at 3–6 h versus at 48 h	Early EN associated with decreased length of stay and mortality (12 versus 8.5%, $p < 0.05$)
Continuous versus bolus enteral nutrition			
MacLeod et al. (96)	Single-center prospective RCT of 164 critically ill adult trauma patients	EN as q 4 h boluses versus continuous drip	Intermittent regimen reached goal quicker with no difference in complications
Glycemic control			
NICE-SUGAR study investigators et al. (97)	Multicenter RCT of 6104 critically ill adults	Intensive glucose control (81–108 mg/dL) versus conventional contol (<180 mg/dL)	Higher mortality (OR 1.14; 95% CI, 1.02–1.28; $p = 0.02$) and more hypoglycemia (6.8 versus 0.5%, $p < 0.001$) in the intensive group

(Continued)

TABLE 2 | Continued

Study	Patient population	Intervention/comparison	Outcomes
Vlasselaers 2009 (98)	Single-center RCT of 317 critically ill infant and 383 critically ill children (700 total)	Intensive normoglycemia with target glucose 50–79 (infant)/70–100 (children) versus target glucose <214 mg/dL	Lower mortality (3 versus 6%, $p = 0.013$) despite more hypoglycemia (25 versus 1%, $p = 0.001$) in the intensive group
Van den Berghe et al. (99)	Single-center RCT of 1200 critically ill adults (medical)	Intensive glucose control (80–110 g/dL) versus conventional control (<180 mg/dL)	No difference in mortality but decreased acute kidney injury (5.9 versus 8.9%, $p = 0.04$), earlier weaning from mechanical ventilation ($p = 0.03$), and shorter hospital stay in intensive group ($p = 0.05$)
Immune modulation			
Glutamine and selenium, antioxidants			
Ziegler et al. (100)	Multicenter RCT of 150 critically ill adults	Alanyl–glutamine dipeptide (0.5 g/kg/d), proportionally replacing amino acids in PN versus standard PN (EN initated as tolerated)	No difference in clinical outcomes
Pérez-Bárcena et al. (101)	Multicenter RCT of 142 critically ill adults (trauma)	L-alanyl–L-glutamine dipeptide (0.5 g/kg body weight/day) supplementation for 5 days versus standard PN	No difference in clinical outcomes
Heyland et al. (102)	Multicenter RCT of 1223 critically ill adults	(L-alanyl–L-glutamine dipeptide at 0.5 g/kg body weight/day PN supplementation and 42.5 g of alanyl–glutamine and glycine–glutamine dipeptides EN supplementation) versus (500 μg of selenium intravenously + 300 μg of selenium, 20 mg of zinc, 10 mg of beta carotene, 500 mg of vitamin E, and 1500 mg of vitamin C orally) versus combination versus placebo	Higher mortality in those receiving glutamine (OR 1.28, CI 1.00–1.64, $p = 0.05$)
Carcillo et al. (103)	Multicenter RCT of 293 critically ill children	Enteral zinc, selenium, glutamine and IV metoclopramide (ZSGM) versus enteral WHEY protein and IV saline up to 28 days of ICU stay	No differences in time until first episode of nosocomial infection/sepsis (median WHEY 13.2 days versus ZSGM 12.1 days, $p = 0.29$) or the rate of nosocomial infection/sepsis (4.83/100 days WHEY versus 4.99/100 days ZSGM, $p = 0.81$)
Andrews et al. (104)	Multicenter RCT of 502 critically ill adults	Parenteral glutamine (20.2 g/day) or selenium (500 μg/day) or both for up to 7 days versus placebo	No affect on new infections or mortality except for a reduction in infections for patients receiving selenium for 5 or more days (OR 0.53, CI 0.30–0.93).
Angstwurm et al. (105)	Multicenter RCT of 189 adults with severe sepsis/SIRS	Selenium as 1000 μg of sodium-selenite over 30 min followed by continuous infusions of 1000 μg daily for 14 days versus placebo	Reduced mortality in the selenium group (OR 0.56; CI 0.32–1.00, $p = 0.049$)
Omega-3 fatty acids alone or in combination			
Grau-Carmona et al. (106)	Multicenter RCT of 159 critically ill adults	Total PN with a lipid emulsion containing 10% fish oil versus a fish oil-free lipid emulsion	Fish oil emulsion associated with decreased nosocomial infections (21.0 versus 37.2%, $p = 0.035$)
Kagan et al. (107)	Single-center RCT of 120 critically ill adults (trauma)	EN enriched with eicosapentaenoic acid, γ-linolenic acid, and antioxidants versus a non-enriched control formula initiated at time of admission	No significant difference in clinical outcomes
van Zanten et al. (108)	Multicenter RCT of 301 intubated adults	EN enriched with glutamine, omega-3 fatty acid, and antioxidants (experimental product, NV Nutricia, Zoetermeer) versus high-protein tube feed (Nutrison Advanced Protison, NV Nutricia, Zoetermeer)	No difference in infection rate and increased 6-month mortality associated with immunomodulatory EN (35 versus 54%, $p = 0.04$)
Jacobs et al. (22)	Multicenter RCT of 26 critically ill children with acute lung injury	EN supplemental with eicosapentaenoic acid, γ-linolenic acid, and antioxidants versus standard EN	Improved biochemical profile
Pontes-Arruda et al. (109)	Multicenter RCT of 115 critically ill adults	Immunomodulator EN with eicosapentaenoic acid and γ-linolenic acid (Oxepa) versus standard EN (Ensure Plus HN)	No significant difference in mortality but immunomodulatory EN associated with decreases in the severity of sepsis, cardiovascular failure, respiratory failure, mechanical ventilation, and length of stay
Radrizzani et al. (110)	Multicenter RCT of 326 critically ill adults	Immunomodulatory EN (Perative, 55% carbohydrate, 25% fat, 21% protein, 1.3 kcal/mL, containing per 100 mL: 0.8 g L-arginine, 0.15 g ω-3 fatty acids, 0.7 g ω-6 fatty acids, 2.9 mg vitamin E, 0.75 mg β-carotene, 2.2 mg zinc, and 7 μg selenium) versus PN (containing 59% carbohydrate, 23% fat, 18% protein, 1.2 kcal/mL)	No difference in mortality. Immunomodulatory EN associated with decreased progression to severe sepsis or septic shock (4.9 versus 13.1%, $p = 0.022$) and shorter ICU length of stay

defined as either undernourished or overnourished at baseline may benefit from a more aggressive nutritional strategy (114). The intensive nutrition in acute lung injury (INTACT) study was designed to deliver >75% of goal energy and protein needs daily to adult ICU patients *via* EN from date of diagnosis of ARDS to hospital discharge as compared with standard nutrition support (**Table 2**) (90). The INTACT study found increased mortality (40 versus 16%, $p = 0.02$) with aggressive nutritional support (85% of estimated energy expenditure) when compared with standard therapy (55% of estimated energy expenditure) and was stopped early (90). While impossible to apply directly to pediatric patients due to their different metabolic needs and ongoing growth and neurocognitive development, these data reinforce the powerful role nutrition exerts on patient outcome and highlight the need for rigorous research to identify the optimal timing and dose of calories and protein, tailored to narrowly defined patient populations.

Individualized nutritional therapies that are "just right" and meet, but do not exceed, needs are currently recommended by ASPEN guidelines for nutritional prescription in critically ill children (50). "Optimal" energy and protein targets remain elusive, and response to nutrition delivery is likely related to baseline nutritional risk and current diagnosis. Increased utilization of non-invasive ventilation (NIV) in pARDS is associated with worse nutritional adequacy, and nutrition-related outcomes for patients managed with NIV are unknown (115). We do not know if potential benefits to NIV are outweighed by risks related to underfeeding. Underfeeding is harmful, but overfeeding is equally harmful. Multiple clinical trials are criticized for comparing very underfed to underfed patients, or for overfeeding patients. At the heart of these controversies lies the difficultly in determining in real-time calorie and protein needs and response to nutritional intervention. Advances in body composition assessments that are practical during pARDS in ultrasound, bioelectrical impedance, CT imaging, and functional outcomes assessments to monitor lean body mass close monitoring of lean body mass during pARDS a possibility, but require further study (116–119).

ROUTE OF NUTRITION

Evidence for Gastric versus Post-pyloric Feeds

The decision to prescribe gastric or post-pyloric EN has limited evidence to provide guidance. A study of 74 critically ill children randomly assigned to gastric or post-pyloric feeds demonstrated no difference in complications, and patients receiving post-pyloric feeds received more of their prescribed calories (120). A large meta-analysis of adult patients with severe traumatic brain injury demonstrated a decreased risk of pneumonitis with post-pyloric feeds (121). Other researchers found an increased risk of gastrointestinal complications when post-pyloric feeds were used in septic patients or patients on epinephrine (**Table 1**) (37, 122). Institution-based policies regarding verification of enteral feeding tube position, particularly for post-pyloric feeds, may result in significant delays in initiation of feeds. No studies, so far, have specifically evaluated gastric versus post-pyloric feeds in the setting of pARDS.

Evidence Regarding Parenteral Nutrition

Current standard practice in the US is to reserve PN for situations in which EN fails or is not possible. This practice is rooted in retrospective evidence linking PN to increased risks of sepsis and mortality when compared with EN alone (3). Unfortunately, the evidence to guide clinical decisions is limited by current practice patterns. Because PN is reserved for the sicker patient who cannot tolerate EN, retrospective studies are likely confounded by variables that predict both increased PN use and mortality. The Pediatric Early versus Late Parenteral Nutrition in Intensive Care Unit (PEPaNIC) study was an international, multicenter, randomized, and controlled trial comparing early versus late initiation of PN in critically ill children (**Table 2**) (123). The PEPaNIC Trial tested the relationship between early and later PN supplementation in 1440 children from newborn to 17 years of age and found no difference in mortality between the two groups (84). This study was not limited to children with pARDS. A significantly increased rate of hospital-acquired infections (18.5 versus 10.7%) was present in patients in the early PN group as compared with the late PN group (84). However, characteristics of the study design limit the generalizability of this study to pARDS patients. The macronutrient dose was not controlled in the study, and central line utilization was not reported in experimental and control groups. The study patients were heterogeneous, and not exclusive to pARDS. Questions remain whether early PN is of benefit in pARDS. The potential benefit and/or harm from early PN is unclear, and the current clinical focus is to provide sufficient energy and protein preferentially by the enteral route until further studies are completed.

Research in neonatal intensive care unit supports the early use of at least low rates of EN to support bowel health in combination with PN to meet metabolic needs with the added advantage of fewer interruptions in nutrient delivery when PN is used (124). The use of this combination therapy, beginning with the first hours to days of life in preterm infants, has been associated with improved growth, improved neurodevelopment, improved EN tolerance, and decreased morbidity at both intermediate (18 months) and long-term (5 year) follow-up (30, 58, 59, 125). It remains unclear if older or term infants with ARDS might benefit from a similar early PN strategy with regard to short-term clinical and long-term neurocognitive outcomes. Research in the adult patient population have demonstrated mixed results with regard to days of mechanical ventilation and morbidity, such as infection and renal insufficiency (78, 86, 88). This is consistent with previous literature suggesting improved outcomes with calorie restriction in the adult population (78). Given the ongoing growth and development of pediatric patients, it is reasonable to question whether combination therapy with EN and PN in children with pARDS will see similar benefits to those demonstrated in the NICU population. Despite the results of the PEPaNIC study, equipoise remains in the pARDS population. The optimal macronutrient dose, timing, and formulation of EN and PN support has yet to be elucidated as increasing evidence demonstrates links between the immune system, homeostasis, and nutritional intake (121, 126–129).

Barriers to Nutritional Support

Barriers to adequate EN can be broadly categorized as medical contraindication, prescriber discomfort, and frequent interruption (7, 9, 130, 131). Subjective rather than objective decision-making continues regarding decisions to initiate, advance, or maintain EN. Medical contraindications can include a need for volume restriction, hemodynamic instability, and ill-defined feeding intolerance. Studies in hemodynamically unstable adults requiring vasopressors demonstrated lower mortality with early EN (132). While large database studies do not demonstrate increase in adverse intestinal outcomes in children fed enterally while on vasoactive infusions, children with hemodynamic instability who do experience complications of EN have worse outcomes than children not fed by the enteral route (38, 122). Provider concerns regarding complications of EN in the setting of hemodynamic instability are warranted (122). Research is needed to further clarify the risks of EN while on vasoactive infusions, to identify optimal dosing strategies in the setting of hemodynamic instability, and to develop biomarkers to monitor safety of EN so that we might minimize risk, minimize unnecessary practice variation, and maximizing EN to patients at low risk of intestinal complications.

Feeding intolerance is the most frequent cause of interruption to EN, particularly in the current practice environment of deferring PN in marked preference for full EN. There is immense variability in clinician assessment of feeding intolerance and frequently used clinical criteria, such as bowel sounds, abdominal exam, gastric residual volumes, and lactate levels have not been validated (9, 130, 133, 134). Feeding intolerance occurs in 43–57% of critically ill children (9, 135). Even the definition of feeding intolerance is widely variable, and the natural history of bowel function in critical illness is yet to be fully elucidated (136, 137). Delayed gastric emptying and poor intestinal motility are causes of feeding intolerance, and, if left untreated, are impediments to achievement of goal EN. Delayed gastric emptying occurs in up to 50% percent of critically ill children, yet remains under recognized as a source of feeding intolerance (138). Promotility agents are commonly used for both gastric and intestinal dysmotility during pediatric critical illness, but only erythromycin and metoclopramide are currently approved in the US. Newer promotility agents, such as cholecystokinin receptor antagonists, ghrelin, and methylnaltrexone, in the setting of opioid-induced dysmotility, require further research in children with pARDS, but show promise to improve EN tolerance (138, 139). The development of validated tools for the diagnosis and monitoring of feeding intolerance represents an opportunity to significantly improve care in PICU patients by decreasing barriers to nutritional support. Biomarker-based guidelines for the initiation, advancement, and maintenance of EN are under development (140). Depending on hospital policies and local practice patterns, procedures are also a frequent cause of held EN and interruption of nutritional support despite an absence of data to guide these decisions (9). NIV and intensive therapies, such as extracorporeal membrane oxygenation, are in particular associated with nutritional interruption (141, 142). In adult ICU's, improved nutritional adequacy is reported when volume-based daily feeds are ordered, rather than an hourly rate (143). Volume-based orders accommodate 4–6 h of NPO status daily with the volume of EN delivered over 18–20 h, but larger studies are needed to understand the clinical outcome of a volume-based EN strategy in pARDS. A currently enrolling clinical trial, continuous versus bolus nasogastric feeding for mechanically ventilated pediatric patients (Clinical Trials ID: NCT02566070), will evaluate feeding intolerance and nutritional adequacy with two gastric feeding strategies. Consideration should be given to early initiation of a bowel regimen to prevent constipation and subsequent feeding intolerance while avoiding diarrhea and malabsorption. Implementation of an early EN guideline improved percent of goal energy and protein achieved in multiple retrospective studies, likely due to perceived emphasis on nutrition in a particular PICU (144, 145).

Glycemic Control

Literature in the adult population demonstrated compelling early evidence for significant decreases in morbidity and mortality with tight glycemic control (146). Subsequent research has demonstrated no benefit, but these results are drawn into question by large differences in mean glucose level and the use of point-of-care glucose testing rather than the arterial blood gas analysis used in the initial study (147–149). The negative impact of poor glycemic control is supported by current pediatric research, but the ideal target for blood glucose ranges has yet to be established (98, 150). The Heart And Lung Failure – Pediatric INsulin Titration (HALF-PINT) trial (Clinical Trials ID: NCT01565941) is a multicenter, randomized clinical treatment trial comparing effectiveness of tight glycemic control to a target range of 80–110 mg/dL versus a target range of 150–180 mg/dL.

THE GUT AS THE MOTOR FOR ARDS

There are many research opportunities to improve nutritional supplementation for critically ill patients in general as well as specifically within the framework of pARDS. Emerging research continues to demonstrate the role of gut dysfunction in the development of ARDS (13, 151). Deitch proposed the "gut lymph" hypothesis, whereby, the injured gut allows translocation of bacteria and bacterial products and liberates cytokines and chemokines, which act *via* the lymphatic duct to activate alveolar macrophages and contribute to pathogenesis of ARDS (152). Clark and Coopersmith proposed the "intestinal crosstalk" theory whereby the intestinal microbiota, immune system, and intestinal epithelial barrier interact and, when dysregulated, worsen systemic inflammation (153–155). Loss of balance in this "crosstalk" may lead to ARDS and is supported by emerging animal and human data examining the microbiome in critical illness. Modulation of intestinal barrier function and microbiome remain novel targets to improve outcomes in pARDS.

Several minimally invasive plasma biomarkers show promise in guiding initiation, titration, and continuation of EN by objectively assessing intestinal epithelial structure and function as well as assessing for the translocation of bacteria and bacterial products (**Table 3**) (156–158). The intestinal epithelial barrier is a single-cell monolayer tasked with competing roles to absorb nutrients, interact with commensal organisms, and limit entrance of pathogens and their products (**Figure 2**) (159, 160). It is the largest surface in the body in contact with the external environment. Intestinal barrier dysfunction is associated with the pathogenesis of multiple organ dysfunction, translocation of bacteria and endotoxin, and loss of remote organ immune function (19, 159, 161). Enteral feeding of at least 15% of goal calories restores intestinal barrier function in murine models of critical illness (69). The minimum dose of EN required to maintain intestinal barrier function in children with pARDS is unknown. Biomarkers to monitor intestinal barrier function could guide provider decisions regarding the minimum necessary dose of enteral feeding. In a study of 20 children after cardiopulmonary bypass, biomarker concentrations were associated with symptoms of feeding intolerance (140). Biomarker-based decision rules for initiation, advancement, and maintenance of EN represent an opportunity to reduce practice variation and improve success in achieving and maintaining nutritional goals. The development of biomarkers to accurately and easily measure the catabolic and anabolic balance of the metabolic system is another area of ongoing research which will assist clinicians to more accurately develop nutritional prescriptions (46).

TABLE 3 | Minimally invasive plasma biomarker candidates to assess intestinal barrier function.

Biomarker	Site specificity	Relevant data
Intestinal fatty acid-binding protein (I-FABP or FABP2)	Enterocytes of the small and large intestine	Plasma concentration correlates with histological phases of enterocyte injury after ischemia-reperfusion and is a marker of acute enterocyte damage (156, 157). Predictive of poor outcome if elevated after refeeding infants with NEC (158)
Liver fatty acid-binding protein (L-FABP)	Enterocytes of the small and large intestine, hepatocytes	Plasma concentration discriminates infants with sepsis versus NEC (162)
Claudin 3	Apical tight junction complex	Strong correlation between plasma claudin 3 and enterocyte tight junction loss in rat hemorrhagic shock model, human necrotizing enterocolitis (163, 164). Ubiquitous in lung tight junctions but lung injury does not cause elevation in plasma levels
Citrulline	Mature enterocytes of small intestine, colon	Manufactured in mitochondria of mature enterocytes. Validated as a biomarker for functional enterocyte mass in short bowel syndrome, HIV patients, stem cell transplant patients, graft-versus-host disease, and in children after bowel resection (165–171)
Trefoil Factor 3	Intestinal goblet and mucin cells	Differentiates between surgical and non-surgical NEC in preterm infants and assess disease activity in inflammatory bowel disease (162, 172)

NEC, necrotizing enterocolitis; HIV, human immunodeficiency virus.

INTESTINAL MICROBIOME MAY SHAPE IMMUNE RESPONSES

Technological advances in computing power and analytic techniques over the last decade make the study of the human microbiome possible (173). In the human body, bacterial cells exceed human cells in number and perform many essential functions, such as production of short chain fatty acids and vitamins (vitamin K), which aid the human host (174). The developmental maturation of the human microbiome is poorly understood, but it reaches adult patterns by 2–4 years of age (175). Dysbiosis occurs when the symbiotic relationship between human and microbial populations is disturbed and may result in reduced microbiome diversity. Reduced microbiome diversity during infancy, a critical time period during microbiome development, may have lasting consequences on the development of several chronic diseases (176). Murine models where antibiotics are provided during infancy, demonstrate rapid and permanent alteration of metabolic phenotype *via* transient reduction in intestinal microbiome diversity (176–178). In contrast, an increased microbiome diversity in human infants enhances maturation of the intestinal mucosal immune system, which can influence LPS responsiveness at 1 year of age in humans (179). Thus, normal metabolic and immune imprinting by essential "keystone" microbes, which can be altered by early antibiotic exposures, may have long-term consequences on immune response to critical illness and risk of chronic illness. This emerging field has the potential to shift our targets with regard to control of both acute and chronic inflammation from modulation of human cells to modulation of the bacterial within us. The gastrointestinal microbiota is implicated in control of inflammation in the lung (180). Diet is a potent determinant of intestinal microbiome diversity and, in murine models, trumps genetic background (181). Carmody et al., demonstrated, in a murine model, that rapid changes in diet resulted in rapid shifts in microbial composition (181). As diet is an essential determinant of microbiome diversity and alters lung inflammation, dietary manipulation of the gastrointestinal microbiome may be a new target for treatment of pARDS. We do not know how medical diets alter the intestinal microbiome during pARDS, nor do we understand the short or long-term consequences of nutritional, probiotic, or pre-biotic interventions.

IMMUNONUTRITION

Immunonutrition is well tolerated and results in improved pro-inflammatory cytokine profiles, but is not associated with clear clinical outcome benefits (182). While small single-center studies of isolated pharmaconutrients showed promise, multiple combination nutritional and pharmacologic additives in critically ill adults aimed at modulating the inflammatory and immune response have not shown benefits (**Table 2**) (183, 184). Specific supplements that have been explored include several antioxidants, arginine, glutamine, metoclopramide, ω-3 fatty acids, zinc, and selenium (103, 185–190). The randomized comparative effectiveness pediatric critical illness stress-induced immune suppression (CRISIS) prevention trial examined the effect in critically ill children of daily enteral zinc, selenium, glutamine,

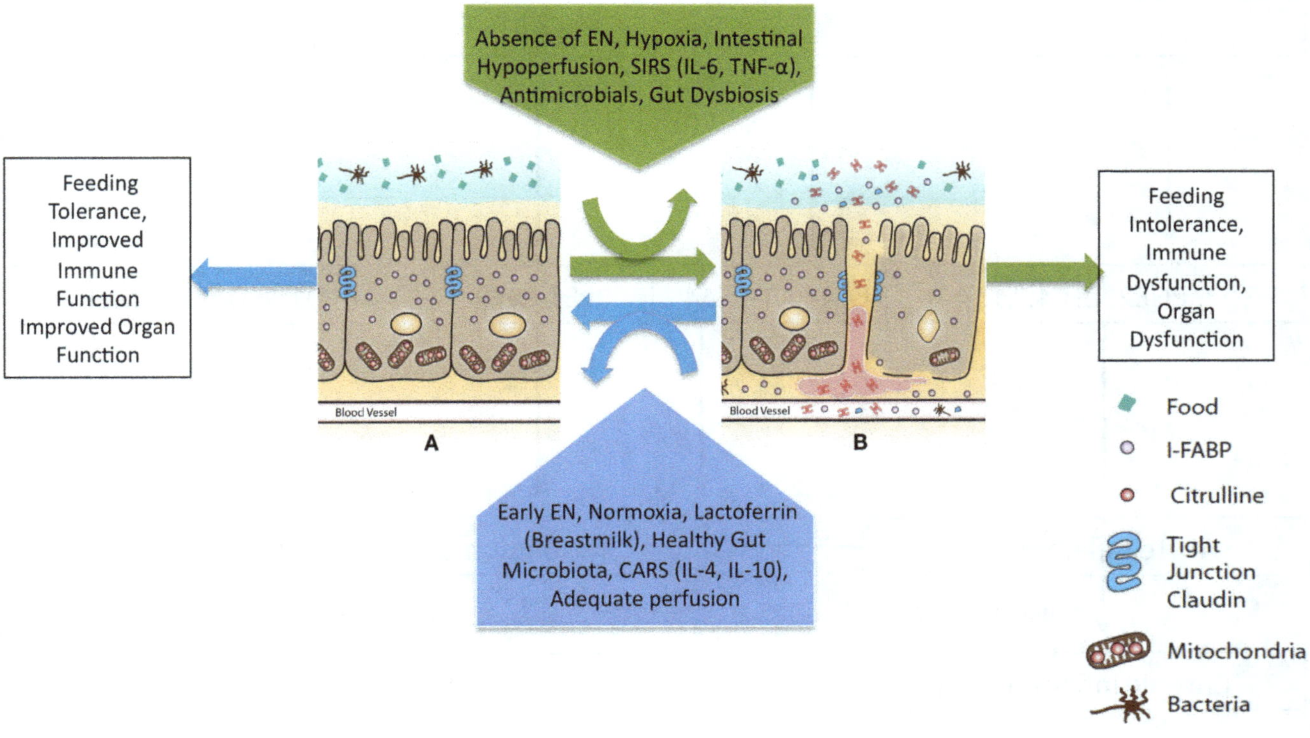

FIGURE 2 | Theoretical framework to maintain intestinal barrier dysfunction in pARDS. EN, enteral nutrition; SIRS, systemic inflammatory response syndrome; CARS, compensatory anti-inflammatory response syndrome. Primary determinants of intestinal barrier function are the apical tight junction complex and the intestinal epithelial cells. Modifiable clinical factors known to modulate intestinal barrier function include EN and antimicrobials. Specific targets for perfusion and oxygenation to improve intestinal barrier funct on in the setting of pARDS are unknown. The balance of forces will lead to intestinal barrier **(A)** function or **(B)** dysfunction and a downstream clinical phenotype with either improved or worsened remote organ (lung) function.

and IV metoclopramide on incidence of nosocomial infections. No difference was seen between the two groups, and the trial was stopped early due to futility (103). Multiple combination nutritional and pharmacologic additives in critically ill adults aimed at modulating the inflammatory and immune response have been trialed, but have generally not shown any benefits (50, 191). The optimal formulation of lipids is an area of active research with continued focus on the role of ω-3 polyunsaturated fatty acids (PUFAs).

OMEGA-3 POLYUNSATURATED FATTY ACIDS

The use of ω-3 PUFAs as a nutritional adjuvant have evidence suggesting they may reduce the pro-inflammatory state in ARDS, but a recent systematic review and meta-analysis looking specifically at ARDS patients in the adult ICU found no benefit in clinical outcomes (107, 192–197). The rationale for ω-3 PUFAs is that they may be beneficial in ARDS as they would compete with ω-6 PUFAs, decrease the synthesis of pro-inflammatory eicosanoids, increase production of anti-inflammatory lipid mediators, such as resolvins and protectins, decrease in chemotaxis, decrease reactive oxygen species (ROS) and pro-inflammatory cytokines, and decrease leukocyte binding and activation through decreased expression of adhesion molecules (**Figure 3**) (192).

Jacobs et al. evaluated the feasibility of ω-3 PUFAs (eicosapentaenoic acid + γ-linolenic acid) in children with ALI and ARDS and examined the impact of ω-3 PUFAs on plasma phospholipid fatty acid concentrations (22). They found that delivery of nutrition enriched with eicosapentaenoic acid + γ-linolenic acid was feasible and resulted in an anti-inflammatory fatty acid profile (22). This study is supportive of future work in this area in children. Whether a change in anti-inflammatory fatty acid profile will improve clinical outcomes is unclear, but promising. Methodological challenges in several adult trials limit conclusions regarding ω-3 PUFAs in adult patients with ARDS (192). Specifically, studies are heterogeneous, and, in some, the control diet was pro-inflammatory.

Several ω-3 PUFA-derived mediators are potential targets to resolve the inflammatory response in the setting of pARDS (**Figure 3**). Alveolar edema and neutrophil recruitment and activation are early events in ARDS. Resolvins, protectins, and maresins are lipid-derived mediators, and several resolvins are emerging as potential therapeutic targets for resolution of ARDS (**Figure 3**) (20, 21). These resolvins are derived from the ω-3 PUFAs docosahexaenoic acid (DHA) and eicosapentaenoic acid (EPA). Eickmeier et al. found that aspirin-triggered resolvin D1 reduces mucosal inflammation and promotes resolution in a murine model of acute lung injury (21). Aspirin-triggered RV D1 decreased lung inflammation and promoted acute lung injury

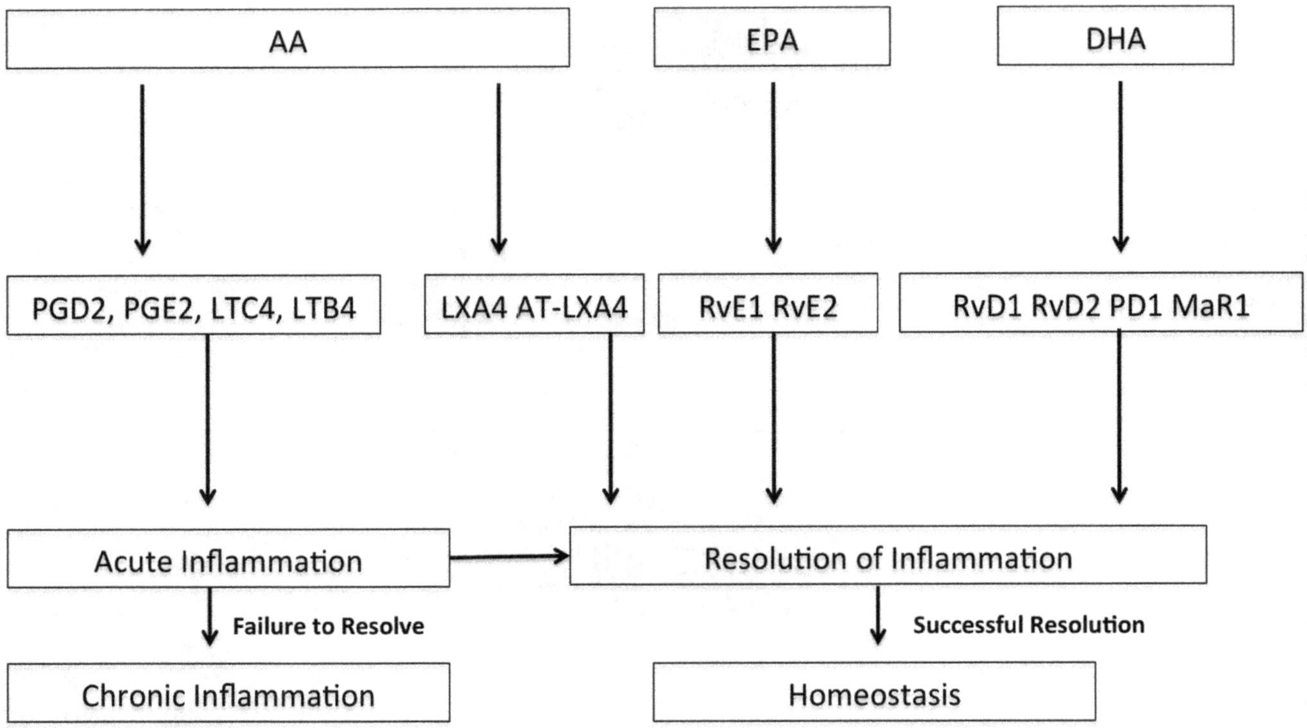

FIGURE 3 | Pathways of selected downstream lipid mediators derived from arachadonic acid (AA), docosahexaenoic acid (DHA), and eicosapentaenoic acid (EPA) for resolution of acute inflammation. DHA and EPA are ω-3 fatty acids. Adapted with permission from Serhan and Petasis (198); PGD2, prostaglandin D2; PGE2, prostaglandin E2; LTC4, leukotriene C4; LTB4, leukotriene B4; LXA4, lipoxin A4; AT-LXA4, aspirin-triggered lipoxin A4; RvE1, resolvin E1; RvE2, resolvin E2; RvD1, resolvin D1, RvD2, resolvin D2; PD1, protectin D1; MaR1, maresin 1.

resolution shortly after injury in an hydrochloric acid model of ARDS by enhancing restitution of barrier integrity, decreasing circulating neutrophil–platelet heterotopic interactions, and regulating inflammatory mediators and nuclear factor-κB (NF-κB) activation (21). Seki et al. found that resolvin E1 protected mice from bacterial pneumonia and acute lung injury with pre-treatment by decreased lung neutrophil accumulation, enhanced microbial clearance, decrease in lung pro-inflammatory mediators, and improved survival (20).

VITAMIN D

Recent evidence suggests an association between vitamin D levels and the risk of ARDS (199–201). Vitamin D deficiency is associated with impaired pulmonary function and increased incidence of viral and bacterial infections and inflammatory disease, including asthma and COPD (202–204). Mechanisms for these associations are unknown, but vitamin D plays a role in macrophage, lymphocyte, and epithelial cell function, critical to ARDS pathophysiology (200, 205).

SUMMARY

There are currently limited data to guide nutritional strategies in the critically ill pediatric patient and an absence of data targeted specifically at pARDS (**Tables 2** and **3**). Current strategies rely on the application of adult data, knowledge of the metabolic derangements caused by critical illness, and knowledge of the nutritional requirements of healthy children. The generally accepted strategy centers on the early identification of need for nutritional supplementation and early initiation of EN targeted toward fulfillment of nutritional goals and implemented by a collaborative, multidisciplinary treatment team. Indirect calorimetry is a recommended adjunct to ensure adequate, but not excessive, nutritional support is supplied. Early prescription of a bowel regimen to limit constipation while avoiding diarrhea is also recommended (50). PN is currently reserved for patients in whom EN is contraindicated or limited, though its routine use as a supplement to EN is an area ripe for research. Before we evaluate the role of immunonutrition to improve outcomes of pARDS, fundamental questions regarding protein and energy requirements during pARDS remain: if delivery should be based on premorbid nutritional risk and if under, normo, or even overfeeding might be beneficial at different stages of illness. Given the mortality benefit of nutritional adequacy on pARDS, it may prove challenging to identify benefits of adjuvant nutritional therapies, unless they are overlaid upon a foundation of adequate macronutrient delivery. Once fundamental questions regarding optimal timing, dose, and route of macronutrient delivery are answered for pARDS, investigations centered on immunonutrition to further improve patient outcomes are appropriate. Systematic investigations to determine the impact of each pharmaconutrient separately and in combination during pARDS are necessary.

In the future, intensivists will likely employ distinct and highly personalized nutritional therapies based on patient premorbid nutritional risk, admission diagnosis, severity of illness, measured energy expenditure, active monitoring of lean body mass, and the composition of patient intestinal microbiome. A select group of high-risk patients are likely to experience benefit from an intensive and personalized, titrated nutritional plan. Long-stay patients, patients with ARDS, sepsis, burns, or preexisting severe malnutrition are most likely to have improved outcomes if nutrition is closely monitored. Intensive nutritional therapies will likely be titrated daily to meet energy and protein needs. Nutritional therapies, monitoring, and impact on meaningful patient outcomes are likely to change dramatically in the next decade as we understand the role of the microbiome in regulating both intestinal health and also the inflammatory response to pARDS. We may require nutritional or "metabolic" teams to precisely tailor metabolic support to meet, but not exceed, energy, protein, and micronutrient needs, preserve lean body mass, the microbiome, the virome, and intestinal barrier functions. Nutrition is fundamental to provision of critical care services, and, with an understanding of the complex role it plays in illness and health, we will be able to design effective clinical trials of nutritional interventions as primary therapies for pARDS.

AUTHOR CONTRIBUTIONS

Dr. BW and Dr. KT contributed equally to the conception, review of literature, writing, and editing of this manuscript. Both authors approve of the final submitted version of this manuscript.

REFERENCES

1. American Academy of Pediatrics, Committee on Nutrition, Barness LA. *Pediatric Nutrition Handbook*. 6th ed. Elk Grove Village, IL: American Academy of Pediatrics (2009).
2. Mehta NM, Bechard LJ, Zurakowski D, Duggan CP, Heyland DK. Adequate enteral protein intake is inversely associated with 60-d mortality in critically ill children: a multicenter, prospective, cohort study. *Am J Clin Nutr* (2015) 102:199–206. doi:10.3945/ajcn.114.104893
3. Mehta NM, Bechard LJ, Cahill N, Wang M, Day A, Duggan CP, et al. Nutritional practices and their relationship to clinical outcomes in critically ill children – an international multicenter cohort study*. *Crit Care Med* (2012) 40:2204–11. doi:10.1097/CCM.0b013e31824e18a8
4. Wong JJ, Han WM, Sultana R, Loh TF, Lee JH. Nutrition delivery affects outcomes in pediatric acute respiratory distress syndrome. *JPEN J Parenter Enteral Nutr* (2016). doi:10.1177/0148607116637937
5. de Neef M, Geukers VG, Dral A, Lindeboom R, Sauerwein HP, Bos AP. Nutritional goals, prescription and delivery in a pediatric intensive care unit. *Clin Nutr* (2008) 27:65–71. doi:10.1016/j.clnu.2007.10.013
6. Hulst J, Joosten K, Zimmermann L, Hop W, van Buuren S, Büller H, et al. Malnutrition in critically ill children: from admission to 6 months after discharge. *Clin Nutr* (2004) 23:223–32. doi:10.1016/S0261-5614(03)00130-4
7. Hulst JM, Joosten KF, Tibboel D, van Goudoever JB. Causes and consequences of inadequate substrate supply to pediatric ICU patients. *Curr Opin Clin Nutr Metab Care* (2006) 9:297–303. doi:10.1097/01.mco.0000222115.91783.71
8. Malakouti A, Sookplung P, Siriussawakul A, Philip S, Bailey N, Brown M, et al. Nutrition support and deficiencies in children with severe traumatic brain injury. *Pediatr Crit Care Med* (2012) 13:e18–24. doi:10.1097/PCC.0b013e31820aba1f
9. Mehta NM, McAleer D, Hamilton S, Naples E, Leavitt K, Mitchell P, et al. Challenges to optimal enteral nutrition in a multidisciplinary pediatric intensive care unit. *JPEN J Parenter Enteral Nutr* (2010) 34:38–45. doi:10.1177/0148607109348065
10. Pollack MM, Ruttimann UE, Wiley JS. Nutritional depletions in critically ill children: associations with physiologic instability and increased quantity of care. *JPEN J Parenter Enteral Nutr* (1985) 9:309–13. doi:10.1177/014860718 5009003309
11. Rendon JL, Choudhry MA. Th17 cells: critical mediators of host responses to burn injury and sepsis. *J Leukoc Biol* (2012) 92:529–38. doi:10.1189/jlb.0212083
12. Ichinohe T, Pang IK, Kumamoto Y, Peaper DR, Ho JH, Murray TS, et al. Microbiota regulates immune defense against respiratory tract influenza A virus infection. *Proc Natl Acad Sci U S A* (2011) 108:5354–9. doi:10.1073/pnas.1019378108
13. Sodhi CP, Jia H, Yamaguchi Y, Lu P, Good M, Egan C, et al. Intestinal epithelial TLR-4 activation is required for the development of acute lung injury after trauma/hemorrhagic shock via the release of HMGB1 from the gut. *J Immunol* (2015) 194:4931–9. doi:10.4049/jimmunol.1402490
14. Galperin C, Gershwin ME. Immunopathogenesis of gastrointestinal and hepatobiliary diseases. *JAMA* (1997) 278:1946–55. doi:10.1001/jama.278.22.1946
15. Kudsk KA. Effect of route and type of nutrition on intestine-derived inflammatory responses. *Am J Surg* (2003) 185:16–21. doi:10.1016/S0002-9610(02)01146-7
16. Janu P, Li J, Renegar KB, Kudsk KA. Recovery of gut-associated lymphoid tissue and upper respiratory tract immunity after parenteral nutrition. *Ann Surg* (1997) 225:707–15; discussion 15–7. doi:10.1097/00000658-199706000-00008
17. Turner JR. Intestinal mucosal barrier function in health and disease. *Nat Rev Immunol* (2009) 9:799–809. doi:10.1038/nri2653
18. Pathan N, Burmester M, Adamovic T, Berk M, Ng KW, Betts H, et al. Intestinal injury and endotoxemia in children undergoing surgery for congenital heart disease. *Am J Respir Crit Care Med* (2011) 184:1261–9. doi:10.1164/rccm.201104-0715OC
19. Fukatsu K, Zarzaur BL, Johnson CD, Lundberg AH, Wilcox HG, Kudsk KA. Enteral nutrition prevents remote organ injury and death after a gut ischemic insult. *Ann Surg* (2001) 233:660–8. doi:10.1097/00000658-200105000-00010
20. Seki H, Fukunaga K, Arita M, Arai H, Nakanishi H, Taguchi R, et al. The anti-inflammatory and proresolving mediator resolvin E1 protects mice from bacterial pneumonia and acute lung injury. *J Immunol* (2010) 184:836–43. doi:10.4049/jimmunol.0901809
21. Eickmeier O, Seki H, Haworth O, Hilberath JN, Gao F, Uddin M, et al. Aspirin-triggered resolvin D1 reduces mucosal inflammation and promotes resolution in a murine model of acute lung injury. *Mucosal Immunol* (2013) 6:256–66. doi:10.1038/mi.2012.66
22. Jacobs BR, Nadkarni V, Goldstein B, Checchia P, Ayad O, Bean J, et al. Nutritional immunomodulation in critically ill children with acute lung injury: feasibility and impact on circulating biomarkers. *Pediatr Crit Care Med* (2013) 14:e45–56. doi:10.1097/PCC.0b013e31827124f3
23. Duggan C, Watkins J, Walker WA. *Nutrition in Pediatrics: Basic Science, Clinical Application*. 4th ed. Hamilton: BC Decker (2008).
24. Mehta NM, Duggan CP. Nutritional deficiencies during critical illness. *Pediatr Clin North Am* (2009) 56:1143–60. doi:10.1016/j.pcl.2009.06.007
25. Graciano AL, Turner DA, editors. *Current Concepts in Pediatric Critical Care*. Mount Prospect, IL: Society of Critical Care Medicine (2015).

26. Bechard LJ, Duggan C, Touger-Decker R, Parrott JS, Rothpletz-Puglia P, Byham-Gray L, et al. Nutritional status based on body mass index is associated with morbidity and mortality in mechanically ventilated critically ill children in the PICU. *Crit Care Med* (2016) 44:1530–7. doi:10.1097/CCM.0000000000001713
27. de Souza Menezes F, Leite HP, Koch Nogueira PC. Malnutrition as an independent predictor of clinical outcome in critically ill children. *Nutrition* (2012) 28:267–70. doi:10.1016/j.nut.2011.05.015
28. Delgado AF, Okay TS, Leone C, Nichols B, Del Negro GM, Vaz FA. Hospital malnutrition and inflammatory response in critically ill children and adolescents admitted to a tertiary intensive care unit. *Clinics (Sao Paulo)* (2008) 63:357–62. doi:10.1590/S1807-59322008000300012
29. Dobbing J, Sands J. Vulnerability of developing brain. IX. The effect of nutritional growth retardation on the timing of the brain growth-spurt. *Biol Neonate* (1971) 19:363–78. doi:10.1159/000240430
30. Ehrenkranz RA, Das A, Wrage LA, Poindexter BB, Higgins RD, Stoll BJ, et al. Early nutrition mediates the influence of severity of illness on extremely LBW infants. *Pediatr Res* (2011) 69:522–9. doi:10.1203/PDR.0b013e318217f4f1
31. Radman M, Mack R, Barnoya J, Castañeda A, Rosales M, Azakie A, et al. The effect of preoperative nutritional status on postoperative outcomes in children undergoing surgery for congenital heart defects in San Francisco (UCSF) and Guatemala City (UNICAR). *J Thorac Cardiovasc Surg* (2014) 147:442–50. doi:10.1016/j.jtcvs.2013.03.023
32. Briassoulis G, Zavras N, Hatzis T. Malnutrition, nutritional indices, and early enteral feeding in critically ill children. *Nutrition* (2001) 17:548–57. doi:10.1016/S0899-9007(01)00578-0
33. Pollack MM, Wiley JS, Holbrook PR. Early nutritional depletion in critically ill children. *Crit Care Med* (1981) 9:580–3. doi:10.1097/00003246-198108000-00005
34. Pollack MM, Wiley JS, Kanter R, Holbrook PR. Malnutrition in critically ill infants and children. *JPEN J Parenter Enteral Nutr* (1982) 6:20–4. doi:10.1177/014860718200600120
35. Prieto MB, Cid JL. Malnutrition in the critically ill child: the importance of enteral nutrition. *Int J Environ Res Public Health* (2011) 8:4353–66. doi:10.3390/ijerph8114353
36. Mikhailov TA, Kuhn EM, Manzi J, Christensen M, Collins M, Brown AM, et al. Early enteral nutrition is associated with lower mortality in critically ill children. *JPEN J Parenter Enteral Nutr* (2014) 38(4):459–66. doi:10.1177/0148607113517903
37. Lopez-Herce J, Santiago MJ, Sanchez C, Mencia S, Carrillo A, Vigil D. Risk factors for gastrointestinal complications in critically ill children with transpyloric enteral nutrition. *Eur J Clin Nutr* (2008) 62:395–400. doi:10.1038/sj.ejcn.1602710
38. Panchal AK, Manzi J, Connolly S, Christensen M, Wakeham M, Goday PS, et al. Safety of enteral feedings in critically ill children receiving vasoactive agents. *JPEN J Parenter Enteral Nutr* (2016) 40(2):236–41. doi:10.1177/0148607114546533
39. Ogden CL, Carroll MD, Curtin LR, McDowell MA, Tabak CJ, Flegal KM. Prevalence of overweight and obesity in the United States, 1999-2004. *JAMA* (2006) 295:1549–55. doi:10.1001/jama.295.13.1549
40. Robinson MK, Mogensen KM, Casey JD, McKane CK, Moromizato T, Rawn JD, et al. The relationship among obesity, nutritional status, and mortality in the critically ill. *Crit Care Med* (2015) 43:87–100. doi:10.1097/CCM.0000000000000602
41. Stapleton RD, Suratt BT. Obesity and nutrition in acute respiratory distress syndrome. *Clin Chest Med* (2014) 35:655–71. doi:10.1016/j.ccm.2014.08.005
42. Mehta NM, Corkins MR, Lyman B, Malone A, Goday PS, Carney LN, et al. Defining pediatric malnutrition: a paradigm shift toward etiology-related definitions. *JPEN J Parenter Enteral Nutr* (2013) 37:460–81. doi:10.1177/0148607113479972
43. Keshen TH, Miller RG, Jahoor F, Jaksic T. Stable isotopic quantitation of protein metabolism and energy expenditure in neonates on- and post-extracorporeal life support. *J Pediatr Surg* (1997) 32:958–62; discussion 62–3. doi:10.1016/S0022-3468(97)90377-8
44. Agus MS, Javid PJ, Piper HG, Wypij D, Duggan CP, Ryan DP, et al. The effect of insulin infusion upon protein metabolism in neonates on extracorporeal life support. *Ann Surg* (2006) 244:536–44. doi:10.1097/01.sla.0000237758.93186.c8
45. Botran M, Lopez-Herce J, Mencia S, Urbano J, Solana MJ, Garcia A. Enteral nutrition in the critically ill child: comparison of standard and protein-enriched diets. *J Pediatr* (2011) 159:27–32. doi:10.1016/j.jpeds.2011.02.001
46. Liebau F, Wernerman J, van Loon LJ, Rooyackers O. Effect of initiating enteral protein feeding on whole-body protein turnover in critically ill patients. *Am J Clin Nutr* (2015) 101:549–57. doi:10.3945/ajcn.114.091934
47. Bechard LJ, Parrott JS, Mehta NM. Systematic review of the influence of energy and protein intake on protein balance in critically ill children. *J Pediatr* (2012) 161(333–9):e1. doi:10.1016/j.jpeds.2012.01.046
48. Goldman HI, Freudenthal R, Holland B, Karelitz S. Clinical effects of two different levels of protein intake on low-birth-weight infants. *J Pediatr* (1969) 74:881–9. doi:10.1016/S0022-3476(69)80222-2
49. Goldman HI, Liebman OB, Freudenthal R, Reuben R. Effects of early dietary protein intake on low-birth-weight infants: evaluation at 3 years of age. *J Pediatr* (1971) 78:126–9. doi:10.1016/S0022-3476(71)80277-9
50. Mehta NM, Compher C, A.S.P.E.N. Board of Directors. A.S.P.E.N. Clinical Guidelines: nutrition support of the critically ill child. *JPEN J Parenter Enteral Nutr* (2009) 33:260–76. doi:10.1177/0148607109333114
51. Coss-Bu JA, Jefferson LS, Walding D, David Y, Smith EO, Klish WJ. Resting energy expenditure in children in a pediatric intensive care unit: comparison of Harris-Benedict and Talbot predictions with indirect calorimetry values. *Am J Clin Nutr* (1998) 67:74–80.
52. Leong AY, Field CJ, Larsen BM. Nutrition support of the postoperative cardiac surgery child. *Nutr Clin Pract* (2013) 28:572–9. doi:10.1177/0884533613497515
53. Mehta NM, Bechard LJ, Dolan M, Ariagno K, Jiang H, Duggan C. Energy imbalance and the risk of overfeeding in critically ill children. *Pediatr Crit Care Med* (2011) 12:398–405. doi:10.1097/PCC.0b013e3181fe279c
54. Briassoulis G, Venkataraman S, Thompson A. Cytokines and metabolic patterns in pediatric patients with critical illness. *Clin Dev Immunol* (2010) 2010:354047. doi:10.1155/2010/354047
55. De Wit B, Meyer R, Desai A, Macrae D, Pathan N. Challenge of predicting resting energy expenditure in children undergoing surgery for congenital heart disease. *Pediatr Crit Care Med* (2010) 11:496–501. doi:10.1097/PCC.0b013e3181ce7465
56. Framson CM, LeLeiko NS, Dallal GE, Roubenoff R, Snelling LK, Dwyer JT. Energy expenditure in critically ill children. *Pediatr Crit Care Med* (2007) 8:264–7. doi:10.1097/01.PCC.0000262802.81164.03
57. Mehta NM, Bechard LJ, Leavitt K, Duggan C. Cumulative energy imbalance in the pediatric intensive care unit: role of targeted indirect calorimetry. *JPEN J Parenter Enteral Nutr* (2009) 33:336–44. doi:10.1177/0148607108325249
58. Franz AR, Pohlandt F, Bode H, Mihatsch WA, Sander S, Kron M, et al. Intrauterine, early neonatal, and postdischarge growth and neurodevelopmental outcome at 5.4 years in extremely preterm infants after intensive neonatal nutritional support. *Pediatrics* (2009) 123:e101–9. doi:10.1542/peds.2008-1352
59. Lucas A, Morley R, Cole TJ. Randomised trial of early diet in preterm babies and later intelligence quotient. *BMJ* (1998) 317:1481–7. doi:10.1136/bmj.317.7171.1481
60. Letton RW, Chwals WJ, Jamie A, Charles B. Early postoperative alterations in infant energy use increase the risk of overfeeding. *J Pediatr Surg* (1995) 30:988–92; discussion 92–3. doi:10.1016/0022-3468(95)90327-5
61. Pons Leite H, Gilberto Henriques Vieira J, Burnow De Carvalho W, Chwals WJ. The role of insulin-like growht factor I, growth hormone, and plasma proteins in surgical outcome of children with congenital heart disease. *Pediatr Crit Care Med* (2001) 2:29–35. doi:10.1097/00130478-200101000-00007
62. Alaedeen DI, Walsh MC, Chwals WJ. Total parenteral nutrition-associated hyperglycemia correlates with prolonged mechanical ventilation and hospital stay in septic infants. *J Pediatr Surg* (2006) 41:239–44; discussion 239–44. doi:10.1016/j.jpedsurg.2005.10.045
63. Long CL, Kinney JM, Geiger JW. Nonsuppressability of gluconeogenesis by glucose in septic patients. *Metabolism* (1976) 25:193–201. doi:10.1016/0026-0495(76)90049-4
64. Powis MR, Smith K, Rennie M, Halliday D, Pierro A. Effect of major abdominal operations on energy and protein metabolism in infants and children. *J Pediatr Surg* (1998) 33:49–53. doi:10.1016/S0022-3468(98)90360-8

65. Srinivasan V. Stress hyperglycemia in pediatric critical illness: the intensive care unit adds to the stress! *J Diabetes Sci Technol* (2012) 6:37–47. doi:10.1177/193229681200600106
66. Van Herpe T, Vanhonsebrouck K, Mesotten D, De Moor B, Van den Berghe G. Glycemic control in the pediatric intensive care unit of Leuven: two years of experience. *J Diabetes Sci Technol* (2012) 6:15–21. doi:10.1177/193229681200600103
67. Feng Y, Ralls MW, Xiao W, Miyasaka E, Herman RS, Teitelbaum DH. Loss of enteral nutrition in a mouse model results in intestinal epithelial barrier dysfunction. *Ann N Y Acad Sci* (2012) 1258:71–7. doi:10.1111/j.1749-6632.2012.06572.x
68. Johnson CD, Kudsk KA, Fukatsu K, Renegar KB, Zarzaur BL. Route of nutrition influences generation of antibody-forming cells and initial defense to an active viral infection in the upper respiratory tract. *Ann Surg* (2003) 237:565–73. doi:10.1097/00000658-200304000-00019
69. Ohta K, Omura K, Hirano K, Kanehira E, Ishikawa N, Kato Y, et al. The effects of an additive small amount of a low residual diet against total parenteral nutrition-induced gut mucosal barrier. *Am J Surg* (2003) 185:79–85. doi:10.1016/S0002-9610(02)01108-X
70. Sacks GS, Kudsk KA. Maintaining mucosal immunity during parenteral feeding with surrogates to enteral nutrition. *Nutr Clin Pract* (2003) 18:483–8. doi:10.1177/0115426503018006483
71. Shankar B, Daphnee DK, Ramakrishnan N, Venkataraman R. Feasibility, safety, and outcome of very early enteral nutrition in critically ill patients: results of an observational study. *J Crit Care* (2015) 30:473–5. doi:10.1016/j.jcrc.2015.02.009
72. Valentine SL, Nadkarni VM, Curley MA, Pediatric Acute Lung Injury Consensus Conference Group. Nonpulmonary treatments for pediatric acute respiratory distress syndrome: proceedings from the Pediatric Acute Lung Injury Consensus Conference. *Pediatr Crit Care Med* (2015) 16:S73–85. doi:10.1097/PCC.0000000000000435
73. Harvey SE, Parrott F, Harrison DA, Bear DE, Segaran E, Beale R, et al. Trial of the route of early nutritional support in critically ill adults. *N Engl J Med* (2014) 371(18):1673–84. doi:10.1056/NEJMoa1409860
74. Charles EJ, Petroze RT, Metzger R, Hranjec T, Rosenberger LH, Riccio LM, et al. Hypocaloric compared with eucaloric nutritional support and its effect on infection rates in a surgical intensive care unit: a randomized controlled trial. *Am J Clin Nutr* (2014) 100:1337–43. doi:10.3945/ajcn.114.088609
75. Choi EY, Park DA, Park J. Calorie intake of enteral nutrition and clinical outcomes in acutely critically ill patients: a meta-analysis of randomized controlled trials. *JPEN J Parenter Enteral Nutr* (2015) 39:291–300. doi:10.1177/0148607114544322
76. Dickerson RN, Boschert KJ, Kudsk KA, Brown RO. Hypocaloric enteral tube feeding in critically ill obese patients. *Nutrition* (2002) 18:241–6. doi:10.1016/S0899-9007(01)00793-6
77. Hart DW, Wolf SE, Herndon DN, Chinkes DL, Lal SO, Obeng MK, et al. Energy expenditure and caloric balance after burn: increased feeding leads to fat rather than lean mass accretion. *Ann Surg* (2002) 235:152–61. doi:10.1097/00000658-200201000-00020
78. Krishnan JA, Parce PB, Martinez A, Diette GB, Brower RG. Caloric intake in medical ICU patients: consistency of care with guidelines and relationship to clinical outcomes. *Chest* (2003) 124:297–305. doi:10.1378/chest.124.1.297
79. Tian F, Wang X, Gao X, Wan X, Wu C, Zhang L, et al. Effect of initial calorie intake via enteral nutrition in critical illness: a meta-analysis of randomised controlled trials. *Crit Care* (2015) 19:180. doi:10.1186/s13054-015-0902-0
80. Dokken M, Rustoen T, Stubhaug A. Indirect calorimetry reveals that better monitoring of nutrition therapy in pediatric intensive care is needed. *JPEN J Parenter Enteral Nutr* (2015) 39:344–52. doi:10.1177/0148607113511990
81. Preiser JC, van Zanten AR, Berger MM, Biolo G, Casaer MP, Doig GS, et al. Metabolic and nutritional support of critically ill patients: consensus and controversies. *Crit Care* (2015) 19:35. doi:10.1186/s13054-015-0737-8
82. Berger MM, Chiolero RL. Hypocaloric feeding: pros and cons. *Curr Opin Crit Care* (2007) 13:180–6. doi:10.1097/MCC.0b013e3280895d47
83. Derde S, Vanhorebeek I, Güiza F, Derese I, Gunst J, Fahrenkrog B, et al. Early parenteral nutrition evokes a phenotype of autophagy deficiency in liver and skeletal muscle of critically ill rabbits. *Endocrinology* (2012) 153:2267–76. doi:10.1210/en.2011-2068
84. Fivez T, Kerklaan D, Mesotten D, Verbruggen S, Wouters PJ, Vanhorebeek I, et al. Early versus late parenteral nutrition in critically ill children. *N Engl J Med* (2016) 374:1111–22. doi:10.1056/NEJMoa1514762
85. Harvey SE, Parrott F, Harrison DA, Bear DE, Segaran E, Beale R, et al. Trial of the route of early nutritional support in critically ill adults. *N Engl J Med* (2014) 371:1673–84. doi:10.1056/NEJMoa1409860
86. Doig GS, Simpson F, Sweetman EA, Finfer SR, Cooper DJ, Heighes PT, et al. Early parenteral nutrition in critically ill patients with short-term relative contraindications to early enteral nutrition: a randomized controlled trial. *JAMA* (2013) 309:2130–8. doi:10.1001/jama.2013.5124
87. Heidegger CP, Berger MM, Graf S, Zingg W, Darmon P, Costanza MC, et al. Optimisation of energy provision with supplemental parenteral nutrition in critically ill patients: a randomised controlled clinical trial. *Lancet* (2013) 381:385–93. doi:10.1016/S0140-6736(12)61351-8
88. Casaer MP, Mesotten D, Hermans G, Wouters PJ, Schetz M, Meyfroidt G, et al. Early versus late parenteral nutrition in critically ill adults. *N Engl J Med* (2011) 365:506–17. doi:10.1056/NEJMoa1102662
89. Arabi YM, Aldawood AS, Haddad SH, Al-Dorzi HM, Tamim HM, Jones G, et al. Permissive underfeeding or standard enteral feeding in critically ill adults. *N Engl J Med* (2015) 372:2398–408. doi:10.1056/NEJMoa1502826
90. Braunschweig CA, Sheean PM, Peterson SJ, Gomez Perez S, Freels S, Lateef O, et al. Intensive nutrition in acute lung injury: a clinical trial (INTACT). *JPEN J Parenter Enteral Nutr* (2015) 39:13–20. doi:10.1177/0148607114528541
91. National Heart, Lung, and Blood Institute Acute Respiratory Distress Syndrome Clinical Trials Network, Rice TW, Wheeler AP, Thompson BT, Steingrub J, Hite RD, et al. Initial trophic vs full enteral feeding in patients with acute lung injury: the EDEN randomized trial. *JAMA* (2012) 307:795–803. doi:10.1001/jama.2012.137
92. Davies AR, Morrison SS, Bailey MJ, Bellomo R, Cooper DJ, Doig GS, et al. A multicenter, randomized controlled trial comparing early nasojejunal with nasogastric nutrition in critical illness. *Crit Care Med* (2012) 40:2342–8. doi:10.1097/CCM.0b013e318255d87e
93. Acosta-Escribano J, Fernández-Vivas M, Grau Carmona T, Caturla-Such J, Garcia-Martinez M, Menendez-Mainer A, et al. Gastric versus transpyloric feeding in severe traumatic brain injury: a prospective, randomized trial. *Intensive Care Med* (2010) 36:1532–9. doi:10.1007/s00134-010-1908-3
94. Hsu CW, Sun SF, Lin SL, Kang SP, Chu KA, Lin CH, et al. Duodenal versus gastric feeding in medical intensive care unit patients: a prospective, randomized, clinical study. *Crit Care Med* (2009) 37:1866–72. doi:10.1097/CCM.0b013e31819ffcda
95. Khorasani EN, Mansouri F. Effect of early enteral nutrition on morbidity and mortality in children with burns. *Burns* (2010) 36:1067–71. doi:10.1016/j.burns.2009.12.005
96. MacLeod JB, Lefton J, Houghton D, Roland C, Doherty J, Cohn SM, et al. Prospective randomized control trial of intermittent versus continuous gastric feeds for critically ill trauma patients. *J Trauma* (2007) 63:57–61. doi:10.1097/01.ta.0000249294.58703.11
97. NICE-SUGAR Study Investigators, Finfer S, Chittock DR, Su SY, Blair D, Foster D, et al. Intensive versus conventional glucose control in critically ill patients. *N Engl J Med* (2009) 360:1283–97. doi:10.1056/NEJMoa0810625
98. Vlasselaers D, Milants I, Desmet L, Wouters PJ, Vanhorebeek I, van den Heuvel I, et al. Intensive insulin therapy for patients in paediatric intensive care: a prospective, randomised controlled study. *Lancet* (2009) 373:547–56. doi:10.1016/S0140-6736(09)60044-1
99. Van den Berghe G, Wilmer A, Hermans G, Meersseman W, Wouters PJ, Milants I, et al. Intensive insulin therapy in the medical ICU. *N Engl J Med* (2006) 354:449–61. doi:10.1056/NEJMoa052521
100. Ziegler TR, May AK, Hebbar G, Easley KA, Griffith DP, Dave N, et al. Efficacy and safety of glutamine-supplemented parenteral nutrition in surgical ICU patients: an American Multicenter Randomized Controlled Trial. *Ann Surg* (2016) 263:646–55. doi:10.1097/SLA.0000000000001487
101. Pérez-Bárcena J, Marsé P, Zabalegui-Pérez A, Corral E, Herrán-Monge R, Gero-Escapa M, et al. A randomized trial of intravenous glutamine supplementation in trauma ICU patients. *Intensive Care Med* (2014) 40:539–47. doi:10.1007/s00134-014-3230-y
102. Heyland D, Muscedere J, Wischmeyer PE, Cook D, Jones G, Albert M, et al. A randomized trial of glutamine and antioxidants in critically ill patients. *N Engl J Med* (2013) 368:1489–97. doi:10.1056/NEJMoa1212722

103. Carcillo JA, Dean JM, Holubkov R, Berger J, Meert KL, Anand KJ, et al. The randomized comparative pediatric critical illness stress-induced immune suppression (CRISIS) prevention trial. *Pediatr Crit Care Med* (2012) 13:165–73. doi:10.1097/PCC.0b013e31823896ae
104. Andrews PJ, Avenell A, Noble DW, Campbell MK, Croal BL, Simpson WG, et al. Randomised trial of glutamine, selenium, or both, to supplement parenteral nutrition for critically ill patients. *BMJ* (2011) 342:d1542. doi:10.1136/bmj.d1542
105. Angstwurm MW, Engelmann L, Zimmermann T, Lehmann C, Spes CH, Abel P, et al. Selenium in intensive care (SIC): results of a prospective randomized, placebo-controlled, multiple-center study in patients with severe systemic inflammatory response syndrome, sepsis, and septic shock. *Crit Care Med* (2007) 35:118–26. doi:10.1097/01.CCM.0000251124.83436.0E
106. Grau-Carmona T, Bonet-Saris A, Garcia-de-Lorenzo A, Sánchez-Alvarez C, Rodríguez-Pozo A, Acosta-Escribano J, et al. Influence of n-3 polyunsaturated fatty acids enriched lipid emulsions on nosocomial infections and clinical outcomes in critically ill patients: ICU lipids study. *Crit Care Med*(2015) 43:31–9.
107. Kagan I, Cohen J, Stein M, Bendavid I, Pinsker D, Silva V, et al. Preemptive enteral nutrition enriched with eicosapentaenoic acid, gamma-linolenic acid and antioxidants in severe multiple trauma: a prospective, randomized, double-blind study. *Intensive Care Med* (2015) 41:460–9. doi:10.1007/s00134-015-3646-z
108. van Zanten AR, Sztark F, Kaisers UX, Zielmann S, Felbinger TW, Sablotzki AR, et al. High-protein enteral nutrition enriched with immune-modulating nutrients vs standard high-protein enteral nutrition and nosocomial infections in the ICU: a randomized clinical trial. *JAMA* (2014) 312:514–24. doi:10.1001/jama.2014.7698
109. Pontes-Arruda A, Martins LF, de Lima SM, Isola AM, Toledo D, Rezende E, et al. Enteral nutrition with eicosapentaenoic acid, gamma-linolenic acid and antioxidants in the early treatment of sepsis: results from a multicenter, prospective, randomized, double-blinded, controlled study: the INTERSEPT study. *Crit Care* (2011) 15:R144. doi:10.1186/cc10267
110. Radrizzani D, Bertolini G, Facchini R, Simini B, Bruzzone P, Zanforlin G, et al. Early enteral immunonutrition vs. parenteral nutrition in critically ill patients without severe sepsis: a randomized clinical trial. *Intensive Care Med* (2006) 32:1191–8. doi:10.1007/s00134-006-0238-y
111. Czapran A, Headdon W, Deane AM, Lange K, Chapman MJ, Heyland DK. International observational study of nutritional support in mechanically ventilated patients following burn injury. *Burns* (2015) 41:510–8. doi:10.1016/j.burns.2014.09.013
112. Peev MP, Yeh DD, Quraishi SA, Osler P, Chang Y, Gillis E, et al. Causes and consequences of interrupted enteral nutrition: a prospective observational study in critically ill surgical patients. *JPEN J Parenter Enteral Nutr* (2015) 39:21–7. doi:10.1177/0148607114526887
113. Weijs PJ, Looijaard WG, Beishuizen A, Girbes AR, Oudemans-van Straaten HM. Early high protein intake is associated with low mortality and energy overfeeding with high mortality in non-septic mechanically ventilated critically ill patients. *Crit Care* (2014) 18:701. doi:10.1186/s13054-014-0701-z
114. Alberda C, Gramlich L, Jones N, Jeejeebhoy K, Day AG, Dhaliwal R, et al. The relationship between nutritional intake and clinical outcomes in critically ill patients: results of an international multicenter observational study. *Intensive Care Med* (2009) 35:1728–37. doi:10.1007/s00134-009-1567-4
115. Canarie MF, Barry S, Carroll CL, Hassinger A, Kandil S, Li S, et al. Risk factors for delayed enteral nutrition in critically Ill children. *Pediatr Crit Care Med* (2015) 16:e283–9. doi:10.1097/PCC.0000000000000527
116. Martinez EE, Smallwood CD, Bechard LJ, Graham RJ, Mehta NM. Metabolic assessment and individualized nutrition in children dependent on mechanical ventilation at home. *J Pediatr* (2015) 166:350–7. doi:10.1016/j.jpeds.2014.09.036
117. Tillquist M, Kutsogiannis DJ, Wischmeyer PE, Kummerlen C, Leung R, Stollery D, et al. Bedside ultrasound is a practical and reliable measurement tool for assessing quadriceps muscle layer thickness. *JPEN J Parenter Enteral Nutr* (2014) 38:886–90. doi:10.1177/0148607113501327
118. Savalle M, Gillaizeau F, Maruani G, Puymirat E, Bellenfant F, Houillier P, et al. Assessment of body cell mass at bedside in critically ill patients. *Am J Physiol Endocrinol Metab* (2012) 303:E389–96. doi:10.1152/ajpendo.00502.2011
119. Sheean PM, Peterson SJ, Gomez Perez S, Troy KL, Patel A, Sclamberg JS, et al. The prevalence of sarcopenia in patients with respiratory failure classified as normally nourished using computed tomography and subjective global assessment. *JPEN J Parenter Enteral Nutr* (2014) 38:873–9. doi:10.1177/0148607113500308
120. Meert KL, Daphtary KM, Metheny NA. Gastric vs small-bowel feeding in critically ill children receiving mechanical ventilation: a randomized controlled trial. *Chest* (2004) 126:872–8. doi:10.1378/chest.126.3.872
121. Wang D, Zheng SQ, Chen XC, Jiang SW, Chen HB. Comparisons between small intestinal and gastric feeding in severe traumatic brain injury: a systematic review and meta-analysis of randomized controlled trials. *J Neurosurg* (2015) 123:1194–201. doi:10.3171/2014.11.JNS141109
122. Lopez-Herce J, Mencia S, Sanchez C, Santiago MJ, Bustinza A, Vigil D. Postpyloric enteral nutrition in the critically ill child with shock: a prospective observational study. *Nutr J* (2008) 7:6. doi:10.1186/1475-2891-7-6
123. Fivez T, Kerklaan D, Verbruggen S, Vanhorebeek I, Verstraete S, Tibboel D, et al. Impact of withholding early parenteral nutrition completing enteral nutrition in pediatric critically ill patients (PEPaNIC trial): study protocol for a randomized controlled trial. *Trials* (2015) 16:202. doi:10.1186/s13063-015-0728-8
124. Denne SC, Poindexter BB. Evidence supporting early nutritional support with parenteral amino acid infusion. *Semin Perinatol* (2007) 31:56–60. doi:10.1053/j.semperi.2007.02.005
125. Evans RA, Thureen P. Early feeding strategies in preterm and critically ill neonates. *Neonatal Netw* (2001) 20:7–18. doi:10.1891/0730-0832.20.7.7
126. Grau-Carmona T, Bonet-Saris A, García-de-Lorenzo A, Sánchez-Alvarez C, Rodríguez-Pozo A, Acosta-Escribano J, et al. Influence of n-3 polyunsaturated fatty acids enriched lipid emulsions on nosocomial infections and clinical outcomes in critically ill patients: ICU lipids study. *Crit Care Med* (2015) 43:31–9. doi:10.1097/CCM.0000000000000612
127. Grintescu IM, Luca Vasiliu I, Cucereanu Badica I, Mirea L, Pavelescu D, Balanescu A, et al. The influence of parenteral glutamine supplementation on glucose homeostasis in critically ill polytrauma patients – a randomized-controlled clinical study. *Clin Nutr* (2015) 34:377–82. doi:10.1016/j.clnu.2014.05.006
128. Najmi M, Vahdat Shariatpanahi Z, Tolouei M, Amiri Z. Effect of oral olive oil on healing of 10-20% total body surface area burn wounds in hospitalized patients. *Burns* (2015) 41:493–6. doi:10.1016/j.burns.2014.08.010
129. Zhang WC, Zheng XJ, Du LJ, Sun JY, Shen ZX, Shi C, et al. High salt primes a specific activation state of macrophages, M(Na). *Cell Res* (2015) 25:893–910. doi:10.1038/cr.2015.87
130. King W, Petrillo T, Pettignano R. Enteral nutrition and cardiovascular medications in the pediatric intensive care unit. *JPEN J Parenter Enteral Nutr* (2004) 28:334–8. doi:10.1177/0148607104028005334
131. Rogers EJ, Gilbertson HR, Heine RG, Henning R. Barriers to adequate nutrition in critically ill children. *Nutrition* (2003) 19:865–8. doi:10.1016/S0899-9007(03)00170-9
132. Khalid I, Doshi P, DiGiovine B. Early enteral nutrition and outcomes of critically ill patients treated with vasopressors and mechanical ventilation. *Am J Crit Care* (2010) 19:261–8. doi:10.4037/ajcc2010197
133. McClave SA, Lukan JK, Stefater JA, Lowen CC, Looney SW, Matheson PJ, et al. Poor validity of residual volumes as a marker for risk of aspiration in critically ill patients. *Crit Care Med* (2005) 33:324–30. doi:10.1097/01.CCM.0000153413.46627.3A
134. Metheny NA, Mills AC, Stewart BJ. Monitoring for intolerance to gastric tube feedings: a national survey. *Am J Crit Care* (2012) 21:e33–40. doi:10.4037/ajcc2012647
135. Meyer R, Harrison S, Sargent S, Ramnarayan P, Habibi P, Labadarios D. The impactofenteralfeedingprotocolsonnutritionalsupportincriticallyillchildren. *J Hum Nutr Diet* (2009) 22:428–36. doi:10.1111/j.1365-277X.2009.00994.x
136. Blaser AR, Starkopf J, Kirsimagi U, Deane AM. Definition, prevalence, and outcome of feeding intolerance in intensive care: a systematic review and meta-analysis. *Acta Anaesthesiol Scand* (2014) 58:914–22. doi:10.1111/aas.12302
137. Smalley N, Vangaveti V. Assessing the bowel function of critically ill children: a pilot study. *Crit Care Resusc* (2014) 16(3):202–5.
138. Martinez EE, Douglas K, Nurko S, Mehta NM. Gastric dysmotility in critically ill children: pathophysiology, diagnosis, and management. *Pediatr Crit Care Med* (2015) 16:828–36. doi:10.1097/PCC.0000000000000493
139. Deane A, Chapman MJ, Fraser RJ, Bryant LK, Burgstad C, Nguyen NQ. Mechanisms underlying feed intolerance in the critically ill: implications for

treatment. *World J Gastroenterol* (2007) 13:3909–17. doi:10.3748/wjg.v13.i29.3909
140. Typpo KV, Larmonier CB, Deschenes J, Redford D, Kiela PR, Ghishan FK. Clinical characteristics associated with postoperative intestinal epithelial barrier dysfunction in children with congenital heart disease. *Pediatr Crit Care Med* (2015) 16:37–44. doi:10.1097/PCC.0000000000000256
141. Reeves A, White H, Sosnowski K, Tran K, Jones M, Palmer M. Energy and protein intakes of hospitalised patients with acute respiratory failure receiving non-invasive ventilation. *Clin Nutr* (2014) 33:1068–73. doi:10.1016/j.clnu.2013.11.012
142. Ridley EJ, Davies AR, Robins EJ, Lukas G, Bailey MJ, Fraser JF, et al. Nutrition therapy in adult patients receiving extracorporeal membrane oxygenation: a prospective, multicentre, observational study. *Crit Care Resusc* (2015) 17:183–9.
143. Haskins IN, Baginsky M, Gamsky N, Sedghi K, Yi S, Amdur RL, et al. A volume-based enteral nutrition support regimen improves caloric delivery but may not affect clinical outcomes in critically ill patients. *JPEN J Parenter Enteral Nutr* (2015). doi:10.1177/0148607115617441
144. Hamilton S, McAleer DM, Ariagno K, Barrett M, Stenquist N, Duggan CP, et al. A stepwise enteral nutrition algorithm for critically ill children helps achieve nutrient delivery goals*. *Pediatr Crit Care Med* (2014) 15:583–9. doi:10.1097/PCC.0000000000000179
145. Joffe A, Anton N, Lequier L, Vandermeer B, Tjosvold L, Larsen B, et al. Nutritional support for critically ill children. *Cochrane Database Syst Rev* (2016) 5:CD005144. doi:10.1002/14651858.CD005144.pub3
146. van den Berghe G, Wouters P, Weekers F, Verwaest C, Bruyninckx F, Schetz M, et al. Intensive insulin therapy in critically ill patients. *N Engl J Med* (2001) 345:1359–67. doi:10.1056/NEJMoa011300
147. Marik PE, Preiser JC. Toward understanding tight glycemic control in the ICU: a systematic review and metaanalysis. *Chest* (2010) 137:544–51. doi:10.1378/chest.09-1737
148. Wiener RS, Wiener DC, Larson RJ. Benefits and risks of tight glucose control in critically ill adults: a meta-analysis. *JAMA* (2008) 300:933–44. doi:10.1001/jama.300.8.933
149. Griesdale DE, de Souza RJ, van Dam RM, Heyland DK, Cook DJ, Malhotra A, et al. Intensive insulin therapy and mortality among critically ill patients: a meta-analysis including NICE-SUGAR study data. *CMAJ* (2009) 180:821–7. doi:10.1503/cmaj.090206
150. Wintergerst KA, Buckingham B, Gandrud L, Wong BJ, Kache S, Wilson DM. Association of hypoglycemia, hyperglycemia, and glucose variability with morbidity and death in the pediatric intensive care unit. *Pediatrics* (2006) 118:173–9. doi:10.1542/peds.2005-1819
151. Sertaridou E, Papaioannou V, Kolios G, Pneumatikos I. Gut failure in critical care: old school versus new school. *Ann Gastroenterol* (2015) 28:309–22.
152. Deitch EA. Gut lymph and lymphatics: a source of factors leading to organ injury and dysfunction. *Ann N Y Acad Sci* (2010) 1207(Suppl 1):E103–11. doi:10.1111/j.1749-6632.2010.05713.x
153. Clark JA, Coopersmith CM. Intestinal crosstalk: a new paradigm for understanding the gut as the "motor" of critical illness. *Shock* (2007) 28:384–93. doi:10.1097/shk.0b013e31805569df
154. Mittal R, Coopersmith CM. Redefining the gut as the motor of critical illness. *Trends Mol Med* (2014) 20:214–23. doi:10.1016/j.molmed.2013.08.004
155. Klingensmith NJ, Coopersmith CM. The gut as the motor of multiple organ dysfunction in critical illness. *Crit Care Clin* (2016) 32:203–12. doi:10.1016/j.ccc.2015.11.004
156. Grootjans J, Thuijls G, Verdam F, Derikx JP, Lenaerts K, Buurman WA. Non-invasive assessment of barrier integrity and function of the human gut. *World J Gastrointest Surg* (2010) 2:61–9. doi:10.4240/wjgs.v2.i3.61
157. Grootjans J, Lenaerts K, Derikx JP, Matthijsen RA, de Bruïne AP, van Bijnen AA, et al. Human intestinal ischemia-reperfusion-induced inflammation characterized: experiences from a new translational model. *Am J Pathol* (2010) 176:2283–91. doi:10.2353/ajpath.2010.091069
158. Reisinger KW, Derikx JP, Thuijls G, van der Zee DC, Brouwers HA, van Bijnen AA, et al. Noninvasive measurement of intestinal epithelial damage at time of refeeding can predict clinical outcome after necrotizing enterocolitis. *Pediatr Res* (2013) 73:209–13. doi:10.1038/pr.2012.160
159. Fukatsu K, Kudsk KA. Nutrition and gut immunity. *Surg Clin North Am* (2011) 91:755–70,vii. doi:10.1016/j.suc.2011.04.007
160. Marchiando AM, Graham WV, Turner JR. Epithelial barriers in homeostasis and disease. *Annu Rev Pathol* (2010) 5:119–44. doi:10.1146/annurev.pathol.4.110807.092135
161. Luo H, Guo P, Zhou Q. Role of TLR4/NF-kappaB in damage to intestinal mucosa barrier function and bacterial translocation in rats exposed to hypoxia. *PLoS One* (2012) 7:e46291. doi:10.1371/journal.pone.0046291
162. Ng EW, Poon TC, Lam HS, Cheung HM, Ma TP, Chan KY, et al. Gut-associated biomarkers L-FABP, I-FABP, and TFF3 and LIT score for diagnosis of surgical necrotizing enterocolitis in preterm infants. *Ann Surg* (2013) 258:1111–8. doi:10.1097/SLA.0b013e318288ea96
163. Thuijls G, Derikx JP, van Wijck K, Zimmermann LJ, Degraeuwe PL, Mulder TL, et al. Non-invasive markers for early diagnosis and determination of the severity of necrotizing enterocolitis. *Ann Surg* (2010) 251:1174–80. doi:10.1097/SLA.0b013e3181d778c4
164. Thuijls G, Derikx JP, de Haan JJ, Grootjans J, de Bruïne A, Masclee AA, et al. Urine-based detection of intestinal tight junction loss. *J Clin Gastroenterol* (2010) 44:e14–9. doi:10.1097/MCG.0b013e31819f5652
165. Bailly-Botuha C, Colomb V, Thioulouse E, Berthe MC, Garcette K, Dubern B, et al. Plasma citrulline concentration reflects enterocyte mass in children with short bowel syndrome. *Pediatr Res* (2009) 65:559–63. doi:10.1203/PDR.0b013e31819986da
166. Crenn P, Messing B, Cynober L. Citrulline as a biomarker of intestinal failure due to enterocyte mass reduction. *Clin Nutr* (2008) 27:328–39. doi:10.1016/j.clnu.2008.02.005
167. Fitzgibbons S, Ching YA, Valim C, Zhou J, Iglesias J, Duggan C, et al. Relationship between serum citrulline levels and progression to parenteral nutrition independence in children with short bowel syndrome. *J Pediatr Surg* (2009) 44:928–32. doi:10.1016/j.jpedsurg.2009.01.034
168. Ioannou HP, Fotoulaki M, Pavlitou A, Efstratiou I, Augoustides-Savvopoulou P. Plasma citrulline levels in paediatric patients with celiac disease and the effect of a gluten-free diet. *Eur J Gastroenterol Hepatol* (2011) 23:245–9. doi:10.1097/MEG.0b013e3283438ad7
169. Piton G, Manzon C, Monnet E, Cypriani B, Barbot O, Navellou JC, et al. Plasma citrulline kinetics and prognostic value in critically ill patients. *Intensive Care Med* (2010) 36:702–6. doi:10.1007/s00134-010-1751-6
170. Diamanti A, Panetta F, Gandullia P, Morini F, Noto C, Torre G, et al. Plasma citrulline as marker of bowel adaptation in children with short bowel syndrome. *Langenbecks Arch Surg* (2011) 396:1041–6. doi:10.1007/s00423-011-0813-8
171. Merlin E, Minet-Quinard R, Pereira B, Rochette E, Auvrignon A, Oudot C, et al. Non-invasive biological quantification of acute gastrointestinal graft-versus-host disease in children by plasma citrulline. *Pediatr Transplant* (2013) 17:683–7. doi:10.1111/petr.12128
172. Hensel KO, Boland V, Postberg J, Zilbauer M, Heuschkel R, Vogel S, et al. Differential expression of mucosal trefoil factors and mucins in pediatric inflammatory bowel diseases. *Sci Rep* (2014) 4:7343. doi:10.1038/srep07343
173. Caporaso JG, Kuczynski J, Stombaugh J, Bittinger K, Bushman FD, Costello EK, et al. QIIME allows analysis of high-throughput community sequencing data. *Nat Methods* (2010) 7:335–6. doi:10.1038/nmeth.f.303
174. Cummings JH, Macfarlane GT. Role of intestinal bacteria in nutrient metabolism. *JPEN J Parenter Enteral Nutr* (1997) 21:357–65. doi:10.1177/0148607197021006357
175. Yatsunenko T, Rey FE, Manary MJ, Trehan I, Dominguez-Bello MG, Contreras M, et al. Human gut microbiome viewed across age and geography. *Nature* (2012) 486:222–7. doi:10.1038/nature11053
176. Cox LM, Yamanishi S, Sohn J, Alekseyenko AV, Leung JM, Cho I, et al. Altering the intestinal microbiota during a critical developmental window has lasting metabolic consequences. *Cell* (2014) 158:705–21. doi:10.1016/j.cell.2014.05.052
177. Cho I, Yamanishi S, Cox L, Methé BA, Zavadil J, Li K, et al. Antibiotics in early life alter the murine colonic microbiome and adiposity. *Nature* (2012) 488:621–6. doi:10.1038/nature11400
178. Tanaka S, Kobayashi T, Songjinda P, Tateyama A, Tsubouchi M, Kiyohara C, et al. Influence of antibiotic exposure in the early postnatal period on the development of intestinal microbiota. *FEMS Immunol Med Microbiol* (2009) 56:80–7. doi:10.1111/j.1574-695X.2009.00553.x

179. Sjögren YM, Tomicic S, Lundberg A, Böttcher MF, Björkstén B, Sverremark-Ekström E, et al. Influence of early gut microbiota on the maturation of childhood mucosal and systemic immune responses. *Clin Exp Allergy* (2009) 39:1842–51. doi:10.1111/j.1365-2222.2009.03326.x
180. Samuelson DR, Welsh DA, Shellito JE. Regulation of lung immunity and host defense by the intestinal microbiota. *Front Microbiol* (2015) 6:1085. doi:10.3389/fmicb.2015.01085
181. Carmody RN, Gerber GK, Luevano JM Jr, Gatti DM, Somes L, Svenson KL, et al. Diet dominates host genotype in shaping the murine gut microbiota. *Cell Host Microbe* (2015) 17:72–84. doi:10.1016/j.chom.2014.11.010
182. Briassoulis G, Filippou O, Kanariou M, Hatzis T. Comparative effects of early randomized immune or non-immune-enhancing enteral nutrition on cytokine production in children with septic shock. *Intensive Care Med* (2005) 31:851–8. doi:10.1007/s00134-005-2631-3
183. Heyland DK, Dhaliwal R, Day AG, Muscedere J, Drover J, Suchner U, et al. REducing Deaths due to OXidative Stress (The REDOXS Study): rationale and study design for a randomized trial of glutamine and antioxidant supplementation in critically-ill patients. *Proc Nutr Soc* (2006) 65:250–63. doi:10.1079/PNS2006505
184. Andrews PJ, Avenell A, Noble DW, Campbell MK, Battison CG, Croal BL, et al. Randomised trial of glutamine and selenium supplemented parenteral nutrition for critically ill patients. Protocol Version 9, 19 February 2007 known as SIGNET (Scottish Intensive care Glutamine or seleNium Evaluative Trial). *Trials* (2007) 8:25. doi:10.1186/1745-6215-8-25
185. Allingstrup M, Afshari A. Selenium supplementation for critically ill adults. *Cochrane Database Syst Rev* (2015) 7:CD003703. doi:10.1002/14651858.CD003703.pub3
186. Barbosa E, Moreira EA, Goes JE, Faintuch J. Pilot study with a glutamine-supplemented enteral formula in critically ill infants. *Rev Hosp Clin Fac Med Sao Paulo* (1999) 54:21–4. doi:10.1590/S0041-87811999000100005
187. Brodska H, Valenta J, Malickova K, Kohout P, Kazda A, Drabek T. Biomarkers in critically ill patients with systemic inflammatory response syndrome or sepsis supplemented with high-dose selenium. *J Trace Elem Med Biol* (2015) 31:25–32. doi:10.1016/j.jtemb.2015.02.005
188. Heyland DK, Dhaliwal R, Drover JW, Gramlich L, Dodek P, Canadian Critical Care Clinical Practice Guidelines Committee. Canadian clinical practice guidelines for nutrition support in mechanically ventilated, critically ill adult patients. *JPEN J Parenter Enteral Nutr* (2003) 27:355–73. doi:10.1177/0148607103027005355
189. Mayes T, Gottschlich MM, Kagan RJ. An evaluation of the safety and efficacy of an anti-inflammatory, pulmonary enteral formula in the treatment of pediatric burn patients with respiratory failure. *J Burn Care Res* (2008) 29:82–8. doi:10.1097/BCR.0b013e31815f594e
190. Tao KM, Li XQ, Yang LQ, Yu WF, Lu ZJ, Sun YM, et al. Glutamine supplementation for critically ill adults. *Cochrane Database Syst Rev* (2014) 9:CD010050. doi:10.1002/14651858.CD010050.pub2
191. Briassoulis G, Filippou O, Hatzi E, Papassotiriou I, Hatzis T. Early enteral administration of immunonutrition in critically ill children: results of a blinded randomized controlled clinical trial. *Nutrition* (2005) 21:799–807. doi:10.1016/j.nut.2004.12.006
192. Garcia de Acilu M, Leal S, Caralt B, Roca O, Sabater J, Masclans JR. The role of omega-3 polyunsaturated fatty acids in the treatment of patients with acute respiratory distress syndrome: a clinical review. *Biomed Res Int* (2015) 2015:653750. doi:10.1155/2015/653750
193. Hall TC, Bilku DK, Al-Leswas D, Neal CP, Horst C, Cooke J, et al. A randomized controlled trial investigating the effects of parenteral fish oil on survival outcomes in critically ill patients with sepsis: a pilot study. *JPEN J Parenter Enteral Nutr* (2015) 39:301–12. doi:10.1177/0148607113518945
194. Hecker M, Linder T, Ott J, Walmrath HD, Lohmeyer J, Vadász I, et al. Immunomodulation by lipid emulsions in pulmonary inflammation: a randomized controlled trial. *Crit Care* (2015) 19:226. doi:10.1186/s13054-015-0933-6
195. Li C, Bo L, Liu W, Lu X, Jin F. Enteral immunomodulatory diet (omega-3 fatty acid, gamma-linolenic acid and antioxidant supplementation) for acute lung injury and acute respiratory distress syndrome: an updated systematic review and meta-analysis. *Nutrients* (2015) 7:5572–85. doi:10.3390/nu7075239
196. Li X, Zhang X, Yang E, Zhang N, Cao S, Zhou Y. Fish oil-supplemented parenteral nutrition could alleviate acute lung injury, modulate immunity, and reduce inflammation in rats with abdominal sepsis. *Nutr Res* (2015) 35:784–91. doi:10.1016/j.nutres.2015.06.008
197. Manzanares W, Langlois PL, Dhaliwal R, Lemieux M, Heyland DK. Intravenous fish oil lipid emulsions in critically ill patients: an updated systematic review and meta-analysis. *Crit Care* (2015) 19:167. doi:10.1186/s13054-015-0888-7
198. Serhan CN, Petasis NA. Resolvins and protectins in inflammation resolution. *Chem Rev* (2011) 111:5922–43. doi:10.1021/cr100396c
199. Onwuneme C, Martin F, McCarthy R, Carroll A, Segurado R, Murphy J, et al. The association of vitamin D status with acute respiratory morbidity in preterm infants. *J Pediatr* (2015) 166:1175.e–80.e. doi:10.1016/j.jpeds.2015.01.055
200. Dancer RC, Parekh D, Lax S, D'Souza V, Zheng S, Bassford CR, et al. Vitamin D deficiency contributes directly to the acute respiratory distress syndrome (ARDS). *Thorax* (2015) 70:617–24. doi:10.1136/thoraxjnl-2014-206680
201. Thickett DR, Moromizato T, Litonjua AA, Amrein K, Quraishi SA, Lee-Sarwar KA, et al. Association between prehospital vitamin D status and incident acute respiratory failure in critically ill patients: a retrospective cohort study. *BMJ Open Respir Res* (2015) 2:e000074. doi:10.1136/bmjresp-2014-000074
202. Parekh D, Thickett DR, Turner AM. Vitamin D deficiency and acute lung injury. *Inflamm Allergy Drug Targets* (2013) 12:253–61. doi:10.2174/18715281113129990049
203. Heulens N, Korf H, Cielen N, De Smidt E, Maes K, Gysemans C, et al. Vitamin D deficiency exacerbates COPD-like characteristics in the lungs of cigarette smoke-exposed mice. *Respir Res* (2015) 16:110. doi:10.1186/s12931-015-0271-x
204. Foong RE, Bosco A, Jones AC, Gout A, Gorman S, Hart PH, et al. The effects of in utero vitamin D deficiency on airway smooth muscle mass and lung function. *Am J Respir Cell Mol Biol* (2015) 53:664–75. doi:10.1165/rcmb.2014-0356OC
205. Nouari W, Ysmail-Dahlouk L, Aribi M. Vitamin D3 enhances bactericidal activity of macrophage against *Pseudomonas aeruginosa*. *Int Immunopharmacol* (2016) 30:94–101. doi:10.1016/j.intimp.2015.11.033

22

Acute Respiratory Distress Syndrome Associated with Clopidogrel in a Young Male Patient

Stephanie M. Roses, Thomas Christianson and Keith Dombrowski*

Department of Neurology, Duke University, Durham, NC, United States

**Correspondence:*
Stephanie M. Roses
stephanie.roses@duke.edu

Background: Clopidogrel is a commonly prescribed antiplatelet drug in patients with stents and histories of arterial vascular disease. It generally has a favorable side effect profile with increasing bleeding risk as the main concern as an adverse event.

Case Presentation: A 19-year-old previously healthy male presented to the neurological intensive care unit with a subarachnoid hemorrhage requiring a flow diverting stent to secure the aneurysm. The patient was stable for 2 weeks and had no changes to management or medication within 48 h of antiplatelet therapy. Within hours of first-time dosing of clopidogrel, the patient experienced a syncopal episode and dyspnea. He was difficult to arouse and using accessory muscles to breath with an otherwise benign exam. He was hypoxic with bibasilar crackles requiring bilevel positive airway pressure (BiPap). Imaging showed bilateral pulmonary edema and he was diagnosed with moderate acute respiratory distress syndrome (ARDS). Infectious, cardiogenic, and contrast-induced ARDS were ruled out. Upon cessation of clopidogrel, his pulmonary function and mental status improved.

Conclusions: This is the first reported case of a young and immunocompetent patient's severe pulmonary edema leading to acute respiratory distress syndrome in association with first- time dosing of clopidogrel.

Keywords: clopidgrel, plavix, ARDS (Acute respiratory distress syndrome), aneurysm, subarachanoid hemorrhage

BACKGROUND

A 19-year-old male with a remote history of asthma was brought to the a university-affiliated tertiary care medical center emergency department by emergency services after he was found obtunded at home. He had an influenza-negative upper respiratory infection, treated with oseltamivir due to flu positive contacts, for 7 days prior to admission. The day prior to admission, he called his parents and reported worst-of-life headache. He stopped responding to messages the next day, and the police department was called. He was found obtunded in his apartment. He was admitted to the intensive care unit with a Hunt-Hess 2, modified Fisher 4, subarachnoid hemorrhage with intraventricular extension secondary to rupture of a bilobed saccular aneurysm of the P2 segment of the right posterior cerebral artery. Hospital day 3 he underwent a right sub-temporal craniotomy for placement of two clips to the aneurysm, leaving a 4 mm residual aneurysm. On hospital day 4, the patient developed symptomatic vasospasm which was supported by Transcranial Doppler data. This resolved with institution of a milrinone infusion, and he remained neurologically intact the following 2 weeks in the intensive care unit. On hospital day 14 he underwent an angiogram to evaluate the residual aneurysm. This revealed a new outpouching of aneurysm adjacent to the clip, needing a flow diverting stent for management.

The patient was subsequently loaded with 150 mg of clopidogrel and started on 75 mg daily. The next morning, the patient reported feeling dizzy and short of breath while walking. Upon return to his room he was somnolent, hypotensive and using accessory muscles to breathe with an oxygen saturation of 75% with bibasilar crackles. He was quickly transitioned to BiPAP with settings as follows: fraction inspired oxygen (FiO2) 60%, inspiratory positive airway pressure 12 mmHg, expiratory positive airway pressure 10 mmHg, and his mental status improved. A norepinephrine infusion (0.01–0.03 mcg/kg/min) was required for roughly 12 h to maintain mean arterial pressure $>$ 65 mm Hg. An arterial blood gas taken after 2 h of BiPAP revealed an arterial partial pressure of oxygen of 61 mmHg, for a P/F ratio (arterial partial pressure of oxygen/fraction inspired oxygen) of 102. On physical exam, the patient was difficult to arouse but was oriented to person, place, time, and situation and otherwise had a benign exam.

The only laboratory abnormality was a white blood cell count of 28.4 K/μL, up from 7.5 K/μL 13 h prior. A chest X-ray showed diffuse bilateral infiltrates without cardiomegaly (see **Figure 1**).

The patient was started on vancomycin and ceftriaxone for a presumed pneumonia. CTA chest revealed significant pulmonary edema without a focal consolidation or pulmonary embolism (see **Figures 2**, **3**). A transthoracic echocardiogram was normal and unchanged from previous study 15 days prior with fully mobile and normal valves, normal chamber diameters and volumes, a calculated ejection fraction of 57%, and positive saline contrast study. Sputum, blood, and urine cultures had no growth. Clopidogrel was the only recent intervention so it was discontinued. Within 21 h the leukocytosis dropped to 12.3 K/μL and antibiotics were stopped.

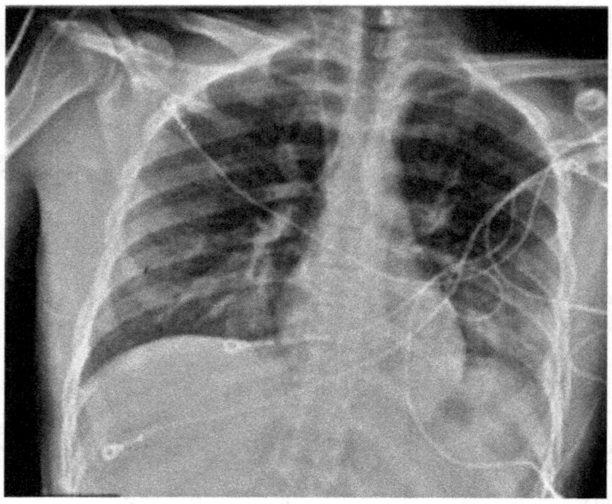

FIGURE 1 | Chest radiograph immediately following syncopal episode and hypoxia.

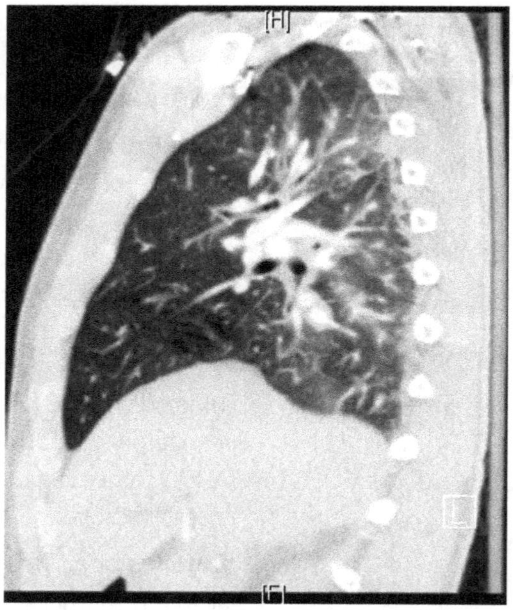

FIGURE 2 | High resolution CT sagittal view of left lung and right heart border. It showed intralobular septal thickening with ground glass opacities consistent with pulmonary edema. Bilateral lower lobe bronchial wall thickening with bronchial debris and consolidative opacities were present. It did not show evidence of pulmonary embolus.

DISCUSSION AND CONCLUSIONS

Infectious Disease was originally consulted and agreed that an infectious etiology was likely. However, the next day the consulting team doubted their initial assessment as the patient's course rapidly improved in a manner not consistent with nosocomial pneumonia. His white blood cell count dropped from 28 to 12.3 K/μL 12 h after antibiotics were administered with no growth on blood or sputum culture. Afebrile the entire hospitalization, he showed no signs of infection besides radiographic chest findings and leukocytosis which occur together in many inflammatory processes, including ARDS. The leukocytosis with left shift and 88.6% neutrophils was attributed to stress demargination. There were no measured eosinophils.

The patient met Berlin criteria for moderate ARDS, though only 2 mm Hg above the severe ARDS cut-off (**Table 1**). The lack of hemoptysis and radiographic evidence did not support interstitial respiratory hemorrhage. His normal cardiac function and chemistries did not support fluid overload or heart failure. Allergy and Immunology were consulted in light of the possibility that this idiopathic ARDS was directly associated with the only addition to intervention within 72 h of symptom onset: Clopidogrel administration several hours before his flash pulmonary edema. We also considered contrast-induced ARDS but the patient tolerated multiple contrast loads prior to and

Abbreviations: BiPap, Bilevel positive airway pressure; ARDS, acute respiratory distress syndrome; CTA, contrast tomography angiography; CT, contrast tomography.

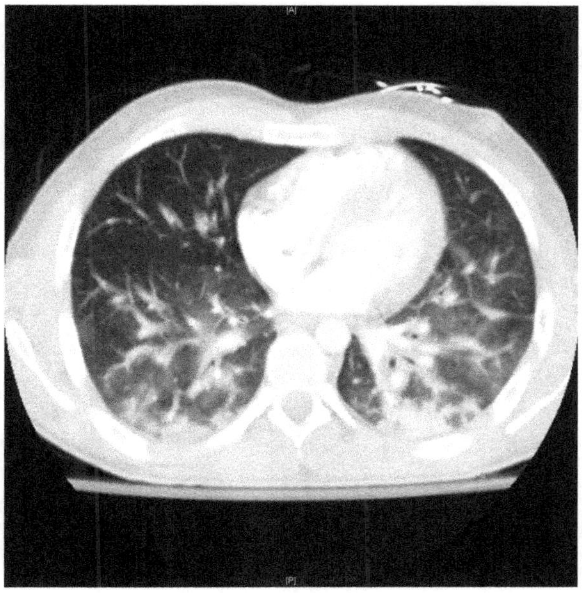

FIGURE 3 | High resolution coronal view of lungs through the lung window showing bilateral intralobular septal thickening with ground glass opacities, bronchial wall thickening and consolidative opacities.

TABLE 1 | Acute respiratory distress syndrome (1).

Timing	Within 1 week of known clinical insult or new or worsening respiratory symptoms
Chest imaging	Bilateral opacities- not fully explained by effusions, lobar/lung collapse, or nodules on chest radiograph or CT
Origin of edema	Respiratory failure not fully explained by cardiac failure or fluid overload
	Need objective assessment (e.g., Echocardiography) to exclude hydrostatic edema if no risk factor present
OXYGENATION	
Mild	200 mm Hg $<$ PaO$_2$ / FiO$_2$ $\leq$ 300 mm Hg with PEEP or CPAP 5 em H$_2$0
Moderate	100 mm Hg $<$ PaO$_2$ / FiO$_2$ $\leq$ 200 mm Hg with PEEP or CPAP 5 em H$_2$0
Severe	PaO$_2$ / FiO$_2$ $\leq$ 100 mm Hg with PEEP5 em H$_2$0

after this event without issue. Fat embolism was unlikely since he was 2 weeks removed from the last invasive intervention and the patient had a benign skin exam throughout his hospitalization, normal hemoglobin, and normal platelet numbers. Air embolism was unlikely again because he was so far removed from surgery and no there was no evidence of focal tissue damage in the heart, lungs, or brain. While changes in mental status and alertness are not part of the Berlin Definition of ARDS, it is a common symptom of hypoxemia and not specific to any diagnosis on the differential.

Known adverse reactions to clopidogrel and its derivative, ticlodipine, include thrombotic thrombocytopenic purpura and hemorrhage. Typical allergic reactions to clopidogrel include pruritic macular, erythematous, confluent rash starting on the trunk or face, angioedema, and anaphylaxis. ARDS and pulmonary edema are not reported in the Federal Drug Administration's overview of clopidogrel and meta-analyses of associated clinical trials (2, 3). In the CAPRIE trial, fewer patients reported dyspnea in the clopidogrel with aspirin group than the placebo with aspirin group, with no difference in attrition in either group (4). In a meta-analysis, antiplatelet therapy in critically ill patients was associated with lower incidence of ARDS, particularly in those with predisposing conditions such as high-risk surgery, trauma, pneumonia, and sepsis (5). This meta-analysis looked at a broad spectrum of antiplatelet therapies and not just clopidogrel or ticlodipine.

Clopidogrel is metabolized via two main pathways in the liver. Eighty-five percentage of circulating metabolites arise from an esterase-mediated hydrolysis of clopidogrel into inactive compounds.

The CYP450 enzyme pathways metabolize the remaining clopidogrel into its active thiol metabolite over two steps. *In vivo*, the CYP450 enzyme pathway is mediated by CYP3A4, CYP2C19, CYP1A2, and CYP2B6. There are known differences in clopidogrel metabolism leading to adverse events in those with variants of the CYP2C19 enzyme, though none reported are non-cardiogenic pulmonary edema (6–8). The active thiol metabolite rapidly and irreversibly binds platelet receptors, inhibiting platelet aggregation. While unchanged clopidogrel has a serum peak at 45 min, the active thiol compound's half-life is 6 h after a single 75 mg oral dose.

There exist known variants in CYP450 enzymes that lead to differences in individual metabolism of drugs in these pathways, especially noted in CYP2C19 variants. Caucasian populations show an increased risk of adverse events and reduced platelet response in poor metabolizers. In the Ashkenazi Jewish population, such as our patient, unique combinations of ultra-rapid metabolizer and poor metabolizer alleles have been described with little clinical data (9–13). However, proponents of pharmacogenetics do suggest that in certain cases, like that of a patient with a personal or family history of unusual drug reactions, genetic testing may help determine which antiplatelet therapy is most appropriate (10, 14).

Our patient's rapid improvement more closely fit with clearance of clopidogrel, with a 6 h half-life. According to the Naranjo adverse drug reactions probability scale criteria, our patient's score of 7 means it is probable that clopidogrel caused his ARDS (see **Table 2**) (15). He quickly improved after discontinuation of clopidogrel and, once stable, was placed on prasugrel with no difficulties. He successfully underwent his planned drug-eluting stent placement and was discharged shortly thereafter.

The only previous case report of non-cardiogenic pulmonary edema possibly due to clopidogrel administration was in an elderly gentleman in Turkey in 2007 (16). Within 48 h of angioplasty and clopidogrel initiation, a 71 year-old otherwise healthy patient was admitted for shortness of breath with dyspnea, tachycardia, and widely distributed pulmonary rales bilaterally. Arterial blood gas showed normal blood pH and normal partial pressure of carbon dioxide with low partial pressure of oxygen (57 mm Hg) and oxygen saturation (91%). Chest radiograph demonstrated diffuse bilateral interstitial and alveolar infiltrates with bilateral pleural effusion. High resolution CT ruled out pulmonary embolus but did show

TABLE 2 | Naranjo Adverse Drug Reaction Probability Scale (14).

To assess the adverse drug reaction, please answer the following questionnaire and give the pertinent score	Yes	No	Do not know
1. Are there previous conclusive reports on this drug reaction?	**1**	0	0
2. Did the adverse event occur after the suspected drug was administered?	**2**	−1	0
3. Did the adverse reaction improve when the drug was discontinued or a specific antagonist was administered?	**1**	0	0
4. Did the adverse reaction reappear when the drug was re-administered?	2	−1	**0**
5. Are there alternative causes (other than the drug) that could have on their own caused the reaction?	−1	**2**	0
6. Did the reaction reappear when a placebo was given?	−1	1	**0**
7. Was the drug detected in the blood (or other fluids) in concentrations known to be toxic?	1	0	**0**
8. Was the reaction more severe when the dose was increased or less severe when the dose was decreased?	1	0	**0**
9. Did the patient have a similar reaction to the same or similar drugs in any previous exposure?	1	**0**	0
10. Was the adverse event confirmed by objective evidence?	**1**	0	0
Total	5	2	

This case results in a 7 on the scale, or probable reaction due to the drug in question. The ADR is assigned to a probability category from the total score as follows: "Definite" if the overall score is 9 or higher, "probable" for a score of 5–8, "possible" for 1–4 and "doubtful" if the score is 0. Corresponding scores for this case are bolded.

localized right-sided fluid collection and bilateral ground-glass appearance of the lungs with pleural effusions and minimal pericardial effusion. Echocardiogram, complete blood count, and throat and blood cultures were unchanged from pre-operative exam. Like the present case report, there was no evidence of the typical adverse events associated with clopidogrel like pulmonary interstitial hemorrhage. The day after discontinuation of clopidogrel, the alveolar infiltrations on chest radiograph regressed over 48 h and fully disappeared on the fifth day of withdrawal.

The previous case differs from the current case in the age and medical history of the patient, though the progression of flash pulmonary edema after clopidogrel initiation to oxygen necessity and bilateral opacities without evidence of cardiogenic or fluid overload pulmonary edema is remarkably similar. The lack of other case reports or data supporting clinically significant dyspnea or pulmonary edema suggests this is a rare but potentially fatal complication in a commonly used drug. Neither the current case nor the previous Turkish case of non-cardiogenic pulmonary edema after clopidogrel tested for CYP450 enzyme variants, especially CYP2C19. The likely eastern European descent of both patients with recent genetic evidence of Turkish descent of Ashkenazi Jews in literature (17) prompt the question of whether these reactions are more widespread than reported in certain populations, and further whether these specific populations may benefit from pharmacogenetic analysis in regard to clopidogrel administration as they often do currently for warfarin (18–23).

This case report is limited in its applications to general patient care but it does represent a clinically relevant and severe probable adverse reaction to a commonly used drug. The patient's course surprised neurological intensive care providers, and allergy, immunology, and infectious disease specialists. Future testing of this patient's CYP450 enzymes and drug metabolism has been recommended to his primary care provider in light of his hospital course. This case represents a rare but severe adverse event associated with clopidogrel administration of which providers should be aware.

AUTHOR CONTRIBUTIONS

SR, TC, and KD all provided direct patient care as a medical student, intensive care fellow, and attending physician respectively. All authors analyzed and interpreted data on our patient's severe acute respiratory distress syndrome. SR was a major contributor in writing the manuscript.

REFERENCES

1. Force ADT, Ranieri VM, Rubenfeld GD, Thompson BT, Ferguson ND, Caldwell E, et al. Acute respiratory distress syndrome: the Berlin definition. *JAMA.* (2012) 307:2526–33. doi: 10.1001/jama.2012.5669
2. Food and Drug Administration. *Label - PLAVIX (Clopidogrel bisulphate) Tablets, for Oral Use.* Food and Drug Administration (2016).
3. McQuaid KR, Laine L. Systematic review and meta-analysis of adverse events of low-dose aspirin and clopidogrel in randomized controlled trials. *Am J Med.* (2006) 119:624–38. doi: 10.1016/j.amjmed.2005.10.039
4. Committee CS. A randomised, blinded, trial of clopidogrel versus aspirin in patients at risk of ischaemic events (CAPRIE). CAPRIE Steering Committee. *Lancet.* (1996) 348:1329–39.
5. Wang Y, Zhong M, Wang Z, Song J, Wu W, Zhu D. The preventive effect of antiplatelet therapy in acute respiratory distress syndrome: a meta-analysis. *Crit Care.* (2018) 22:60. doi: 10.1186/s13054-018-1988-y
6. Liu YP, Hao PP, Zhang MX, Zhang C, Gao F, Zhang Y, et al. Association of genetic variants in CYP2C19 and adverse clinical outcomes after treatment with clopidogrel: an updated meta-analysis. *Thromb Res.* (2011) 128:593–4. doi: 10.1016/j.thromres.2011.07.003

7. Scott SA, Sangkuhl K, Gardner EE, Stein CM, Hulot JS, Johnson JA, et al. Clinical pharmacogenetics implementation consortium guidelines for cytochrome P450-2C19 (CYP2C19) genotype and clopidogrel therapy. *Clin Pharmacol Ther.* (2011) 90:328–32. doi: 10.1038/clpt.2011.132
8. Jang JS, Cho KI, Jin HY, Seo JS, Yang TH, Kim DK, et al. Meta-analysis of cytochrome P450 2C19 polymorphism and risk of adverse clinical outcomes among coronary artery disease patients of different ethnic groups treated with clopidogrel. *Am J Cardiol.* (2012) 110:502–8. doi: 10.1016/j.amjcard.2012.04.020
9. Scott SA, Martis S, Peter I, Kasai Y, Kornreich R, Desnick RJ. Identification of CYP2C19*4B: pharmacogenetic implications for drug metabolism including clopidogrel responsiveness. *Pharmacogenomics J.* (2012) 12:297–305. doi: 10.1038/tpj.2011.5
10. Scott SA, Sangkuhl K, Stein CM, Hulot JS, Mega JL, Roden DM, et al. Clinical pharmacogenetics implementation consortium guidelines for CYP2C19 genotype and clopidogrel therapy: 2013 update. *Clin Pharmacol Ther.* (2013) 94:317–23. doi: 10.1038/clpt.2013.105
11. Martis S, Mei H, Vijzelaar R, Edelmann L, Desnick RJ, Scott SA. Multi-ethnic cytochrome-P450 copy number profiling: novel pharmacogenetic alleles and mechanism of copy number variation formation. *Pharmacogenomics J.* (2013) 13:558–66. doi: 10.1038/tpj.2012.48
12. Sorich MJ, Rowland A, McKinnon RA, Wiese MD. CYP2C19 genotype has a greater effect on adverse cardiovascular outcomes following percutaneous coronary intervention and in Asian populations treated with clopidogrel: a meta-analysis. *Circ Cardiovasc Genet.* (2014) 7:895–902. doi: 10.1161/CIRCGENETICS.114.000669
13. Yang Y, Peter I, Scott SA. Pharmacogenetics in Jewish populations. *Drug Metabol Drug Interact.* (2014) 29:221–33. doi: 10.1515/dmdi-2013-0069
14. Shuldiner AR, Palmer K, Pakyz RE, Alestock TD, Maloney KA, O'Neill C, et al. Implementation of pharmacogenetics: the University of Maryland personalized anti-platelet pharmacogenetics program. *Am J Med Genet C Semin Med Genet.* (2014) 166C:76–84. doi: 10.1002/ajmg.c.31396
15. Naranjo CA, Busto U, Sellers EM, Sandor P, Ruiz I, Roberts EA, et al. A method for estimating the probability of adverse drug reactions. *Clin Pharmacol Ther.* (1981) 30:239–45. doi: 10.1038/clpt.1981.154
16. Erdinler IC, Ucer E, Eksik A, Akyol A, Yazici S. Noncardiogenic pulmonary edema associated with clopidogrel: a serious but unexpected side effect of clopidogrel. *Can J Cardiol.* (2007) 23:478–80. doi: 10.1016/S0828-282X(07)70788-2
17. Das R, Wexler P, Pirooznia M, Elhaik E. Localizing Ashkenazic Jews to primeval villages in the ancient Iranian lands of Ashkenaz. *Genome Biol Evol.* (2016) 8:1132–49. doi: 10.1093/gbe/evw046
18. Schwartz JB. Pharmacogenetics: has it reached the clinic? *J Gend Specif Med.* (2002) 5:13–8.
19. Gottlieb B. Human genome variation and pharmacogenetics. *Hum Mutat.* (2008) 29:453–5. doi: 10.1002/humu.20728
20. Scott SA, Edelmann L, Kornreich R, Desnick RJ. Warfarin pharmacogenetics: CYP2C9 and VKORC1 genotypes predict different sensitivity and resistance frequencies in the Ashkenazi and Sephardi Jewish populations. *Am J Hum Genet.* (2008) 82:495–500. doi: 10.1016/j.ajhg.2007.10.002
21. Dean L. Clopidogrel therapy and CYP2C19 genotype. In: Pratt V, McLeod H, Dean L, Malheiro A, Rubinstein W, editors. *Medical Genetics Summaries.* Bethesda, MD: National Center for Biotechnology Information (NCBI). (2012).
22. Mao L, Jian C, Changzhi L, Dan H, Suihua H, Wenyi T, et al. Cytochrome CYP2C19 polymorphism and risk of adverse clinical events in clopidogrel-treated patients: a meta-analysis based on 23,035 subjects. *Arch Cardiovasc Dis.* (2013) 106:517–27. doi: 10.1016/j.acvd.2013.06.055
23. van Schaik RH, IFCC Task Force on Pharmacogenetics: Prof. Dr. Maurizio Ferrari (IT), Prof. Dr. Michael Neumaier (GER), Prof. Dr. Munir Pirmohamed (UK), Prof. Dr. Henk-Jan Guchelaar (NL), Prof. Dr. Ron van Schaik (NL). Clinical application of pharmacogenetics: where are we now? *EJIFCC.* (2013) 24:105–12.

23

Viral Infection in the Development and Progression of Pediatric Acute Respiratory Distress Syndrome

*Steven Nye, Richard J. Whitley and Michele Kong**

The University of Alabama at Birmingham, Birmingham, AL, USA

Correspondence:
Michele Kong
mkong@peds.uab.edu

Viral infections are an important cause of pediatric acute respiratory distress syndrome (ARDS). Numerous viruses, including respiratory syncytial virus (RSV) and influenza A (H1N1) virus, have been implicated in the progression of pneumonia to ARDS; yet the incidence of progression is unknown. Despite acute and chronic morbidity associated with respiratory viral infections, particularly in "at risk" populations, treatment options are limited. Thus, with few exceptions, care is symptomatic. In addition, mortality rates for viral-related ARDS have yet to be determined. This review outlines what is known about ARDS secondary to viral infections including the epidemiology, the pathophysiology, and diagnosis. In addition, emerging treatment options to prevent infection, and to decrease disease burden will be outlined. We focused on RSV and influenza A (H1N1) viral-induced ARDS, as these are the most common viruses leading to pediatric ARDS, and have specific prophylactic and definitive treatment options.

Keywords: RSV, influenza A virus, H1N1 subtype, ARDS, pediatrics, viral infections

INTRODUCTION

Acute respiratory distress syndrome (ARDS) was first described in 1967 in adults presenting with tachypnea, hypoxemia, and decreased pulmonary compliance (1). Since then, the understanding, diagnosis, and management of ARDS has advanced greatly, with most research performed in adults. For more than two decades, pediatric health-care providers have relied heavily on adult-derived diagnostic criteria (2, 3). In recent years, the Pediatric Acute Lung Injury Consensus Conference (PALICC) has provided age-specific diagnostic and management guidelines for pediatric ARDS (4, 5). With these new pediatric-specific recommendations, future research in pediatric ARDS looks promising, as new areas for investigation have been identified (5).

One area of interest warranting further exploration is the role of viral infection in the development and progression of pediatric ARDS. While some information is available specific to pediatrics, much of our understanding continues to be derivative from adult data. This review outlines what is known about ARDS attributable to viral infections, specifically respiratory syncytial virus (RSV) and influenza A (H1N1) virus, as well as viral-specific treatment options.

EPIDEMIOLOGY OF RSV AND INFLUENZA-INDUCED ARDS

Accurate incidence outcomes reporting for pediatric ARDS are limited by the changing definition for ARDS. Studies using the 1994 American European Consensus Conference (AECC) definition (2) outlined epidemiology and outcomes for both acute lung injury (ALI) and ARDS as separate entities (6). However, both the Berlin definition (3) and the PALICC recommendations (5) no longer identify ALI as a separate entity, instead categorizing ARDS as mild, moderate, or severe. Since these guidelines are recent, few studies have been conducted to determine the incidence of ARDS utilizing these new criteria (7, 8). In addition, management for ARDS has also changed over the years, with improved outcomes demonstrated with lung-protective mechanical ventilation strategies (9, 10).

Pediatric studies conducted using the AECC definition define an incidence ranging from 2.96 to 12.8 per 100,000 children for all causes of ALI/ARDS, with the predominant etiology reported to be secondary to pneumonia, with or without systemic infection (11). In a more recent study, using the Berlin definition, Barreira et al. reported that ARDS accounts for 10% of all PICU admissions, and was associated with a high mortality rate of 24.5% (7). While the overall incidence of respiratory virus infection, in particular RSV and influenza A (H1N1) virus, leading to lower respiratory tract disease is widely studied (12, 13), the frequency of progression to pediatric ARDS has yet to be clearly determined.

Respiratory syncytial virus infection has been recognized as an important cause of lower lung disease. In an earlier study, Dahlem et al. reported 15.9% of ARDS cases due to RSV-related infection, but specific mortality for this group was not reported (14). In a more recent study by Lopez-Fernandez et al., 19.8% of patients admitted to the PICU with ARDS tested positive for RSV, with a reported mortality of 13.7% (15). A 12-year study in the Netherlands by Schene et al. analyzed 155 patients mechanically ventilated for RSV with 129 (83%) patients progressing to ARDS (16). Of those with ARDS, 38% were found to have a bacterial coinfection. The mortality rate was not used as a measure of outcome and therefore not reported.

Since the beginning of the influenza A (H1N1) virus pandemic of 2009, influenza-related respiratory failure has become a notable cause of ARDS (17). During the pandemic and post-pandemic era, it is clear that children are particularly vulnerable to disease even if they had been previously healthy (18). In 2009 alone, more than 43,000 cases were reported, with an estimated 73% of cases occurring in patients less than 24 years of age (13). In previous years, influenza-related pediatric deaths averaged 82 annually but increased to 317 during the 2009 pandemic (19). While post-pandemic studies suggest a decrease in influenza A (H1N1) virus disease severity and burden (20, 21), it continues to be a significant cause of severe illness and pediatric ARDS (22).

In a retrospective analysis of adult patients within the German ARDS network, investigators reported that 32% of ARDS patients were influenza A (H1N1) virus positive (23). In another pediatric study in India, Kinikar et al. reported that 18% of patients hospitalized with confirmed influenza A (H1N1) virus developed ARDS (24). In this study, 9 of the 15 children who died were found to have histologic pulmonary findings reflective of ARDS at autopsy. In Argentina, Farias et al. studied 147 patients admitted with respiratory failure due to influenza A (H1N1) virus and found 118 (80%) met criteria for pediatric ARDS, 45% of whom died within 28 days after PICU admission (25).

The second, less common novel influenza virus, avian influenza A (H5N1) virus, was first identified in 1998 (26) and remains a common cause of severe respiratory disease (27). Kawachi et al. reviewed pediatric patients with ARDS over a 4½-year period in Vietnam and found 12 (32.4%) of the 37 patients to have confirmed infection with the highly pathogenic influenza A (H5N1) virus (28). They described rapid progression of disease to ARDS with nine (75%) resulting in death. Further investigation has led to improved understanding of transmission, predominantly direct avian-to-human transmission with significant risk in handling sick or dead poultry. Type 2 pneumocytes and macrophages are the primary lung target (29).

Together, these studies demonstrate that RSV and influenza virus infection play a role in the development of pediatric ARDS. However, to better understand the disease burden, future studies should seek to more clearly identify the rate of occurrence of primary viral-induced ARDS, as well as incidence of secondary viral-induced lung injury. Furthermore, in patients who have a coinfection with a bacterial pathogen, it may be hard to determine whether the virus or bacteria played the inciting role in the development and progression of pediatric ARDS.

Taken together, the overall mortality attributable to either RSV or influenza is relatively similar; thus, it is more likely the syndrome of ARDS and associated pathology that is responsible for outcome.

OTHER VIRUSES LEADING TO ARDS

While RSV and influenza A (H1N1) virus are the most commonly reported viruses leading to pediatric ARDS, other viral pathogens are worth mentioning. Typically viral infections leading to respiratory failure in the ICU are separated as community acquired and nosocomial (30).

Community acquired viral infections include both seasonal and pandemic pathogens (31). Seasonal viruses most commonly include RSV, non-pandemic influenza, rhinoviruses, parainfluenza, adenovirus, coronaviruses, and human metapneumovirus (hMPV). Seasonal viruses remain the most frequent cause of childhood community acquired pneumonia (32). The most common etiology of pediatric ARDS is primary pneumonia, with or without systemic infection (15). It can then be assumed that viral infections may play an important role in development of pediatric ARDS. However, determining an accurate estimate of the disease burden of viral-induced pediatric ARDS will be difficult, as many simple viral infections can progress to coinfection with the second virus or a bacterial pathogen. As will be detailed below, with the development of multiplex PCR diagnostic platforms that identify multiple viral agents, further insight into coinfections will develop.

A single-center adult study reported seven patients developing ARDS from adenovirus, four of whom died (33). Hung and Lin described a case of a 9-month-old male with adenoviral ARDS requiring extracorporeal membrane oxygenation (ECMO) (34). Hasvold et al. studied adult patients hospitalized with hMPV and discovered progression to ARDS in 19 (14.8%) patients (35). In 2014, an outbreak of enterovirus D68 in the United States led to symptoms of respiratory failure similar to influenza A (H1N1) virus, although less severe (36). While seasonal viruses typically cause severe infection in immunocompromised patients (37), cases of severe disease in immunocompetent patients are becoming increasingly reported (38).

At an international level, community acquired, novel pathogens have been recognized as a significant cause of ARDS in the last 15–20 years (31). In 2015, the World Health Organization (WHO) developed a panel of experts to prioritize emerging pathogens to likely cause severe outbreaks in the near future, and for which little or no preventative or curative treatments are available (39). The list includes two novel coronaviruses, severe acute respiratory syndrome (SARS)-CoV and MERS-CoV, which are widely recognized as noteworthy causes of ARDS.

In 2002, SARS-CoV led to the development of SARS in China (40). Affecting patients of all ages, SARS led to significant mortality worldwide within a few months (41). A large number of infected patients developed severe complications, with 20% developing ARDS (42). However, reported SARS cases have ceased since 2004 as the spread of infection has subsided (43). More recently, the second novel coronavirus, MERS-CoV, led to the Middle East respiratory syndrome (44). Clinical symptoms range from mild upper respiratory symptoms to severe pneumonia and ARDS, septic shock, and multi-organ failure (45) and carry an estimated mortality of 40% (46). This virus continues to be a substantial etiology of ARDS with high mortality as no definitive prevention or treatment other than supportive care has been identified (47).

With the unpredictable nature of epidemics and pandemics, these novel viruses illustrate the need to improve our understanding of viral progression to ARDS in order to advance management and reduce mortality.

Aside from community acquired viral infections, nosocomial infections are an important cause of respiratory illness, and can lead to ARDS in both adults and children. In mechanically ventilated adults, reactivation of latent herpes simplex virus (HSV) in the oropharynx can potentially lead to lower respiratory tract infection and ARDS (48, 49). However, the pathogenicity of reactivated HSV lower respiratory tract infection may not be that straightforward as it remains unclear whether HSV contributes to worsening illness or whether reactivation occurs due to the underlying critical illness (50). Schuller et al. found higher levels of clinical severity and mortality in critically ill immunocompetent adults with HSV-1 infection compared to immunocompromised patients with HSV-1 (51). The true extent of HSV reactivation in critically ill children leading to respiratory illness has yet to be studied. Hennus et al. described two previously healthy children presenting with respiratory failure due to human herpes virus 6 (HHV-6), and later workup revealed an immunodeficiency in both patients (52). A separate pediatric case reported a child with HSV ARDS resulting in need of extracorporeal support (53). These cases illustrate the rare, but possible severe infection and progression to ARDS from HSV-1.

Finally, many seasonal and pandemic viruses are a potential nosocomial infectious risk secondary to either a health-care provider or air-ventilation transmission. In a study over two influenza seasons in Germany, Huzly et al. reported a rate of nosocomial transmission of 24% (2012–2013) and 20% (2013–2014) (54). Specific guidelines are available to help prevent transmission of infectious pathogens through isolation precautions (55). However, Dhar et al. found that an increased number in patients placed on contact isolation led to a decrease in compliance with isolation precautions (56). Decreasing nosocomial transmission within care areas for critically ill patients is an important area for improvement.

DIAGNOSIS OF VIRAL-INDUCED ARDS

The PALICC has recently provided guidelines for diagnosing pediatric ARDS (5). The new guidelines define important diagnostic criteria, including age, timing, origin of edema, imaging, and oxygenation. Patients with perinatal lung disease are excluded, and pARDS criteria must be met within 7 days of a clinical insult. The cause of respiratory failure must not be explained by heart failure or fluid overload, and must be evidenced by new pulmonary infiltrate(s) on chest radiograph consistent with parenchymal disease. Finally, the use of oxygenation index is preferred over the PaO_2:FiO_2 (PF) ratio in determining the severity of pARDS in mechanically ventilated patients, while the PF ratio or SpO_2:FiO_2 (SF) ratio may be used in patients requiring non-invasive ventilation (5). The same clinical guideline is used in the diagnosis of viral-induced pediatric ARDS. Currently, there are several different types of laboratory tests that are commercially available for diagnosis. Most clinical laboratories utilize antigen detection tests, which consist of multiple steps to accurately identify a single virus (57), with or without cell culture.

It is worth noting that over the past 20 years, the development and refinement of real-time reverse transcriptase polymerase chain reaction (RT-PCR) has enhanced the clinician's ability to diagnose an array of viruses rapidly and accurately. Multiplex RT-PCR testing analyzes a single sample for multiple viral agents and subtypes simultaneously, producing sensitive and specific results in a short period of time (58). Even with the 2009 influenza A (H1N1) virus pandemic, the Centers for Disease Control and Prevention (CDC) quickly modified standard PCR assays to detect the new virus (59). A challenge to routine RT-PCR testing in all patients who present with viral symptoms is the prohibitive cost, need for specialized equipment, and the relatively longer time between sampling and availability of results (60). Furthermore, PCRs detect viral genes that are used as a surrogate measurement of whole virions. In some instances, viral gene detection may actually reflect non-replicating, non-infectious virions. Newer rapid point-of-care PCRs are currently being developed, but their implications for clinical decision making remain uncertain (61). In addition, rapid antigen detection tests (RADT) are also available commercially for detection of both RSV and influenza virus infection in the outpatient and emergency department settings (62, 63). However, in a recent study by Moesker et al., RADTs were found to have relatively low sensitivity compared to RT-PCR testing which limits their use for clinical decision making (64). Nonetheless, RADT maybe a valuable tool, especially during an outbreak, because it is a point-of-care test that is easy to use with a rapid turnaround time (65). Since clinical symptoms for different viral respiratory infections are often the same, and with the limitations of our current testing methods, it is critical that clinicians obtain microbiology data early, especially in the risk population (66–69).

TABLE 1 | Clinical risk factors for severe viral respiratory infection.

RSV	Influenza A (H1N1) virus
Age <6 months	Age <5 years
History of prematurity	Chronic lung disease
Chronic lung disease	Congenital heart disease
Congenital heart disease	Immunocompromised conditions
Viral coinfection	

There is also a large variability of disease severity in children infected with RSV or influenza A (H1N1) virus. In RSV infection, development of lower respiratory track disease in premature infants, with or without chronic neonatal lung disease is associated with a significantly higher risk of hospitalization, intensive care unit admission, need for mechanical ventilation, and death (12, 70–73). In a study of 2,147 children with lower respiratory infection due to RSV, Rodriguez et al. reported age less than 6 months, history of prematurity, chronic respiratory disease or congenital heart disease, and coinfection with adenovirus were significant predictors of increased disease severity (74). Similar predictors exist for children infected with influenza A (H1N1) virus, including age less than 5 years, a history of chronic lung disease, congenital heart disease, and immune compromise (**Table 1**) (75). It is therefore prudent that clinicians should conduct laboratory evaluations early in the illness for viral infections in these at-risk populations presenting with respiratory failure and ARDS.

In contrast to clinical predictors of disease severity, the contribution of viral factors to disease burden remains unclear. In RSV infection, although earlier studies suggested no correlation between viral load and disease severity (76, 77) newer findings suggest otherwise. Studies by both DeVincenzo et al. and Houben et al. reported a direct correlation between viral load and disease severity in infants with primary RSV infection (78, 79). El Saleeby et al. also reported that viral load is independently associated with increased risk of patients with RSV requiring prolonged hospitalization or intensive care, or to develop respiratory failure (80). The relevance of viral load in influenza A (H1N1) virus infection is unclear. Launes et al. found that in children who had more than 5 days of symptoms, a higher influenza A (H1N1) viral load at diagnosis correlated with an increased risk of requiring mechanical ventilation (81). Similarly others have found that patients with systemic symptoms and pneumonia had higher viral load when compared to those with uncomplicated upper respiratory tract infections alone (82). As would be expected children have a higher influenza A (H1N1) viral load compared to adults because of less exposure to influenza antigens. However, this finding did not correlate with the occurrence of disease complications (83).

PATHOPHYSIOLOGY AND HISTOLOGY OF RSV AND INFLUENZA A (H1N1) VIRAL-INDUCED ARDS

Both RSV and influenza A (H1N1) virus result in a broad spectrum of disease, ranging from mild upper respiratory symptoms to fulminant respiratory failure and ARDS (59, 84). This high degree of variability may be due to the pathogenicity of the viral pathogen, host immune response, or a combination of both (85).

Human RSV consists of subgroups A and B and primarily infects humans. The RSV genome encodes 11 different proteins involved in transmission, infection, evasion of host response, and replication (86). Infection is typically restricted to respiratory epithelial cells, including both type I and type II alveolar pneumocytes, from the trachea to the level of bronchioles. Infection leads to epithelial and interstitial inflammation with progression to inflammatory infiltrates and epithelial sloughing (87). After infection and viral replication, RSV causes epithelial cells to fuse, forming a syncytium from which the virus spreads from cell to cell (88). Those infected epithelial cells are then destroyed, releasing inflammatory cytokines and chemokines that ultimately attract additional inflammatory cells and degrade capillary integrity (89). Disruption of the alveolar–capillary barrier results in leakage of plasma proteins into interstitial tissue and within the alveoli, finally interfering with surfactant function (90). With an understanding of the pathophysiologic process of RSV, it is no surprise that progression to ARDS is a potential end point.

Aside from viral pathogenicity, host immune-mediated factors also contribute to disease severity. A rapidly progressive area of research is in understanding the role of biomarkers not only in the diagnosis and prognosis of ARDS, but also in potential therapeutic options to alter such biomarkers (91). Inflammatory proteins in the matrix metalloproteinase (MMP) family have been shown to be elevated in pediatric ALI (92) with a specific increase in MMP-9 production in RSV infection. Blocking MMP-9 *in vitro* and *in vivo* resulted in decrease in viral load (93). In addition, activation of several chemokine and interleukin subtypes, as well as tumor necrosis factors, has been shown to positively correlate with severity of illness in children with RSV (94). In their study, Fernandez et al. discovered that higher levels of soluble interleukin-10 (IL-10) positively correlated with both disease severity and duration of supplemental oxygen in infants with acute RSV infection (95). A separate study confirmed this associate with increased levels of IL-10 in nasopharyngeal secretions (96), but the pathogenicity of this correlation has yet to be determined.

Antigenic variability exists with both influenza A (H1N1) virus and the resultant immune-mediated response. Like influenza B and C, influenza A is made up of structural proteins and two groups of surface glycoproteins, hemagglutinin (HA), and neuraminidase (NA). These glycoproteins are responsible for attachment and entry into cells, viral spread throughout the respiratory tract, and are capable of a large degree of variability (97). Waterfowl serve as the largest natural reservoir for influenza A subtypes (98). The avian-to-human leap can occur through direct transmission (99) or, alternatively, through pigs (100). Although transmission from pigs to humans is a rare event, it occurred in the 1918 pandemic (101) a small outbreak in New Jersey in 1976 (102) and the most recent pandemic of influenza A (H1N1) starting in 2009 (103).

Influenza A (H1N1) virus primarily targets alveolar epithelial cells that serve as first-line defense against respiratory infections (104). Histological evaluation of 100 fatal cases of influenza A (H1N1) virus infection revealed diffuse alveolar damage with inflammation, fibrosis and edema, disruption of surfactant production, and detection of viral antigens throughout the lung parenchyma (105). Like RSV, this pathogenic can process rapidly progresses to refractory hypoxemia and ARDS (106).

In addition to viral pathogenicity, disease severity of influenza A (H1N1) virus infection is also closely associated with host response (107). In both healthy patients and those with comorbidities, influenza A (H1N1) virus can lead to an exaggerated inflammatory response with dysregulation of local and systemic chemokine and cytokine production (108, 109). In a study specifically in the pediatric population, Takano et al. found a positive correlation with disease severity and elevated levels of serum interferon gamma, several interleukin types, and monocyte chemoattractant protein-1 (MCP-1) (110). Some studies suggest that these elevations may be adequate immune response to infection (111), but further exploration of the inflammatory response in influenza A (H1N1) virus infection is likely to yield development of potential interventions to prevent disease progression to ARDS.

TREATMENT OPTIONS AVAILABLE FOR RSV AND INFLUENZA A (H1N1) VIRAL-INDUCED ARDS

The treatment of ARDS has significantly evolved over the past several decades. Perhaps the greatest improvement in management developed from studies involving lung-protective ventilation (9). Other interventions such as inhaled nitric oxide (112), fluid management (113), use of steroids (114), and prone positioning (115) are being further investigated and validated. However, specific treatment for RSV infection remains lacking. Despite the substantial short and long-term morbidity and mortality associated with RSV disease in children, the current management for RSV infection consists of supportive care, in the form of oxygen supplementation, adequate hydration, and mechanical ventilation for those who develop respiratory failure. Multiple therapeutic strategies have been explored with very limited success, and a vital need remains for an effective disease treatment.

Interventions for either virus can be separated into primary prevention of infection, typically through vaccination, and reduction of infectious burden once transmission has already taken place.

Primary prevention through vaccination continues to be a major area of research and potential advancement for both RSV and influenza A (H1N1) virus. To date, no RSV vaccine has proven efficacious. While significant research has been devoted to vaccine development, major obstacles specific to RSV, such as young age of infection, lack of persistent immunity, and poorly validated animal models make it difficult to find an effective and safe solution (116). One current prospect, Medi-534, a live-attenuated, intranasal vaccine providing protection against both RSV and parainfluenza 3, although safe in children ages 1–9, has yet to show a beneficial immunogenic response in infants (117). Other more recent advances continue to focus on live-attenuated vaccines, as well as chimeric live vectors (118), with varying antibody response between children (119, 120).

While vaccine development continues, prophylactic use of polyclonal RSV intravenous immunoglobulin (RespiGam) or human anti-F monoclonal antibodies (palivizumab and motavizumab – which is not yet licensed for use) in high-risk infants has been shown to reduce the risk of RSV-associated acute lower respiratory tract infections and disease severity (121). Palivizumab is a human, monoclonal antibody targeted to block viral infected cells from fusing with adjacent cells (122). Palivizumab has been shown to be most effective in high-risk populations, specifically premature infants and those with chronic lung disease or congenital heart disease (123). The use of palivizumab as treatment for RSV infection in mechanically ventilated pediatric patients has not been shown to be effective (124). Furthermore, studies have also shown that palivizumab prophylaxis in these patients has a limited effect on the total disease burden of RSV infection, including overall RSV-related hospital admissions and resource utilization (12, 125). Although not approved for use in the United States, motavizumab, the second-generation derivative of palivizumab, decreased viral load compared with placebo (126). However, in a more recent study of hospitalized RSV infected infants treated with motavizumab or placebo, no antiviral effect was demonstrated (127). Furthermore, both therapies produce only temporary, passive immunity (128).

The 2009 influenza A (H1N1) virus was a novel strain, leaving children and young adults with little if any preexisting antibodies and without adequate protection with the seasonal influenza vaccine alone (129). A new influenza A (H1N1) virus vaccine was rapidly developed and has subsequently been shown to be safe and effective at providing adequate immunological response (130, 131). One post-pandemic study showed a correlation with higher rates of influenza A (H1N1) virus infection, compared with other influenza types, along with increased ICU admissions for countries with limited numbers of the population having received influenza A (H1N1) virus vaccination (132).

In addition to general supportive care, the second goal of therapy in viral infection focuses on reducing the infectious burden and, theoretically, subsequent viral sequelae. Currently, inhaled ribavirin is the only approved antiviral treatment for RSV infection in children (133) but its use is associated with potential teratogenicity, and its efficacy remains uncertain (134). Ribavirin directly and indirectly inhibits replication of both DNA and RNA viruses, including RSV (135). Studies in infants found a decrease in mortality and respiratory deterioration, and a decrease in days of hospitalization and days of mechanical ventilation in ventilated infants (136). Luo et al. reported an adult case of severe RSV infection progressing to ARDS that was successfully treated with inhaled ribavirin (137), but overall effectiveness in treatment of viral pediatric ARDS has yet to be determined. In addition to its use in RSV, ribavirin has also been used in treatment of severe influenza A (H1N1) virus infection (138). Ribavirin can be given orally but is typically aerosolized when used for respiratory viral infections. However, safety considerations regarding potential teratogenicity and exposure to health-care workers during administration (134) limit its use. The American Academy of Pediatrics does not recommend the routine use of ribavirin to treat RSV infection, reserving its use for patients with potentially life-threatening disease (139). Several small molecule inhibitors that interfere with RSV F protein (MDT-637 and JNJ-2408068) (140) have been identified, including the GS-5806 that was recently evaluated in a challenge safety study of healthy adults (141). In this study by DeVincenzo et al., treatment resulted in decreased viral burden and severity of clinical disease. The use of these small molecule inhibitors in the context of pediatric subjects who develop ARDS remains untested at this point.

Neuraminidase inhibitors (which prevent the release of influenza virions), including oral oseltamivir, inhaled zanamivir and laninamivir, and parenteral peramivir, remain first-line interventions for influenza. Only oseltamivir, peramivir, and zanamivir are available in the United States. Perhaps the most widely used, oseltamivir results in a significant decrease in duration of symptoms as well as severity of illness with early treatment (<48 h of symptoms) (142). Use of oseltamivir in severe cases of influenza A (H1N1) has become standard practice (24, 143), although some studies have shown increased resistance (144). Randolph et al. conducted a retrospective study of 838 children admitted to the PICU with confirmed influenza A (H1N1) infection (145). Overall, 564 (67.3%) required mechanical ventilation, but the rate of progression to ARDS was not reported. Although 88% were treated with oseltamivir, there was no association with improved mortality. Farias et al. found a reduced mortality in patients with PARDS from influenza A (H1N1) if oseltamivir was administered within the first 24 h (25).

While further studies are needed to look at the effectiveness of antiviral medications in the treatment of viral-induced ARDS, in recent years, investigators are also focusing on the potential benefits of immune modulation. With enhancement in research surrounding viral pathogenicity and host immune response, potential targets of intervention will hopefully be identified.

Aside from viral-specific therapies, ECMO has been utilized as rescue therapy for severe respiratory failure in pediatrics for more than 20 years, with more than 50% survival (146). The overall use of ECMO for treatment of ARDS has increased with improvement in mortality (147). The recent PALICC recommendations conclude that ECMO should be considered for treatment of pARDS when lung-protective strategies have failed, when the cause of respiratory failure is thought to be reversible, or when the child may be suitable for lung transplantation (148).

The use of ECMO in pediatric respiratory failure due to RSV is well reported (149, 150). In their retrospective review of 151 children requiring mechanical ventilation for RSV bronchiolitis, Flamant et al. reported the use of ECMO in 14 patients (151). In this study, the median duration of ECMO was 12.5 (5–18) days with a survival rate of 71.4%. On the other hand, the use of ECMO in pARDS due to influenza A (H1N1) virus is sparsely reported (152, 153) and most of our understanding stems from adult studies. In a study in Australia and New Zealand during the 2009 influenza A (H1N1) pandemic, 68 adult patients with influenza-induced ARDS were treated with ECMO (154). The median duration of ECMO was 10 (7–15) days. When the report was submitted, 48 (71%) patients had survived to ICU discharge, with 14 deaths and 6 patients remaining in the ICU, 2 of whom remained on ECMO. In their study in the United Kingdom during the same pandemic, Noah et al. discovered a decrease in mortality for patients with ARDS due to influenza A (H1N1) who were referred and transferred to an ECMO center compared with matched non-ECMO-referred patients (155). In this study, 69 patients received ECMO with a mortality rate of 14.4%. Expanded use of ECMO within the pediatric population for influenza A (H1N1) virus induced ARDS has yet to be investigated. However, the use of ECMO in refractory cases or RSV or influenza A (H1N1) virus induced ARDS should be considered when applicable.

CONCLUSION

While it is clear that viral infections are an important cause of pediatric ARDS, the exact disease burden remains unknown. With more definitive diagnostic criteria, clinicians now have a wide array of research possibilities regarding pediatric ARDS, both retrospective and prospective. Further studies to expand our understanding of viral-induced pediatric ARDS will be of great benefit, both in understanding the epidemiology and viral-specific treatment options available. In addition, an improved comprehension of viral transmission, pathogenicity, and host response will be particularly important in times of pandemics, either from known or novel viruses. Finally, continued efforts in prevention and treatment of viral infections will likely be of greatest advantage to decrease viral progression to pediatric ARDS.

AUTHOR CONTRIBUTIONS

SN, RW, and MK contributed to the conception, writing, and final edits of this manuscript.

REFERENCES

1. Ashbaugh DG, Bigelow DB, Petty TL, Levine BE. Acute respiratory distress in adults. *Lancet* (1967) 2:319–23. doi:10.1016/S0140-6736(67)90168-7
2. Bernard GR, Artigas A, Brigham KL, Carlet J, Falke K, Hudson L, et al. The American-European consensus conference on ARDS. Definitions, mechanisms, relevant outcomes, and clinical trial coordination. *Am J Respir Crit Care Med* (1994) 149:818–24. doi:10.1164/ajrccm.149.3.7509706
3. Ranieri VM, Rubenfeld GD, Thompson BT, Ferguson ND, Caldwell E, Fan E, et al. Acute respiratory distress syndrome: the Berlin definition. *JAMA* (2012) 307:2526–33. doi:10.1001/jama.2012.5669
4. Thomas NJ, Jouvet P, Willson D. Acute lung injury in children – kids really aren't just "little adults". *Pediatr Crit Care Med* (2013) 14:429–32. doi:10.1097/PCC.0b013e31827456aa
5. Pediatric Acute Lung Injury Consensus Conference Group. Pediatric acute respiratory distress syndrome: consensus recommendations from the pediatric acute lung injury consensus conference. *Pediatr Crit Care Med* (2015) 16:428–39. doi:10.1097/PCC.0000000000000350

6. Sweatt AJ, Levitt JE. Evolving epidemiology and definitions of the acute respiratory distress syndrome and early acute lung injury. *Clin Chest Med* (2014) 35:609–24. doi:10.1016/j.ccm.2014.08.002
7. Barreira ER, Munoz GO, Cavalheiro PO, Suzuki AS, Degaspare NV, Shieh HH, et al. Epidemiology and outcomes of acute respiratory distress syndrome in children according to the Berlin definition: a multicenter prospective study. *Crit Care Med* (2015) 43:947–53. doi:10.1097/CCM.0000000000000866
8. De Luca D, Piastra M, Chidini G, Tissieres P, Calderini E, Essouri S, et al. The use of the Berlin definition for acute respiratory distress syndrome during infancy and early childhood: multicenter evaluation and expert consensus. *Intensive Care Med* (2013) 39:2083–91. doi:10.1007/s00134-013-3110-x
9. Ventilation with lower tidal volumes as compared with traditional tidal volumes for acute lung injury and the acute respiratory distress syndrome. The Acute Respiratory Distress Syndrome Network. *N Engl J Med* (2000) 342:1301–8. doi:10.1056/NEJM200005043421801
10. Kallet RH, Jasmer RM, Pittet JF, Tang JF, Campbell AR, Dicker R, et al. Clinical implementation of the ARDS network protocol is associated with reduced hospital mortality compared with historical controls. *Crit Care Med* (2005) 33:925–9. doi:10.1097/01.CCM.0000162382.59289.9C
11. Erickson S, Schibler A, Numa A, Nuthall G, Yung M, Pascoe E, et al. Acute lung injury in pediatric intensive care in Australia and New Zealand: a prospective, multicenter, observational study. *Pediatr Crit Care Med* (2007) 8:317–23. doi:10.1097/01.PCC.0000269408.64179.FF
12. Hall CB, Weinberg GA, Iwane MK, Blumkin AK, Edwards KM, Staat MA, et al. The burden of respiratory syncytial virus infection in young children. *N Engl J Med* (2009) 360:588–98. doi:10.1056/NEJMoa0804877
13. Jhung MA, Swerdlow D, Olsen SJ, Jernigan D, Biggerstaff M, Kamimoto L, et al. Epidemiology of 2009 pandemic influenza A (H1N1) in the United States. *Clin Infect Dis* (2011) 52(Suppl 1):S13–26. doi:10.1093/cid/ciq008
14. Dahlem P, van Aalderen WM, Hamaker ME, Dijkgraaf MG, Bos AP. Incidence and short-term outcome of acute lung injury in mechanically ventilated children. *Eur Respir J* (2003) 22:980–5. doi:10.1183/09031936.03.00003303
15. Lopez-Fernandez Y, Azagra AM, de la Oliva P, Modesto V, Sanchez JI, Parrilla J, et al. Pediatric acute lung injury epidemiology and natural history study: incidence and outcome of the acute respiratory distress syndrome in children. *Crit Care Med* (2012) 40:3238–45. doi:10.1097/CCM.0b013e318260caa3
16. Schene KM, van den Berg E, Wosten-van Asperen RM, van Rijn RR, Bos AP, van Woensel JB. FiO_2 predicts outcome in infants with respiratory syncytial virus-induced acute respiratory distress syndrome. *Pediatr Pulmonol* (2014) 49:1138–44. doi:10.1002/ppul.22974
17. Blank R, Napolitano LM. Epidemiology of ARDS and ALI. *Crit Care Clin* (2011) 27:439–58. doi:10.1016/j.ccc.2011.05.005
18. Carr S. Seasonal and pandemic influenza: an overview with pediatric focus. *Adv Pediatr* (2012) 59:75–93. doi:10.1016/j.yapd.2012.04.016
19. Cox CM, Blanton L, Dhara R, Brammer L, Finelli L. 2009 Pandemic influenza A (H1N1) deaths among children – United States, 2009-2010. *Clin Infect Dis* (2011) 52(Suppl 1):S69–74. doi:10.1093/cid/ciq011
20. Rao S, Torok MR, Bagdure D, Cunningham MA, Williams JT, Curtis DJ, et al. A comparison of H1N1 influenza among pediatric inpatients in the pandemic and post pandemic era. *J Clin Virol* (2015) 71:44–50. doi:10.1016/j.jcv.2015.07.308
21. Wong KK, Jain S, Blanton L, Dhara R, Brammer L, Fry AM, et al. Influenza-associated pediatric deaths in the United States, 2004-2012. *Pediatrics* (2013) 132:796–804. doi:10.1542/peds.2013-1493
22. Pariani E, Martinelli M, Canuti M, Jazaeri Farsani SM, Oude Munnink BB, Deijs M, et al. Influenza and other respiratory viruses involved in severe acute respiratory disease in northern Italy during the pandemic and postpandemic period (2009-2011). *Biomed Res Int* (2014) 2014:241298. doi:10.1155/2014/241298
23. Topfer L, Menk M, Weber-Carstens S, Spies C, Wernecke KD, Uhrig A, et al. Influenza A (H1N1) vs non-H1N1 ARDS: analysis of clinical course. *J Crit Care* (2014) 29:340–6. doi:10.1016/j.jcrc.2013.12.013
24. Kinikar AA, Kulkarni RK, Valvi CT, Mave V, Gupte N, Khadse S, et al. Predictors of mortality in hospitalized children with pandemic H1N1 influenza 2009 in Pune, India. *Indian J Pediatr* (2012) 79:459–66. doi:10.1007/s12098-011-0578-7
25. Farias JA, Fernandez A, Monteverde E, Vidal N, Arias P, Montes MJ, et al. Critically ill infants and children with influenza A (H1N1) in pediatric intensive care units in Argentina. *Intensive Care Med* (2010) 36:1015–22. doi:10.1007/s00134-010-1853-1
26. Claas EC, Osterhaus AD, van Beek R, De Jong JC, Rimmelzwaan GF, Senne DA, et al. Human influenza A H5N1 virus related to a highly pathogenic avian influenza virus. *Lancet* (1998) 351:472–7. doi:10.1016/S0140-6736(97)11212-0
27. Beigel JH, Farrar J, Han AM, Hayden FG, Hyer R, de Jong MD, et al. Avian influenza A (H5N1) infection in humans. *N Engl J Med* (2005) 353:1374–85. doi:10.1056/NEJMra052211
28. Kawachi S, Luong ST, Shigematsu M, Furuya H, Phung TT, Phan PH, et al. Risk parameters of fulminant acute respiratory distress syndrome and avian influenza (H5N1) infection in Vietnamese children. *J Infect Dis* (2009) 200:510–5. doi:10.1086/605034
29. Abdel-Ghafar AN, Chotpitayasunondh T, Gao Z, Hayden FG, Nguyen DH, de Jong MD, et al. Update on avian influenza A (H5N1) virus infection in humans. *N Engl J Med* (2008) 358:261–73. doi:10.1056/NEJMra0707279
30. Luyt CE, Combes A, Nieszkowska A, Trouillet JL, Chastre J. Viral infections in the ICU. *Curr Opin Crit Care* (2008) 14:605–8. doi:10.1097/MCC.0b013e32830f1e12
31. Luyt CE, Combes A, Trouillet JL, Nieszkowska A, Chastre J. Virus-induced acute respiratory distress syndrome: epidemiology, management and outcome. *Presse Med* (2011) 40:e561–8. doi:10.1016/j.lpm.2011.05.027
32. Wang M, Cai F, Wu X, Wu T, Su X, Shi Y. Incidence of viral infection detected by PCR and real-time PCR in childhood community-acquired pneumonia: a meta-analysis. *Respirology* (2015) 20:405–12. doi:10.1111/resp.12472
33. Sun B, He H, Wang Z, Qu J, Li X, Ban C, et al. Emergent severe acute respiratory distress syndrome caused by adenovirus type 55 in immunocompetent adults in 2013: a prospective observational study. *Crit Care* (2014) 18:456. doi:10.1186/s13054-014-0456-6
34. Hung KH, Lin LH. Adenovirus pneumonia complicated with acute respiratory distress syndrome: a case report. *Medicine* (2015) 94:e776. doi:10.1097/MD.0000000000000776
35. Hasvold J, Sjoding M, Pohl K, Cooke C, Hyzy RC. The role of human metapneumovirus in the critically ill adult patient. *J Crit Care* (2016) 31:233–7. doi:10.1016/j.jcrc.2015.09.035
36. Rao S, Messacar K, Torok MR, Rick AM, Holzberg J, Montano A, et al. Enterovirus D68 in critically ill children: a comparison with pandemic H1N1 influenza. *Pediatr Crit Care Med* (2016) 17(11):1023–31. doi:10.1097/PCC.0000000000000922
37. Carrigan DR. Adenovirus infections in immunocompromised patients. *Am J Med* (1997) 102:71–4. doi:10.1016/S0002-9343(97)00015-6
38. Hakim FA, Tleyjeh IM. Severe adenovirus pneumonia in immunocompetent adults: a case report and review of the literature. *Eur J Clin Microbiol Infect Dis* (2008) 27:153–8. doi:10.1007/s10096-007-0416-z
39. World Health Organization. Blueprint for R&D preparedness and response to public health emergencies due to highly infectious pathogens. *Workshop on Prioritization of Pathogens*. (2015). Available from: http://www.who.int/medicines/ebola-treatment/WHO-list-of-top-emerging-diseases/en
40. Ksiazek TG, Erdman D, Goldsmith CS, Zaki SR, Peret T, Emery S, et al. A novel coronavirus associated with severe acute respiratory syndrome. *N Engl J Med* (2003) 348:1953–66. doi:10.1056/NEJMoa030781
41. Peiris JS, Yuen KY, Osterhaus AD, Stohr K. The severe acute respiratory syndrome. *N Engl J Med* (2003) 349:2431–41. doi:10.1056/NEJMra032498
42. Peiris JS, Chu CM, Cheng VC, Chan KS, Hung IF, Poon LL, et al. Clinical progression and viral load in a community outbreak of coronavirus-associated SARS pneumonia: a prospective study. *Lancet* (2003) 361:1767–72. doi:10.1016/S0140-6736(03)13412-5
43. Wang M, Yan M, Xu H, Liang W, Kan B, Zheng B, et al. SARS-CoV infection in a restaurant from palm civet. *Emerg Infect Dis* (2005) 11:1860–5. doi:10.3201/eid1112.041293
44. de Wit E, van Doremalen N, Falzarano D, Munster VJ. SARS and MERS: recent insights into emerging coronaviruses. *Nat Rev Microbiol* (2016) 14:523–34. doi:10.1038/nrmicro.2016.81
45. WHO Mers-Cov Research Group. State of knowledge and data gaps of Middle East respiratory syndrome coronavirus (MERS-CoV) in humans. *PLoS Curr* (2013) 5. doi:10.1371/currents.outbreaks.0bf719e352e7478f8ad85fa30127ddb8

46. Zumla A, Hui DS, Perlman S. Middle East respiratory syndrome. *Lancet* (2015) 386:995–1007. doi:10.1016/S0140-6736(15)60454-8
47. Khalid I, Alraddadi BM, Dairi Y, Khalid TJ, Kadri M, Alshukairi AN, et al. Acute management and long-term survival among subjects with severe Middle East respiratory syndrome coronavirus pneumonia and ARDS. *Respir Care* (2016) 61:340–8. doi:10.4187/respcare.04325
48. Bruynseels P, Jorens PG, Demey HE, Goossens H, Pattyn SR, Elseviers MM, et al. Herpes simplex virus in the respiratory tract of critical care patients: a prospective study. *Lancet* (2003) 362:1536–41. doi:10.1016/S0140-6736(03)14740-X
49. Luyt CE, Combes A, Deback C, Aubriot-Lorton MH, Nieszkowska A, Trouillet JL, et al. Herpes simplex virus lung infection in patients undergoing prolonged mechanical ventilation. *Am J Respir Crit Care Med* (2007) 175:935–42. doi:10.1164/rccm.200609-1322OC
50. Simoons-Smit AM, Kraan EM, Beishuizen A, Strack van Schijndel RJ, Vandenbroucke-Grauls CM. Herpes simplex virus type 1 and respiratory disease in critically-ill patients: real pathogen or innocent bystander? *Clin Microbiol Infect* (2006) 12:1050–9. doi:10.1111/j.1469-0691.2006.01475.x
51. Schuller D, Spessert C, Fraser VJ, Goodenberger DM. Herpes simplex virus from respiratory tract secretions: epidemiology, clinical characteristics, and outcome in immunocompromised and nonimmunocompromised hosts. *Am J Med* (1993) 94:29–33. doi:10.1016/0002-9343(93)90116-7
52. Hennus MP, van Montfrans JM, van Vught AJ, Tesselaar K, Boelens JJ, Jansen NJ. Life-threatening human herpes virus-6 infection in early childhood: presenting symptom of a primary immunodeficiency? *Pediatr Crit Care Med* (2009) 10:e16–8. doi:10.1097/PCC.0b013e31819bb956
53. Ryan DP, Doody DP. Treatment of acute pulmonary failure with extracorporeal support: 100% survival in a pediatric population. *J Pediatr Surg* (1992) 27:1111–6. doi:10.1016/0022-3468(92)90570-W
54. Huzly D, Kurz S, Ebner W, Dettenkofer M, Panning M. Characterisation of nosocomial and community-acquired influenza in a large university hospital during two consecutive influenza seasons. *J Clin Virol* (2015) 73:47–51. doi:10.1016/j.jcv.2015.10.016
55. Siegel JD, Rhinehart E, Jackson M, Chiarello L. 2007 guideline for isolation precautions: preventing transmission of infectious agents in health care settings. *Am J Infect Control* (2007) 35:S65–164. doi:10.1016/j.ajic.2007.10.007
56. Dhar S, Marchaim D, Tansek R, Chopra T, Yousuf A, Bhargava A, et al. Contact precautions: more is not necessarily better. *Infect Control Hosp Epidemiol* (2014) 35:213–21. doi:10.1086/675294
57. Stockton J, Ellis JS, Saville M, Clewley JP, Zambon MC. Multiplex PCR for typing and subtyping influenza and respiratory syncytial viruses. *J Clin Microbiol* (1998) 36:2990–5.
58. Boivin G, Cote S, Dery P, De Serres G, Bergeron MG. Multiplex real-time PCR assay for detection of influenza and human respiratory syncytial viruses. *J Clin Microbiol* (2004) 42:45–51. doi:10.1128/JCM.42.1.45-51.2004
59. Dawood FS, Jain S, Finelli L, Shaw MW, Lindstrom S, Garten RJ, et al. Emergence of a novel swine-origin influenza A (H1N1) virus in humans. *N Engl J Med* (2009) 360:2605–15. doi:10.1056/NEJMoa0903810
60. Schutten M, van Baalen C, Zoeteweij P, Fraaij P. The influenza virus: disease, diagnostics, and treatment. *MLO Med Lab Obs* (2013) 45:38–40.
61. Tuttle R, Weick A, Schwarz WS, Chen X, Obermeier P, Seeber L, et al. Evaluation of novel second-generation RSV and influenza rapid tests at the point of care. *Diagn Microbiol Infect Dis* (2015) 81:171–6. doi:10.1016/j.diagmicrobio.2014.11.013
62. Chartrand C, Leeflang MM, Minion J, Brewer T, Pai M. Accuracy of rapid influenza diagnostic tests: a meta-analysis. *Ann Intern Med* (2012) 156:500–11. doi:10.7326/0003-4819-156-7-201204030-00403
63. Principi N, Esposito S. Antigen-based assays for the identification of influenza virus and respiratory syncytial virus: why and how to use them in pediatric practice. *Clin Lab Med* (2009) 29:649–60. doi:10.1016/j.cll.2009.07.006
64. Moesker FM, van Kampen JJ, Aron G, Schutten M, van de Vijver DA, Koopmans MP, et al. Diagnostic performance of influenza viruses and RSV rapid antigen detection tests in children in tertiary care. *J Clin Virol* (2016) 79:12–7. doi:10.1016/j.jcv.2016.03.022
65. World Health Organization. *WHO Recommendations on the Use of Rapid Testing for Influenza Diagnosis*. Geneva: WHO (2005).
66. Adams O, Weis J, Jasinska K, Vogel M, Tenenbaum T. Comparison of human metapneumovirus, respiratory syncytial virus and rhinovirus respiratory tract infections in young children admitted to hospital. *J Med Virol* (2015) 87:275–80. doi:10.1002/jmv.24025
67. Kusel MM, de Klerk NH, Holt PG, Kebadze T, Johnston SL, Sly PD. Role of respiratory viruses in acute upper and lower respiratory tract illness in the first year of life: a birth cohort study. *Pediatr Infect Dis J* (2006) 25:680–6. doi:10.1097/01.inf.0000226912.88900.a3
68. Stranak Z, Saliba E, Kosma P, Posfay-Barbe K, Yunis K, Farstad T, et al. Predictors of RSV LRTI hospitalization in infants born at 33 to 35 weeks gestational age: a large multinational study (PONI). *PLoS One* (2016) 11:e0157446. doi:10.1371/journal.pone.0157446
69. Weisman L. Populations at risk for developing respiratory syncytial virus and risk factors for respiratory syncytial virus severity: infants with predisposing conditions. *Pediatr Infect Dis J* (2003) 22:S33–7. doi:10.1097/01.inf.0000053883.08663.e5
70. Purcell K, Fergie J. Driscoll Children's Hospital respiratory syncytial virus database: risk factors, treatment and hospital course in 3308 infants and young children, 1991 to 2002. *Pediatr Infect Dis J* (2004) 23:418–23. doi:10.1097/01.inf.0000126273.27123.33
71. Yuksel B, Greenough A. Birth weight and hospital readmission of infants born prematurely. *Arch Pediatr Adolesc Med* (1994) 148:384–8. doi:10.1001/archpedi.1994.02170040050008
72. Stevens TP, Sinkin RA, Hall CB, Maniscalco WM, McConnochie KM. Respiratory syncytial virus and premature infants born at 32 weeks' gestation or earlier: hospitalization and economic implications of prophylaxis. *Arch Pediatr Adolesc Med* (2000) 154:55–61.
73. McCormick J, Tubman R. Readmission with respiratory syncytial virus (RSV) infection among graduates from a neonatal intensive care unit. *Pediatr Pulmonol* (2002) 34:262–6. doi:10.1002/ppul.10169
74. Rodriguez DA, Rodriguez-Martinez CE, Cardenas AC, Quilaguy IE, Mayorga LY, Falla LM, et al. Predictors of severity and mortality in children hospitalized with respiratory syncytial virus infection in a tropical region. *Pediatr Pulmonol* (2014) 49:269–76. doi:10.1002/ppul.22781
75. Chen Y, Shang S, Tang Y, Zhang C, Tong M, Dai Y. Clinical features of severe influenza A (H1N1) virus infection. *Indian J Pediatr* (2013) 80:97–101. doi:10.1007/s12098-012-0784-y
76. Wright PF, Gruber WC, Peters M, Reed G, Zhu Y, Robinson F, et al. Illness severity, viral shedding, and antibody responses in infants hospitalized with bronchiolitis caused by respiratory syncytial virus. *J Infect Dis* (2002) 185:1011–8. doi:10.1086/339822
77. Legg JP, Hussain IR, Warner JA, Johnston SL, Warner JO. Type 1 and type 2 cytokine imbalance in acute respiratory syncytial virus bronchiolitis. *Am J Respir Crit Care Med* (2003) 168:633–9. doi:10.1164/rccm.200210-1148OC
78. DeVincenzo JP, El Saleeby CM, Bush AJ. Respiratory syncytial virus load predicts disease severity in previously healthy infants. *J Infect Dis* (2005) 191:1861–8. doi:10.1086/430008
79. Houben ML, Coenjaerts FE, Rossen JW, Belderbos ME, Hofland RW, Kimpen JL, et al. Disease severity and viral load are correlated in infants with primary respiratory syncytial virus infection in the community. *J Med Virol* (2010) 82:1266–71. doi:10.1002/jmv.21771
80. El Saleeby CM, Bush AJ, Harrison LM, Aitken JA, Devincenzo JP. Respiratory syncytial virus load, viral dynamics, and disease severity in previously healthy naturally infected children. *J Infect Dis* (2011) 204:996–1002. doi:10.1093/infdis/jir494
81. Launes C, Garcia-Garcia JJ, Jordan I, Selva L, Rello J, Munoz-Almagro C. Viral load at diagnosis and influenza A H1N1 (2009) disease severity in children. *Influenza Other Respir Viruses* (2012) 6:e89–92. doi:10.1111/j.1750-2659.2012.00383.x
82. Li CC, Wang L, Eng HL, You HL, Chang LS, Tang KS, et al. Correlation of pandemic (H1N1) 2009 viral load with disease severity and prolonged viral shedding in children. *Emerg Infect Dis* (2010) 16:1265–72. doi:10.3201/eid1608.091918
83. Redlberger-Fritz M, Hirk S, Buchinger D, Haberl R, Hell M, Perkmann-Nagele N, et al. Distinct differences in clinical manifestation and viral laboratory parameters between children and adults with influenza A(H1N1) pdm09 infection – a retrospective comparative analysis. *J Med Virol* (2014) 86:1048–55. doi:10.1002/jmv.23912
84. Hammer J, Numa A, Newth CJ. Acute respiratory distress syndrome caused by respiratory syncytial virus. *Pediatr Pulmonol* (1997) 23:176–83. doi:10.1002/(SICI)1099-0496(199703)23:3<176::AID-PPUL2>3.0.CO;2-M

85. Collins PL, Graham BS. Viral and host factors in human respiratory syncytial virus pathogenesis. *J Virol* (2008) 82:2040–55. doi:10.1128/JVI.01625-07
86. Collins PL, Fearns R, Graham BS. Respiratory syncytial virus: virology, reverse genetics, and pathogenesis of disease. *Curr Top Microbiol Immunol* (2013) 372:3–38. doi:10.1007/978-3-642-38919-1_1
87. Johnson JE, Gonzales RA, Olson SJ, Wright PF, Graham BS. The histopathology of fatal untreated human respiratory syncytial virus infection. *Mod Pathol* (2007) 20:108–19. doi:10.1038/modpathol.3800725
88. Villenave R, Thavagnanam S, Sarlang S, Parker J, Douglas I, Skibinski G, et al. In vitro modeling of respiratory syncytial virus infection of pediatric bronchial epithelium, the primary target of infection in vivo. *Proc Natl Acad Sci U S A* (2012) 109:5040–5. doi:10.1073/pnas.1110203109
89. van Schaik SM, Welliver RC, Kimpen JL. Novel pathways in the pathogenesis of respiratory syncytial virus disease. *Pediatr Pulmonol* (2000) 30:131–8. doi:10.1002/1099-0496(200008)30:2<131::AID-PPUL8>3.0.CO;2-S
90. Dargaville PA, South M, McDougall PN. Surfactant abnormalities in infants with severe viral bronchiolitis. *Arch Dis Child* (1996) 75:133–6. doi:10.1136/adc.75.2.133
91. Orwoll BE, Sapru A. Biomarkers in pediatric ARDS: future directions. *Front Pediatr* (2016) 4:55. doi:10.3389/fped.2016.00055
92. Kong MY, Gaggar A, Li Y, Winkler M, Blalock JE, Clancy JP. Matrix metalloproteinase activity in pediatric acute lung injury. *Int J Med Sci* (2009) 6:9–17. doi:10.7150/ijms.6.9
93. Kong MY, Whitley RJ, Peng N, Oster R, Schoeb TR, Sullender W, et al. Matrix metalloproteinase-9 mediates RSV infection in vitro and in vivo. *Viruses* (2015) 7:4230–53. doi:10.3390/v7082817
94. Tabarani CM, Bonville CA, Suryadevara M, Branigan P, Wang D, Huang D, et al. Novel inflammatory markers, clinical risk factors and virus type associated with severe respiratory syncytial virus infection. *Pediatr Infect Dis J* (2013) 32:e437–42. doi:10.1097/INF.0b013e3182a14407
95. Fernandez JA, Tapia L, Palomino MA, Larranaga C, Pena M, Jaramillo H. Plasma interferon-gamma, interleukin-10 and soluble markers of immune activation in infants with primary adenovirus (ADV) and respiratory syncytial virus (RSV) infection. *Eur Cytokine Netw* (2005) 16:35–40.
96. Vieira RA, Diniz EM, Ceccon ME. Correlation between inflammatory mediators in the nasopharyngeal secretion and in the serum of children with lower respiratory tract infection caused by respiratory syncytial virus and disease severity. *J Bras Pneumol* (2010) 36:59–66. doi:10.1590/S1806-37132010000100011
97. Aras S, Aiyar A, Amedee AM, Gallaher WR. Molecular character of influenza A/H1N1 2009: implications for spread and control. *Indian J Microbiol* (2009) 49:339–47. doi:10.1007/s12088-009-0060-7
98. Webster RG, Bean WJ, Gorman OT, Chambers TM, Kawaoka Y. Evolution and ecology of influenza A viruses. *Microbiol Rev* (1992) 56:152–79.
99. Manz B, Schwemmle M, Brunotte L. Adaptation of avian influenza A virus polymerase in mammals to overcome the host species barrier. *J Virol* (2013) 87:7200–9. doi:10.1128/JVI.00980-13
100. Ma W, Kahn RE, Richt JA. The pig as a mixing vessel for influenza viruses: human and veterinary implications. *J Mol Genet Med* (2008) 3:158–66.
101. Johnson NP, Mueller J. Updating the accounts: global mortality of the 1918-1920 "Spanish" influenza pandemic. *Bull Hist Med* (2002) 76:105–15. doi:10.1353/bhm.2002.0022
102. Gaydos JC, Top FH Jr, Hodder RA, Russell PK. Swine influenza a outbreak, Fort Dix, New Jersey, 1976. *Emerg Infect Dis* (2006) 12:23–8. doi:10.3201/eid1201.050965
103. CDC. Swine influenza A (H1N1) infection in two children – Southern California, March-April 2009. *MMWR Morb Mortal Wkly Rep* (2009) 58:400–2.
104. Travanty E, Zhou B, Zhang H, Di YP, Alcorn JF, Wentworth DE, et al. Differential susceptibilities of human lung primary cells to H1N1 influenza viruses. *J Virol* (2015) 89:11935–44. doi:10.1128/JVI.01792-15
105. Shieh WJ, Blau DM, Denison AM, Deleon-Carnes M, Adem P, Bhatnagar J, et al. 2009 pandemic influenza A (H1N1): pathology and pathogenesis of 100 fatal cases in the United States. *Am J Pathol* (2010) 177:166–75. doi:10.2353/ajpath.2010.100115
106. Perez-Padilla R, de la Rosa-Zamboni D, Ponce de Leon S, Hernandez M, Quinones-Falconi F, Bautista E, et al. Pneumonia and respiratory failure from swine-origin influenza A (H1N1) in Mexico. *N Engl J Med* (2009) 361:680–9. doi:10.1056/NEJMoa0904252
107. Kido H. Influenza virus pathogenicity regulated by host cellular proteases, cytokines and metabolites, and its therapeutic options. *Proc Jpn Acad Ser B Phys Biol Sci* (2015) 91:351–68. doi:10.2183/pjab.91.351
108. Cheng XW, Lu J, Wu CL, Yi LN, Xie X, Shi XD, et al. Three fatal cases of pandemic 2009 influenza A virus infection in Shenzhen are associated with cytokine storm. *Respir Physiol Neurobiol* (2011) 175:185–7. doi:10.1016/j.resp.2010.11.004
109. Tiwari N, Kapoor P, Dhole TN. Antibody and inflammatory response-mediated severity of pandemic 2009 (pH1N1) influenza virus. *J Med Virol* (2014) 86:1034–40. doi:10.1002/jmv.23877
110. Takano T, Tajiri H, Kashiwagi Y, Kimura S, Kawashima H. Cytokine and chemokine response in children with the 2009 pandemic influenza A (H1N1) virus infection. *Eur J Clin Microbiol Infect Dis* (2011) 30:117–20. doi:10.1007/s10096-010-1041-9
111. Dessing MC, van der Sluijs KF, Florquin S, van der Poll T. Monocyte chemoattractant protein 1 contributes to an adequate immune response in influenza pneumonia. *Clin Immunol* (2007) 125:328–36. doi:10.1016/j.clim.2007.08.001
112. Hunt JL, Bronicki RA, Anas N. Role of inhaled nitric oxide in the management of severe acute respiratory distress syndrome. *Front Pediatr* (2016) 4:74. doi:10.3389/fped.2016.00074
113. Wiedemann HP, Wheeler AP, Bernard GR, Thompson BT, Hayden D, deBoisblanc B, et al. Comparison of two fluid-management strategies in acute lung injury. *N Engl J Med* (2006) 354:2564–75. doi:10.1056/NEJMoa062200
114. Steinberg KP, Hudson LD, Goodman RB, Hough CL, Lanken PN, Hyzy R, et al. Efficacy and safety of corticosteroids for persistent acute respiratory distress syndrome. *N Engl J Med* (2006) 354:1671–84. doi:10.1056/NEJMoa051693
115. Guerin C, Reignier J, Richard JC, Beuret P, Gacouin A, Boulain T, et al. Prone positioning in severe acute respiratory distress syndrome. *N Engl J Med* (2013) 368:2159–68. doi:10.1056/NEJMoa1214103
116. Graham BS. Biological challenges and technological opportunities for respiratory syncytial virus vaccine development. *Immunol Rev* (2011) 239:149–66. doi:10.1111/j.1600-065X.2010.00972.x
117. Gomez M, Mufson MA, Dubovsky F, Knightly C, Zeng W, Losonsky G. Phase-I study MEDI-534, of a live, attenuated intranasal vaccine against respiratory syncytial virus and parainfluenza-3 virus in seropositive children. *Pediatr Infect Dis J* (2009) 28:655–8. doi:10.1097/INF.0b013e318199c3b1
118. Karron RA, Buchholz UJ, Collins PL. Live-attenuated respiratory syncytial virus vaccines. *Curr Top Microbiol Immunol* (2013) 372:259–84. doi:10.1007/978-3-642-38919-1_13
119. Karron RA, Luongo C, Thumar B, Loehr KM, Englund JA, Collins PL, et al. A gene deletion that up-regulates viral gene expression yields an attenuated RSV vaccine with improved antibody responses in children. *Sci Transl Med* (2015) 7:312ra175. doi:10.1126/scitranslmed.aac8463
120. Liang B, Surman S, Amaro-Carambot E, Kabatova B, Mackow N, Lingemann M, et al. Enhanced neutralizing antibody response induced by respiratory syncytial virus prefusion F protein expressed by a vaccine candidate. *J Virol* (2015) 89:9499–510. doi:10.1128/JVI.01373-15
121. Geevarghese B, Simoes EA. Antibodies for prevention and treatment of respiratory syncytial virus infections in children. *Antivir Ther* (2012) 17:201–11. doi:10.3851/IMP2061
122. Johnson S, Oliver C, Prince GA, Hemming VG, Pfarr DS, Wang SC, et al. Development of a humanized monoclonal antibody (MEDI-493) with potent in vitro and in vivo activity against respiratory syncytial virus. *J Infect Dis* (1997) 176:1215–24. doi:10.1086/514115
123. Homaira N, Rawlinson W, Snelling TL, Jaffe A. Effectiveness of palivizumab in preventing RSV hospitalization in high risk children: a real-world perspective. *Int J Pediatr* (2014) 2014:571609. doi:10.1155/2014/571609
124. Helmink BJ, Ragsdale CE, Peterson EJ, Merkel KG. Comparison of intravenous palivizumab and standard of care for treatment of respiratory syncytial virus infection in mechanically ventilated pediatric patients. *J Pediatr Pharmacol Ther* (2016) 21:146–54. doi:10.5863/1551-6776-21.2.146
125. Prais D, Danino D, Schonfeld T, Amir J. Impact of palivizumab on admission to the ICU for respiratory syncytial virus bronchiolitis: a national survey. *Chest* (2005) 128:2765–71. doi:10.1378/chest.128.4.2765

126. Lagos R, DeVincenzo JP, Munoz A, Hultquist M, Suzich J, Connor EM, et al. Safety and antiviral activity of motavizumab, a respiratory syncytial virus (RSV)-specific humanized monoclonal antibody, when administered to RSV-infected children. *Pediatr Infect Dis J* (2009) 28:835–7. doi:10.1097/INF.0b013e3181a165e4
127. Ramilo C, Lagos R, Saez-Llorens X, Suzich J, Wang CK, Jensen KM, et al. Motavizumab treatment of infants hospitalized with respiratory syncytial virus infection does not decrease viral load or severity of illness. *Pediatr Infect Dis J* (2014) 33:703–9. doi:10.1097/INF.0000000000000240
128. Wegzyn C, Toh LK, Notario G, Biguenet S, Unnebrink K, Park C, et al. Safety and effectiveness of palivizumab in children at high risk of serious disease due to respiratory syncytial virus infection: a systematic review. *Infect Dis Ther* (2014) 3:133–58. doi:10.1007/s40121-014-0046-6
129. CDC. Serum cross-reactive antibody response to a novel influenza A (H1N1) virus after vaccination with seasonal influenza vaccine. *MMWR Morb Mortal Wkly Rep* (2009) 58:521–4.
130. Mallory RM, Malkin E, Ambrose CS, Bellamy T, Shi L, Yi T, et al. Safety and immunogenicity following administration of a live, attenuated monovalent 2009 H1N1 influenza vaccine to children and adults in two randomized controlled trials. *PLoS One* (2010) 5:e13755. doi:10.1371/journal.pone.0013755
131. Zhu FC, Wang H, Fang HH, Yang JG, Lin XJ, Liang XF, et al. A novel influenza A (H1N1) vaccine in various age groups. *N Engl J Med* (2009) 361:2414–23. doi:10.1056/NEJMoa0908535
132. Cuesta JG, Aavitsland P, Englund H, Gudlaugsson O, Hauge SH, Lyytikainen O, et al. Pandemic vaccination strategies and influenza severe outcomes during the influenza A(H1N1)pdm09 pandemic and the post-pandemic influenza season: the Nordic experience. *Euro Surveill* (2016) 21(16). doi:10.2807/1560-7917.ES.2016.21.16.30208
133. Smith DW, Frankel LR, Mathers LH, Tang AT, Ariagno RL, Prober CG. A controlled trial of aerosolized ribavirin in infants receiving mechanical ventilation for severe respiratory syncytial virus infection. *N Engl J Med* (1991) 325:24–9. doi:10.1056/NEJM199107043250105
134. Krilov LR. Safety issues related to the administration of ribavirin. *Pediatr Infect Dis J* (2002) 21:479–81. doi:10.1097/00006454-200205000-00037
135. Sidwell RW, Huffman JH, Khare GP, Allen LB, Witkowski JT, Robins RK. Broad-spectrum antiviral activity of Virazole: 1-beta-D-ribofuranosyl-1,2,4-triazole-3-carboxamide. *Science* (1972) 177:705–6. doi:10.1126/science.177.4050.705
136. Ventre K, Randolph AG. Ribavirin for respiratory syncytial virus infection of the lower respiratory tract in infants and young children. *Cochrane Database Syst Rev* (2007) CD000181. doi:10.1002/14651858.CD000181.pub3
137. Luo YH, Huang CY, Yang KY, Lee YC. Inhaled ribavirin therapy in adult respiratory syncytial virus-induced acute respiratory distress syndrome. *Arch Bronconeumol* (2011) 47:315–7. doi:10.1016/j.arbres.2010.12.002
138. Kang SJ, Park KH, Kee SJ, Shin JH, Jung SI, Kwon YS, et al. Virological clearance rate of high-dose oseltamivir or triple-combination antiviral therapy in complicated 2009 pandemic influenza A (H1N1) infection. *Jpn J Infect Dis* (2013) 66:425–7. doi:10.7883/yoken.66.425
139. American Academy of Pediatrics. Respiratory syncytial virus. In: Kimberlin DW, Brady MT, Jackson MA, Long SS, editors. *Red Book®: 2015 Report of the Committee on Infectious Diseases*. Elk Grove Village, IL: American Academy of Pediatrics (2015). p. 667–76.
140. Douglas JL, Panis ML, Ho E, Lin KY, Krawczyk SH, Grant DM, et al. Small molecules VP-14637 and JNJ-2408068 inhibit respiratory syncytial virus fusion by similar mechanisms. *Antimicrob Agents Chemother* (2005) 49:2460–6. doi:10.1128/AAC.49.6.2460-2466.2005
141. DeVincenzo JP, Whitley RJ, Mackman RL, Scaglioni-Weinlich C, Harrison L, Farrell E, et al. Oral GS-5806 activity in a respiratory syncytial virus challenge study. *N Engl J Med* (2014) 371:711–22. doi:10.1056/NEJMoa1401184
142. Hayden FG, Treanor JJ, Fritz RS, Lobo M, Betts RF, Miller M, et al. Use of the oral neuraminidase inhibitor oseltamivir in experimental human influenza: randomized controlled trials for prevention and treatment. *JAMA* (1999) 282:1240–6. doi:10.1001/jama.282.13.1240
143. Teke T, Coskun R, Sungur M, Guven M, Bekci TT, Maden E, et al. 2009 H1N1 influenza and experience in three critical care units. *Int J Med Sci* (2011) 8:270–7. doi:10.7150/ijms.8.270
144. Thorlund K, Awad T, Boivin G, Thabane L. Systematic review of influenza resistance to the neuraminidase inhibitors. *BMC Infect Dis* (2011) 11:134. doi:10.1186/1471-2334-11-134
145. Randolph AG, Vaughn F, Sullivan R, Rubinson L, Thompson BT, Yoon G, et al. Critically ill children during the 2009-2010 influenza pandemic in the United States. *Pediatrics* (2011) 128:e1450–8. doi:10.1542/peds.2011-0774
146. Green TP, Moler FW, Goodman DM. Probability of survival after prolonged extracorporeal membrane oxygenation in pediatric patients with acute respiratory failure. Extracorporeal life support organization. *Crit Care Med* (1995) 23:1132–9. doi:10.1097/00003246-199506000-00021
147. Natt BS, Desai H, Singh N, Poongkunran C, Parthasarathy S, Bime C. Extracorporeal membrane oxygenation for ARDS: national trends in the United States 2008-2012. *Respir Care* (2016) 61:1293–8. doi:10.4187/respcare.04760
148. Dalton HJ, Macrae DJ. Extracorporeal support in children with pediatric acute respiratory distress syndrome: proceedings from the pediatric acute lung injury consensus conference. *Pediatr Crit Care Med* (2015) 16:S111–7. doi:10.1097/PCC.0000000000000439
149. Khan JY, Kerr SJ, Tometzki A, Tyszczuk L, West J, Sosnowski A, et al. Role of ECMO in the treatment of respiratory syncytial virus bronchiolitis: a collaborative report. *Arch Dis Child Fetal Neonatal Ed* (1995) 73:F91–4. doi:10.1136/fn.73.2.F91
150. Steinhorn RH, Green TP. Use of extracorporeal membrane oxygenation in the treatment of respiratory syncytial virus bronchiolitis: the national experience, 1983 to 1988. *J Pediatr* (1990) 116:338–42. doi:10.1016/S0022-3476(05)80676-6
151. Flamant C, Hallalel F, Nolent P, Chevalier JY, Renolleau S. Severe respiratory syncytial virus bronchiolitis in children: from short mechanical ventilation to extracorporeal membrane oxygenation. *Eur J Pediatr* (2005) 164:93–8. doi:10.1007/s00431-004-1580-0
152. Streng A, Prifert C, Weissbrich B, Liese JG. Continued high incidence of children with severe influenza A(H1N1)pdm09 admitted to paediatric intensive care units in Germany during the first three post-pandemic influenza seasons, 2010/11-2012/13. *BMC Infect Dis* (2015) 15:573. doi:10.1186/s12879-015-1293-1
153. Tokuhira N, Shime N, Inoue M, Kawasaki T, Sakurai Y, Kurosaka N, et al. Mechanically ventilated children with 2009 pandemic influenza A/H1N1: results from the National Pediatric Intensive Care Registry in Japan. *Pediatr Crit Care Med* (2012) 13:e294–8. doi:10.1097/PCC.0b013e31824fbb10
154. Davies A, Jones D, Bailey M, Beca J, Bellomo R, Blackwell N, et al. Extracorporeal membrane oxygenation for 2009 influenza A(H1N1) acute respiratory distress syndrome. *JAMA* (2009) 302:1888–95. doi:10.1001/jama.2009.1535
155. Noah MA, Peek GJ, Finney SJ, Griffiths MJ, Harrison DA, Grieve R, et al. Referral to an extracorporeal membrane oxygenation center and mortality among patients with severe 2009 influenza A(H1N1). *JAMA* (2011) 306:1659–68. doi:10.1001/jama.2011.1471

24

Pediatric Acute Respiratory Distress Syndrome: Fluid Management in the PICU

Sarah A. Ingelse[1], Roelie M. Wösten-van Asperen[1], Joris Lemson[2], Joost G. Daams[3], Reinout A. Bem[1] and Job B. van Woensel[1]*

[1] Pediatric Intensive Care Unit, Academic Medical Center, Emma Children's Hospital, Amsterdam, Netherlands, [2] Pediatric Intensive Care Unit, Radboud University Medical Center, Nijmegen, Netherlands, [3] Medical Library, Academic Medical Center, University of Amsterdam, Amsterdam, Netherlands

***Correspondence:**
Sarah A. Ingelse
s.a.ingelse@amc.uva.nl

The administration of an appropriate volume of intravenous fluids, while avoiding fluid overload, is a major challenge in the pediatric intensive care unit. Despite our efforts, fluid overload is a very common clinical observation in critically ill children, in particular in those with pediatric acute respiratory distress syndrome (PARDS). Patients with ARDS have widespread damage of the alveolar–capillary barrier, potentially making them vulnerable to fluid overload with the development of pulmonary edema leading to prolonged course of disease. Indeed, studies in adults with ARDS have shown that an increased cumulative fluid balance is associated with adverse outcome. However, age-related differences in the development and consequences of fluid overload in ARDS may exist due to disparities in immunologic response and body water distribution. This systematic review summarizes the current literature on fluid imbalance and management in PARDS, with special emphasis on potential differences with adult patients. It discusses the adverse effects associated with fluid overload and the corresponding possible pathophysiological mechanisms of its development. Our intent is to provide an incentive to develop age-specific fluid management protocols to improve PARDS outcomes.

Keywords: PARDS, fluid balance, management, critical care, children, lung edema

INTRODUCTION

Pediatric acute respiratory distress syndrome (PARDS) is one of the most challenging disease entities in the pediatric intensive care unit (PICU). PARDS was recently defined by the Pediatric Acute Lung Injury Consensus Conference (PALICC) group as acute-onset hypoxic respiratory failure with new infiltrate(s) on chest radiography not fully explained by cardiac failure or fluid overload (1). This definition is based on the Berlin ARDS definition (2), with several adaptations to more adequately adhere to ARDS specifically occurring in children. Importantly, this includes the use of pulse-oximetry derived data to obtain the SpO_2/FiO_2 (S/F) ratio and oxygen saturation index (OSI) in the many patients in whom PaO_2 measurements are unavailable. Of note, due to the relative novelty of the PALICC definition, the articles included in this review still employ the Berlin or older AECC definition of ARDS.

Patients with PARDS form a heterogeneous population within the PICU. This is due to the large age distribution, as PARDS affects infants to adolescents, and the variety of underlying triggers, such as pneumonia, sepsis, trauma, and aspiration. Importantly, differences in the pathophysiology between PARDS and adult ARDS are likely. This is best illustrated by the lower incidence (2.0–12.8/100,000 person-years versus 17.9–81.0/100,000 person-years) and lower mortality (18–35% versus 27–45%) of ARDS in children as compared with adults (1). Although there are potential age-related differences in lung immune and injury responses (3–5), the precise similarities and disparities in the pathophysiological mechanisms between PARDS and adult ARDS are not fully known. At the same time, the development of treatment strategies for PARDS leans heavily on adult ARDS studies and Bayesian approaches (6), as to circumvent lack of power in pediatric studies. It is needless to say that treating children with modalities tested in adults, while the current literature suggests important differences may exist between PARDS and adult ARDS, is highly undesirable. Further exploration of the specific age-related characteristics in relation to outcomes and treatments of PARDS is therefore highly needed.

Appropriate fluid management has become an important non-pulmonary treatment in the current "best practice" care of adult patients with ARDS. To prevent aggravation of lung edema, it is now generally recommended to avoid positive cumulative fluid balance and treat fluid overload after initial hemodynamic stabilization. Several studies in adult ARDS patients have studied the effect of a restrictive fluid management protocol (7). Most importantly, in the NHLBI Fluid and Catheter Treatment Trial (FACTT), it was demonstrated that an early restrictive fluid management protocol in adults with ARDS was effective in preventing fluid overload, which was associated with improved oxygenation and shorter duration of mechanical ventilation and ICU stay (8). This appears in line with the current adult literature on sepsis, which suggests that although early goal-directed therapy including (aggressive) fluid resuscitation is generally beneficial, it does not always lead to reduced mortality (9–11), and may even be associated with longer hospitalization and higher organ failure scores (11). Hence early fluid resuscitation is most likely beneficial, whereas early fluid overload is not. Several studies in a variety of populations of critically ill children, including those in the general PICU, post heart surgery, and those receiving renal replacement therapy, have also shown a positive association between early fluid overload and adverse outcome (12–17).

In this manuscript, we review the literature on the adverse effects of fluid overload with emphasis on potential physiological differences in fluid homeostasis between children and adults. In addition, we summarize the current evidence for a restrictive fluid management protocol specifically in PARDS by a systematic literature review.

AGE AND FLUID OVERLOAD

In adults, multiple studies in patients with ARDS have indicated higher cumulative fluid balance is associated with worse disease outcome. There is an evident inverse correlation between number of ventilator-free days (VFDs) and cumulative fluid balance (18–23). In two randomized controlled trials comparing conservative and liberal fluid treatment, patients in the conservative fluid treatment arm were shown to have higher number of VFDs (8, 18). The correlation with mortality seems more ambiguous. Mortality has been shown to correlate with increasing cumulative fluid balance (21–23), but controversially not to a restrictive fluid treatment (8, 18). In one of the above mentioned trials, lung injury scores and oxygenation indices were also assessed, which both were significantly better when patients received a more restrictive fluid treatment. Consequently, these patients spent an average of 2.5 days less on ventilation as compared with patients treated in the liberal arm (8).

As mentioned above, there are distinct differences in incidence and outcome between adult ARDS and PARDS. As fluid overload is an important and much prevalent aspect of this disease entity, we deem it likely that physiological differences between adults and children in fluid homeostasis influence the progression and outcome of PARDS. Differences in fluid homeostasis exist between children and adults. In humans, aging is associated with a decrease in total body water (TBW) (24). The TBW exists of extracellular (ECW) and intracellular water (ICW). An often used measure to describe fluid compartments is the ECW/TBW ratio. With aging, the TBW declines from approximately 70% of body weight in infants to 60% in elderly (25). The ECW/TBW ratio initially decreases in childhood, but increases again after adulthood due to a relative increase of the ECW. While the lower ECW/TBW ratio in (young) children, together with a high metabolic rate and insensible loss, is a risk for dehydration, vice versa elderly with a higher ECW/TBW ratio may be more prone for fluid overload. For example, in elderly patients suffering from congestive heart failure, fluid overload is predominantly reflected by an increase in ECW (26). In addition, compensation mechanisms by means of redistribution of water between intracellular and extracellular compartments during fluid loss or overload may vary between children, adults, and elderly (27).

In critically ill children, including those with PARDS, it is likely, although yet hypothetical, that age-dependent changes in ICW and ECW as described above alter their susceptibility for adverse effects in end organs during fluid overload. For example, young children have a large brain to intracranial volume ratio as compared with adults, possibly making them relatively vulnerable to encephalopathy as a result of brain edema by excess of water. This is for example illustrated by the higher susceptibility for cerebral edema accompanying diabetic ketoacidosis in children when compared with adults (28, 29). In the lungs, extravascular water content normalized for body weight, and thus TBW, is higher in children as compared with adults, although it is age-independent when indexed for height (30). One could hypothesize that the relative large lung mass to body weight renders children less prone for development of lung edema by increased hydrostatic pressure during fluid overload. In addition, the rate of alveolar fluid clearance (AFC), which is important for the resolution of lung edema, may differ between children and adults. For example, regulation of expression of the epithelial sodium channel (ENaC), one of the essential epithelial channels for fluid clearance, appears age-dependent in the lungs and kidneys (31–33). ENaC is known to increase shortly before birth, and is implicated to decrease with aging. This indicates that children might have higher expression of ENaC than adults, possibly making them less vulnerable to develop lung edema. Similar age-dependent effects of keratinocyte growth factor on AFC have been suggested (34). Indeed, studies in animal models have indicated juveniles to be less prone to develop lung edema compared with their adult or senescent equivalents (4). Unfortunately, the relative paucity of human and animal studies comparing data from the whole age-spectrum with regard to mechanisms and effects of fluid overload at this point makes it undesirable to elaborate beyond speculation.

ADVERSE EFFECTS OF FLUID OVERLOAD

Fluid overload in children with PARDS, and more broadly in all critically ill patients, may have an adverse effect on clinical outcome by leading to interstitial edema resulting in impaired oxygenation and perfusion of several tissues in the human body. Increased hydrostatic pressure as a consequence of intravascular fluid challenge is a major mechanism of this increase in extravascular water content. However, the development of interstitial edema by fluid overload is not solely due to heightened hydrostatic pressure as explained by the Starling forces (35). In addition, it may be explained by the proinflammatory response of the endothelium to increasing intravascular pressure with mechanical stress, which by itself adds to further leakage of proteins and fluid (35–37). Lately, interest is given to a specific part of the endothelium; the glycocalyx. The glycocalyx is a layer lining the luminal side of the endothelium, which consists of a complex web of membrane-bound proteoglycans, glycoproteins, and glycosaminoglycans (GAGs) (38). Degradation of the glycocalyx with shedding of components such as GAGs into the circulation leads to activation of proinflammatory and coagulation pathways resulting in increased endothelial permeability (39, 40). Interestingly, recent studies suggest that intravascular fluid overload may also cause glycocalyx degradation; however, the extent and clinical importance of this effect is yet unclear (41, 42).

Fluid overload can have deleterious consequences for many end organs. In patients with PARDS, the lungs appear particularly affected and the aggravation of lung edema is therefore considered a key mechanism of adverse outcome by fluid overload. Extravascular accumulation of protein-rich edema in the lungs is a hallmark of PARDS and occurs by disruption of the alveolar–capillary barrier. The principal proinflammatory, cell death, and proteolytic and coagulation pathways underlying this increased lung permeability have been reviewed elsewhere (43, 44). As a consequence of this increased alveolar–capillary permeability, patients with PARDS are likely to develop lung edema at a lower hydrostatic pressure threshold as is suggested by early studies in dogs (45, 46). In addition, increased systemic venous pressure as a consequence of fluid loading diminishes the lymphatic drainage, which also decreases the absorption rate of lung edema (47). Importantly, in children with acute respiratory failure, including PARDS, the extravascular lung water content, as measured by hemodynamic volumetric monitoring, correlates with both the extent of fluid overload and lung permeability, and is predictive of survival and duration of mechanical ventilation (48).

Other tissues, especially encapsulated organs such as the kidneys and liver, may be specifically prone for adverse effects of fluid overload by lower perfusion pressures. This could be explained by the capsule acting as an unyielding shield leading to a type of compartment syndrome (49–51). For example, a number of studies have shown that a high cumulative fluid balance is associated with the development of acute kidney injury (AKI) in critically ill patients (52–56). In particular, in the setting of ongoing oliguria despite hemodynamic stabilization, fluid overload may be harmful (49). Moreover, the healing of skin and other tissues, as well as the incidence of gastro-intestinal complications such as ileus, after surgery are negatively affected by interstitial edema resulting from fluid overload (57, 58).

EFFECT OF FLUID OVERLOAD IN PARDS

In summary, fluid overload may be associated with negative outcome in critically ill children including those with PARDS, although important differences between children and adults in susceptibility and pathophysiology may exist. In order to address the current evidence that advocates or would support a restrictive fluid management specifically in PARDS, we performed a systematic review as described below. An overview of the search, screening and selection process of the studies can be found in **Figure 1**. Due to heterogeneity of the data, a meta-analysis was not deemed possible. The systematic literature search and critical appraisal are presented in the supplemental material of this manuscript.

Overview of Included Studies

All studies included in this systematic review were part of a prospective or retrospective observational cohort or *post hoc* analysis. **Table 1** holds the descriptions of the included studies. The correlations found between fluid balance and outcomes were broadly similar across the included articles. **Table 2** provides a summary of the overall findings.

Mortality was one of the primary outcomes in this systematic review and was reported in most of the included studies. Flori et al. showed that mortality was associated with increasing cumulative fluid balance (grouped in sets of 10 ml/kg/day) in both bivariate and multivariate regression (OR 1.12, 95% CI 1.06–1.20, $p < 0.001$ and 1.08, 95% CI 1.01–1.15, $p = 0.02$, respectively) (59). Valentine et al. examined the same association in critically ill children with acute lung injury (ALI) according to the AECC definition of ALI (60). A trend of difference in cumulative fluid balance between survivors and non-survivors was found ($p = 0.11$). In the *post hoc* analysis by Willson et al. the increased cumulative fluid balance (as averaged per meter squared of body surface) was associated with in-hospital mortality on days 1–7 ($p < 0.001$) in children with ALI/ARDS (61). Hu et al. examined children with acute hypoxemic respiratory failure (AHRF) in China (62). A subgroup of these patients ($n = 306$, 66%) was identified according to the AECC criteria of ARDS. With regard to fluid data, they showed that non-survivors of AHRF had higher median fluid balances, although this was statistically not significant ($p = 0.079$). The mortality of patients with a daily fluid balance ≤10 ml/kg/day was lower than the group with a balance of >10 ml/kg/day ($p = 0.049$). There were no fluid data presented of only the ARDS subgroup. The last included study by Randolph et al. on the relation between weaning duration and fluid balance in mechanically ventilated children in the PICU held no data on mortality (63).

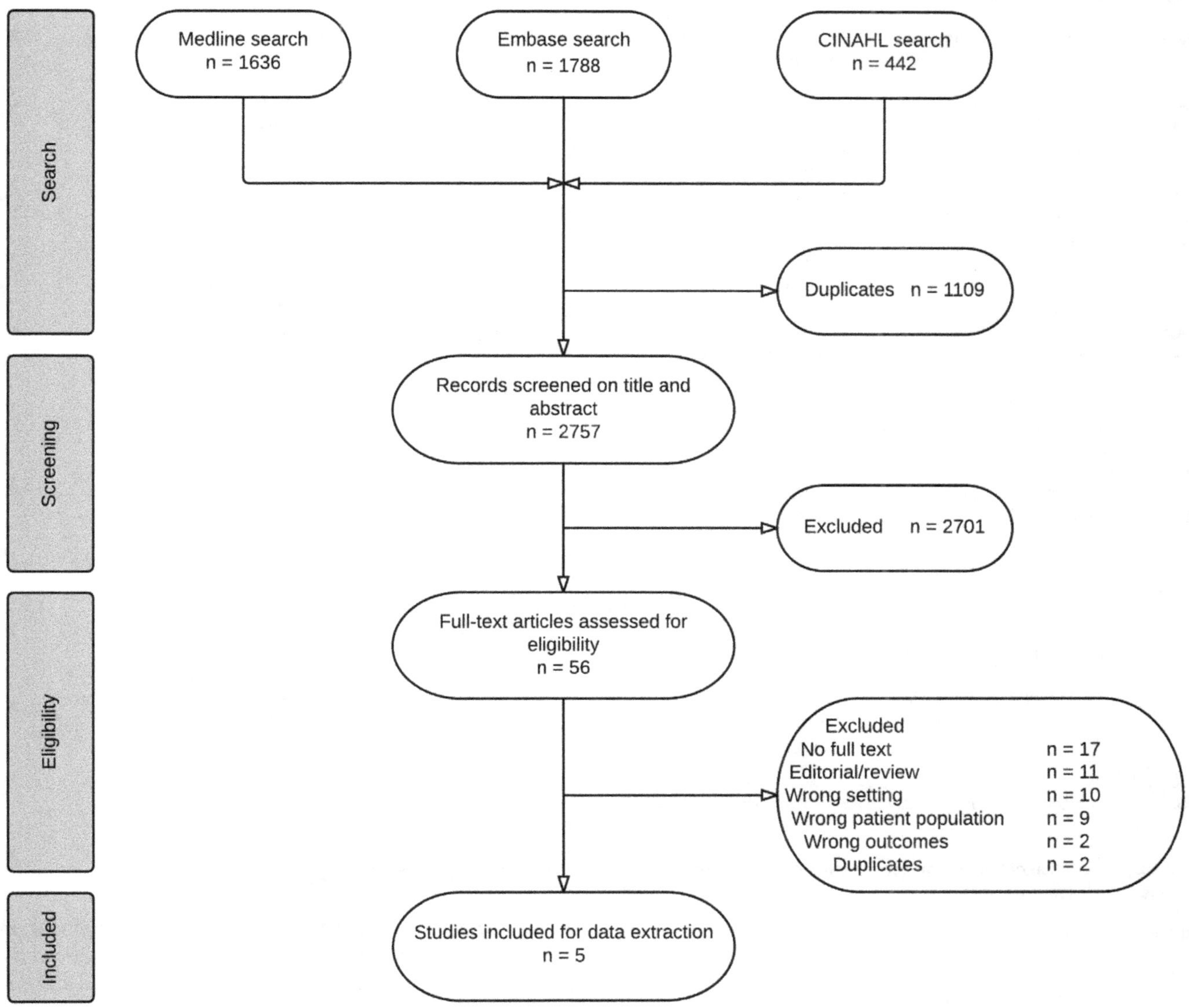

FIGURE 1 | **Flow chart of selection process.**

The other primary and important outcome measure was the number of VFDs measured at day 28 after admission or duration of ventilation. VFDs were used in three of the five included studies (59–61) and in all three fewer VFDs were associated with higher cumulative fluid balance. Valentine et al. reported that in days 2–4 of admission in the PICU, a higher cumulative fluid balance was associated with fewer VFDs ($p = 0.01$, 0.01, and 0.05 for days 2, 3, and 4, respectively) (60). Likewise, Willson et al. found the number of VFDs to be significantly inversely related to fluid balance ($p < 0.001$) (61). The study of Randolph et al. looked at fluid balance during weaning of ventilation and at the time of extubation (63). Their primary outcome was extubation success and secondary outcome was duration of weaning. Fluid balance was assessed at the time when an extubation readiness test (ERT) was performed or at the time of extubation, thus late in the course of disease. Cumulative fluid balance was neither at time of ERT nor at time of extubation associated with successful extubation ($p = 0.56$ and $p = 0.77$, respectively). Duration of weaning showed a non-significant relation with higher cumulative fluid balances at ERT (Hazard ratio 0.94, 95% CI 0.87–1.00, $p = 0.06$); however, it was (marginally) significant when predicted by the cumulative fluid balance values at extubation (Hazard ratio 0.94, 95% CI 0.87–1.00, $p = 0.051$). An important note to be taken into account when comparing the study of Randolph et al. to the others is that ARDS was not defined explicitly or analyzed separately.

One study found that a higher cumulative fluid balance showed a trend of an association with longer duration of stay in the PICU and hospital (61). This outcome was not addressed in other studies. These authors also compared the oxygenation

TABLE 1 | Summary of included articles.

Study	Design	Outcome measure	Variable measure	Subjects	Definition ARDS	Outcome	NOS total
Flori et al. (59)	*Post hoc* analysis of a prospective observational study	PICU mortality, VFDs	Cumulative fluid balance in 10 ml/kg/day increments	313 children with ALI	ALI according to AECC definition	OR 1.08 ($p = 0.02$) mortality with increasing cumulative FB, VFDs ($p = 0.02$)	8
Valentine et al. (60)	Multicenter, retrospective cohort study	VFDs	Cumulative fluid balance and fluid overload (%)	168 children meeting ALI criteria	ALI according to AECC definition	Increasing cumulative FB at day 2–4 associated with fewer VFDs ($p = 0.01$/$p = 0.01$/$p = 0.05$). Cumulative fluid balance was not associated with mortality ($p = 0.11$)	7
Willson et al. (61)	*Post hoc* analysis of pediatric arm of prospective, randomized, placebo-controlled trial	In-hospital mortality, duration of MV, PICU, and hospital LoS, VFDs, OSI	Cumulative fluid balance	110 children with direct ALI/ARDS	ALI/ARDS according to AECC definition	Cumulative FB was associated with mortality ($p < 0.001$), VFDs ($p < 0.001$), PICU-free days ($p = 0.14$), and hospital-free days ($p = 0.06$). OSI increase of 0.52/l/m^2 increase FB ($p = 0.011$)	8
Hu et al. (62)	Prospective study in 26 PICUs	Incidence, mortality and burden of AHRF and ARDS	Daily fluid balance	461 patients with AHRF, of which 306 (66%) ARDS	AHRF: $PaO_2 \leq 50$ mmHg or $PaO_2/FiO_2 \leq 250$ mmHg for ≥ 6 h, needing $FiO_2 > 30\%$ and PEEP >2 cm H_2O to maintain $PaO_2 > 60$ mmHg or $SpO_2 > 90\%$. ALI/ARDS according to AECC definition	In AHRF: non-survivors had higher median FB ($p = 0.079$). Mortality of FB ≤10 ml/kg/day lower than >10 ($p = 0.049$). No specific ARDS data	6
Randolph et al. (63)	Prospective clinical trial	Extubation success (use of ERT) and duration of weaning	Cumulative fluid balance at extubation and start weaning	301 children with mechanical ventilation >24 h	No mention of ARDS definition	No relation cumulative FB with successful extubation. Duration of weaning with cumulative FB at ERT (HR 0.94, $p = 0.06$) and at extubation (HR 0.94, $p = 0.051$). No ARDS data only	7

PICU, pediatric intensive care unit; ALI, acute lung injury; AECC, American-European consensus conference; VFDs, ventilator-free days; MV, mechanical ventilation; LoS, length of stay; OSI, oxygenation saturation index; FB, fluid balance; AHRF, acute hypoxemic respiratory failure; ERT, extubation readiness test.

TABLE 2 | Description of findings on correlation between cumulative fluid balance and clinical outcomes.

Outcome	Results	
Mortality	Significant association in three out of four studies in which mortality was assessed	
	Flori	$p = 0.02$
	Willson	$p < 0.001$
	Hu	$p = 0.079$
	Stratified in ≤10 or >10 ml/kg/day	$p = 0.049$
	Valentine	$p = 0.11$
VFDs	Significant association in three out of three studies in which VFDs were assessed	
	Flori	$p = 0.02$
	Valentine	$p = 0.01$
	Willson	$p < 0.001$
Oxygenation failure	Significant association in 1 out of 1 study in which degree of oxygenation failure was assessed	
	Willson	$p = 0.011$
Other	Willson	
	PICU-free days	$p = 0.14$
	Hospital-free days	$p = 0.06$
	Randolph	
	CFB at extubation associated with duration of weaning	$p = 0.051$

saturation index (OSI) and fluid balance and found that for every liter per meter square body surface increase in fluid balance, the OSI increased with 0.52 point ($p = 0.011$) (61).

CLINICAL IMPLICATIONS

Fluid overload early in PARDS progression seems to have a major impact on recovery. In particular *early* fluid overload is of main interest, as this seems to negatively affect clinical outcome. Late fluid overload may have a more modest effect on outcome (63), potentially because the cumulative fluid balance curve flattens out after the first few days of admission. Children with other causes of critical illness, such as shock or post-cardiac surgery, have shown the same trend of effect (56, 64). Likewise, in the general PICU population, early fluid overload is associated with longer duration of mechanical ventilation and worse oxygenation (13). The peak of illness, which is usually at or a few days after admission, coincides with the presence of early fluid overload. During this period of critical illness, one could speculate that children are especially vulnerable to the effects of fluid overload. Even more so, the positive fluid balance might enhance inflammatory processes (65), which may contribute to the association with adverse outcomes seen mainly in this first period. Vice versa, inflammation in itself could also worsen fluid accumulation by causing (endothelial) tissue damage (e.g., to the glycocalyx) and increasing permeability in the lungs. For pediatric critical care specialists, it is important to realize that children with PARDS appear particularly vulnerable for developing fluid overload already in the early phase of admission (15, 60). In order to prevent and/or adequately handle early fluid overload in daily practice, it is important to be very aware of the significance of this phenomenon. In particular, fluid treatment should probably be tailored more to the actual needs of patients, taking into account fluid responsiveness not only during resuscitation but also with regard to maintenance fluid therapy during the recovery phase (66).

Even though prevention is always more desirable than treatment, fluid overload is a common problem and needs to be treated. Fluid overload could be partially caused by an excess of fluid treatment or nutrients, which is an important pointer to base new fluid protocols on. To treat fluid overload, critically ill patients, both children and adults, often receive diuretics. In the population of critically ill children, furosemide has been shown to effectively achieve diuresis (67). In the particular setting of hypoproteinemic adult patients with ALI, treatment with the combination of furosemide and albumin improved oxygenation, hemodynamics, and fluid balance (19, 20). In animal models of ALI, furosemide also improved lung injury scores and oxygenation (68). The downside to diuretics is that patients are prone to become drug resistant, in which case increased amounts of the drug, a change of the administration route, or more drugs are needed. Moreover, loop diuretics such as furosemide are not compatible with all drugs, which must be taken into account when prescribing them (69).

Another more invasive method of reducing fluid overload is continuous renal replacement therapy (CRRT) (70). In multiple distinct populations of critically ill children, greater fluid overload at start of CRRT has been associated with mortality, even after adjusting for disease severity (14, 71–74). It is suggested that an earlier start of CRRT may result in better outcome as survivors have significantly less days in the PICU prior to start of CRRT than non-survivors do (71, 74). Sutherland et al. discuss the possibility of a threshold for CRRT initiation. For example, based on the recommendation by the American College of Critical Care Medicine, a threshold of >10% fluid overload is suggested for "an intervention" (14, 75). It seems that the choice of using CRRT to treat fluid overload can be defended; however, the optimal timing for initiation still remains to be elucidated and potential complications should be taken into account.

Although fluid restriction could be one of the strategies to prevent or overcome fluid overload, it is at the same time one of the main impeding factors in achieving energy requirements (76). Accomplishing sufficient nutrition is particularly important to prevent nutritional depletion, muscle wasting, and decreased immune function (70, 76) and is associated with better outcome (77). The development of clear fluid and nutritional protocols will be greatly beneficial in achieving optimal balance in both strategies. A Bayesian statistical approach could be the key to designing a randomized controlled trial in children with enough power to adequately assess the optimal fluid (and nutritional) protocol in children with PARDS. The gross effect of fluid overload seems similar in children and adults; however, the *size* of the effect cannot be readily compared due to the nature of the retrospective studies in children and lack of prospective randomized trials.

CONCLUSION

Pediatric acute respiratory distress syndrome is a complex disease entity in need of multimodal therapy, of which fluid treatment is a major component. The current literature on fluid balance in PARDS is sparse but demonstrates that fluid overload is associated with worsening clinical outcome, such as fewer VFDs and worse oxygenation. Varying evidence was found on the relation with mortality and increasing fluid balance. In particular, *early* fluid overload was found to be of main influence. However, definite evidence by randomizing liberal versus restrictive fluid treatment in PARDS is lacking. This systematic review indicates the overall effect of fluid overload on outcomes is rather similar to the effect seen in adults; however, the size of effect cannot be compared at this time. Given the accumulating evidence for differences in (patho) physiology and outcome between children with PARDS and adults with ARDS, as well as known differences in fluid homeostasis related to aging, further study of the effects of specific tailor made fluid maintenance strategies in PARDS is highly warranted. In particular, the place for early diuretic and renal replacement therapy in order to limit fluid overload need to be explored. Further studies are needed to determine whether development of specific age-related fluid management protocols, taking into account all aspects of PARDS, is essential for optimal treatment of this patient group.

AUTHOR CONTRIBUTIONS

SI designed the review, conceptualized the systematic literature search, conducted the eligibility screening, assessed the quality of selected studies, extracted data from the selected studies, and drafted the initial manuscript. RA conceptualized the design of the review and critically revised the manuscript. JD conceptualized and performed the systematic literature search and critically revised the manuscript. JL conceptualized the design of the review and critically revised the manuscript. RB designed the review, conducted the eligibility screening, assessed the quality of selected studies, supervised the data extraction, collaborated in drafting the initial manuscript and critically revised the manuscript. JW designed the review, supervised the literature search and data collection, and critically revised the manuscript.

REFERENCES

1. Khemani RG, Smith LS, Zimmerman JJ, Erickson S, Pediatric Acute Lung Injury Consensus Conference Group. Pediatric acute respiratory distress syndrome: definition, incidence, and epidemiology: proceedings from the pediatric acute lung injury consensus conference. *Pediatr Crit Care Med* (2015) **16**(5 Suppl 1):S23–40. doi:10.1097/PCC.0000000000000432
2. Ranieri VM, Rubenfeld GD, Thompson BT, Ferguson ND, Caldwell E, Fan E, et al. Acute respiratory distress syndrome: the Berlin definition. *JAMA* (2012) **307**(23):2526–33. doi:10.1001/jama.2012.5669
3. Sapru A, Flori H, Quasney MW, Dahmer MK, Pediatric Acute Lung Injury Consensus Conference Group. Pathobiology of acute respiratory distress syndrome. *Pediatr Crit Care Med* (2015) **16**(5 Suppl 1):S6–22. doi:10.1097/PCC.0000000000000431
4. Schouten LR, Schultz MJ, van Kaam AH, Juffermans NP, Bos AP, Wosten-van Asperen RM. Association between maturation and aging and pulmonary responses in animal models of lung injury: a systematic review. *Anesthesiology* (2015) **123**(2):389–408. doi:10.1097/ALN.0000000000000687
5. Bem RA, Bos AP, Matute-Bello G, van Tuyl M, van Woensel JB. Lung epithelial cell apoptosis during acute lung injury in infancy. *Pediatr Crit Care Med* (2007) **8**(2):132–7. doi:10.1097/01.PCC.0000269376.51877.12
6. Schoenfeld DA, Hui Z, Finkelstein DM. Bayesian design using adult data to augment pediatric trials. *Clin Trials* (2009) **6**(4):297–304. doi:10.1177/1740774509339238
7. Roch A, Guervilly C, Papazian L. Fluid management in acute lung injury and ards. *Ann Intensive Care* (2011) **1**(1):16. doi:10.1186/2110-5820-1-16
8. Wiedemann HP, Wheeler AP, Bernard GR, Thompson BT, Hayden D, deBoisblanc B, et al. Comparison of two fluid-management strategies in acute lung injury. *N Engl J Med* (2006) **354**(24):2564–75. doi:10.1056/NEJMoa062200
9. Peake SL, Delaney A, Bailey M, Bellomo R, Cameron PA, Cooper DJ, et al. Goal-directed resuscitation for patients with early septic shock. *N Engl J Med* (2014) **371**(16):1496–506. doi:10.1056/NEJMoa1404380
10. Yealy DM, Kellum JA, Huang DT, Barnato AE, Weissfeld LA, Pike F, et al. A randomized trial of protocol-based care for early septic shock. *N Engl J Med* (2014) **370**(18):1683–93. doi:10.1056/NEJMoa1401602
11. Mouncey PR, Osborn TM, Power GS, Harrison DA, Sadique MZ, Grieve RD, et al. Trial of early, goal-directed resuscitation for septic shock. *N Engl J Med* (2015) **372**(14):1301–11. doi:10.1056/NEJMoa1500896
12. Seguin J, Albright B, Vertullo L, Lai P, Dancea A, Bernier PL, et al. Extent, risk factors, and outcome of fluid overload after pediatric heart surgery*. *Crit Care Med* (2014) **42**(12):2591–9. doi:10.1097/CCM.0000000000000517
13. Sinitsky L, Walls D, Nadel S, Inwald DP. Fluid overload at 48 hours is associated with respiratory morbidity but not mortality in a general PICU: retrospective cohort study*. *Pediatr Crit Care Med* (2015) **16**(3):205–9. doi:10.1097/PCC.0000000000000318
14. Sutherland SM, Zappitelli M, Alexander SR, Chua AN, Brophy PD, Bunchman TE, et al. Fluid overload and mortality in children receiving continuous renal replacement therapy: the prospective pediatric continuous renal replacement therapy registry. *Am J Kidney Dis* (2010) **55**(2):316–25. doi:10.1053/j.ajkd.2009.10.048
15. Arikan AA, Zappitelli M, Goldstein SL, Naipaul A, Jefferson LS, Loftis LL. Fluid overload is associated with impaired oxygenation and morbidity in critically ill children. *Pediatr Crit Care Med* (2012) **13**(3):253–8. doi:10.1097/PCC.0b013e31822882a3
16. Hazle MA, Gajarski RJ, Yu S, Donohue J, Blatt NB. Fluid overload in infants following congenital heart surgery. *Pediatr Crit Care Med* (2013) **14**(1):44–9. doi:10.1097/PCC.0b013e3182712799
17. Soler YA, Nieves-Plaza M, Prieto M, Garcia-De Jesus R, Suarez-Rivera M. Pediatric risk, injury, failure, loss, end-stage renal disease score identifies acute kidney injury and predicts mortality in critically ill children: a prospective study. *Pediatr Crit Care Med* (2013) **14**(4):e189–95. doi:10.1097/PCC.0b013e3182745675
18. Grissom CK, Hirshberg EL, Dickerson JB, Brown SM, Lanspa MJ, Liu KD, et al. Fluid management with a simplified conservative protocol for the acute respiratory distress syndrome*. *Crit Care Med* (2015) **43**(2):288–95. doi:10.1097/CCM.0000000000000715
19. Martin GS, Mangialardi RJ, Wheeler AP, Dupont WD, Morris JA, Bernard GR. Albumin and furosemide therapy in hypoproteinemic patients with acute lung injury. *Crit Care Med* (2002) **30**(10):2175–82. doi:10.1097/00003246-200210000-00001
20. Martin GS, Moss M, Wheeler AP, Mealer M, Morris JA, Bernard GR. A randomized, controlled trial of furosemide with or without albumin in hypoproteinemic patients with acute lung injury. *Crit Care Med* (2005) **33**(8):1681–7. doi:10.1097/01.CCM.0000171539.47006.02
21. Rosenberg AL, Dechert RE, Park PK, Bartlett RH; NIH NHLBI ARDS Network. Review of a large clinical series: association of cumulative fluid balance on outcome in acute lung injury: a retrospective review of the ARDSnet tidal volume study cohort. *J Intensive Care Med* (2009) **24**(1):35–46. doi:10.1177/0885066608329850
22. Sakr Y, Vincent JL, Reinhart K, Groeneveld J, Michalopoulos A, Sprung CL, et al. High tidal volume and positive fluid balance are associated with worse outcome in acute lung injury. *Chest* (2005) **128**(5):3098–108. doi:10.1378/chest.128.5.3098
23. Simmons RS, Berdine GG, Seidenfeld JJ, Prihoda TJ, Harris GD, Smith JD, et al. Fluid balance and the adult respiratory distress syndrome. *Am Rev Respir Dis* (1987) **135**(4):924–9. doi:10.1164/arrd.1987.135.4.924
24. Aloia JF, Vaswani A, Flaster E, Ma R. Relationship of body water compartments to age, race, and fat-free mass. *J Lab Clin Med* (1998) **132**(6):483–90. doi:10.1016/S0022-2143(98)90126-3
25. Tai R, Ohashi Y, Mizuiri S, Aikawa A, Sakai K. Association between ratio of measured extracellular volume to expected body fluid volume and renal outcomes in patients with chronic kidney disease: a retrospective single-center cohort study. *BMC Nephrol* (2014) **15**:189. doi:10.1186/1471-2369-15-189
26. Sergi G, Lupoli L, Volpato S, Bertani R, Coin A, Perissinotto E, et al. Body fluid distribution in elderly subjects with congestive heart failure. *Ann Clin Lab Sci* (2004) **34**(4):416–22.
27. Morgan AL, Sinning WE, Weldy DL. Age effects on body fluid distribution during exercise in the heat. *Aviat Space Environ Med* (2002) **73**(8):750–7.
28. Edge JA. Cerebral oedema during treatment of diabetic ketoacidosis: are we any nearer finding a cause? *Diabetes Metab Res Rev* (2000) **16**(5):316–24. doi:10.1002/1520-7560(2000)9999:9999<::AID-DMRR143>3.0.CO;2-R
29. Rosenbloom AL. Intracerebral crises during treatment of diabetic ketoacidosis. *Diabetes Care* (1990) **13**(1):22–33. doi:10.2337/diacare.13.1.22
30. Nusmeier A, Cecchetti C, Blohm M, Lehman R, van der Hoeven J, Lemson J. Near-normal values of extravascular lung water in children. *Pediatr Crit Care Med* (2015) **16**(2):e28–33. doi:10.1097/PCC.0000000000000312
31. Tian Y, Riazi S, Khan O, Klein JD, Sugimura Y, Verbalis JG, et al. Renal ENaC subunit, Na-K-2Cl and Na-Cl cotransporter abundances in aged, water-restricted F344 x Brown Norway rats. *Kidney Int* (2006) **69**(2):304–12. doi:10.1038/sj.ki.5000076
32. Tiwari S, Li L, Riazi S, Halagappa VK, Ecelbarger CM. Sex and age result in differential regulation of the renal thiazide-sensitive NaCl cotransporter and the epithelial sodium channel in angiotensin II-infused mice. *Am J Nephrol* (2009) **30**(6):554–62. doi:10.1159/000252776
33. Voilley N, Lingueglia E, Champigny G, Mattei MG, Waldmann R, Lazdunski M, et al. The lung amiloride-sensitive Na+ channel: biophysical properties, pharmacology, ontogenesis, and molecular cloning. *Proc Natl Acad Sci U S A* (1994) **91**(1):247–51. doi:10.1073/pnas.91.1.247
34. Smith LS, Zimmerman JJ, Martin TR. Mechanisms of acute respiratory distress syndrome in children and adults: a review and suggestions for future research. *Pediatr Crit Care Med* (2013) **14**(6):631–43. doi:10.1097/PCC.0b013e318291753f
35. Staub NC. Pulmonary edema: physiologic approaches to management. *Chest* (1978) **74**(5):559–64. doi:10.1378/chest.74.5.559
36. Calfee CS, Gallagher D, Abbott J, Thompson BT, Matthay MA; NHLBI ARDS Network. Plasma angiopoietin-2 in clinical acute lung injury: prognostic and pathogenetic significance. *Crit Care Med* (2012) **40**(6):1731–7. doi:10.1097/CCM.0b013e3182451c87
37. Kuebler WM, Ying X, Singh B, Issekutz AC, Bhattacharya J. Pressure is proinflammatory in lung venular capillaries. *J Clin Invest* (1999) **104**(4):495–502. doi:10.1172/JCI6872
38. Woodcock TE, Woodcock TM. Revised starling equation and the glycocalyx model of transvascular fluid exchange: an improved paradigm for prescribing

intravenous fluid therapy. *Br J Anaesth* (2012) **108**(3):384–94. doi:10.1093/bja/aer515
39. Schmidt EP, Yang Y, Janssen WJ, Gandjeva A, Perez MJ, Barthel L, et al. The pulmonary endothelial glycocalyx regulates neutrophil adhesion and lung injury during experimental sepsis. *Nat Med* (2012) **18**(8):1217–23. doi:10.1038/nm.2843
40. Yang Y, Schmidt EP. The endothelial glycocalyx: an important regulator of the pulmonary vascular barrier. *Tissue Barriers* (2013) **1**(1):23494. doi:10.4161/tisb.23494
41. Chappell D, Bruegger D, Potzel J, Jacob M, Brettner F, Vogeser M, et al. Hypervolemia increases release of atrial natriuretic peptide and shedding of the endothelial glycocalyx. *Crit Care* (2014) **18**(5):538. doi:10.1186/s13054-014-0538-5
42. Guidet B, Ait-Oufella H. Fluid resuscitation should respect the endothelial glycocalyx layer. *Crit Care* (2014) **18**(6):707. doi:10.1186/s13054-014-0707-6
43. Matthay MA, Ware LB, Zimmerman GA. The acute respiratory distress syndrome. *J Clin Invest* (2012) **122**(8):2731–40. doi:10.1172/JCI60331
44. Ware LB, Matthay MA. The acute respiratory distress syndrome. *N Engl J Med* (2000) **342**(18):1334–49. doi:10.1056/NEJM200005043421806
45. Guyton AC. Interstitial fluid presure. II. Pressure-volume curves of interstitial space. *Circ Res* (1965) **16**:452–60. doi:10.1161/01.RES.16.5.452
46. Prewitt RM, McCarthy J, Wood LD. Treatment of acute low pressure pulmonary edema in dogs: relative effects of hydrostatic and oncotic pressure, nitroprusside, and positive end-expiratory pressure. *J Clin Invest* (1981) **67**(2):409–18. doi:10.1172/JCI110049
47. Laine GA, Allen SJ, Katz J, Gabel JC, Drake RE. Effect of systemic venous pressure elevation on lymph flow and lung edema formation. *J Appl Physiol (1985)* (1986) **61**(5):1634–8.
48. Lubrano R, Cecchetti C, Elli M, Tomasello C, Guido G, Di Nardo M, et al. Prognostic value of extravascular lung water index in critically ill children with acute respiratory failure. *Intensive Care Med* (2011) **37**(1):124–31. doi:10.1007/s00134-010-2047-6
49. Besen BA, Gobatto AL, Melro LM, Maciel AT, Park M. Fluid and electrolyte overload in critically ill patients: an overview. *World J Crit Care Med* (2015) **4**(2):116–29. doi:10.5492/wjccm.v4.i2.116
50. Damman K, van Deursen VM, Navis G, Voors AA, van Veldhuisen DJ, Hillege HL. Increased central venous pressure is associated with impaired renal function and mortality in a broad spectrum of patients with cardiovascular disease. *J Am Coll Cardiol* (2009) **53**(7):582–8. doi:10.1016/j.jacc.2008.08.080
51. Stone HH, Fulenwider JT. Renal decapsulation in the prevention of post-ischemic oliguria. *Ann Surg* (1977) **186**(3):343–55. doi:10.1097/00000658-197709000-00012
52. Neyra JA, Li X, Yessayan L, Adams-Huet B, Yee J, Toto RD, et al. Dipstick albuminuria and acute kidney injury recovery in critically ill septic patients. *Nephrology* (2015). doi:10.1111/nep.12637
53. Palmieri T, Lavrentieva A, Greenhalgh DG. Acute kidney injury in critically ill burn patients. Risk factors, progression and impact on mortality. *Burns* (2010) **36**(2):205–11. doi:10.1016/j.burns.2009.08.012
54. Bagshaw SM, Cruz DN. Fluid overload as a biomarker of heart failure and acute kidney injury. *Contrib Nephrol* (2010) **164**:54–68. doi:10.1159/000313721
55. Macedo E, Bouchard J, Soroko SH, Chertow GM, Himmelfarb J, Ikizler TA, et al. Fluid accumulation, recognition and staging of acute kidney injury in critically-ill patients. *Crit Care* (2010) **14**(3):R82. doi:10.1186/cc9004
56. Hassinger AB, Wald EL, Goodman DM. Early postoperative fluid overload precedes acute kidney injury and is associated with higher morbidity in pediatric cardiac surgery patients. *Pediatr Crit Care Med* (2014) **15**(2):131–8. doi:10.1097/PCC.0000000000000043
57. Brandstrup B, Tonnesen H, Beier-Holgersen R, Hjortso E, Ording H, Lindorff-Larsen K, et al. Effects of intravenous fluid restriction on postoperative complications: comparison of two perioperative fluid regimens: a randomized assessor-blinded multicenter trial. *Ann Surg* (2003) **238**(5):641–8. doi:10.1097/01.sla.0000094387.50865.23
58. Macafee DA, Allison SP, Lobo DN. Some interactions between gastrointestinal function and fluid and electrolyte homeostasis. *Curr Opin Clin Nutr Metab Care* (2005) **8**(2):197–203. doi:10.1097/00075197-200503000-00015
59. Flori HR, Church G, Liu KD, Gildengorin G, Matthay MA. Positive fluid balance is associated with higher mortality and prolonged mechanical ventilation in pediatric patients with acute lung injury. *Crit Care Res Pract* (2011) **2011**:854142. doi:10.1155/2011/854142
60. Valentine SL, Sapru A, Higgerson RA, Spinella PC, Flori HR, Graham DA, et al. Fluid balance in critically ill children with acute lung injury. *Crit Care Med* (2012) **40**(10):2883–9. doi:10.1097/CCM.0b013e31825bc54d
61. Willson DF, Thomas NJ, Tamburro R, Truemper E, Truwit J, Conaway M, et al. The relationship of fluid administration to outcome in the pediatric calfactant in acute respiratory distress syndrome trial. *Pediatr Crit Care Med* (2013) **14**(7):666–72. doi:10.1097/PCC.0b013e3182917cb5
62. Hu X, Qian S, Xu F, Huang B, Zhou D, Wang Y, et al. Incidence, management and mortality of acute hypoxemic respiratory failure and acute respiratory distress syndrome from a prospective study of Chinese paediatric intensive care network. *Acta Paediatr* (2010) **99**(5):715–21. doi:10.1111/j.1651-2227.2010.01685.x
63. Randolph AG, Forbes PW, Gedeit RG, Arnold JH, Wetzel RC, Luckett PM, et al. Cumulative fluid intake minus output is not associated with ventilator weaning duration or extubation outcomes in children. *Pediatr Crit Care Med* (2005) **6**(6):642–7. doi:10.1097/00130478-200511000-00027
64. Bhaskar P, Dhar AV, Thompson M, Quigley R, Modem V. Early fluid accumulation in children with shock and ICU mortality: a matched case-control study. *Intensive Care Med* (2015) **41**(8):1445–53. doi:10.1007/s00134-015-3851-9
65. Avila-Diaz M, Ventura MD, Valle D, Vicente-Martinez M, Garcia-Gonzalez Z, Cisneros A, et al. Inflammation and extracellular volume expansion are related to sodium and water removal in patients on peritoneal dialysis. *Perit Dial Int* (2006) **26**(5):574–80.
66. Marik PE. Fluid responsiveness and the six guiding principles of fluid resuscitation. *Crit Care Med* (2015). doi:10.1097/CCM.0000000000001483
67. Miller JL, Thomas AN, Johnson PN. Use of continuous-infusion loop diuretics in critically ill children. *Pharmacotherapy* (2014) **34**(8):858–67. doi:10.1002/phar.1443
68. Reising CA, Chendrasekhar A, Wall PL, Paradise NF, Timberlake GA, Moorman DW. Continuous dose furosemide as a therapeutic approach to acute respiratory distress syndrome (ARDS). *J Surg Res* (1999) **82**(1):56–60. doi:10.1006/jsre.1998.5513
69. Martin SJ, Danziger LH. Continuous infusion of loop diuretics in the critically ill: a review of the literature. *Crit Care Med* (1994) **22**(8):1323–9. doi:10.1097/00003246-199408000-00017
70. Valentine SL, Nadkarni VM, Curley MA; Pediatric Acute Lung Injury Consensus Conference G. Nonpulmonary treatments for pediatric acute respiratory distress syndrome: proceedings from the pediatric acute lung injury consensus conference. *Pediatr Crit Care Med* (2015) **16**(5 Suppl 1):S73–85. doi:10.1097/PCC.0000000000000435
71. Foland JA, Fortenberry JD, Warshaw BL, Pettignano R, Merritt RK, Heard ML, et al. Fluid overload before continuous hemofiltration and survival in critically ill children: a retrospective analysis. *Crit Care Med* (2004) **32**(8):1771–6. doi:10.1097/01.CCM.0000132897.52737.49
72. Goldstein SL, Somers MJ, Baum MA, Symons JM, Brophy PD, Blowey D, et al. Pediatric patients with multi-organ dysfunction syndrome receiving continuous renal replacement therapy. *Kidney Int* (2005) **67**(2):653–8. doi:10.1111/j.1523-1755.2005.67121.x
73. Hayes LW, Oster RA, Tofil NM, Tolwani AJ. Outcomes of critically ill children requiring continuous renal replacement therapy. *J Crit Care* (2009) **24**(3):394–400. doi:10.1016/j.jcrc.2008.12.017
74. Selewski DT, Cornell TT, Lombel RM, Blatt NB, Han YY, Mottes T, et al. Weight-based determination of fluid overload status and mortality in pediatric intensive care unit patients requiring continuous renal replacement therapy. *Intensive Care Med* (2011) **37**(7):1166–73. doi:10.1007/s00134-011-2231-3
75. Brierley J, Carcillo JA, Choong K, Cornell T, Decaen A, Deymann A, et al. Clinical practice parameters for hemodynamic support of pediatric and neonatal septic shock: 2007 update from the American College of Critical Care Medicine. *Crit Care Med* (2009) **37**(2):666–88. doi:10.1097/CCM.0b013e31819323c6
76. Rogers EJ, Gilbertson HR, Heine RG, Henning R. Barriers to adequate

nutrition in critically ill children. *Nutrition* (2003) **19**(10):865–8. doi:10.1016/S0899-9007(03)00170-9

77. Mehta NM, Bechard LJ, Zurakowski D, Duggan CP, Heyland DK. Adequate enteral protein intake is inversely associated with 60-d mortality in critically ill children: a multicenter, prospective, cohort study. *Am J Clin Nutr* (2015) **102**(1):199–206. doi:10.3945/ajcn.114.104893

25

Pediatric Acute Respiratory Distress Syndrome: Fibrosis versus Repair

Daniel Im[1], *Wei Shi*[2] *and Barbara Driscoll*[2*]

[1] Pediatric Critical Care Medicine, Department of Pediatrics, The Saban Research Institute, Children's Hospital Los Angeles, University of Southern California, Los Angeles, CA, USA, [2] Developmental Biology and Regenerative Medicine Program, Department of Surgery, The Saban Research Institute, Children's Hospital Los Angeles, University of Southern California, Los Angeles, CA, USA

***Correspondence:**
Barbara Driscoll
bdriscoll@chla.usc.edu

Clinical and basic experimental approaches to pediatric acute lung injury (ALI), including acute respiratory distress syndrome (ARDS), have historically focused on acute care and management of the patient. Additional efforts have focused on the etiology of pediatric ALI and ARDS, clinically defined as diffuse, bilateral diseases of the lung that compromise function leading to severe hypoxemia within 7 days of defined insult. Insults can include ancillary events related to prematurity, can follow trauma and/or transfusion, or can present as sequelae of pulmonary infections and cardiovascular disease and/or injury. Pediatric ALI/ARDS remains one of the leading causes of infant and childhood morbidity and mortality, particularly in the developing world. Though incidence is relatively low, ranging from 2.9 to 9.5 cases/100,000 patients/year, mortality remains high, approaching 35% in some studies. However, this is a significant decrease from the historical mortality rate of over 50%. Several decades of advances in acute management and treatment, as well as better understanding of approaches to ventilation, oxygenation, and surfactant regulation have contributed to improvements in patient recovery. As such, there is a burgeoning interest in the long-term impact of pediatric ALI/ARDS. Chronic pulmonary deficiencies in survivors appear to be caused by inappropriate injury repair, with fibrosis and predisposition to emphysema arising as irreversible secondary events that can severely compromise pulmonary development and function, as well as the overall health of the patient. In this chapter, the long-term effectiveness of current treatments will be examined, as will the potential efficacy of novel, acute, and long-term therapies that support repair and delay or even impede the onset of secondary events, including fibrosis.

Keywords: acute lung injury, pediatric pulmonary fibrosis, lung injury repair, pediatric lung inflammation, pediatric respiratory distress syndrome, surfactant therapy

INTRODUCTION

Since first described by Ashbaugh and colleagues in 1967 as "Adult Respiratory Distress Syndrome in Children," Pediatric Acute Respiratory Distress Syndrome (Pediatric ARDS) has been recognized as a distinct syndrome, with hallmarks and outcomes that differ from those of patients suffering from adult ARDS or neonatal RDS (1–3). Pediatric ARDS is a syndrome of non-cardiogenic pulmonary edema with clinical hallmarks including hypoxemia, bilateral radiographic opacities, increased venous admixture, decreased functional residual capacity, increased physiological deadspace, and decreased lung compliance. Early studies singled out lung surfactant deficiency that can be caused by a large variety of pulmonary and extra-pulmonary insults as an underlying factor in Pediatric ARDS, but the pathophysiology has since been recognized as much more complex (3). Key precipitating events are (1) activation of an unruly inflammatory milieu, which leads to (2) injury to the alveolar epithelial-endothelial permeability barrier, followed by (3) impaired alveolar fluid clearance. This fundamental change in pulmonary homeostasis can be caused by injury to either the alveolar or the capillary epithelium (4). The time course of lung structural damage in Pediatric ARDS has been classically thought to occur in three phases: an inflammatory exudative phase, characterized by diffuse alveolar injury with necrosis of alveolar type I cells, increase in vascular permeability, and an influx of inflammatory cells; a proliferative phase, starting approximately 72 h after the initial insult and lasting approximately 7 days, associated with alveolar epithelial type II (AEC2) repair; mesenchymal cell (interstitial fibroblast and myofibroblast) migration, proliferation, and secretion of extracellular matrix proteins, such as collagen; and a fibrotic phase, characterized by significant upregulation of collagen synthesis and chronic remodeling (4–10). Conventional treatments include ventilatory support, fluid clearance, and/or, in the most extreme cases, extra-corporeal membrane oxygenation (ECMO). Exogenous surfactant administration, prone positioning, and anti-inflammatory approaches, including administration of corticosteroids, may also be used, though consensus on the efficacy of these therapies is not universal, especially in children, for whom data are sparse (3, 11–14). Pediatric survivors with a history of ARDS exhibit pulmonary function characteristic of restrictive lung disease, though the severity of this functional deficit may fade over time, indicating a capacity for repair in a significant subset of patients. It has come to be understood that the timeline of disease progression in Pediatric ARDS is not as clearly as demarcated as originally described and outcomes can vary, dependent on both individual response and course of treatment. In this chapter, the complex cellular and molecular events that determine whether outcome features a more reparative or a more fibrotic profile will be examined. A better understanding of how fibrosis is precipitated and how repair might be facilitated in pediatric patients is critical for addressing the pulmonary fibrotic outcome of Pediatric ARDS, which is associated worldwide with significant levels of morbidity and mortality.

PATHOPHYSIOLOGY AND OUTCOMES: PEDIATRIC ARDS VERSUS ADULT ARDS AND NEONATAL RDS

Classically, Neonatal RDS has been described as a disease of lung immaturity with consequent surfactant insufficiency, which responds well to supplementary surfactant treatment. This approach has substantially changed outcomes for premature newborns and is one of the great success stories of modern neonatal medicine. In contrast, treatment of adult ARDS with supplementary surfactant has not been as successful (15–18). Studies by Willson and colleagues on pediatric patients show that children, while not as responsive as neonates, are still much more responsive to surfactant replacement therapy than adults. In a number of studies, Pediatric ARDS patients show improvement following administration of synthetic exogenous surfactants, particularly when the formula is stabilized (19–22). These differences in response are presumably due to the etiology of the syndrome in neonatal versus pediatric versus adult patients. In neonata patients suffering from prematurity, surfactant therapy not only supports pulmonary function but may also aid in lung maturation. In pediatric and adult lung, in which lungs have matured or are in the latter stages of maturing and which have no prior surfactant compromise, exogenous surfactant may acutely support lung function, but may not have as striking an impact on already mature epithelium. Although ARDS patients do suffer from diminished surfactant levels due to trauma to the surfactant secreting AEC2 population and/or sequestration of surfactant by substances present following edema or inflammation, the pathophysiology of the syndrome is clearly more complex than can be ascribed to this loss. Pediatric ARDS can occur in children with no pre-existing illnesses, but occurrence and mortality are both significantly higher in those with serious underlying conditions, including oncologic diagnoses and especially immune deficiency (23). The syndrome in children also differs from adult disease in outcome, again pointing to potential, underlying differences in pathophysiology. Overall mortality in Pediatric ARDS patients is much lower than that for adult patients. In fact, a subset of pediatric patients show a remarkable capacity for repair, whereas in Adult ARDS survivors, lung function is more often reduced long-term, with permanent alveolar simplification and fibrosis presumably due to regenerative failure. While pediatric survivors can be compromised by exertional dyspnea, hypoxemia, and, in some cases, persistent peripheral airway disease, these patients as a whole appear to possess a notable capacity to recover alveolar units destroyed by trauma (24–26).

Pediatric ARDS develops following a broad range of injuries, when breakdown of the alveolar permeability barrier leads to an influx of proteins and fluids across lung epithelium and endothelium and accumulation of protein-rich inflammatory fluid in the normally fluid-free alveolar space. Altered alveolar permeability and fluid accumulation occur in the setting of inflammation, featuring inappropriate activation of leukocytes and platelets, and uncontrolled activation of coagulation pathways. Solutes and large molecules, such as albumin, enter the alveolar space, creating a highly proteinaceous edema. Significant concentrations of cytokines [e.g., interleukin (IL)-1, IL-8, and tumor necrosis factor (TNF)-α] and lipid mediators (e.g., leukotriene B4) are also present. In response to pro-inflammatory mediators, leukocytes – especially neutrophils – migrate into the pulmonary interstitium and alveoli (4). The presence of protein, fibrinogen, and fibrin degradation products in the edema fluid due to impairment of alveolar fluid clearance leads to surfactant degradation and a subsequent increase in alveolar surface tension. A resulting fall in pulmonary compliance and increased alveolar instability ultimately lead to areas of atelectasis and significant pulmonary dysfunction.

Following acute lung injury (ALI), not only inflammatory cytokines but also growth-promoting agents, especially in pediatric patients that are still developing (e.g., PDGF, TGF-α, TGF-β), are released systemically and locally, as well as activated in the disrupted alveolar structure, which initiate repair processes in response to the injury. It appears that in a subset of pediatric patients, this response can occur swiftly in response to trauma. One retrospective study showed that Pediatric ARDS survivors that exhibit immediate, positive changes in response to treatment over the first 3 days following onset have much faster, more complete reparative outcomes compared to those who do not respond as quickly (27). How a slower response to treatment might contribute to fibrosis in survivors is still under investigation. Inappropriate mesenchymal cell proliferation and extracellular matrix production (known downstream responses to TGF-α and TGF-β, in particular) due to severe or repeated epithelial cell damage have been shown in both animal models and in human patients to eventually evolve into alveolar fibrosis (28, 29). As intra-alveolar fibrosis evolves, infiltrating leukocytes decrease and are replaced by increased numbers of mononuclear phagocytes within the alveolar wall and airspace. Additionally, a variety of signals that are capable of stimulating alveolar macrophage growth factor release (e.g., endotoxin, activated complement components) are present in the distal lung under most of the circumstances associated with acute pediatric lung injury. It may be that slower patient responses allow a cascade of signaling events to occur that promotes long-term, pro-fibrotic remodeling. Though this hypothesis has yet to be completely tested, multiple studies in animal models and on cadaveric human tissue have demonstrated potential mechanisms and intervention points for the development of fibrosis following ALI resulting in Pediatric ARDS.

This fibroproliferative response, which precludes alveolar repair, is regulated by many factors (30, 31). Madtes et al. described a role for the epithelial and mesenchymal cell mitogen transforming growth factor (TGF)-α in the fibroproliferative response in ARDS and have shown that significant levels of TGF-α and procollagen peptide (PCP) III, a biological marker of fibroproliferation, are present in the BAL fluid of ARDS patients. Armstrong et al. noted that BAL fluid from patients with ARDS showed an early shift in the balance between type I collagen synthesis and degradation by collagenase, which favors development of fibrosis (32). As early as 36 h following the onset of injury, this fibrotic phase begins with extensive remodeling of sparsely cellular and collagenous tissue within the distal lung (30). Early morphologic examination of the lungs of patients that die from ALI reveals a common anatomic theme, in which a marked accumulation of mesenchymal cells and their connective tissue products appear in the alveolar airspace and in the walls of intra-acinal microvessels, i.e., an acute fibroproliferative response (33). On gross examination, the lungs of patients with ARDS appear heavy and edematous. The surface appears violaceous and hemorrhagic fluid exudes from the cut pleural surface (4). Microscopically, within hours of the onset of lung injury, the air-lung interface is denuded as type 1 epithelial cells (AEC1) die; within a few days after the inciting injury, there are intra-alveolar accumulations of mesenchymal cells, macrophages, and inflammatory cells (33–35). The interstitium becomes expanded with an increasing number of mesenchymal cells and numerous collagen fibrils and elastic fibers (35). The epithelial basement membrane becomes compromised with gaps of denuded areas, leaving the disrupted interstitium in direct communication with the alveolar airspace. Hyaline membranes form in the absence of alveolar epithelium. Vascular obliteration by microthrombi and fibrocellular proliferation also occurs. Activated myofibroblasts from the interstitium migrate into the alveolar airspace through the gaps in the compromised basement membrane and attach to the luminal surface of the damaged basement membrane (36). While presumably an attempt at repair, blockage of further damage, and/or a valiant effort to prevent drowning due to vascular leak, once myofibroblasts proliferate and persist, the excessive production of abnormal extracellular matrices ultimately obliterates the gas exchange unit. Immunohistochemical studies have shown increased amounts of fibronectin in the airspaces of ARDS patients. Biochemical analysis has also shown an accumulation of collagens type I and III in the expanded interstitium, with type III collagen predominantly present in the early stages following lung injury and type I collagen present at a later stage (36, 37).

Thus, the fibrotic phase of Pediatric ARDS is identified by the deposition of excess collagen and other extracellular matrix material and is associated with intra-alveolar, alveolar septal wall and alveolar ductal fibrosis as there is an attempt by the body to recreate the alveolar basement membrane that overlies collapsed and atelectatic regions of the lung (30, 38). Together, these pathologic changes result in the impaired lung physiology characteristic of Pediatric ARDS, which includes decreased functional residual capacity, diminished compliance accompanied by an increase in the work of breathing, increased deadspace and shunt fraction, and impaired gas exchange (39–41). The persistence of fibrosis in adult ARDS survivors has been documented to 2 years or more, by biopsy (25). Data on pediatric ARDS survivors show much more potential for repair, though this has mainly been demonstrated indirectly, by follow up that includes spirometry. Conversely, pediatric patients that respond poorly to initial treatments, even if they do not succumb, exhibit a problematic course of recovery that may require prolonged ventilation that can last much longer than that administered to quickly responding pediatric patients and adult survivors (23, 42). Unfortunately, this mechanical intervention has a well-known capacity to feed forward to create further injury via mechanical stretch and mesenchymal activation, thereby exacerbating the development of fibrosis.

MECHANICAL VENTILATOR ASSOCIATED FIBROSIS

It is important to consider the role of mechanical ventilation in the development of fibrosis in Pediatric ARDS patients. Protective mechanical ventilation is considered the most important supportive therapy for pediatric patients with ARDS. This approach was first validated by a multicenter randomized trial on Adult ARDS patients conducted by the ARDS Network under the auspices of the National Institutes of Health (43). Subsequent trials for Pediatric ARDS patients have generated some equivocal data, but the general agreement in the field is that ventilator support, including high-frequency oscillating ventilation (HFOV), especially if applied early in the disease course, has a beneficial impact (11, 12, 42). However, mechanical ventilation can also induce or aggravate lung injury, referred to as ventilator-induced lung injury (VILI) (5), to which the smaller, still maturing lungs of children can be particularly susceptible. The level of antioxidants, a critical component of lung homeostasis, can be compromised in Pediatric ARDS by alterations in both cell populations and the balance of proteins and water in interstitial spaces, leading to increased susceptibility to oxygen toxicity induced by forced ventilation. Pro-inflammatory and profibrotic responses may become persistent or uncontrolled during mechanical ventilation. Notably, recent ventilation strategies aimed at decreasing lung stretch has significantly decreased mortality (11, 12). However, the morbidity of mechanical ventilation remains as ventilation at high transpulmonary pressures leads to "barotrauma" and alveolar overdistention leads to "volutrauma," both characterized by increased alveolar-capillary leak and pulmonary edema (44, 45). Repeated opening and collapsing of delicate alveolar spaces at abnormally high pressures contributes to injury via a mechanism called "atelectrauma" (46). In all, there is an emerging evidence demonstrating that barotrauma, volutrauma, and/or atelectrauma from mechanical ventilation influence the course of lung remodeling in experimental models, which provide insight into the pathologies observed in over-ventilated Pediatric ARDS patients (47, 48).

In isolated rat lung and in lung parenchymal strips, mechanical stretch results in enhanced PCPIII expression. Application of recruitment maneuvers associated with atelectasis has also been shown to increase PCPIII expression in animal models of ARDS. In open-chest rabbits, mechanical ventilation with a high-positive end expiratory pressure led to greater gene expression of PCPIII, procollagen IV, fibronectin, and TGF-β1, the classical growth factor for fibrosis formation (49–51). In contrast, ventilation with a low PEEP did not stimulate expression of these genes. Furthermore, mechanical ventilation causes injury not only by structural disruption of the lung but also by induction of inflammatory responses associated with mediator release, which can worsen lung injury and potentially cause systemic organ dysfunction (52–55). The physical forces generated during mechanical ventilation can induce the release and/or activation of cytokines, chemokines, and growth factors in lungs, which together with inflammatory cell recruitment, may play a significant role in the progression from injury to fibroproliferation in pediatric patients. This altered condition in the lung presumably impacts any ability to repair. It can also alter the homeostatic profile and function of the lung even after repair, making once-damaged lungs especially vulnerable to further injury. Taken together, these studies suggest that atelectasis and alveolar overdistention due to mechanical ventilation are harmful and can lead to or exacerbate the development of fibrosis, while careful ventilation management in responsive patients, can support repair.

REPAIR

Pediatric lungs in general have a substantial potential for repair and recovery after ARDS. In major treatment centers, a majority of pediatric patients recover from ARDS. In community treatment settings, as well as globally, this percentage is lower, however, indicating that a critical, early time frame exists for effective intervention. This hypothesis is reinforced by the observation that pediatric patients that respond rapidly to treatment and/or recover by 6 months following the initial insult often recover completely (23). However, pediatric lung injury can have divergent outcomes, with the appearance of fibrosing alveolitis in some patients versus others with seemingly equivalent degrees of lung injury that resolve the inflammation without evidence of fibrosis. The underlying molecular basis of these different outcomes is unclear. Tissue repair involves a variety of mechanisms including edema reabsorption, resolution of inflammation, and cell proliferation in order to repopulate the alveolar epithelium. Strategies that support these natural mechanisms of repair are currently under study using both animal models and clinical trials (**Table 1**). Unfortunately, few of these present data on long-term outcomes for Pediatric ARDS patients. Thus, a better understanding of the mechanisms underlying repair in the juvenile lung, and

TABLE 1 | Pediatric ARDS Therapies (NB: impact on repair versus fibrosis as a long-term outcome is currently unknown, even for animal studies, for all treatments).

Therapy	Data from animal models (adult or neonatal)	Data from *pediatric* pilot and experimental studies and clinical trials	In use routinely or experimentally in *pediatric* patients
Ventilatory support	(56–58)	(3, 11, 12, 43, 59–61)	Yes[b]
Fluid clearance	(62)	(59, 63–65)	Yes[a,b]
ECMO	(66)	(67, 68)	Yes[b]
Surfactant replacement therapy using synthetic and animal-derived surfactants, ±inhaled nitric oxide	(57, 69–77), reviewed in Ref. (16)	(19–21, 78–92) reviewed in Ref. (16, 22)	Yes[a,c,d]
Corticosteroids and other anti-inflammatories and fluid clearance agents	(93–95)	(96)[e,f]	Yes[a,c]
Gene therapy for fluid clearance and anti-inflammatory impact	(97–105), reviewed in Ref. (106)	ND[e]	No
Mesenchymal (or other) stem cells	Reviewed in Ref. (107)	ND[e]	No
Growth factors (epidermal and fibroblast growth factor family members)	(108–113)	ND	No

[a] *Used in conjunction with ventilatory support.*
[b] *Recommended by the Pediatric Acute Lung Injury Consensus Conference Group.*
[c] *Not recommended by the Pediatric Acute Lung Injury Consensus Conference Group but may be considered in severe cases.*
[d] *Clinical trials have curtailed use of certain synthetic surfactants that have shown lesser efficacy than animal-derived surfactants.*
[e] *Trials, safety, pilot, or experimental studies performed in adult patients; few or no studies in pediatric patients.*
[f] *Trials, safety, pilot, or experimental studies performed in neonatal or premature patients; few or no studies in pediatric patients.*

how they may be supported by conventional and experimental therapies, is highly warranted.

The inflammatory response in ARDS is a complex sequence of events that requires the interplay between several immune mediators (114, 115). In the most reparative scenario, anti-inflammatory cytokines (e.g., IL-10) are released as a negative feedback mechanism. When pro-inflammatory pathways are downregulated, these anti-inflammatory mediators can then decrease cytokine expression. Although anti-inflammatory mediators are involved in limiting inflammation, there are also pro-resolution mediators that act to mitigate inflammation and restore tissue homeostasis without causing immune suppression. Pro-resolution mediators include several classes of signaling molecules generated from polyunsaturated fatty acids: lipoxins, resolvins, and protectins (4). These agents appear to signal the recruitment of macrophages, the phagocytosis of apoptoic neutrophils, and the secretion of molecules that can act as anti-inflammatory agents at later stages of recovery, such as IL-10 and TGF-β. Apoptosis of inflammatory cells, mainly neutrophils, has also been shown when pro-survival signals such as granulocyte-colony stimulating factor (G-CSF), disappear. Alveolar macrophages have also been shown to play a role in this phase by engulfing apoptotic cells (114). Therefore, modulation of the inflammatory milieu using corticosteroids, direct administration of anti-inflammatory cytokines, or administration of recombinant viruses or modified stem cells that secrete immunomodulatory molecules have all been proposed to address this aspect of Pediatric ARDS. As yet, with the exception of steroid administration, these approaches have yet to move beyond the experimental phase.

The regeneration of the alveolar structure requires the proliferation and differentiation of AEC2 progenitors into AEC1 pneumocytes (116). It was recently established that the oxygen environment has a significant impact on AEC2 stem cell capacity during development, which may also occur following injury (117). This may particularly hold true in the case of Pediatric ARDS, where oxygenation is disrupted by trauma and artificially modulated by ventilation. Repair of the epithelium is a complex process that involves epithelial cell spreading and migration, as well as proliferation and differentiation of the stem cell population. It is this critical response that may underlie the difference between Pediatric and Adult ARDS patients in their capacity for both initial recovery and long-term return to normal lung function. Given the more robust nature of chronologically younger stem cells, therapeutic approaches that support stem cell function should be a priority for pediatric patients as newer treatments are developed. During the early stages of epithelial repair, epithelial progenitor cells migrate along the underlying matrix that is, in turn, remodeled during the repair process. Growth factors (EGF, KGF, and HGF) that act through tyrosine-kinase receptors, promote cell proliferation (116), and exogenous administration of KGF *in vivo* has been shown to speed this process [(118–120), reviewed in Ref. (121)]. Multiple other molecules that support lung progenitor cells have been extensively studied, *ex vivo*, in isolated primary human and animal cells in culture and in non-transformed human lung cell lines. These include chemokine receptors, anti-inflammatory ILs, eicosinoids, modulators of integrins, and matrix metalloproteinases (MMPs) to aid spreading and wound closure while blocking excessive collagen deposition, modulation of Rho GTPases and MAP kinases, modulation of STAT, PTEN, and PI3 kinase signaling, all critical for a broad range of stem cell functions, modulators of epithelial-mesenchymal transition, including Wnt1, TGF-ß, and E-cadherin (121). As yet, few of these attempts to modify and/or support epithelial stem cell-directed repair have been translated to even comprehensive *in vivo* studies, and clinical trials have yet to be achieved. Likewise, use of gene therapy or modified stem cell therapy approaches that modulate the function of these molecules and pathways within the context of Pediatric ARDS are still highly speculative approaches, with limited data available from laboratory studies and contraindications from experimental adult human trials (106). Additional studies have attempted to determine the regenerative capacity of subsets of endogenous progenitor cells in the absence of exogenous support, though these studies too are at a very early stage and recapitulation using human lung stem cell and progenitor populations has been slow. Endogenous progenitor cells include both resident epithelial and mesenchymal stem cells and bone marrow-derived mesenchymal cells. Recent studies in rodent models suggest that there may be other lung progenitor cells involved in the repair of the lung epithelium, including club cells, integrin α6β4 alveolar epithelial cells, and Scgb1a1-expressing cells and AEC1 themselves (122–124). However, the majority of data to date on lung epithelial response to injury has been generated by focusing on the role of AEC2. AEC2 classically represent the resident stem cells that can proliferate after injury and transdifferentiate into AEC1. In experimental models, AEC2 have been shown to migrate, proliferate, and differentiate into AEC1 (125). A recently developed experimental mouse model of extreme (>80%) AEC2 depletion that results, at both acute and long-term follow up stages, in a distal lung that phenotypically resembles that of ARDS patients that suffer fibrotic outcomes, indicating the essential role for these cells in alveolar homeostasis (126). Furthermore, newer data show that if this depletion is induced in juvenile mice, repair is more robust and outcome is much more favorable. These data indicate that resident distal lung stem cell populations harbor highly functional stem cells capable of efficient repair under favorable circumstances.

In addition to its stem cell capacity, the AEC2 population also plays a critical role in surfactant production. Though surfactant therapy is often considered an acute response to the problem of surfactant deficiency that occurs within the early stages of ARDS, there are experimental data to show that the presence of surfactant itself is critical for maintaining AEC2 homeostasis (127–129). Additional data from animal models and studies using isolated patient cells indicate that a robust, functional AEC2 population and the presence of normal surfactant levels function as a defense against development of fibrosis (130–133). Thus, surfactant therapy for Pediatric ARDS, while it has still not achieved the level of success when used for Neonatal RDS, is still considered a promising and important mechanism for supporting repair (16, 22), particularly when used in conjunction with standard ventilation approaches. This is especially true for ARDS caused by direct pulmonary insults (infection, trauma, radiation, drowning, toxin exposure), where the pulmonary epithelium, including AEC2 is the main target, versus indirect causes (sepsis, burns, shock, transfusions), where damage to the alveolar capillary epithelium may play a greater role. Thus, this latter variety of Pediatric ARDS may not be as responsive to alveolar epithelial supportive therapy (21, 78).

Interestingly, there is also evidence that populations of pulmonary and even extra-pulmonary-derived stem cells that are present in the circulation in response to ARDS may play a role in alveolar regeneration. Lung mesenchymal cells are activated after lung injury and, in addition to collagen synthesis, may secrete growth factors and modulate the immune system by secreting anti-inflammatory cytokines (134). Clinical observations indicate the presence of endothelial progenitor cells post-ALI that may contribute to repair, though findings so far have been limited to adult and neonatal patients and to animal models (107). In contrast, a study by Bui and colleagues pediatric patients being treated by ECMO, including some suffering from Pediatric ARDS, showed that distinctive populations of stem-like cells of hematopoietic, mesenchymal, and epithelial lineages could be isolated from ECMO circuits, indicating that novel stem-like cell populations may be mobilized into the circulation by severe lung injury (135). Interestingly, the lineage prevalence and stem-like characteristics of these cells differed with patient age, again supporting the observation that pediatric ARDS patients respond in ways unique to their chronological age, in ways that differ from Neonatal RDS and Adult ARDS patients. An additional finding from this study was that a significant number of stem-like cells, especially those exhibiting characteristics of epithelial progenitors, were isolated from ECMO circuits very early in course of treatment, which correlates with the observation that those patients that respond quickly to treatment exhibit better outcomes. Taken together, these data indicate that early interventions that support endogenous stem cell function and take advantage of the patients' own response to pulmonary insult should be a focus of future treatments. In addition, conventional treatments that support reparative outcomes should also be more thoroughly investigated and augmented where possible.

One conventional treatment that impacts surfactant function, as well as the general integrity of the alveolar space, is fluid reduction. In order to restore normal respiratory function post-injury, collagen scars formed to preserve alveolar integrity and prevent drowning due to edema caused by vascular leak. These scars must be processed and removed by MMPs, a family of enzymes that digest extracellular fibers (136). One of the most important sources of MMPs is inflammatory cells, such as neutrophils and macrophages. Thus, ironically, the inflammatory response that can cause acute injury is important during resolution stages for adequate lung repair. MMPs represent one of the links between these two phenomena of inflammation and repair. MMPs are upregulated during the repair process and appear to be involved in facilitating cellular migration and the remodeling of the ECM (121). Studies in animal and tissue culture models indicate that migration and proliferation of epithelial progenitor cells are regulated by soluble factors released in response to lung injury. These factors include members of the epidermal growth factor family (EGF and TGF-α) and fibroblast growth factor family (HGF, KGF, FGF-10). Once the alveolar permeability barrier is re-established, removal of lung edema occurs via movement of water out of the airspaces through aquaporins (water channels) in AEC2, which is driven by the active transport of sodium and chloride through specific epithelial cell ion channels (eNAC and CFTR) (101, 106, 137–140). This endogenous repair function can be augmented by mechanical suction, with or without saline lavage (140, 141). More recent studies have focused on pharmacological stimulation of epithelial ion channels, though these studies, again, are still at the experimental stage.

SUMMARY

Since identification of the pathways involved in lung injury, most of the literature has been focused on the use of therapies aimed at truncating the inflammatory response. However, recent studies have, and future studies should, focus on enhancing the repair process. Using approaches that address both acute inflammation and support repair in combination has also been given recent consideration, as each may address particular pathways that contribute to shifting long-term outcomes from pro-fibrotic to pro-repair (16, 142, 143). While Pediatric ARDS survivors exhibit an obstructive disease phenotype, at least during the acute phase and within the first year following recovery, significant long-term improvement in some patients has been documented. It is therefore imperative to consider bold strategies that could support repair during this period. A variety of approaches have been suggested, ranging from the use of biocompatible materials or cells to bolster remodeling to the therapeutic use of mediators aimed at promoting normal cell proliferation, migration, and differentiation. Because the mechanisms that cause tissue disruption and inflammation in the early phase of lung injury also contribute to repair and matrix remodeling later on, a fundamental key to future therapy is impeding the onset of fibrosis. Thus, therapies that disrupt pro-inflammatory pathways, such as MMP inhibition, may have a prophylactic value. Growth factors, exogenous stem cells, or drugs that promote matrix remodeling could also improve both the short- and long-term prognosis of patients with ARDS. Knowledge of the mediators involved in tissue repair and re-establishment of normal development and lung homeostasis could lead to new therapeutic strategies being applied of pediatric patients after the initial insult has been controlled. In fact, given the much higher potential for regeneration and repair in children, future experimental and clinical studies should be directed toward therapies for these patients that support effective repair, proper regeneration, and a return to homeostasis.

AUTHOR CONTRIBUTIONS

DI drafted the paper and added additional research. WS contributed to the writing of the paper and added additional research. BD wrote the abstract, contributed to the writing of the paper, and contributed initial and additional research.

REFERENCES

1. Ashbaugh DG, Bielow DB, Petty TL, Levine BE. Acute respiratory distress in adults. *Lancet* (1967) **2**:319–23. doi:10.1016/S0140-6736(67)90168-7
2. Paulson TE, Spear RM, Peterson BM. New concepts in the treatment of children with acute respiratory distress syndrome. *J Pediatr* (1995) **127**:163–75. doi:10.1016/S0022-3476(95)70291-1
3. Cornfield DN. Acute respiratory distress syndrome in children: physiology and management. *Curr Opin Pediatr* (2013) **25**:338–43. doi:10.1097/MOP.0b013e328360bbe7
4. Sapru A, Flori H, Quasney MW, Dahmer MK, Pediatric Acute Lung Injury Consensus Conference Group. Pathobiology of acute respiratory distress syndrome. *Pediatr Crit Care Med* (2015) **16**:S6–22. doi:10.1097/PCC.0000000000000431
5. Cabrera-Benitez NE, Laffey JG, Parotto M, Spieth PM, Villar J, Zhang H, et al. Mechanical ventilation-associated lung fibrosis in acute respiraotry distress syndrome. *Anesthesiology* (2014) **121**:189–98. doi:10.1097/ALN.0000000000000264
6. Pastor CM, Matthay MA, Frossard JL. Pancreatitis-associated acute lung injury: new insights. *Chest* (2003) **124**:2341–51. doi:10.1378/chest.124.6.2341
7. Rocco PR, Negri EM, Kurtz PM, Vasconcellos FP, Silva GH, Capelozzi VL, et al. Lung tissue mechanics and extracellular matrix remodeling in acute lung injury. *Am J Respir Crit Care Med* (2001) **164**:1067–71. doi:10.1164/ajrccm.164.6.2007062
8. Zapol WM, Trelstad RL, Coffey JW, Tsai I, Salvador RA. Pulmonary fibrosis in severe acute respiratory failure. *Am Rev Respir Dis* (1979) **119**:547–54.
9. Raghu G, Striker LJ, Hudson LD, Striker GE. Extracellular matrix in normal and fibrotic human lungs. *Am Rev Respir Dis* (1985) **131**:281–9.
10. Curley GF, Contreras M, Higgins B, O'Kane C, McAuley DF, O'Toole D, et al. Evolution of the inflammatory and fibroproliferative responses during resolution and repair after ventilator-induced lung injury in the rat. *Anesthesiology* (2011) **115**:1022–32. doi:10.1097/ALN.0b013e31823422c9
11. Pediatric Acute Lung Injury Consensus Conference Group. Pediatric acute respiratory distress syndrome: consensus recommendations from the pediatric acute lung injury consensus conference. *Pediatr Crit Care Med* (2015) **5**:428–39. doi:10.1097/PCC.0000000000000350
12. Tamburro RF, Kneyber MCJ, Pediatric Acute Lung Injury Consensus Conference Group. Pulmonary specific ancillary treatment for pediatric acute respiratory distress syndrome: proceedings from the pediatric acute lung injury consensus conference. *Pediatr Crit Care Med* (2015) **16**:S61–72. doi:10.1097/PCC.0000000000000434
13. Schneider J, Sweberg T. Acute respiratory failure. *Crit Care Clin* (2013) **29**:167–83. doi:10.1016/j.ccc.2012.12.004
14. Mok YH, Lee JH, Rehder KJ, Turner DA. Adjunctive treatments in pediatric acute respiratory distress syndrome. *Expert Rev Respir Med* (2014) **8**:703–16. doi:10.1586/17476348.2014.948854
15. Taeusch HW. Treatment of acute (adult) respiratory distress syndrome: the Holy Grail of surfactant therapy. *Biol Neonate* (2000) **77**:2–8. doi:10.1159/000047050
16. Raghavendran K, Willson D, Notter RH. Surfactant therapy of ALI and ARDS. *Crit Care Clin* (2011) **27**:525–59. doi:10.1016/j.ccc.2011.04.005
17. Anzueto A, Baughman RP, Guntupalli KK, Weg JG, Wiedemann HP, Raventós AA, et al. Aerosolized surfactant in adults with sepsis-induced acute respiratory distress syndrome. *N Engl J Med* (1996) **334**:1417–21. doi:10.1056/NEJM199605303342201
18. Gregory TJ, Steinberg KP, Spragg R, Gadek JE, Hyers TM, Longmore WJ, et al. Bovine surfactant therapy for patients with acute respiratory distress syndrome. *Am J Respir Crit Care Med* (1997) **155**:109–31. doi:10.1164/ajrccm.155.4.9105072
19. Willson DF, Jiao JH, Bauman LA, Zaritsky A, Craft H, Dockery K, et al. Calf lung surfactant extract in acute hypoxemic respiratory failure in children. *Crit Care Med* (1996) **24**:1316–22. doi:10.1097/00003246-199608000-00008
20. Willson DF, Bauman LA, Zaritsky A, Dockery K, James RL, Stat M, et al. Instillation of calf lung surfactant extract (calfactant) is beneficial in pediatric acute hypoxemic respiratory failure. *Crit Care Med* (1999) **27**:188–95. doi:10.1097/00003246-199901000-00050
21. Willson DF, Thomas NJ, Markovitz BP, Bauman LA, DiCarlo JV, Pon S, et al. Effect of exogenous surfactant (calfactant) in pediatric acute lung injury. *JAMA* (2005) **293**:470–6. doi:10.1001/jama.293.4.470
22. Willson DF, Chess PR, Notter RH. Surfactant for pediatric acute lung injury. *Pediatr Clin North Am* (2008) **55**:545–62. doi:10.1016/j.pcl.2008.02.016
23. Redding GJ. Current concepts in adult respiratory distress syndrome in children. *Curr Opin Pediatr* (2001) **13**:261–6. doi:10.1097/00008480-200106000-00009
24. Fanconi S, Kraemer R, Weber J, Tschaeppeler H, Pfenninger J. Long-term sequelae in children surviving adult respiratory distress syndrome. *J Pediatr* (1985) **106**:218–22. doi:10.1016/S0022-3476(85)80290-0
25. Elliot CG, Morris AH, Cengiz M. Pulmonary function and exercise gas exchange in survivors of adult respiratory distress syndrome. *Am Rev Respir Dis* (1981) **123**:492–5.
26. Elliott CG, Rasmusson Y, Crapo RO. Prediction of pulmonary function abnormalities after ARDS. *Am Rev Respir Dis* (1987) **135**:634–8.
27. Ben-Abraham R, Moreh O, Auger-ten A, Vardi A, Harel R, Barzilay Z, et al. Adapting prognostic respiratory variables of ARDS in children to small-scale community needs. *J Crit Care* (1999) **14**:120–4. doi:10.1016/S0883-9441(99)90024-2
28. Snyder LS, Hertz MI, Harmon KR, Bitterman PB. Failure of lung repair following acute lung injury: regulation of the fibroproliferative response (part 2). *Chest* (1990) **98**:989–93. doi:10.1378/chest.98.3.733
29. Sporn MB, Robert AB. Peptide growth factors in inflammation, tissue repair, and cancer. *J Clin Invest* (1986) **78**:329–32. doi:10.1172/JCI112580
30. Schwarz MA. Acute lung injury: cellular mechanisms and derangements. *Paediatr Respir Rev* (2001) **2**:3–9. doi:10.1053/prrv.2000.0095
31. Madtes DK, Rubenfeld G, Klima LD, Milberg JA, Steinberg KP, Martin TR, et al. Elevated transforming growth factor-alpha levels in bronchoalveolar lavage fluid of patients with acute respiratory distress syndrome. *Am J Respir Crit Care Med* (1998) **158**:424–30. doi:10.1164/ajrccm.158.2.9711112
32. Armstrong L, Thickett DR, Mansell JP, Ionescu M, Hoyle E, Billinghurst RC, et al. Changes in collagen turnover in early acute respiratory distress syndrome. *Am J Respir Crit Care Med* (1999) **160**:1910–5. doi:10.1164/ajrccm.160.6.9811084
33. Snyder LS, Hertz MI, Harmon KR, Bitterman PB. Failure of lung repair following acute lung injury: regulation of the fibroproliferative response (part 1). *Chest* (1990) **98**:733–8. doi:10.1378/chest.98.4.989
34. Pietra GG, Rüttner JR, Wüst W, Glinz W. The lung after trauma and shock – fine structure of the alveolar capillary barrier in 23 autopsies. *J Trauma* (1981) **21**:454.
35. Schnells G, Voigt WH, Redl H, Schlag G, Glatzl A. Electron-microscopic investigation of lung biopsies in patients with post-traumatic respiratory insufficiency. *Acta Chir Scand* (1980) **499**:9.
36. Fukuda Y, Ishizaki M, Masuda Y, Kimura G, Kawanami O, Masugi Y. The role of intraalveolar fibrosis in the process of pulmonary structural remodeling in patients with diffuse alveolar damage. *Am J Pathol* (1987) **126**:171–82.
37. Shoemaker CT, Reiser KM, Goetzman BW, Last JA. Elevated ratios of type I/III collagen in the lungs of chronically ventilated neonates with respiratory distress. *Pediatr Res* (1984) **18**:1176–80. doi:10.1203/00006450-198411000-00025
38. Kuhn C III, Boldt J, King TE Jr, Crouch E, Vartio T, McDonald JA. An immunohistochemical study of architectural remodeling and connective tissue synthesis in pulmonary fibrosis. *Am Rev Respir Dis* (1989) **140**:1693–703. doi:10.1164/ajrccm/140.6.1693
39. Ware LB, Matthay MA. The acute respiratory distress syndrome. *N Engl J Med* (2000) **342**:1334–49. doi:10.1056/NEJM200005043421806
40. ARDS Definition Task Force, Ranieri VM, Rubenfeld GD, Thompson BT, Ferguson ND, Caldwell E, et al. Acute respiratory distress ssyndrome: the Berlin definition. *JAMA* (2012) **307**:2526–33. doi:10.1016/j.medin.2012.08.010
41. Fein A, Grossman RF, Jones JG, Overland E, Pitts L, Murray JF, et al. The value of edema fluid protein measurement in patients with pulmonary edema. *Am J Med* (1979) **67**:32–8. doi:10.1016/0002-9343(79)90066-4
42. Prodhan P, Noviski N. Pediatric acute hypoxemic respiratory failure: management of oxygenation. *J Intensive Care Med* (2004) **19**:140–53. doi:10.1177/0885066604263859
43. The Acute Respiratory Distress Syndrome Network. Ventilation with lower tidal volumes as compared with traditional tidal volumes for acute lung injury

and the respiratory distress syndrome. *N Engl J Med* (2000) **342**:1301–8. doi:10.1056/NEJM200005043421801

44. Ricard JD, Dreyfuss D, Saumon G. Ventilator-induced lung injury. *Curr Opin Crit Care* (2002) **8**:12–20. doi:10.1097/00075198-200202000-00003
45. Pecchiari M, Monaco A, Koutsoukou A, D'Angelo E. Plasma membrane disruptions with different modes of injurious mechanical ventilation in normal rat lungs. *Crit Care Med* (2012) **40**:869–75. doi:10.1097/CCM.0b013e318232da2b
46. Slutsky AS. Lung injury caused by mechanical ventilation. *Chest* (1999) **116**:9S–15S. doi:10.1378/chest.116.suppl_1.9S-a
47. Copland IB, Reynaud D, Pace-Asciak C, Post M. Mechanotransduction of stretch-induced prostanoid release by fetal lung epithelial cells. *Am J Physiol Lung Cell Mol Physiol* (2006) **291**:L487–95. doi:10.1152/ajplung.00510.2005
48. Torday JS, Torres E, Rehan VK. The role of fibroblast transdifferentiation in lung epithelial cell proliferation, differentiation, and repair in vitro. *Pediatr Pathol Mol Med* (2003) **22**:189–207. doi:10.1080/15227950307732
49. Parker JC, Breen EC, West JB. High vascular and airway pressures increase interstitial protein mRNA expression in isolated rat lungs. *J Appl Physiol* (1997) **83**:1697–705.
50. Garcia CS, Rocco PR, Facchinetti LD, Lassance RM, Caruso P, Deheinzelin D, et al. What increases type III procollagen mRNA levels in lung tissue: stress induced by changes in force or amplitude? *Respir Physiol Neurobiol* (2004) **144**:59–70. doi:10.1016/j.resp.2004.07.023
51. Rocco PR, Dos Santos C, Pelosi P. Lung parenchyma remodeling in acute respiratory distress syndrome. *Minerva Anestesiol* (2009) **75**:730–40.
52. Tatler AL, Jenkins G. TGF-beta activation and lung fibrosis. *Proc Am Thorac Soc* (2012) **9**:130–6. doi:10.1513/pats.201201-003AW
53. Tremblay LN, Slutsky AS. Pathogenesis of ventilator-induced lung injury: trials and tribulations. *Am J Physiol Lung Cell Mol Physiol* (2005) **288**:L596–8. doi:10.1152/ajplung.00438.2004
54. Riva DR, Oliveira MB, Rzezinski AF, Rangel G, Capelozzi VL, Zin WA, et al. Recruitment maneuver in pulmonary and extrapulmonary experimental acute lung injury. *Crit Care Med* (2008) **36**:1900–8. doi:10.1097/CCM.0b013e3181760e5d
55. Steimback PW, Oliveira GP, Rzezinski AF, Silva PL, Garcia CS, Rangel G, et al. Effects of frequency and inspiratory plateau pressure during recruitment meanoeuvres on lung and distal organs in acute lung injury. *Intensive Care Med* (2009) **35**:1120–8. doi:10.1007/s00134-009-1439-y
56. Zucker A, Holm BA, Wood LDH, Crawford G, Ridge K, Sznajder IA. Exogenous surfactant with PEEP reduces pulmonary edema and improves lung function in canine aspiration pneumonitis. *J Appl Physiol* (1992) **73**:679–86.
57. Lutz CJ, Picone A, Gatto LA, Paskanik A, Landas S, Nieman G. Exogenous surfactant and positive end-expiratory pressure in the treatment of endotoxin-induced lung injury. *Crit Care Med* (1998) **26**:1379–89. doi:10.1097/00003246-199808000-00025
58. Desai LP, Sinclair SE, Chapman KE, Hassid A, Waters CM. High tidal volume mechanical ventilation with hyperoxia alters alveolar type II cell adhesion. *Am J Physiol Lung Cell Mol Physiol* (2007) **293**:L769–78. doi:10.1152/ajplung.00127.2007
59. Randolph AG. Management of acute lung injury and acute respiratory distress syndrome in children. *Crit Care Med* (2009) **37**:2448–54. doi:10.1097/CCM.0b013e3181aee5dd
60. Turi JL, Cheifetz IM. *Acute Respiratory Failure. Resuscitation and Stabilization of the Critically ill Child.* London: Springer (2009).
61. Marraro GA. Innovative practices of ventilatory support with pediatric patients. *Pediatr Crit Care Med* (2003) **4**:8–20. doi:10.1097/00130478-200301000-00003
62. Kobayashi T, Ganzuka M, Taniguchi J, Nitta K, Murakami S. Lung lavage and surfactant replacement for hydrochloric acid aspiration in rabbits. *Acta Anaesthesiol Scand* (1990) **34**:216–21. doi:10.1111/j.1399-6576.1990.tb03073.x
63. Arikan AA, Zappitelli M, Goldstein SL, Naipaul A, Jefferson LS, Loftis LL. Fluid overload is associated with impaired oxygenation and morbidity in critically ill children. *Pediatr Crit Care Med* (2012) **13**:253. doi:10.1097/PCC.0b013e31822882a3
64. Flori HR, Church G, Liu KD, Gildengorin G, Matthay MA. Positive fluid balance is associated with higher mortality and prolonged mechanical ventilation in pediatric patients with acute lung injury. *Crit Care Res Pract* (2011) **2011**:854142. doi:10.1155/2011/854142
65. Foland JA, Fortenberry JD, Warshaw BL, Pettignano R, Merritt RK, Heard ML, et al. Fluid overload before continuous hemofiltration and survival in critically ill children: a retrospective analysis. *Crit Care Med* (2004) **32**:1771. doi:10.1097/01.CCM.0000132897.52737.49
66. Möller JC, Reiss I, Schaible TF, Kohl M, Göpel W, Fischer T, et al. Oxygenation and lung morphology in a rabbit pediatric ARDS-model under high peak pressure ventilation plus nitric oxide and surfactant compared with veno-venous ECMO. *Int J Artif Organs* (1999) **22**:747–53.
67. O'Rourke PP, Stolar CJ, Zwischenberger JB, Snedecor SM, Bartlett RH. Extracorporeal membrane oxygenation: support for overwhelming pulmonary failure in the pediatric population. Collective experience from the extracorporeal life support organization. *J Pediatr Surg* (1993) **28**:523–8. doi:10.1016/0022-3468(93)90610-W
68. Haines NM, Rycus PT, Zwischenberger JB, Bartlett RH, Undar A. Extracorporeal Life Support Registry Report 2008: neonatal and pediatric cardiac cases. *ASAIO J* (2009) **55**:111–6. doi:10.1097/MAT.0b013e318190b6f7
69. Matalon S, Holm BA, Notter RH. Mitigation of pulmonary hyperoxic injury by administration of exogenous surfactant. *J Appl Physiol* (1987) **62**:756–61.
70. Loewen GM, Holm BA, Milanowski L, Wild LM, Notter RH, Matalon S. Alveolar hyperoxic injury in rabbits receiving exogenous surfactant. *J Appl Physiol* (1989) **66**:1987–92.
71. Nieman G, Gatto L, Paskanik A, Yang B, Fluck R, Picone A. Surfactant replacement in the treatment of sepsis-induced adult respiratory distress syndrome in pigs. *Crit Care Med* (1996) **24**:1025–33. doi:10.1097/00003246-199606000-00024
72. Lutz C, Carney D, Finck C, Picone A, Gatto L, Paskanik A, et al. Aerosolized surfactant improves pulmonary function in endotoxin-induced lung injury. *Am J Respir Crit Care Med* (1998) **158**:840–5. doi:10.1164/ajrccm.158.3.9801089
73. Eijking EP, van Daal GJ, Tenbrinck R, Luyenduijk A, Sluiters JF, Hannappel E, et al. Effect of surfactant replacement on *Pneumocystis carinii* pneumonia in rats. *Intensive Care Med* (1990) **17**:475–8. doi:10.1007/BF01690770
74. Sherman MP, Campbell LA, Merritt TA, Long WA, Gunkel JH, Curstedt T, et al. Effect of different surfactants on pulmonary group B streptococcal infection in premature rabbits. *J Pediatr* (1994) **125**:939–47. doi:10.1016/S0022-3476(05)82013-X
75. Tashiro K, Li W-Z, Yamada K, Matsumoto Y, Kobayashi T. Surfactant replacement reverses respiratory failure induced by intratracheal endotoxin in rats. *Crit Care Med* (1995) **23**:149–56. doi:10.1097/00003246-199501000-00024
76. Karamanoukian HL, Glick PL, Wilcox DL, Rossman JE, Morin FC, Holm BA. Pathophysiology of congenital diaphragmatic hernia VII: inhaled nitric oxide requires exogenous surfactant therapy in the lamb model of CDH. *J Pediatr Surg* (1995) **30**(1):1–4. doi:10.1016/0022-3468(95)90596-0
77. Gommers D, Hartog A, van't Veen A, Lachmann B. Improved oxygenation by nitric oxide is enhanced by prior lung reaeration with surfactant, rather than positive end-expiratory pressure, in lung-lavaged rabbits. *Crit Care Med* (1997) **25**(11):1868–73. doi:10.1097/00003246-199711000-00027
78. Spragg RG, Lewis JF, Wurst W, Hafner D, Baughman RP, Wewers MD, et al. Treatment of acute respiratory distress syndrome with recombinant surfactant protein C surfactant. *Am J Respir Crit Care Med* (2003) **167**:1562–6. doi:10.1164/rccm.200207-782OC
79. Günther A, Schmidt R, Harodt J, Schmehl T, Walmrath D, Ruppert C, et al. Bronchoscopic administration of bovine natural surfactant in ARDS and septic shock: impact on biophysical and biochemical surfactant properties. *Eur Respir J* (2002) **10**:797–804. doi:10.1183/09031936.02.00243302
80. Walmrath D, Gunther A, Ghofrani HA, Schermuly R, Schnedier T, Grimminger F, et al. Bronchoscopic surfactant administration in patients with severe adult respiratory distress syndrome and sepsis. *Am J Respir Crit Care Med* (1996) **154**:57–62. doi:10.1164/ajrccm.154.1.8680699
81. Lopez-Herce J, de Lucas N, Carrillo A, Bustinza A, Moral R. Surfactant treatment for acute respiratory distress syndrome. *Arch Dis Child* (1999) **80**:248–52. doi:10.1136/adc.80.3.248
82. Hermon MM, Golej J, Burda G, Boigner H, Stoll E, Vergesslich K, et al. Surfactant therapy in infants and children: three years experience in a pediatric intensive care unit. *Shock* (2002) **17**:247–51. doi:10.1097/00024382-200204000-00001
83. Herting E, Moller O, Schiffman JH, Robertson B. Surfactant improves oxygenation in infants and children with pneumonia and acute respiratory distress

syndrome. *Acta Paediatr* (2002) **91**:1174–8. doi:10.1111/j.1651-2227.2002.tb00124.x

84. Moller JC, Schaible T, Roll C, Schiffmann JH, Bindl L, Schrod L, et al. Treatment with bovine surfactant in severe acute respiratory distress syndrome in children: a randomized multicenter study. *Intensive Care Med* (2003) **29**:437–46.
85. Pappert D, Busch T, Gerlach H, Lewandowski K, Radermacher P, Rossaint R. Aerosolized prostacyclin versus inhaled nitric oxide in children with severe acute respiratory distress syndrome. *Anesthesiology* (1995) **82**:1507–11. doi:10.1097/00000542-199506000-00020
86. Day RW, Guarin M, Lynch JM, Vernon DD, Mean JM. Inhaled nitric oxide in children with severe lung disease: results of acute and prolonged therapy with two concentrations. *Crit Care Med* (1996) **24**:215–21. doi:10.1097/00003246-199602000-00006
87. Demirakça S, Dötsch J, Knothe C, Magsaam J, Reiter HL, Bauer J, et al. Inhaled nitric oxide in neonatal and pediatric acute respiratory distress syndrome: dose response, prolonged inhalation, and weaning. *Crit Care Med* (1996) **24**:1913–9. doi:10.1097/00003246-199611000-00024
88. Okamoto K, Hamaguchi M, Kukita I, Kikuta K, Sato T. Efficacy of inhaled nitric oxide in children with ARDS. *Chest* (1998) **114**:827–33. doi:10.1378/chest.114.3.827
89. Sokol J, Jacobs SE, Bohn D. Inhaled nitric oxide for acute hypoxic respiratory failure in children and adults: a meta-analysis. *Anesth Analg* (2003) **97**:989–98. doi:10.1213/01.ANE.0000078819.48523.26
90. Seger N, Soll R. Animal derived surfactant extract for treatment of respiratory distress syndrome. *Cochrane Database Syst Rev* (2009) **2**:CD007836. doi:10.1002/14651858.CD007836
91. Duffett M, Choong K, Ng V, Randolph A, Cook DJ. Surfactant therapy for acute respiratory failure in children: a systematic review and meta-analysis. *Crit Care* (2007) **11**:R66. doi:10.1186/cc5944
92. Dobyns EL, Cornfield DN, Anas NG, Fortenberry JD, Tasker RC, Lynch A, et al. Multicenter randomized controlled trial of the effects of inhaled nitric oxide therapy on gas exchange in children with acute hypoxemic respiratory failure. *J Pediatr* (1999) **134**:406–12. doi:10.1016/S0022-3476(99)70196-4
93. Schlag G, Strohmaier W. Experimental aspiration trauma: comparison of steroid treatment versus exogenous natural surfactant. *Exp Lung Res* (1993) **19**:397–405. doi:10.3109/01902149309064354
94. McAllister F, Ruan S, Steele C, Zheng M, McKinley L, Ulrich L, et al. CXCR3 and IFN protein-10 in *Pneumocystis* pneumonia. *J Immunol* (2006) **177**(3):1846–54. doi:10.4049/jimmunol.177.3.1846
95. Ruan S, McKinley L, Zheng M, Rudner X, D'Souza A, Kolls JK, et al. Interleukin-12 and host defense against murine *Pneumocystis* pneumonia. *Infect Immun* (2008) **76**(5):2130–7. doi:10.1128/IAI.00065-08
96. Dahlem P, van Aalderen WM, de Neef M, Dijkgraaf MG, Bos AP. Randomized controlled trial of aerosolized prostacyclin therapy in children with acute lung injury. *Crit Care Med* (2004) **32**:1055–60. doi:10.1097/01.CCM.0000120055.52377.BF
97. Factor P, Saldias F, Ridge K, Dumasius V, Zabner J, Jaffe HA, et al. Augmentation of lung liquid clearance via adenovirus-mediated transfer of a Na, K-ATPase beta1 subunit gene. *J Clin Invest* (1998) **102**(7):1421–30. doi:10.1172/JCI3214
98. Factor P, Dumasius V, Saldias F, Brown LA, Sznajder JI. Adenovirus-mediated transfer of an Na+/K+-ATPase beta1 subunit gene improves alveolar fluid clearance and survival in hyperoxic rats. *Hum Gene Ther* (2000) **11**(16):2231–42. doi:10.1089/104303400750035753
99. Ridge KM, Olivera WG, Saldias F, Azzam Z, Horowitz S, Rutschman DH, et al. Alveolar type 1 cells express the alpha2 Na, K-ATPase, which contributes to lung liquid clearance. *Circ Res* (2003) **92**(4):453–60. doi:10.1161/01.RES.0000059414.10360.F2
100. Adir Y, Welch LC, Dumasius V, Factor P, Sznajder JI, Ridge KM. Overexpression of the Na-K-ATPase alpha2-subunit improves lung liquid clearance during ventilation-induced lung injury. *Am J Physiol Lung Cell Mol Physiol* (2008) **294**(6):L1233–7. doi:10.1152/ajplung.00076.2007
101. Mutlu GM, Sznajder JI. Mechanisms of pulmonary edema clearance. *Am J Physiol Lung Cell Mol Physiol* (2005) **289**(5):L685–95. doi:10.1152/ajplung.00247.2005
102. Otterbein LE, Kolls JK, Mantell LL, Cook JL, Alam J, Choi AM. Exogenous administration of heme oxygenase-1 by gene transfer provides protection against hyperoxia-induced lung injury. *J Clin Invest* (1999) **103**(7):1047–54. doi:10.1172/JCI5342
103. Hashiba T, Suzuki M, Nagashima Y, Suzuki S, Inoue S, Tsuburai T, et al. Adenovirus-mediated transfer of heme oxygenase-1 cDNA attenuates severe lung injury induced by the influenza virus in mice. *Gene Ther* (2001) **8**(19):1499–507. doi:10.1038/sj.gt.3301540
104. Inoue S, Suzuki M, Nagashima Y, Suzuki S, Hashiba T, Tsuburai T, et al. Transfer of heme oxygenase 1 cDNA by a replication-deficient adenovirus enhances interleukin 10 production from alveolar macrophages that attenuates lipopolysaccharide-induced acute lung injury in mice. *Hum Gene Ther* (2001) **12**(8):967–79. doi:10.1089/104303401750195926
105. Buff SM, Yu H, McCall JN, Caldwell SM, Ferkol TW, Flotte TR, et al. IL-10 delivery by AAV5 vector attenuates inflammation in mice with *Pseudomonas* pneumonia. *Gene Ther* (2010) **17**(5):567–76. doi:10.1038/gt.2010.28
106. Lin X, Dean DA. Gene therapy for ALI/ARDS. *Crit Care Clin* (2011) **27**:705–18. doi:10.1016/j.ccc.2011.04.002
107. Rafat N, Tonshoff B, Bierhaus A, Beck GC. Endothelial progenitor cells in regeneration after acute lung injury do they play a role? *Am J Respir Cell Mol Biol* (2013) **48**:399–405. doi:10.1165/rcmb.2011-0132TR
108. Verghese GM, McCormick-Shannon K, Mason RJ, Matthay MA. Hepatocyte growth factor and keratinocyte growth factor in the pulmonary edema fluid of patients with acute lung injury. Biologic and clinical significance. *Am J Respir Crit Care Med* (1998) **158**:386–94. doi:10.1164/ajrccm.158.2.9711111
109. Erjefalt JS, Erjefalt I, Sundler F, Persson CG. In vivo restitution of airway epithelium. *Cell Tissue Res* (1995) **281**:305–16. doi:10.1007/BF00583399
110. Ulich TR, Yi ES, Longmuir K, Yin S, Biltz R, Morris CF, et al. Keratinocyte growth factor is a growth factor for type II pneumocytes in vivo. *J Clin Invest* (1994) **93**:1298–306. doi:10.1172/JCI117086
111. Atabai K, Ishigaki M, Geiser T, Ueki I, Matthay MA, Ware LB. Keratinocyte growth factor can enhance alveolar epithelial repair by nonmitogenic mechanisms. *Am J Physiol Lung Cell Mol Physiol* (2002) **283**:L163–9. doi:10.1152/ajplung.00396.2001
112. Fehrenbach H, Kasper M, Koslowski R, Pan T, Schuh D, Muller M, et al. Alveolar epithelial type II cell apoptosis in vivo during resolution of keratinocyte growth factor-induced hyperplasia in the rat. *Histochem Cell Biol* (2000) **114**:49–61.
113. Fehrenbach H, Kasper M, Tschernig T, Pan T, Schuh D, Shannon JM, et al. Keratinocyte growth factor-induced hyperplasia of rat alveolar type II cells in vivo is resolved by differentiation into type I cells and by apoptosis. *Eur Respir J* (1999) **14**:534–44. doi:10.1034/j.1399-3003.1999.14c10.x
114. Gonzalez-Lopez A, Albaiceta GM. Repair after acute lung injury: molecular mechanisms and therapeutic opportunities. *Crit Care* (2012) **16**:209. doi:10.1186/cc11224
115. Bhatia M, Moochhala S. Role of inflammatory mediators in the pathophysiology of acute respiratory distress syndrome. *J Pathol* (2004) **202**:145–56. doi:10.1002/path.1491
116. Kubo H. Molecular basis of lung tissue regeneration. *Gen Thorac Cardiovasc Surg* (2011) **59**:231–44. doi:10.1007/s11748-010-0757-x
117. Yee M, Gelein R, Mariani TJ, Lawrence BP, O'Reilly MA. The oxygen environment at birth specifies the population of alveolar epithelial stem cells in the adult lung. *Stem Cells* (2016). doi:10.1002/stem.2330
118. Panos RJ, Rubin JS, Csaky KG, Aaronson SA, Mason RJ. Keratinocyte growth factor and hepatocyte growth factor/scatter factor are heparin-binding growth factors for alveolar type II cells in fibroblast-conditioned medium. *J Clin Invest* (1993) **92**:969–77. doi:10.1172/JCI116673
119. Panos RJ, Bak PM, Simonet WS, Rubin JS, Smith LJ. Intratracheal instillation of keratinocyte growth factor decreases hyperoxia-induced mortality in rats. *J Clin Invest* (1995) **96**:2026–33. doi:10.1172/JCI118250
120. Panos RJ, Patel R, Bak PM. Intratracheal administration of hepatocyte growth factor/scatter factor stimulates rat alveolar type II cell proliferation in vivo. *Am J Respir Cell Mol Biol* (1996) **15**:574–81. doi:10.1165/ajrcmb.15.5.8918364
121. Crosby LM, Waters CM. Epithelial repair mechanisms in the lung. *Am J Physiol Lung Cell Mol Physiol* (2010) **298**:L715–31. doi:10.1152/ajplung.00361.2009
122. Chapman HA, Li X, Alexander JP, Brumwell A, Lorizio W, Tan K, et al. Integrin α6β4 identifies an adult distal lung epithelial population with regenerative potential in mice. *J Clin Invest* (2011) **121**:2855–62. doi:10.1172/JCI57673
123. Zheng D, Limmon GV, Yin L, Leung NH, Yu H, Chow VT, et al. Regeneration of alveolar type I and II cells from Scgb1a1-expressing cells following severe

pulmonary damage induced by bleomycin and influenza. *PLoS One* (2012) 7:e48451. doi:10.1371/journal.pone.0048451
124. Jain R, Barkauskas CE, Takeda N, Bowie EJ, Aghajanian H, Wang Q, et al. Plasticity of Hopx(+) type I alveolar cells to regenerate type II cells in the lung. *Nat Commun* (2015) **6**:6727. doi:10.1038/ncomms7727
125. Barkauskas CE, Cronce MJ, Rackley CR, Bowie EJ, Keene DR, Stripp BR, et al. Type 2 alveolar cells are stem cells in adult lung. *J Clin Invest* (2013) **123**(7):3025–36. doi:10.1172/JCI68782
126. Garcia O, Hiatt MJ, Lundin A, Lee J, Reddy R, Navarro S, et al. Targeted type 2 alveolar cell depletion provides a dynamic functional model for lung injury repair. *Am J Respir Cell Mol Biol* (2016) **54**(3):319–30. doi:10.1165/rcmb.2014-0246OC
127. Engstrom PC, Holm BA, Matalon S. Surfactant replacement attenuates the increase in alveolar permeability in hyperoxia. *J Appl Physiol* (1989) **67**:688–93.
128. Novotny WE, Hudak BB, Matalon S, Holm BA. Hyperoxic lung injury reduces exogenous surfactant clearance in vitro. *Am J Respir Crit Care Med* (1995) **151**:1843–7. doi:10.1164/ajrccm.151.6.7767528
129. Mulugeta S, Nureki S, Beers MF. Lost after translation: insights from pulmonary surfactant for understanding the role of alveolar epithelial dysfunction and cellular quality control in fibrotic lung disease. *Am J Physiol Lung Cell Mol Physiol* (2015) **309**:L507–25. doi:10.1152/ajplung.00139.2015
130. Selman M, Pardo A. Role of epithelial cells in idiopathic pulmonary fibrosis: from innocent targets to serial killers. *Proc Am Thorac Soc* (2006) **3**(4):364–72. doi:10.1513/pats.200601-003TK
131. Buckley S, Shi W, Xu W, Frey MR, Moats R, Pardo A, et al. Increased alveolar soluble annexin V promotes lung inflammation and fibrosis. *Eur Respir J* (2015) **46**(5):1417–29. doi:10.1183/09031936.00002115
132. Yanagi S, Tsubouchi H, Miura A, Matsumoto N, Nakazato M. Breakdown of epithelial barrier integrity and overdrive activation of alveolar epithelial cells in the pathogenesis of acute respiratory distress syndrome and lung fibrosis. *Biomed Res Int* (2015) **2015**:573210. doi:10.1155/2015/573210
133. Cai Y, Yoneda M, Tomita T, Kurotani R, Okamoto M, Kido T, et al. Transgenically-expressed secretoglobin 3A2 accelerates resolution of bleomycin-induced pulmonary fibrosis in mice. *BMC Pulm Med* (2015) **15**:72. doi:10.1186/s12890-015-0065-4
134. Lindsay CD. Novel therapeutic strategies for acute lung injury induced by lung damaging agents: the potential role of growth factors as treatment options. *Hum Exp Toxicol* (2011) **30**:701–24. doi:10.1177/0960327110376982
135. Bui KCT, Senadheera D, Wang X, Hendrickson B, Friedlich P, Lutzko C. Recovery of multipotent progenitors from the peripheral blood of patients requiring extracorporeal membrane oxygenation support. *Am J Respir Crit Care Med* (2010) **181**:226–37. doi:10.1164/rccm.200812-1901OC
136. Davey A, McAuley DF, O'Kane CM. Matrix metalloproteinases in acute lung injury: mediators of injury and drivers of repair. *Eur Respir J* (2011) **389**:959–70. doi:10.1183/09031936.00032111
137. Matthay MA, Ware LB, Zimmerman GA. The acute respiratory distress syndrome. *J Clin Invest* (2012) **122**:2731–40. doi:10.1172/JCI60331
138. Ware LB. Pathophysiology of acute lung injury and the acute respiratory distress syndrome. *Semin Respir Crit Care Med* (2006) **27**:337–49. doi:10.1055/s-2006-948288
139. Liu KD, Matthay MA. Advances in critical care for the nephrologist: acute lung injury/ARDS. *Clin J Am Soc Nephrol* (2008) **3**(2):578–86. doi:10.2215/CJN.01630407
140. Budinger GR, Sznajder JI. The alveolar-epithelial barrier: a target for potential therapy. *Clin Chest Med* (2006) **27**(4):655–69. doi:10.1016/j.ccm.2006.06.007
141. Smith LS, Zimmerman JJ, Martin TR. Mechanisms of acute respiratory distress syndrome in children and adults: a review and suggestions for future research. *Pediatr Crit Care Med* (2013) **14**:631–43. doi:10.1097/PCC.0b013e318291753f
142. Raghavendran K, Pryhuber GS, Chess PR, Davidson BA, Knight PR, Notter RH. Pharmacotherapy of acute lung injury and acute respiratory distress syndrome. *Curr Med Chem* (2008) **15**:1911–24. doi:10.2174/092986708785132942
143. Pryhuber GS, D'Angio CT, Finkelstein JN, Notter RH. Combined-modality therapies for lung injury. In: Notter RH, Finkelstein JN, Holm BA, editors. *Lung injury: Mechanisms, pathophysiology, and therapy*. Boca Raton: Taylor Francis Group, Inc (2005). p. 779–838.

26

Role of Inhaled Nitric Oxide in the Management of Severe Acute Respiratory Distress Syndrome

Juliette Lucinda Hunt[1]*, Ronald A. Bronicki[2] and Nick Anas[1]

[1] CHOC Children's Hospital, Orange, CA, USA, [2] Texas Children's Hospital, Houston, TX, USA

****Correspondence:***
Juliette Lucinda Hunt
jhunt@choc.org

To date, there have been several systematic reviews with meta-analysis that have shown no reduction in mortality with the use of inhaled nitric oxide (iNO) in patients with acute respiratory distress syndrome (ARDS). Importantly, these reports fail to make a distinction between the pediatric and adult patient. The number of adult patients in these reviews are far greater than the number of pediatric patients, which makes it difficult to interpret the data regarding the role of iNO on the pediatric population. Extrapolating data from the adult population to the pediatric population is complicated as we know that physiology and the body's response to disease can be different between adult and pediatric patients. iNO has been demonstrated to improve outcomes in term and near-term infants with hypoxic respiratory failure associated with pulmonary hypertension. Recently, Bronicki et al. published a prospective randomized control trial investigating the impact of iNO on the pediatric patient population with acute respiratory failure. In this study, a benefit of decreased duration of mechanical ventilation and an increased rate of ECMO-free survival was demonstrated in patients who were randomized to receiving iNO, suggesting that there may be benefit to the use of iNO in pediatric ARDS (PARDS) that has not been demonstrated in adults. iNO has repeatedly been shown to transiently improve oxygenation in all age groups, and yet neonates and pediatric patients have shown improvement in other outcomes that have not been seen in adults. The mechanism that explains improvement with the use of iNO in these patient populations are not well understood but does not appear to be solely a result of sustained improvement in oxygenation. There are physiologic studies that suggest alternative mechanisms for explaining the positive effects of iNO, such as platelet aggregation inhibition and reduction in systemic inflammation. Hence, the role of iNO by various mechanisms and in various age groups warrants further investigation.

Keywords: pediatric acute respiratory distress syndrome, inhaled nitric oxide, pulmonary hypertension, mechanisms of action, clinical trials

INTRODUCTION

In many review articles of acute respiratory distress syndrome (ARDS), the conclusion that the use of iNO does not reduce mortality continues to be perpetuated. Most often, the references for this conclusion are the systematic reviews with meta analysis by Adhikari et al. (1, 2) and Afshari et al. (3) These are well conducted systematic reviews; however, the conclusion made from these studies as it pertains to pediatric ARDS (PARDS) could be challenged.

Analysis of these influential systemic reviews reveals that the number of pediatric studies and overall number of pediatric patients are small. In fact, there are only three pediatric studies on this matter included. The number of pediatric studies are too few to determine the effect of iNO on PARDS outcome.

However, the extrapolation of this adult data to pediatrics has been widely accepted, and there has been inadequate investigation on the subject in pediatrics since these systematic reviews were published. Most have taken for granted that the answer regarding the benefit of iNO in PARDS exists when in fact the question as it applies to pediatrics has never scientifically been evaluated.

The other limitation to understanding the full impact of iNO has been the primary emphasis on its mechanism of action as a selective pulmonary vasodilator in improving V/Q matching and the outcome of mortality. Focusing on the effect of iNO by only this mechanism and this outcome may minimize its therapeutic importance. For example, Nitric oxide (NO) has a variety of effects on the immune system and immune regulation. This could be of particular interest in the context of ARDS, a disease whose pathology is largely a result of the immune response. Some studies in neonates have demonstrated that the incidence of chronic lung disease, a disease that results from an inflammatory process, could be attenuated with the use of iNO (4–6). These findings are important as they give evidence of the effects of iNO that we might be underestimating.

Until we have more pediatric specific data on ARDS and iNO, we are left reviewing what has been learned about ARDS, NO, and iNO from the laboratory and from adults. Equipped with the understanding that the pathology of ARDS and the response to ARDS are likely different between pediatrics and adults and that the mechanisms of iNO are diverse, pediatric practitioners should be challenging the notions that we have accepted from the adult data by re-examining the many properties of iNO and bringing new, important pediatric specific research to the forefront.

PATHOPHYSIOLOGY AND EPIDEMIOLOGY OF ARDS AND PARDS

One of the hallmarks of ARDS is hypoxemia. In this disease state, inflammation leads to injury of the pulmonary capillary endothelium and the alveolar epithelium, which results in permeability and accumulation of polymorphonuclear cells, erythrocytes, platelets, and water in the airspaces (7). Pulmonary edema and inactivation of surfactant result in intrapulmonary shunting and thus hypoxemia.

One of the practice changing results from the ARDS Network study was the reduced mortality in adult patients with ARDS who were randomized to a low tidal volume ventilation strategy (8). The explanation for why mortality is significantly improved with lower tidal volume is not known, but one theory is the reduction in the inflammatory response induced by a lower tidal volume. Ranieri et al. found that patients with ARDS ventilated with a lower tidal volume had a decrease in inflammatory cells and cytokines in their BAL and plasma (9). The association between inflammation and tidal volume, or stretching of the respiratory system, became known as biotrauma (10). This concept emphasizes the significant role the immune system plays in the pathogenesis of ARDS.

Interestingly, although impaired oxygenation is a hallmark of the disease, therapies that have led to improved oxygenation, including iNO, have failed to show a significant reduction in mortality outcome (11). Perhaps the lack of demonstrable mortality benefit is because patients with ARDS often die of multi-system organ failure (MSOF) rather than hypoxemia (12, 13). The presence of MSOF in ARDS is likely due to the host immune response. With damage to the alveolar-capillary barrier, inflammatory cells and cytokines can enter the general circulation and illicit a systemic inflammatory response than can lead to the impairment of multiple organs (14). In this scenerio, the lung becomes the source of inflammation and not solely the target of inflammation.

From an epidemiological standpoint, most studies show that ARDS is less common in children than in adults and that the mortality rate of children is less than adults (15). Sepsis is the most common risk factor in adults with concomitant MSOF as compared to children in whom pulmonary infections are the most common risk factor (16). And perhaps it is the increased MSOF in adults compared to children that explains the difference in mortality risk between these populations. This is an important distinction as we begin to further explore the potential therapeutic benefits of iNO and the possibility that there may be a difference on the impact on adults and children. As a lung-selective therapy, it has been thought that iNO is unlikely to improve overall survival when most adult patients dying from ARDS suffer from multiple organ failure (17). However, since children are more likely to have pneumonia than multi-organ failure, a lung-selective therapy, such as iNO, could provide more of a survival benefit in children than in adults.

Smith and colleagues provide a review of the pathophysiology of ARDS in children and adults (18). The point that the lungs are still developing and growing in children compared to adults is an important distinction emphasized in this paper, particularly because the response to infection and injury are likely different based on the milieu of growth factors, gene expression, and protein expression at various stages of lung development. They also emphasize that the innate immune response is different between children and adults. Infants have impaired clearance of the pathogen and less of the pro inflammatory response, which may be injurious to the lungs. In contrast, adults can clear the pathogen but suffer injury from the inflammatory response itself. The content of surfactant between patients with ARDS and PARDS is also different (19, 20), which may account for difference in benefit in the use of exogenous surfactant between children and adults with ARDS (21) and may also suggest that there is a difference in the injury to the alveolar epithelium between these groups.

Understanding the pathology of ARDS is important as it illustrates potential mechanisms for therapeutic interventions. Additionally, highlighting the differences between ARDS and PARDS, exemplifies that the disease state is not the same in all age groups, and hence the response to therapies, particularly iNO, may be different.

HISTORY OF NO AND iNO

Since its discovery only a few decades ago, inhaled nitric oxide (iNO) has fascinated many in the field of critical care and medicine in general. Its potential benefits, limited evidence of proven benefit, but ongoing use as a rescue medication continue to be the focus of research and debate.

Nitric oxide gained much notoriety within the scientific community when it was declared the Molecule of the Year by Science in 1992. It was 6 years later that the individuals credited with its discovery, Ferid Murad, Robert Furchgott, and Louis Ignarro were awarded the Nobel prize for Physiology and Medicine in 1998.

In 1993, Rossaint et al. published a landmark article in the New England Journal of Medicine that described the role of iNO in Acute Respiratory Distress Syndrome (ARDS) in reducing pulmonary artery pressures and increasing arterial oxygenation by improving V/Q mismatch without precipitating systemic hypotension (22).

Rossaint's paper was followed by many important studies including several focused on the neonatal population, which showed definitive benefit of iNO in this patient population. In 1997, the Neonatal Inhaled Nitric Oxide Study Group (NINOS) showed that iNO was beneficial in full-term and nearly full-term infants with hypoxic respiratory failure by demonstrating that the use of iNO reduced the use of extracorporeal membrane oxygenation (ECMO) (23, 24). In 1998, the I-NO/PPHN study group showed that early use of iNO in term infants with persistent pulmonary hypertension (PPHN) had an acute and sustained improvement in oxygenation and a reduction in ECMO use that did not reach statistical significance (25).

In December 1999, The US Food and Drug Administration (FDA) approved the use of INOmax (nitric oxide) for inhalation for the treatment of "term and near-term (>34 weeks) neonates with hypoxic respiratory failure associated with clinical or echocardiographic evidence of pulmonary hypertension where it improves oxygenation and reduces the need for extracorporeal membrane oxygenation" (26). To date, this remains the only licensed indication for the use for iNO.

In August 2000, the American Academy of Pediatrics published a statement on the conditions in which iNO should be used, which endorsed the FDA indications of the use of iNO for newborns with hypoxic respiratory failure (27).

The sole commercial manufacturer of INOmax at the time of FDA approval was INO Therapeutics. In March 2007, INO Therapeutics and Ikaria merged, and INOmax was then exclusively supplied by Ikaria until April of 2015, when Mallinckrodt Pharmaceuticals acquired Ikaria, Inc. Mallinckrodt Pharmaceuticals now maintains the many patents on the INOMAX drug label and INOMAX delivery system, five of which provide protection until 2029 and another five that provide protection until 2031.

MECHANISMS OF NO AND iNO

Nitric oxide is composed of two atoms that form a gaseous molecule. It is found naturally in the atmosphere and produced in various parts of the body. The enzyme nitric oxide synthase (NOS) converts L-arginine to nitric oxide. There are multiple isoforms of nitric oxide synthase (NOS). nNOS is the neuronal form that is involved in neurotransmission. iNOS is an inducible form involved in the immune response. eNOS is the endothelial nitric oxide synthase isoform, which is the form that is active in healthy vascular endothelial cells (28).

eNOS produces NO that acts specifically on endothelial smooth muscle cells. NO penetrates the cell membrane, which binds to the soluble guanylyl cyclase and activates it forming cGMP. cGMP binds to the cGMP-dependent protein kinase. The activated protein kinase then affixes to ionic channels of the cell membrane and the sarcoplasmic reticulum, which has the effect of decreasing the influx of calcium to the cell, increasing the ejection of calcium from the cell, sequestering the calcium within the sarcoplasmic reticulum, and decreasing calcium mobilization. The net effect of these reactions makes less calcium available for depolarization and contraction, which leads to smooth muscle relaxation (29).

With the understanding of NO's ability to relax endothelial smooth muscle, multiple laboratory studies were performed to assess the effect of inhaled NO on the pulmonary vasculature (30, 31). In 1991, Frostell et al. demonstrated in lamb models that iNO could produce pulmonary vasodilation by reversing hypoxic pulmonary vasoconstriction or thromboxane-induced pulmonary hypertension without causing systemic hypotension

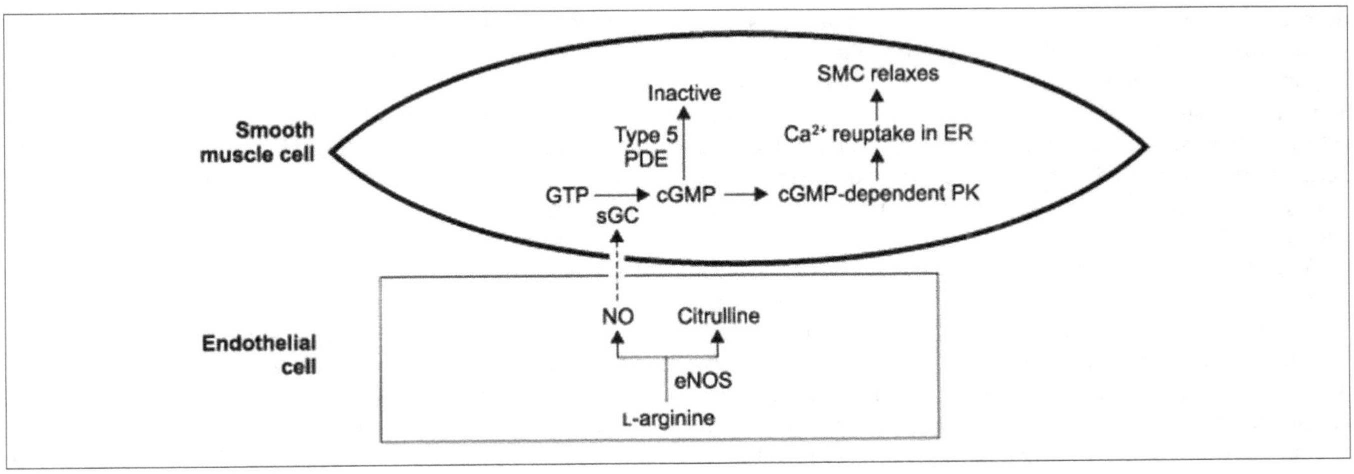

(30). The mechanism similar to that of eNOS is the most likely explanation of how iNO leads to this effect. The inhaled NO is delivered directly to the pulmonary vascular endothelial cells causing the endothelial smooth muscle relaxation of the pulmonary vasculature. The pulmonary vasodilation reduces intrapulmonary shunting when lung disease is present, which allows for increased ventilation/perfusion (V/Q) matching and improved oxygenation.

Nitric oxide is known to have a multitude of other effects on various cells in the body as well. Yet, it is commonly believed that when delivered by inhalation, the effect of nitric oxide is limited to the lungs. As NO is exposed to the bloodstream, it binds rapidly and with a high affinity to hemoglobin, which then inactivates it (32). This is the explanation for why iNO leads to pulmonary vasodilation without causing significant systemic vasodilation or hypotension. It is worth noting, however, that there are some studies to suggest that NO bioactivity may actually reach distant organs even when delivered by inhalation. The implications of this is even less well understood that even further limits our true appreciation of the impact of iNO.

In addition to its effect on endothelial smooth muscle, NO also affects platelet activity. It has been observed *in vitro* that NO activates the guanylate cyclase inside platelets, which increases intraplatelet cGMP. The resulting activation of cGMP-dependent protein kinase here causes a reduction in fibrinogen biding to glycoprotein GP IIb/IIIa, which induces partial inhibition of platelet aggregation (33, 34).

Considering that activation and accumulation of platelets is observed in the alveolar tissues of patients with ARDS (35), and given the effect NO has on platelet aggregation, Samama et al. investigated whether iNO could inhibit platelet aggregation in patients with ARDS (34). They found that the six patients studied showed a significant improvement in oxygenation, significant decrease in pulmonary artery pressure, and a significant decrease in *ex vivo* platelet aggregation after iNO administration without a change in their Ivy bleeding time. They concluded that the improvement in arterial oxygenation and pulmonary circulation are associated with a significant inhibition of platelet aggregation.

Nitric oxide has also been noted to have a number of potentially important effects on the immune system and has been implicated in a variety of mechanisms (36). NO has been shown to alter the balance between T helper (Th)1 and Th2 cells. In particular, NO decreases Th1 proliferation and IL-2 synthesis but increases IL-4 synthesis from Th2 cells. By decreasing Th1 and increasing Th2 responses, NO may inhibit the inflammatory response to viral and bacterial infections. Additionally, NO has an effect on leukocyte adhesion and recruitment to sites of infection. NO has also been reported to have a direct effect on a variety of organisms by directly inhibiting the growth of some viruses, bacteria, parasites, and fungi (37).

As previously stated, ventilator-induced lung injury results in an increase in systemic inflammatory mediators (biotrauma). With the above understanding of the many ways, NO can affect immune regulation and the potential impact of iNO in ARDS is intriguing. Kinsella et al. looked at the effects of iNO on pulmonary hemodynamics, gas exchange, pulmonary edema, and lung myeloperoxidase (MPO) activity, as a marker of lung neutrophil accumulation in extremely premature lambs (38). They studied lambs exposed to iNO and compared them to controls. They found that the lambs exposed to iNO had improved gas exchange but did not have an increase in their lung weight or permeability to albumin after several hours of mechanical ventilation. They also found that the iNO exposed lambs had a reduction in the MPO activity by 79%. They concluded that low dose iNO can augment pulmonary blood flow without worsening pulmonary edema and can decrease lung neutrophil accumulation, which may reduce lung injury. These findings support iNO's properties as both a pulmonary vasodilator and immune modulator.

In 2000, The Clinical Inhaled Nitric Oxide Research Group (CINRGI) showed that low-dose iNO therapy for PPHN of the newborn could decrease the need for ECMO in these neonates (5). Additionally, this study showed that the group that received low dose iNO also had less chronic lung disease when compared to controls. This work was followed by Schreiber et al. who also demonstrated that treatment with iNO decreased the incidence of chronic lung disease and death among preterm infants with respiratory distress syndrome (6). The finding that chronic lung disease is decreased with the use of iNO, suggests that the benefit of iNO likely extends beyond just pulmonary vasodilation. As chronic lung disease is caused at least in part by irritation and inflammation of the neonatal lungs, the impact of the use of iNO may be a result of iNO's effect on the immune response to lung injury.

ARDS AND iNO IN ADULTS

As mentioned above, the use of iNO for adult patients with ARDS began in 1993 when Rossaint et al. showed improved oxygenation in this patient population (22). Subsequent studies would also show that oxygenation was improved when iNO was used in adult patients with ARDS but demonstrated that there was no decrease in morbidity and mortality. The lack of survival benefit then called into question the true advantage of using iNO, especially given that in some adults iNO use may increase renal impairment (3, 39).

A number of systematic reviews with meta-analysis have since been conducted to try to answer the question of whether iNO reduces mortality in patients with ARDS. These meta-analysis have looked at available randomized control trials (RCTs) in which there were data on iNO use, ARDS and mortality. In 2007, Adhikari published his first systemic review of 12 RCTs that met inclusion criteria which included a total of 1237 patient with ARDS (1). Of the RCTs included two of them were done with the pediatric population and accounted for only 132 of the total number of patients. The authors of this review found no significant effect of iNO on hospital mortality or number of ventilator-free days. They concluded that iNO had a short lived improvement on oxygenation that conferred no survival benefit. In 2014, Adhikari et al. updated their previous search and analyzed the data from the systemic review to determine if a survival benefit with iNO use could be demonstrated when the patients with ARDS were divided into severe versus mild-moderate ARDS (2). This review had 9 RCTs and 1142 patients that met inclusion criteria. In this review, there were no RCTs with only pediatric patients and only one study that included pediatric patients of which there were only three children. The conclusion from this review was that iNO does not reduce mortality in adults and children with ARDS, regardless of the degree of hypoxemia. Additionally, it should be noted, that many of these trials used a wide range of iNO levels, several of them using 5–10 ppm.

In 2011, Afshari et al. also undertook a systemic review with meta analysis in which they included 14 RCTs with 1303 patients (3). This review included three pediatric studies with a total of 164 pediatric patients. Ten of the studies had a high risk of bias. These authors found no statistically significant effect of iNO on duration of ventilation, ventilator-free days, or on length of stay in the intensive care unit and hospital. They also concluded that iNO results in a transient improvement in oxygenation but does not reduce mortality and may be harmful as it increases the risk of renal impairment in adults.

ARDS AND iNO IN PEDIATRICS

To date, there are no published systemic reviews with meta analysis comprised exclusively of pediatric RCTs investigating the effect of iNO on PARDS. This is not surprising since the findings from the aforementioned systemic reviews reveal a very limited number of eligible pediatric RCTs on the topic. Of those pediatric RCTs that were included, individually they were small in number with study designs that limit the ability to draw conclusions on how iNO impacts the outcome of PARDS.

By including such a small number of pediatric patients in the above systematic reviews with such a larger number of adult studies and much larger number of adult patients it: (1) may diminish the impact and true findings from the pediatric studies and (2) allows the authors to apply conclusions generated largely by adult data to both adult and pediatric patients which may not be valid.

Of the three pediatric RCTs in the aforementioned systemic reviews, only one study was multi-centered which included 7 centers and 108 pediatric patients (40). This multi-center study was a double-blinded, randomized, placebo-controlled trial, which looked at oxygenation as an end-point. The study allowed for cross-over of the placebo group with treatment failure, which made assessment of other endpoints (mortality, duration of ventilation) difficult. The results from this study showed that iNO improved oxygenation at 12 and 24 h, but by 72 h, there was no difference in oxygenation. Interestingly, immunocompromised patients and those patients with more severe oxygenation impairment appeared to have a more sustained improvement in oxygenation.

The other two pediatric RCTs were single-centered studies. The study by Day et al. included 24 pediatric patients and also allowed for cross-over of the placebo group with treatment failure again making a conclusion on outcome differences impossible (41). The third study was conducted by Ibrahim and El-Mohamady and they collected data on 32 pediatric patients for only 24 h to assess the outcome on oxygenation, they did not collect data on other outcomes (42).

The first RCT to evaluate outcomes other than oxygenation in patients with PARDS that received iNO was published in 2014 (43). In this study, Bronicki et al. enrolled 55 pediatric patients in a prospective, randomized placebo-controlled trial that showed a significant reduction in duration of mechanical ventilation and a significantly greater rate of ECMO-free survival. There was a trend toward improved overall 28-day survival that did not meet statistical significance. There was a significant improvement in the oxygenation index of those patient receiving iNO at 12 h, but no difference between the oxygenation index of both groups at 24 h. An important feature of this study is that it suggests that there were benefits to the pediatric patients that received iNO, which did not correlate to a sustained improvement in oxygenation.

The Pediatric Acute Lung Injury Consensus Conference Group was formed in 2012 to better establish the definition for pediatric ARDS and to provide recommendations for management. Their first consensus recommendations for were published in 2015 (44), and the following was their recommendation specifically about iNO and PARDS:

> "Inhaled nitric oxide is not recommended for routine use in PARDS. However, its use may be considered in patients with documented pulmonary hypertension or severe right ventricular dysfunction. In addition, it may be considered in severe cases of PARDS as a rescue from or bridge to extracorporeal life support. When used, assessment of benefit must be undertaken promptly and serially to minimize toxicity and to eliminate continued use without established effect. Finally, future study is needed to better define its role, if any, in the treatment of PARDS." The Group was in strong agreement about this recommendation.

The recommendations by the group indicate that iNO may by considered for severe ARDS but ultimately that more data needs to be collected to understand its role in pediatric ARDS.

WHERE DO WE GO FROM HERE?

Santschi et al. illustrated that there is wide practice variability in the management in PARDS (45). In the discussion of their paper, they estimated that in order to conduct an international clinical trial to assess a reduction in mortality in PARDS that it would take 60 PICUs and about 4 years to recruit the 800 patients needed. Additionally, RCTs call for the limitation of co-founders that would force us to individually investigate every aspect of management as it pertains to PARDS when the reality is that most patients receive a combination of therapies. The resources it would require to accomplish studies in this fashion are not realistic.

With the challenges of using mortality as an outcome measure in pediatric trials, perhaps alternative outcome metrics in PARDS should be considered and evaluated such as a health related quality of life metric validated in pediatrics, the PedsQL™ Scale (46). As it pertains to the impact of iNO in particular, perhaps we should be looking at how it impacts the Pediatric Multiple Organ Dysfunction Score (P-MODS) (47). As previously stated, ARDS is often not present in isolation and the effects of iNO may spread beyond the lungs in a way that could effect the P-MODS, which could potentially have an additional impact on the PedsQL™ scale.

But likely the most important pursuit is the path toward personalized and precision medicine, an emerging reality with the rapid evolution of genomic medicine. Although ARDS is a disease state with a common histology and pathophysiology, the exact manifestation and the response to therapies, such as iNO, are likely much more individualized than we will ever gather from studying the population as a whole with our tradition approaches. Wong and colleagues have done important work in the field of genomics and septic shock (48). Among his groups, important contributions are the ability for subclass stratification that identifies high risk patients with septic shock based on inflammatory response and genomic profiling. This identification has already been shown to allow for therapy-related clinical decision making particularly as it applies to the use of corticosteroids in septic shock (49). Wong and colleagues have demonstrated a path for similar work that could be done to link individual genomics with ARDS. This could allow for a stratification scheme to identify individuals whose genetic profile might benefit from iNO therapy and the discovery of the true impact of iNO in ARDS might truly be realized. This might prove to be the most worthwhile endeavor to truly understand the impact of iNO.

CONCLUSION

As we continue to strive to improve our management of ARDS, it is important to acknowledge that although the disease may look similar from patient to patient that it is likely not the same disease in everyone. The pathology, the pathophysiology and the response to therapy may be quite varied not just by the age of the patient but by other individual characteristics of the patients as well. So although the RCTs and the systemic reviews of iNO and ARDS have helped to guide the management in adults, we should be cautious about extrapolating that data to all patients with ARDS. Perhaps further exploring the impact of iNO on inflammation, coagulation, and applying genomics will provide further insight to the very varied disease of ARDS and the patient populations that are effected by it. The story of iNO, a molecule whose discovery was only within the past 30 years, is still young.

AUTHOR CONTRIBUTIONS

JH: majority of original writing. RB: contributed to the outline of the paper with significant direction toward resources used. NA: major editing and some of the original writing.

REFERENCES

1. Adhikari NK, Burns KE, Friedrich JO, Granton JT, Cook DJ, Meade MO. Effect of nitric oxide on oxygenation and mortality in acute lung injury: systematic review and meta-analysis. *BMJ* (2007) 334(7597):779. doi:10.1136/bmj.39139.716794.55
2. Adhikari NK, Dellinger RP, Lundin S, Payen D, Vallet B, Gerlach H, et al. Inhaled nitric oxide does not reduce mortality in patients with acute respiratory distress syndrome regardless of severity: systematic review and meta-analysis. *Crit Care Med* (2014) 42(2):404–12. doi:10.1097/CCM.0b013e3182a27909
3. Afshari A, Brok J, Møller AM, Wetterslev J. Inhaled nitric oxide for acute respiratory distress syndrome and acute lung injury in adults and children: a systematic review with meta-analysis and trial sequential analysis. *Anesth Analg* (2011) 112(6):1411–21. doi:10.1213/ANE.0b013e31820bd185
4. Ballard RA, Truog WE, Cnaan A, Martin RJ, Ballard PL, Merrill JD, et al. Inhaled nitric oxide in preterm infants undergoing mechanical ventilation. *N Engl J Med* (2006) 355:343–53. doi:10.1056/NEJMoa061088
5. Clark RH, Kueser TJ, Walker MW, Southgate WM, Huckaby JL, Perez JA, et al. Low-dose nitric oxide therapy for persistent pulmonary hypertension of the newborn. Clinical Inhaled Nitric Oxide Research Group. *N Engl J Med* (2000) 342(7):469–74. doi:10.1056/NEJM200002173420704
6. Schreiber MD, Gin-Mestan K, Marks JD, Huo D, Lee G, Srisuparp P. Inhaled nitric oxide in premature infants with the respiratory distress syndrome. *N Engl J Med* (2003) 349:2099–107. doi:10.1056/NEJMoa031154
7. PiantadosiCA,SchwartzDA.Theacuterespiratorydistresssyndrome.*AnnIntern Med* (2004) 141(6):460–70. doi:10.7326/0003-4819-141-6-200409210-00012
8. Network ARDS. Ventilation with lower tidal volumes as compared with traditional tidal volumes for acute lung injury and the acute respiratory distress syndrome. *N Engl J Med* (2000) 342:1301–8. doi:10.1056/NEJM200005043421801
9. Ranieri VM, Suter PM, Tortorella C, De Tullio R, Dayer JM, Brienza A, et al. Effect of mechanical ventilation on inflammatory mediators in patients with acute respiratory distress syndrome: a randomized controlled trial. *JAMA* (1999) 282(1):54–61. doi:10.1001/jama.282.1.54
10. Tremblay LN, Slutsky AS. Ventilator-induced lung injury: from barotraumas to biotrauma. *Proc Assoc Am Physicians* (1998) 110:482–8.
11. Gattinoni L, Tognoni G, Pesenti A, Taccone P, Mascheroni D, Labarta V, et al. Effect of prone positioning on the survival of patients with acute respiratory failure. *N Engl J Med* (2001) 345(8):568–73. doi:10.1056/NEJMoa010043
12. Doyle RL, Szaflarski N, Modin GW, Wiener-Kronish JP, Matthay MA. Identification of patients with acute lung injury. Predictors of mortality. *Am J Respir Crit Care Med* (1995) 152(6 Pt 1):1818–24. doi:10.1164/ajrccm.152.6.8520742
13. Montgomery AB, Stager MA, Carrico CJ, Hudson LD. Causes of mortality in patients with the adult respiratory distress syndrome. *Am Rev Respir Dis* (1985) 132(3):485–9.
14. Slutsky AS, Tremblay LN. Multiple system organ failure. *Am J Respir Crit Care Med* (1998) 157(6):1721–5. doi:10.1164/ajrccm.157.6.9709092
15. Zimmerman JJ, Akhtar SR, Caldwell E, Rubenfeld GD. Incidence and outcomes of pediatric acute lung injury. *Pediatrics* (2009) 124(1):87–95. doi:10.1542/peds.2007-2462
16. Rubenfeld GD, Caldwell E, Peabody E, et al. Prevalence and outcomes of acute lung injury. *N Engl J Med* (2005) 353:1685–93. doi:10.1056/NEJMoa050333
17. Ichinose F, Roberts JD Jr, Zapol WM. Inhaled nitric oxide: a selective pulmonary vasodilator: current uses and therapeutic potential. *Circulation* (2004) 109:3106–11. doi:10.1161/01.CIR.0000134595.80170.62
18. Smith LS, Zimmerman JJ, Martin TR. Mechanisms of acute respiratory distress syndrome in children and adults: a review and suggestions for future research. *Pediatr Crit Care Med* (2013) 14(6):631–43. doi:10.1097/PCC.0b013e318291753f
19. Greene KE, Wright JR, Steinberg KP, Ruzinski JT, Caldwell E, Wong WB, et al. Serial changes in surfactant-associated proteins in lung and serum before and after onset of ARDS. *Am J Respir Crit Care Med* (1999) 160(6):1843–50. doi:10.1164/ajrccm.160.6.9901117
20. LeVine AM, Lotze A, Stanley S, Stroud C, O'Donnell R, Whitsett J, et al. Surfactant content in children with inflammatory lung disease. *Crit Care Med* (1996) 24(6):1062–7. doi:10.1097/00003246-199606000-00029

21. Duffett M, Choong K, Ng V, Randolph A, Cook DJ. Surfactant therapy for acute respiratory failure in children: a systematic review and meta-analysis. *Crit Care* (2007) 11(3):R66. doi:10.1186/cc5944
22. Rossaint R, Falke KJ, Lopez F, Slama K, Pison U, Zapol WM. Inhaled nitric oxide for the adult respiratory distress syndrome. *N Engl J Med* (1993) 328:399–405. doi:10.1056/NEJM199302113280605
23. Neonatal Inhaled Nitric Oxide Study Group. Inhaled nitric oxide in full-term and nearly full-term infants with hypoxic respiratory failure. *N Engl J Med* (1997) 336:597–604. doi:10.1056/NEJM199702273360901
24. Roberts JD Jr, Fineman JR, Morin FC, Shaul PW, Rimar S, Schreiber MD, et al. Inhaled nitric oxide and persistent pulmonary hypertension of the newborn. *N Engl J Med* (1997) 336:605–10. doi:10.1056/NEJM199702273360902
25. Davidson D, Barefield ES, Kattwinkel J, Dudell G, Damask M, Straube R, et al. Inhaled nitric oxide for the early treatment of persistent pulmonary hypertension of the term newborn: a randomized, double-masked, placebo-controlled, dose-response, multicenter study. The I-NO/PPHN Study Group. *Pediatrics* (1998) 101(3 Pt 1):325–34. doi:10.1542/peds.101.3.325
26. *Approval Letter by US Food and Drug Administration on the FDA website*. Available from: http://www.accessdata.fda.gov/drugsatfda_docs/nda/99/20845_INOmax_Approv.pdf
27. American Academy of Pediatrics Committee on Fetus and Newborn. Use of inhaled nitric oxide. *Pediatrics* (2000) 106(2 Pt 1):344–5. doi:10.1542/peds.106.2.344
28. Alderton WK, Cooper CE, Knowles RG. Nitric oxide synthases: structure, function and inhibition. *Biochem J* (2001) 357(Pt 3):593–615. doi:10.1042/0264-6021:3570593
29. Katz I. *Inhaled Nitric Oxide: Therapeutic Uses And Potential Hazards*. Glenview, IL: PCCSU (Vol. 25, Lesson 22) (2012).
30. Frostell C, Fratacci MD, Wain JC, Jones R, Zapol WM. Inhaled nitric oxide. A selective pulmonary vasodilator reversing hypoxic pulmonary vasoconstriction [published correction appears in Circulation. 1991;84: 2212]. *Circulation* (1991) 83:2038–47. doi:10.1161/01.CIR.83.6.2038
31. Roberts JD Jr, Chen TY, Kawai N, Wain J, Dupuy P, Shimouchi A, et al. Inhaled nitric oxide reverses pulmonary vasoconstriction in the hypoxic and acidotic newborn lamb. *Circ Res* (1993) 72:246–54. doi:10.1161/01.RES.72.2.246
32. Joshi MS, Ferguson TB Jr, Han TH, Hyduke DR, Liao JC, Rassaf T, et al. Nitric oxide is consumed, rather than conserved, by reaction with oxyhemoglobin under physiological conditions. *Proc Natl Acad Sci U S A* (2002) 99(16):10341–6. doi:10.1073/pnas.152149699
33. Radomski MW, Moncada S. Regulation of vascular homeostasis by nitric oxide. *Thromb Haemost* (1993) 70(1):36–41.
34. Samama CM, Diaby M, Fellahi JL, Mdhafar A, Eyraud D, Arock M, et al. Inhibition of platelet aggregation by inhaled nitric oxide in patients with acute respiratory distress syndrome. *Anesthesiology* (1995) 83(1):56–65. doi:10.1097/00000542-199507000-00007
35. Idell S, Maunder R, Fein AM, Switalska HI, Tuszynski GP, McLarty J, et al. Platelet-specific alpha-granule proteins and thrombospondin in bronchoalveolar lavage in the adult respiratory distress syndrome. *Chest* (1989) 96:1125–32. doi:10.1378/chest.96.5.1125
36. Mannick JB. Immunoregulatory and antimicrobial effects of nitrogen oxides. *Proc Am Thorac Soc* (2006) 3:161–5. doi:10.1513/pats.200505-048BG
37. Bogdan C. Nitric oxide and the immune response. *Nat Immunol* (2001) 2:907–16. doi:10.1038/ni1001-907
38. Kinsella JP, Parker TA, Galan H, Sheridan BC, Halbower AC, Abman SH. Effects of inhaled nitric oxide on pulmonary edema and lung neutrophil accumulation in severe experimental hyaline membrane disease. *Pediatr Res* (1997) 41:457–63. doi:10.1203/00006450-199704000-00002
39. Ruan S-Y, Huang T-M, Wu H-Y, Wu H-D, Yu C-J, Lai M-S. Inhaled nitric oxide therapy and risk of renal dysfunction: a systematic review and meta-analysis of randomized trials. *Crit Care* (2015) 19(1):137. doi:10.1186/s13054-015-0880-2
40. Dobyns EL, Cornfield DN, Anas NG, Fortenberry JD, Tasker RC, Lynch A, et al. Multicenter randomized controlled trial of the effects of inhaled nitric oxide therapy on gas exchange in children with acute hypoxemic respiratory failure. *J Pediatr* (1999) 134:406–12. doi:10.1016/S0022-3476(99)70196-4
41. Day RW, Allen EM, Witte MK. A randomized, controlled study of the 1-hour and 24-hour effects of inhaled nitric oxide therapy in children with acute hypoxemic respiratory failure. *Chest* (1997) 112(5):1324–31. doi:10.1378/chest.112.5.1324
42. Ibrahim TS, El-Mohamady HS. Inhaled nitric oxide and prone position: how far they can improve oxygenation in pediatric patients with acute respiratory distress syndrome? *J Med Sci* (2007) 7:390–5. doi:10.3923/jms.2007.390.395
43. Bronicki RA, Fortenberry J, Schreiber M, Checchia PA, Anas NG. Multicenter randomized controlled trial of inhaled nitric oxide for pediatric acute respiratory distress syndrome. *J Pediatr* (2015) 166(2):365–9.e1. doi:10.1016/j.jpeds.2014.10.011
44. Pediatric Acute Lung Injury Consensus Conference Group. Pediatric acute respiratory distress syndrome: consensus recommendations from the Pediatric Acute Lung Injury Consensus Conference. *Pediatr Crit Care Med* (2015) 16(5):428–39. doi:10.1097/PCC.0000000000000350
45. Santschi M, Jouvet P, Leclerc F, Gauvin F, Newth CJ, Carroll CL, et al. Acute lung injury in children: therapeutic practice and feasibility of international clinical trials. *Pediatr Crit Care Med* (2010) 11(6):681–9. doi:10.1097/PCC.0b013e3181d904c0
46. Varni JW, Seid M, Kurtin P. PedsQL™ 4.0: reliability and validity of the Pediatric Quality of Life Inventory™ Version 4.0 Generic Core Scales in healthy and patient populations. *Med Care* (2001) 39(8):800–12. doi:10.1097/00005650-200108000-00006
47. Graciano AL, Balko JA, Rahn DS, Ahmad N, Giroir BP. The Pediatric Multiple Organ Dysfunction Score (P-MODS): development and validation of an objective scale to measure the severity of multiple organ dysfunction in critically ill children. *Crit Care Med* (2005) 33(7):1484–91. doi:10.1097/01.CCM.0000170943.23633.47
48. Wong HR. Genome-wide expression profiling in pediatric septic shock. *Pediatr Res* (2013) 73(4 Pt 2):564–9. doi:10.1038/pr.2013.11
49. Wong HR, Cvijanovich NZ, Anas N, Allen GL, Thomas NJ, Bigham MT, et al. Developing a clinically feasible personalized medicine approach to pediatric septic shock. *Am J Respir Crit Care Med* (2015) 191(3):309–15. doi:10.1164/rccm.201410-1864OC

Permissions

All chapters in this book were first published by Frontiers; hereby published with permission under the Creative Commons Attribution License or equivalent. Every chapter published in this book has been scrutinized by our experts. Their significance has been extensively debated. The topics covered herein carry significant findings which will fuel the growth of the discipline. They may even be implemented as practical applications or may be referred to as a beginning point for another development.

The contributors of this book come from diverse backgrounds, making this book a truly international effort. This book will bring forth new frontiers with its revolutionizing research information and detailed analysis of the nascent developments around the world.

We would like to thank all the contributing authors for lending their expertise to make the book truly unique. They have played a crucial role in the development of this book. Without their invaluable contributions this book wouldn't have been possible. They have made vital efforts to compile up to date information on the varied aspects of this subject to make this book a valuable addition to the collection of many professionals and students.

This book was conceptualized with the vision of imparting up-to-date information and advanced data in this field. To ensure the same, a matchless editorial board was set up. Every individual on the board went through rigorous rounds of assessment to prove their worth. After which they invested a large part of their time researching and compiling the most relevant data for our readers.

The editorial board has been involved in producing this book since its inception. They have spent rigorous hours researching and exploring the diverse topics which have resulted in the successful publishing of this book. They have passed on their knowledge of decades through this book. To expedite this challenging task, the publisher supported the team at every step. A small team of assistant editors was also appointed to further simplify the editing procedure and attain best results for the readers.

Apart from the editorial board, the designing team has also invested a significant amount of their time in understanding the subject and creating the most relevant covers. They scrutinized every image to scout for the most suitable representation of the subject and create an appropriate cover for the book.

The publishing team has been an ardent support to the editorial, designing and production team. Their endless efforts to recruit the best for this project, has resulted in the accomplishment of this book. They are a veteran in the field of academics and their pool of knowledge is as vast as their experience in printing. Their expertise and guidance has proved useful at every step. Their uncompromising quality standards have made this book an exceptional effort. Their encouragement from time to time has been an inspiration for everyone.

The publisher and the editorial board hope that this book will prove to be a valuable piece of knowledge for researchers, students, practitioners and scholars across the globe.

List of Contributors

Ling Liu, Yue Yu, Xiaoting Xu, Qin Sun, Haibo Qiu and Yi Yang
Jiangsu Provincial Key Laboratory of Critical Care Medicine, Department of Critical Care Medicine, Zhongda Hospital, School of Medicine, Southeast University, Nanjing, China

Davide Chiumello
SC Anesthesia and Resuscitation, San Paolo Hospital—University Campus, ASST Santi Paolo e Carlo, Milan, Italy
Department of Health Sciences, University of Milan, Milan, Italy
Coordinated Research Center of Respiratory Insufficiency, University of Milan, Milan, Italy

Pien Swart and Frederique Paulus
Department of Intensive Care, Amsterdam University Medical Center, Location 'Academic Medical Center', Amsterdam, Netherlands

Sunny G. L. H. Nijbroek
Department of Intensive Care, Amsterdam University Medical Center, Location 'Academic Medical Center', Amsterdam, Netherlands
Department of Anaesthesiology, Amsterdam University Medical Center, Location 'Academic Medical Center', Amsterdam, Netherlands

Ary Serpa Neto
Department of Intensive Care, Amsterdam University Medical Center, Location 'Academic Medical Center', Amsterdam, Netherlands
Australian and New Zealand Intensive Care Research Centre, Monash University, Melbourne, VIC, Australia
Department of Critical Care Medicine, Hospital Israelita Albert Einstein, São Paulo, Brazil

Marcus J. Schultz
Department of Intensive Care, Amsterdam University Medical Center, Location 'Academic Medical Center', Amsterdam, Netherlands
Mahidol Oxford Tropical Medicine Research Unit (MORU), Mahidol University, Bangkok, Thailand
Nuffield Department of Medicine, University of Oxford, Oxford, United Kingdom

Jianhua Sun, Na Cui, Wen Han, Qi Li, Zunzhu Li, Wei Cheng, Hongbo Luo and Mingxi Zhao
Department of Critical Care Medicine, State Key Laboratory of Complex Severe and Rare Diseases, Peking Union Medical College Hospital, Peking Union Medical College, Chinese Academy of Medical Science, Beijing, China

Hao Wang
Department of Critical Care Medicine, Beijing Jishuitan Hospital, Beijing, China

Baoli Wang
Department of Burn Surgery, The First Affiliated Hospital of Naval Medical University, Shanghai, China
Department of Burns and Plastic Surgery, General Hospital of Central Theater Command of Chinese People's Liberation Army, Shanghai, China
Research Unit of Key Techniques for Treatment of Burns and Combined Burns and Trauma Injury, Chinese Academy of Medical Sciences, Shanghai, China

Wei Chenru, Yong Jiang, Lunyang Hu, He Fang, Feng Zhu, Qing Yu, Banghui Zhu, Guosheng Wu and Yu Sun
Department of Burn Surgery, The First Affiliated Hospital of Naval Medical University, Shanghai, China

Zhaofan Xia
Department of Burn Surgery, The First Affiliated Hospital of Naval Medical University, Shanghai, China
Research Unit of Key Techniques for Treatment of Burns and Combined Burns and Trauma Injury, Chinese Academy of Medical Sciences, Shanghai, China

Jing Li, Jing Zhang, Qingfei Hao, Yanna Du, Jie Lu, Haoming Chen and Xiuyong Cheng
Department of Neonatology, The First Affiliated Hospital of Zheng Zhou University, Zhengzhou, China

Wei Cheng, Jiahui Zhang, Dongkai Li, Guangxu Bai and Jianwei Chen
State Key Laboratory of Complex Severe and Rare Diseases, Department of Critical Care Medicine, Peking Union Medical College Hospital, Chinese Academy of Medical Science and Peking Union Medical College, Beijing, China

Carmen M. Hernández-Cárdenas, Carlos Torruco-Sotelo, Felipe Jurado, Héctor Serna-Secundino, Cristina Aguilar, José G. García-Olazarán, Diana Hernández-García and Gustavo Lugo-Goytia
Respiratory Intensive Care Unit, Instituto Nacional de Enfermedades Respiratorias Ismael Cosío Villegas, Mexico City, Mexico

José Alberto Choreño-Parra
Laboratory of Immunobiology and Genetics, Instituto Nacional de Enfermedades Respiratorias Ismael Cosío Villegas, Mexico City, Mexico
Escuela Nacional de Ciencias Biológicas, Instituto Politécnico Nacional, Mexico City, Mexico

Eduardo M. Choreño-Parra
Posgrado en Ciencias Biológicas, Universidad Nacional Autónoma de México, Mexico City, Mexico

Joaquín Zúñiga
Laboratory of Immunobiology and Genetics, Instituto Nacional de Enfermedades Respiratorias Ismael Cosío Villegas, Mexico City, Mexico
Tecnologico de Monterrey, Escuela de Medicina y Ciencias de la Salud, Mexico City, Mexico

Silvia Mikolajcikova, Katarina Matasova Sr. and Mirko Zibolen
Clinic of Neonatology, Jessenius Faculty of Medicine, Comenius University and University Hospital, Martin, Slovakia

Zora Lasabova
Department of Molecular Biology and Genomics, Jessenius Faculty of Medicine, Comenius University, Martin, Slovakia

Veronika Holubekova and Maria Skerenova
Biomedical Centre Martin, Jessenius Faculty of Medicine, Comenius University, Martin, Slovakia

Jana Zibolenova
Department of Public Health, Jessenius Faculty of Medicine, Comenius University, Martin, Slovakia

Andrea Calkovska
Department of Physiology, Jessenius Faculty of Medicine, Comenius University, Martin, Slovakia

Sébastien Gibot, Marie Conrad, Guilhem Courte and Aurélie Cravoisy
Service de Réanimation Médicale, Hôpital Central, CHRU, Nancy, France

Hong-Jie Jhou
Department of Neurology, Changhua Christian Hospital, Changhua, Taiwan
School of Medicine, Kaohsiung Medical University, Kaohsiung, Taiwan

Po-Huang Chen
Department of General Medicine, National Defense Medical Center, Tri-Service General Hospital, Taipei, Taiwan
Department of Internal Medicine, National Defense Medical Center, Tri-Service General Hospital, Taipei, Taiwan

Liang-Jun Ou-Yang
Department of Physical Medicine and Rehabilitation, Chang Gung Memorial Hospital, Taoyuan, Taiwan

Chin Lin
School of Public Health, National Defense Medical Center, Taipei, Taiwan
Department of Research and Development, National Defense Medical Center, Taipei, Taiwan

Shih-En Tang
Division of Pulmonary and Critical Care Medicine, Department of Internal Medicine, National Defense Medical Center, Tri-Service General Hospital, Taipei, Taiwan
National Defense Medical Center, Graduate Institute of Aerospace and Undersea Medicine, Taipei, Taiwan

Cho-Hao Lee
Division of Hematology and Oncology Medicine, Department of Internal Medicine, National Defense Medical Center, Tri-Service General Hospital, Taipei, Taiwan

Xudong Duan and Jiujun Li
Department of Pediatrics, Shengjing Hospital of China Medical University, Shenyang, China
Plateau Medical Research Center of China Medical University, Shenyang, China

Long Chen and Yuan Shi
Department of Neonatology, Children's Hospital Affiliated Chongqing Medical University, Chongqing, China

Xianyang Chen
BaoFeng Key Laboratory of Genetics and Metabolism, Beijing, China
Zhongguancun Biological and Medical Big Data Center, Beijing, China

Teng Xue
Zhongguancun Biological and Medical Big Data Center, Beijing, China
Zhongyuanborui (Hengqin, Zhuhai) Key Laboratory of Genetics and Metabolism, Zhuhai, China

Chongde Liu and Xiaorong Wang
Department of Neonatology, Qinghai Women and Children's Hospital, Xining, China

Quanfang Qiu, Zhen Yu and Bacuozhen Qiang
Department of Pediatrics, Lhasa People's Hospital, Lhasa, China

Hong Wu and Tianqi Wu
Department of Pediatrics, People's Hospital of Tibet, Tibet, China

Lihong Zhang
Department of Pediatrics, Linzhi People's Hospital, Tibet, China

Zhangsheng Chen
Center of Pediatrics, Zhujiang Hospital, Southern Medical University, Guangzhou, China

Dobje Jigme
Department of Pediatrics, Naqu People's Hospital, Tibet, China

Aili Xu and Zhuoga Mima
Department of Pediatrics, Shigatse People's Hospital, Tibet, China

Zhen Da and Min Ren
Department of Pediatrics, Second People's Hospital of Tibet, Tibet, China

Deji Gesang and Zhaxi Pubu
Department of Pediatrics, Shannan People's Hospital, Tibet, China

Chun Li and Yanchao Lv
Department of Pediatrics, Changdu People's Hospital, Tibet, China

Haoquan Zhou and Xue Zhang
Department of Pediatrics, The First Affiliated Hospital of University of Science and Technology of China, Hefei, China
Division of Life Science and Medicine, University of Science and Technology of China, Hefei, China

Zhuoma Dawa and Wujin Gongjue
Department of Pediatrics, People's Hospital of Ali District, Tibet, China

Li Wang, Li Wu and Xuelian Li
Department of Pediatrics, Daping Hospital, Third Military Medical University, Chongqing, China

Jing Zhou, Zhimin Lin, Xiumei Deng, Baiyun Liu, Yu Zhang, Yongxin Zheng, Haichong Zheng, Yingzhi Wang, Yan Lai, Weixiang Huang, Xiaoqing Liu, Weiqun He, Yuanda Xu, Yimin Li and Yongbo Huang
State Key Laboratory of Respiratory Disease, National Clinical Research Center for Respiratory Disease, Guangzhou Institute of Respiratory Health, The First Affiliated Hospital of Guangzhou Medical University, Guangzhou, China

Ling Sang
State Key Laboratory of Respiratory Disease, National Clinical Research Center for Respiratory Disease, Guangzhou Institute of Respiratory Health, The First Affiliated Hospital of Guangzhou Medical University, Guangzhou, China
Guangzhou Laboratory, Guangdong, China

Renato Fraga Righetti, Samantha Torres Grams, Wesla Neves da Silva Costa, Leandro Teixeira Saraiva, Isabel Chateaubriand Diniz de Salles and Wellington Pereira Yamaguti
Hospital Sírio-Libanês, São Paulo, Brazil

Honoré Papalia, Anais Samonini, E. Gras and Clotilde des Robert
Neonatal Unit, Hospital University La Conception, APHM, Marseille, France

Christophe Buffat
Laboratory of Biochemistry and Molecular Biology, Hospital University la Conception, APHM, Marseille, France

Jean-Francois Landrier
Aix-Marseille University, INSERM, INRAE, C2VN, Marseille, France

Vanessa Pauly
EA 3279, CEReSS—Health Service Research and Quality of Life Center, Public Health and Medical Information Department, APHM, Marseille, France

Farid Boubred
Neonatal Unit, Hospital University La Conception, APHM, Marseille, France
Aix-Marseille University, INSERM, INRAE, C2VN, Marseille, France

Li-Juan Yi, Min Chen, Jin-Mei Lei and Na Xiao
Nursing Department, Hunan Traditional Chinese Medical College, Zhuzhou, China

Xu Tian and Maria F. Jiménez-Herrera
Nursing Department, Universitat Rovira i Virgili, Tarragona, Spain

Takeshi Tanaka
Infection Control and Education Center, Nagasaki University Hospital, Nagasaki, Japan

Masahiko Moris
Department of Paediatrics, University of Oxford, Oxford, United Kingdom

Masato Tashiro and Koichi Izumikawa
Infection Control and Education Center, Nagasaki University Hospital, Nagasaki, Japan
Department of Infectious Diseases, Nagasaki University Graduate School of Biomedical Sciences, Nagasaki, Japan

Ting You, Xiao-Chen Liu and Lu-Quan Li
Department of Neonatology, National Clinical Research Center for Child Health and Disorders, Ministry of Education Key Laboratory of Child Development and Disorders, Chongqing Key Laboratory of Pediatrics, Children's Hospital of Chongqing Medical University, Chongqing, China

Yan-Rong Zhou
Jiulongpo People's Hospital of Chongqing, Chongqing, China

Lijun Tang and Lianhua Chen
Department of Anesthesiology, Shanghai General Hospital of Nanjing Medical University, Shanghai, China

Xiao Zhao, Shitong Li, Lina Huang, Jinbao Li and Shiwei Huang
Department of Anesthesiology, Shanghai General Hospital, Shanghai Jiao Tong University, Shanghai, China

Nadir Yehya
Department of Anesthesiology and Critical Care Medicine, Children's Hospital of Philadelphia, University of Pennsylvania, Philadelphia, PA, USA

Neal J. Thomas
Department of Pediatrics and Public Health Science, Division of Pediatric Critical Care Medicine, Penn State Hershey Children's Hospital, Hershey, PA, USA

Bryan Wilson
Department of Emergency Medicine, University of Arizona College of Medicine, Tucson, AZ, USA

Katri Typpo
Department of Pediatrics, Steele Children's Research Center, University of Arizona College of Medicine, Tucson, AZ, USA

Stephanie M. Roses, Thomas Christianson and Keith Dombrowski
Department of Neurology, Duke University, Durham, NC, United States

Steven Nye, Richard J. Whitley and Michele Kong
The University of Alabama at Birmingham, Birmingham, AL, USA

Sarah A. Ingelse, Roelie M. Wösten-van Asperen, Reinout A. Bem and Job B. van Woensel
Pediatric Intensive Care Unit, Academic Medical Center, Emma Children's Hospital, Amsterdam, Netherlands

Joris Lemson
Pediatric Intensive Care Unit, Radboud University Medical Center, Nijmegen, Netherlands

Joost G. Daams
Medical Library, Academic Medical Center, University of Amsterdam, Amsterdam, Netherlands

Daniel Im
Pediatric Critical Care Medicine, Department of Pediatrics, The Saban Research Institute, Children's Hospital Los Angeles, University of Southern California, Los Angeles, CA, USA

Wei Shi and Barbara Driscoll
Developmental Biology and Regenerative Medicine Program, Department of Surgery, The Saban Research Institute, Children's Hospital Los Angeles, University of Southern California, Los Angeles, CA, USA

Juliette Lucinda Hunt and Nick Anas
CHOC Children's Hospital, Orange, CA, USA

Ronald A. Bronicki
Texas Children's Hospital, Houston, TX, USA

Index